Backyard Poultry Medicine and Surgery

Backyard Poultry Medicine and Surgery

A Guide for Veterinary Practitioners

Second Edition

Edited by

Cheryl B. Greenacre, DVM, DABVP-Avian, DABVP-ECM
University of Tennessee's College of Veterinary Medicine in Knoxville, Tennessee, USA

Teresa Y. Morishita, DVM, MPVM, MS, PhD, DACPV
Western University College of Veterinary Medicine in Pomona, California, USA

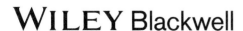

This second edition first published 2021
© 2021 John Wiley & Sons, Inc.

Edition History
John Wiley and Sons, Inc. (1e, 2015)

Blackwell Publishing was acquired by John Wiley & Sons in February 2007. Blackwell's publishing program has been merged with Wiley's global Scientific, Technical and Medical business to form Wiley-Blackwell.

The right of Cheryl B. Greenacre and Teresa Y. Morishita to be identified as the authors of the editorial material in this work has been asserted in accordance with law.

Registered Office
John Wiley & Sons, Inc., 111 River Street, Hoboken, NJ 07030, USA

Editorial Office
111 River Street, Hoboken, NJ 07030, USA

For details of our global editorial offices, customer services, and more information about Wiley products visit us at www.wiley.com.

Wiley also publishes its books in a variety of electronic formats and by print-on-demand. Some content that appears in standard print versions of this book may not be available in other formats.

Library of Congress Cataloging-in-Publication Data

Names: Greenacre, Cheryl B., editor. | Morishita, Teresa Y., editor.
Title: Backyard poultry medicine and surgery : a guide for veterinary
   practitioners / edited by Cheryl B. Greenacre, Teresa Y. Morishita.
Description: Second edition. | Hoboken, NJ : Wiley-Blackwell, 2021. |
   Includes bibliographical references and index.
Identifiers: LCCN 2020020808 (print) | LCCN 2020020809 (ebook) | ISBN 9781119511755
   (paperback) | ISBN 9781119511779 (adobe pdf) | ISBN 9781119511762 (epub)
Subjects: MESH: Poultry | Poultry Diseases | Animal Husbandry–methods |
   Veterinary Medicine–methods | United States
Classification: LCC SF487.8.A1 (print) | LCC SF487.8.A1 (ebook) | NLM SF
   487.8.A1 | DDC 636.5–dc23
LC record available at https://lccn.loc.gov/2020020808
LC ebook record available at https://lccn.loc.gov/2020020809

Cover Design: Wiley
Cover Images: Courtesy of Ashley Hanna, Marcie Logsdon, John Mattoon and Dr. Cheryl Greenacre

Set in 9.5/12.5pt STIXTwoText by SPi Global, Pondicherry, India

This book is dedicated to several people: my parents who taught me through example to be a lifelong learner and a keen observer; my supportive husband of over 30 years who has always been there challenging me to be my best, and to our two children whom we love very much; and Dr. Branson Ritchie for providing me a start in the wonderful field of avian medicine and his willingness to share his knowledge.

Cheryl B. Greenacre

I dedicate this book to my parents, Yasuyuki and Doris Sai Kuk Morishita, for their love, laughter, support, guidance, and encouragement throughout my life; and to my dear P for being there for me. You are all the wind beneath my wings.

Teresa Y. Morishita

Contents

Contributors   *x*
Foreword   *xiii*
Preface   *xv*
Acknowledgments   *xvii*
About the Companion Website   *xix*

Section 1   General Care   *1*

1   **Laws and Regulations Governing Backyard Poultry in the United States**   *3*
J. Bruce Nixon

2   **Common Breeds of Backyard Poultry**   *23*
Lillian Gerhardt and Cheryl B. Greenacre

3   **Basic Housing and Management**   *45*
Darrin Karcher

4   **Anseriforme Husbandry and Management**   *56*
M. Scott Echols

5   **Biosecurity**   *107*
Teresa Y. Morishita and Theodore Derksen

6   **Backyard Poultry Nutrition**   *117*
Todd J. Applegate and Justin Fowler

Section 2   Initial Examinations   *131*

7   **Anatomy and Physiology**   *133*
Wael Khamas and Josep Rutllant-Labeaga

8 Physical Examination *159*
Cheryl B. Greenacre

9 Radiographic Evaluation of Normal and Common Diseases *173*
Ashley L. Hanna, Marcie L. Logsdon and John S. Mattoon

Section 3 Diseases *193*

10 Zoonotic Diseases *195*
Marcy J. Souza

11 Parasitic Diseases *206*
Richard Gerhold

12 Respiratory Diseases *218*
Richard M. Fulton

13 Avian Influenza and Viscerotropic Velogenic (Exotic) Newcastle Disease *229*
Richard M. Fulton

14 Musculoskeletal Diseases *234*
Cheryl B. Greenacre

15 Dermatological Diseases *259*
Angela Lennox

16 Reproductive Diseases *275*
Eric Gingerich and Daniel Shaw

17 Gastrointestinal and Hepatic Diseases *289*
Teresa Y. Morishita and Robert E. Porter, Jr

18 Cardiovascular Diseases *317*
Hugues Beaufrère and Marina Brash

Section 4 Specialized Care and Surgery *341*

19 Emergency and Critical Care *343*
Jennifer E. Graham and Elizabeth A. Rozanski

20 Toxicology *368*
Marieke H. Rosenbaum and Cheryl B. Greenacre

21 Soft Tissue Surgery *381*
M. Scott Echols

22 Chicken Behavior *434*
Christine Calder and Julia Albright

Section 5   Diagnosis of Disease *455*

23 Euthanasia *457*
Cheryl B. Greenacre

24 Egg Diagnostics *462*
Teresa Y. Morishita, Josep Rutllant-Labeaga and Darrin Karcher

25 How to Perform a Necropsy *477*
Jarra Jagne and Elizabeth Buckles

26 Diagnostic Laboratory Sampling *504*
Rocio Crespo and H.L. Shivaprasad

27 Interpretation of Laboratory Results and Values *515*
Rocio Crespo and H.L. Shivaprasad

Section 6   Treatment and Prevention of Disease *533*

28 Regulatory Considerations for Medication Use in Poultry *535*
Lisa Tell, Tara Marmulak and Krysta Martin

29 Commonly Used Medications *562*
Cheryl B. Greenacre

30 Vaccination of Poultry *584*
Robert Porter

Index *594*

Contributors

Julia Albright, MA, DVM, DACVB
Associate Professor, Behavior
Department of Small Animal Clinical Sciences
College of Veterinary Medicine
University of Tennessee, Knoxville
Knoxville, Tennessee

Todd J. Applegate, PhD
Department Head and Professor
Department of Poultry Science
College of Agriculture and Environmental
Sciences
University of Georgia
Athens, Georgia

Hugues Beaufrère, Dr Med Vet, PhD, DACZM,
DABVP (Avian), DECZM (Avian)
Assistant Professor, Avian and Exotic Medicine
Department of Clinical Studies
Ontario Veterinary College
University of Guelph
Guelph, Ontario, Canada

Marina Brash, DVM, DVSc, DACVP
Animal Health Laboratory
Ontario Veterinary College
University of Guelph
Guelph, Ontario, Canada

Elizabeth Buckles, DVM, PhD, DACVP
Associate Clinical Professor
Department of Biomedical Sciences
Cornell University
College of Veterinary Medicine
Ithaca, New York

Christine Calder, DVM, DACVB
Maine Veterinary Medical Center
Emergency and Specialty Hospital
Behavior Department
Scarborough, Maine

Rocio Crespo, DVM, MS, DVSc, DACPV
Professor
Poultry Health Management
North Carolina State University
College of Veterinary Medicine
Raleigh, North Carolina

Theodore Derksen, MS, DVM
College of Veterinary Medicine
Western University of Health
Sciences
Pomona, California

M. Scott Echols, DVM, DABVP (Avian)
Associate Veterinarian
Co-Founder
Mobile Avian Surgical Services
The Medical Center for Birds
Oakley, California

Justin Fowler, PhD
Assistant Professor
Department of Poultry Science
College of Agriculture and Environmental
Sciences
University of Georgia
Athens, Georgia

Richard M. Fulton, DVM, PhD, DACVP
Professor, Avian Diseases
Department of Pathobiology and Diagnostic
Investigation
Diagnostic Center for Population and Animal
Health
College of Veterinary Medicine
Michigan State University
Lansing, Michigan

Lillian Gerhardt, LVMT
Senior Veterinary Technician, Avian and
Zoological Medicine Service
Department of Small Animal Clinical Sciences
College of Veterinary Medicine
University of Tennessee, Knoxville
Knoxville, Tennessee

Richard Gerhold, DVM, PhD
Associate Professor, Parasitology
Department of Biomedical and Diagnostic
Sciences
University of Tennessee
College of Veterinary Medicine
Knoxville, Tennessee

Eric Gingerich, DVM
Technical Services Specialist-Poultry
Zionsville, Indiana

**Jennifer E. Graham, DVM, DABVP (Avian, DABVP
(Exotic Companion Mammal)), DACZM**
Associate Professor of Zoological Companion
Animal Medicine
Department of Clinical Sciences
Cummings School of Veterinary Medicine at
Tufts University
North Grafton, Massachusetts

**Cheryl B. Greenacre, DVM, DABVP (Avian),
DABVP (Exotic Companion Mammal)**
Professor and Section Head, Avian and
Zoological Medicine Service
Department of Small Animal Clinical Sciences
College of Veterinary Medicine
University of Tennessee, Knoxville
Knoxville, Tennessee

Ashley L. Hanna, DVM
Clinical Assistant Professor, Diagnostic
Imaging
Department of Veterinary Clinical Sciences
College of Veterinary medicine
Washington State University
Pullman, Washington

Jarra Jagne, DVM, DACPV
Senior Extension Associate
Department of Population Medicine and
Diagnostic Sciences
Cornell University
College of Veterinary Medicine
Ithaca, New York

Darrin Karcher, PhD
Associate Professor
Poultry Extension Specialist
Purdue University
West Lafayette, Indiana

Wael Khamas, DVM, PhD
Professor of Anatomy and Embryology
College of Veterinary Medicine
Western University of Health Sciences
Pomona, California

**Angela Lennox, DVM, DABVP (Avian), DABVP
(Exotic Companion Mammal), ECZM-SA**
Avian and Exotic Animal Clinic of
Indianapolis
Indianapolis, Indiana

Marcie L. Logsdon, DVM
Clinical Instructor, Exotics
Department of Veterinary Clinical Sciences
College of Veterinary Medicine
Washington State University
Pullman, Washington

Tara Marmulak
Veterinary Teaching Hospital, College
of Veterinary Medicine and Biomedical
Sciences
Colorado State University
Fort Collins, Colorado

Krysta Martin, PharmD, FSVHP
Veterinary Medicine
Medicine & Epidemiology
School of Veterinary Medicine
University of California
Davis, California

John S. Matoon, DVM, DACVR
Clinical Professor, Diagnostic Imaging
Department of Veterinary Clinical Sciences
College of Veterinary Medicine
Washington State University
Pullman, Washington

Teresa Y. Morishita, DVM, MPVM, PhD, DACPV
Professor, Poultry Medicine and
Food Safety
College of Veterinary Medicine
Western University of Health Sciences
Pomona, California

J. Bruce Nixon, DVM
Owner, Texas Avian & Exotic Hospital
Grapevine, Texas

Robert E. Porter Jr, DVM, PhD, DACVP, DACPV
Clinical Professor
Veterinary Diagnostic Laboratory
St. Paul, Minnesota

Marieke H. Rosenbaum, DVM, MPH, MS
Research Assistant Professor
Department of Infectious Disease and Global
Health
Cummings School of Veterinary Medicine at
Tufts University
North Grafton, Massachusetts

Elizabeth A. Rozanski, DVM, DACVIM, DACVECC
Associate Professor
Department of Clinical Sciences
Cummings School of Veterinary Medicine at
Tufts University
North Grafton, Massachusetts

Josep Rutllant-Labeaga, DVM, PhD
Year 2 Curriculum Director and Professor
Anatomy and Embryology
College of Veterinary Medicine
Western University of Health Sciences
Pomona, California

Daniel Shaw, DVM, PhD, ACVP, ACPV
Department of Veterinary Pathobiology
College of Veterinary Medicine
University of Missouri-Columbia
Veterinary Medical Diagnostic Laboratory
Columbia, Missouri

H. L. Shivaprasad, MS, DVSc, PhD
Professor, Clinical Diagnostic Pathology
California Animal Health and Food Safety
Laboratory System
Fresno, California

Marcy J. Souza, DVM, MPH, MPPA, DABVP-Avian, DACVPM
Professor and Director of Veterinary Public
Health
Department of Biomedical and Diagnostic
Sciences
University of Tennessee
College of Veterinary Medicine
Knoxville, Tennessee

Lisa Tell, DVM, DABVP (Avian), DACZM
Professor
Medicine & Epidemiology
School of Veterinary Medicine
University of California
Davis, California

Foreword

Chickens, simply stated, are cool. They represent, in many ways, what modern-day companion avian medical practice is all about. The richness of the human–animal bond and the unique challenges of medical and surgical diagnosis and treatment are both attractive and sometimes intimidating to veterinary healthcare providers. The deep rewards for veterinarians, staff, and the owners of the birds that are achieved with our collective efforts to help these unique and sentient animals, all mixed in and stirred well together, in essence amount to exactly what companion avian practice is and should be.

As a reflection of this, backyard poultry overall constitute a significant portion of the caseload for healthy, growing avian practices worldwide. In our own avian species-exclusive practice as an example, the domestic chicken represents the third most common single species that we provide veterinary care for, based on numbers of patient accessions as well as revenues generated. The reasons for this in part originates from the drive by the public who own, care for, and care about the birds in their stewardship and who are asking for good quality veterinary care for their birds when needed. The days of avian practice being represented by merely exotic or nondomestic avian species are gone.

A part of our ability to provide good care comes from familiarity with the species that we are treating. Compassion and true interest in the birds are essential for successful healthcare to be delivered. Other key factors that influence our ability to provide good care include our familiarity with good avian medical principles and the sometimes-unique or varying ways these principles are applied to the species at hand. Not only has avian practice changed to fundamentally include backyard poultry species, it has also changed in regards to the need for taxon-specific references that are up to date and practical and can rapidly meet the need to access appropriate information with which to provide accurate healthcare.

This text provides the readers with all of this needed information and more. Drs Greenacre and Morishita are to be commended for their efforts with this second edition of *Backyard Poultry Medicine and Surgery – A Guide for Veterinary Practitioners* to continue to bring timely, up to date, accurate and appropriate information which veterinarians can use. This edition, as did the first, effectively crosses the lines between production poultry medicine and companion bird medicine, which is so relevant for practitioners who see these birds in need of medical care. This text should be readily available on your library shelf, for quick reference when you see poultry in practice. Not only can your familiarity with the breeds and the animals themselves including anatomy and physiology be enriched, but the medical aspects of diagnosis, appropriate therapeutics, surgery, and more can be rapidly located. An excellent addition is the section focused on emergency medicine and critical care. Many backyard poultry are presented for veterinary care in emergency departments and practices around the country and beyond, and any veterinarian in such a potential situation would greatly benefit from having this reference on their shelf. The crossover between backyard poultry as food animal species and companion animals is clarified, keeping the reader appraised of public health and regulatory considerations that are directly relevant to the bigger picture as well. The editors have assembled an excellent cast of contributors that have all combined to bring you the best information, all between two covers of this book.

This reference is an essential tool for any practice that may be presented with backyard poultry species for medical care. It is also a key for veterinarians who hope to expand and broaden their scope of their current avian medical caseload, consistent with current times and trends that can unlock a treasure trove of rewards, personally and professionally.

Brian Speer, DVM, DABVP (Avian Practice),
DECZM (Avian)
Medical Center for Birds, Oakley,
California, USA

Preface

In the five years since the first edition of *Backyard Poultry Medicine and Surgery – A Guide for Veterinary Practitioners*, the number of backyard poultry presenting to veterinarians for individual or small flock care has expanded exponentially. Practitioners are increasingly being asked to care for backyard poultry and are seeking practical information on husbandry, medicine, and surgery in order to provide state-of-the-art medical care for their patients. The diseases and care of backyard flocks is different than that of commercial broilers, breeders, or layers, and information on their care can be found in scattered resources such as texts on commercial poultry, agricultural extension information, state and federal government websites, laybooks, and websites.

This book describes diseases of backyard poultry organized by body systems so that it is practical for use by veterinarians providing individual or small flock care, unlike other books that are organized by name of disease or causative organism. This book is especially useful in the initial stages of creating a differential disease listing based on the presenting clinical signs and provides information on treatment of individual or small-flock birds, whereas many other books currently available were created to solve large-flock problems in a commercial setting.

Both of us have each worked with backyard poultry for longer than 25 years. Teresa has experience in both the backyard and commercial poultry settings, has worked with youth groups such as 4H, and is a diplomate of the American College of Poultry Veterinarians. Cheryl has experience in the backyard poultry setting while working in an academic avian and zoological medicine position and is a diplomate of the American Board of Veterinary Practitioners-Avian Practice. It was a common long-time goal of ours to create a practical book on poultry medicine for veterinary practitioners by bringing together information and expertise from varied resources and from respected authors reflecting a broad background of expertise and interests from both the commercial poultry setting and the avian practitioner setting. Our authors are among the most respected in their field and encompass a broad range of specialists.

We are proud to present this second edition of *Backyard Poultry Medicine and Surgery – A Guide for Veterinary Practitioners* to our colleagues and readers. The chapters familiar to you from the first edition have been expanded and updated including chapters describing common diseases of various body systems (gastrointestinal, hepatic, respiratory, integumentary, reproductive, cardiovascular, and musculoskeletal) and chapters on laws and regulations, breeds, husbandry, nutrition, Anseriformes, anatomy, physiology, performing a physical examination, zoonosis, biosecurity, parasitology, interpreting and performing diagnostic testing, egg diagnostics, vaccination, regulatory considerations for medication use, and surgical techniques, as well as chapters on economically important diseases such as avian influenza and exotic (virulent) Newcastle disease. Based on feedback from our readers, the second edition has been greatly improved by the addition of six new chapters written by experts in their respective fields: (i) Radiology – an extensive chapter on both normal and abnormal radiographic findings; (ii) Behavior – written by two board certified behaviorists; (iii) Toxicology – including zoonotic concerns of lead toxicity; (iv) How to Perform a Necropsy – a practical "How To" with great pictures; (v) Emergency Procedures – a thorough description of individual patient care; and (vi) Euthanasia – explains how to follow the American Veterinary Medical Association's Guidelines. Last, but not least, there is an expanded chapter on Commonly Used Medications – a formulary of commonly used medications including label and extra-label uses.

The chapters on laws and regulations that govern backyard poultry care, ownership, and treatment will help the reader intelligently field questions from their clientele and understand important concepts such as the difference between prohibited drug use and extra-label drug use. The reader is provided the tools for determining and understanding appropriate drug use in backyard chickens and is provided a list of commonly used labeled and extra-label drugs used in backyard poultry. In the "Regulatory Considerations for the Use of

Medications in Poultry" chapter, the reader is referred to extensive and thorough formularies and websites. There is information on all aspects of backyard poultry care including fundamental information on anatomy and physiology, nutrition, housing, biosecurity, vaccines, and how to identify common breeds; specific information such as how to perform and interpret an echocardiogram, fecal examinations, egg diagnostics, and understanding and interpreting serological and other diagnostic tests; and a chapter dedicated on how to perform simple and complex surgeries. There is also a chapter specific for the diseases of waterfowl such as ducks, geese, and swans, although all chapters include information on all poultry such as turkeys, quail, pheasants, and other birds.

We hope you find the extra efforts taken to provide a practical approach to veterinary care of backyard poultry offered in this second edition useful. Please visit the website to view many extras including links to references and videos such as how to perform a physical examination, how to give intramuscular and subcutaneous injections, stance and attitude of chickens with Marek's disease, respiratory disease symptoms, endoscopic retrieval of coins from a duck ventriculus, physical therapy in action, and watching a chick hatch!

Cheryl B. Greenacre and Teresa Y. Morishita

Acknowledgments

Books are usually a collaborative effort, and this one is no exception. Many people have directly or indirectly been involved in making this book a reality. I am thankful for a solid base in avian medicine from my veterinary education at the University of Georgia that included an entire course in poultry medicine taught by Dr. Richard (Dick) Davis as well as an entire course in companion and wild avian medicine taught by Dr. Branson Ritchie. I learned a lot from the experience and knowledge gained during my internship, residency, and academic careers in avian medicine, and I learned from clients who brought me their birds asking for state-of-the-art care. I also learned from all the interns, residents, and students I have taught along the way.

I thank each contributing author for their precious time and the hard work that went into writing these outstanding chapters. This book was a group effort, and we did it! This book also benefitted from the many generous people who gave permission for their pictures to be used in this book. Thank you. I also thank our University of Tennessee College of Veterinary Medicine Librarian, Ann Viera, for the continuous stream of all things poultry she has sent my way over the past several years, including books, pamphlets, journal and news articles, websites, people, and even her own chickens. I also thank the wonderful staff at Wiley for all their support, especially Erica Judisch, who encouraged us to write the book, and Susan Engelken and Purvi Patel, for making the book so much better.

The idea of writing this book stemmed from the need for a practical backyard poultry resource for practitioners organized by body systems to aid in the diagnosis of disease. I am very grateful that Dr. Teresa Morishita agreed to be co-editor for this book, because she contributed her invaluable knowledge, expertise, and contacts in both the commercial and backyard poultry medicine fields to make this book what we both wanted it to be. It has been a pleasure working with her on this project with the common goal of providing the best care possible for backyard poultry and their owners.

**Cheryl Benham Greenacre, DVM,
DABVP-Avian, DABVP-Exotic
Companion Mammal**

There is the Japanese saying *Okage sama de* which is translated as "I am what I am because of you." I am so grateful to all the individuals whom I have encountered on my life journey, whether for a brief moment or for an extended part of my journey. I am what I am because of all these individuals who gave me their time, thoughts, and resources. Their guidance and mentorship have been immeasurable. Of course, there are the rocks in my life, like my grandfather, Anthony H.L., who introduced me to caring for animals and teaching me how to raise my pet chickens and geese; my parents, for their never-ending love, support, and encouragement to reach for my dreams; and my immediate and extended *ohana*, including my *hanai* brother Tom Kwai and *hanai* sister Moina Elizabeth, and Josep Rutllant for always being there for me. Then, there are my many teachers, advisors, and mentors during my educational years, from kindergarten to high school, undergraduate, graduate, and professional school, who have led me to become the person I am today and to a career that I enjoy. Every step of the way, there were individuals who helped me. There are also my mentors who helped me throughout my career with sage advice and encouragement, for having faith in me, and by providing the opportunities to grow professionally. I cannot list every individual as that alone would fill an entire book. I am thankful for all of them and am grateful to have had them on my journey of life. I am who I am today due to all the individuals who believed in and encouraged me to soar for my dreams and took me under their wing. I definitely have a flock with me.

There is no doubt that like life, this book is what it is today due to the efforts of our many contributors, some who have been with us since the first edition and some new contributors who became part of our team; to our colleagues, students, and clients who relayed to us the need for such a book and provided their reviews and candid comments to make this second edition even better; to my co-editor Dr. Cheryl Greenacre, for her vision and tenacity to get this major project accomplished and for her invitation to join her on this amazing book-writing journey; and of course, to the staff at Wiley, especially Erica Judisch, who encouraged and believed in our dream book, and to Susan Engelken and Purvi Patel, who have helped fine tune and polish our final product. I would also like to acknowledge the dedication and efforts of Anh Doan, Deborah Ann Harris, and Chris Vander Veen, who have assisted me in completing this second edition. This book is what it is because of all of them. We each have so much impact on the lives of others we encounter on our daily life journey. Let us spread positivity, kindness, and encouragement in our daily interactions with others as when we are blessed; it is important to share our blessings with others. So, we want to take this moment to share this book with all of you. Together we can all play an important role in keeping our backyard poultry flocks healthy. Much gratitude and aloha to all!

Teresa Y. Morishita, DVM, MPVM, PhD, Dipl. ACPV

About the Companion Website

This book is accompanied by a companion website:

www.wiley.com/go/greenacre/medicine

The website includes:

- Power Point images of all figures from the book for downloading
- Reference lists from the book for downloading
- Web-exclusive videos

Section 1

General Care

1

Laws and Regulations Governing Backyard Poultry in the United States

J. Bruce Nixon

Texas Avian & Exotic Hospital, Grapevine, TX, USA

Introduction

When a veterinarian is presented with the task of caring for a client's backyard flock, many daunting obstacles will eventually become evident, including questions of legal and regulatory requirements and obligations. While the appropriateness of whether to extend your professional services to these clients is a personal choice, legal requirements of the veterinarian and your client are mandatory. Violations of law may have criminal consequences, and regulatory violations may carry punishments of fines and/or reprimands. It is even possible for a client to have their backyard flock depopulated and/or quarantined against their will. As in almost every area of modern veterinary practice, civil liability is always a threat.

For the veterinarian, there is no substantial legal requirement specific to practicing on poultry other than state licensure. Providing standard of care to backyard poultry is the primary issue of concern, and this determination falls squarely within each state's veterinary licensing body. While backyard flocks are gaining in popularity with a concurrent rise in the number of veterinarians seeing such patients, these relationships are still relatively rare within a given practice area, even in major metropolitan cities. If a standard of care complaint is lodged with a state licensing board, its members must decide whose standards you will be held against. For instance, if a small flock under your care succumbs to Marek disease, any commercial poultry veterinarian would consider it standard practice to have had a vaccination protocol in place. While it would seem unreasonable to hold a veterinarian who occasionally practices on small flocks to such a standard, it is not an impossible scenario. Even if the licensing authority dismisses such a complaint, a client is still free to sue for civil damages. This sort of risk is ever present in modern society, however, and hopefully will not dissuade those inclined to enter this new and growing area of veterinary medicine.

It might also be helpful for the veterinarian to know exactly who would be defined as a specialist, or expert, in poultry, backyard or otherwise. Unquestionably, boarded members of the American College of Poultry Veterinarians are considered veterinary poultry specialists, and most members spend their careers managing poultry. They work in academia, government, industry, and the private sector. Most of these veterinarians are also

Backyard Poultry Medicine and Surgery: A Guide for Veterinary Practitioners, Second Edition.
Edited by Cheryl B. Greenacre and Teresa Y. Morishita.
Companion website: www.wiley.com/go/greenacre/medicine

members of the American Association of Avian Pathologists. Because most of these veterinarians are working with large, commercial flocks, they may not be readily accessible to most backyard poultry enthusiasts. Many veterinarians working with the occasional backyard chicken may not even be aware of their existence. It is obvious that their assistance, when sought, can be invaluable.

The American Board of Veterinary Practitioners (ABVP) also board certifies specialists in the field of avian medicine and surgery. These veterinarians are bona fide experts for all avian species, including chickens. Veterinarians who are ABVP (avian) boarded specialists are largely found in private practices devoted to companion animal care, although they are certainly also found in academia, government, and industry.

The largest veterinary avian community (by membership) is the Association of Avian Veterinarians (AAV). Its membership is primarily composed of veterinarians working with companion birds but is by no means confined to it. In fact, there is no avian family that is excluded by AAV. Historically, psittacine birds have comprised a very large percentage of the species seen by AAV members, but members have always worked with passerines (finches, canaries), ratites (ostriches), Columbiformes (pigeons), and others. Backyard chicken care is a rapidly growing topic within the AAV.

The more common legal issues for the practitioner involves our role as an advisor to our clients, informing them of their own legal responsibilities. Many clients will enthusiastically and quickly form their own backyard flock and invest a substantial amount of time and financial resources into their new hobby without a moment's thought that they may have already grossly violated the law. To the best of our ability, it is our professional duty to at least provide them with some guidance on applicable laws, much as we inform clients of leash laws and local ordinances that may forbid certain types of pets.

Homeowners and Neighborhood Associations

Covenants, conditions, and restrictions (CC&Rs) are limitations and rules placed on a group of homes by a builder, developer, neighborhood association, or homeowners association (HOA). Most established neighborhoods and subdivisions and practically all townhomes and condominiums have CC&Rs. This is the first place for a prospective backyard poultry client to look for obstacles. When clients purchase a home in a covenant-protected community, they enter into a contract with the HOA or neighborhood association. The owner agrees to be bound by the restrictions contained in the community's governing documents, which include the declaration of CC&Rs that are recorded with the clerk's office of the county in which that community is located. Those restrictions are legally binding on all property owners in the community.

Even when a town, city, or county adopts an ordinance allowing backyard flocks, such permissiveness does NOT negate the contractual agreement between the owner and the association. So even if your client lives in a city that expressly allows (even encourages!) small backyard flocks, a prohibiting clause within the client's CC&Rs will take precedence and the client will not be able to proceed with establishing their flock. The more restrictive rule applies, and HOAs can and do exist in rural settings, even within land zoned for agricultural use. Also, if the homeowner is seeking to build a coop, they must first comply with requirements for preapproval of construction of enclosures with the HOA before obtaining any necessary building permits from the city or county.

Some HOAs are extremely active, whereas others seem to be almost nonexistent in reality. These neighborhood associations usually have no real policing powers but can appeal to civil courts to force compliance on an uncooperative member. Monetary penalties can show up as a lien when a property is sold. On the other hand, HOA rules can be the easiest and least complicated to amend or create. A simple appeal directly to the HOA board or a letter of support from the neighbors bordering a potential small coop is often all that is needed to gain permission. Another common tactic is for homeowners to get themselves elected to the HOA board, which can be surprisingly easy to accomplish. Once elected, it is a simple matter to add poultry issues to the agenda and only a majority of the existing board members need be convinced of the need for a rule change.

Renters should also note that although their lease may not specifically prohibit chickens, the owner of the property is bound by any such agreement and subsequently anyone occupying the property is bound by the same. Even a willing and accepting landlord may not be aware of such restrictions and a renter should ask for a copy of HOA rules rather than risk the demolition of a newly constructed coop and re-homing of just-bought chicks.

Are Backyard Chickens Pets or Farm Animals?

Because many municipal officials and members of HOA's lack agricultural knowledge, they lack a basis for understanding whether chickens can peacefully coexist with their constituents in a cosmopolitan area [1]. Few things excite people as greatly as the goings-on in their neighborhood. It is often the case that the set of rules that apply to backyard chickens is determined by whether chickens are defined as pets or livestock, as some may believe that chicken raising and other agricultural practices involving animals simply have no place in the modern city. Some cities define chickens as domestic animals or pets and thus subject them to the same enclosure and nuisance regulations as other domestic animals like cats and dogs [2]. Other cities specifically define poultry as farm animals [3], and hence they are subject to the same laws and regulations that apply to cattle and swine. Some owners may be shocked to find that their hometown outlaws chickens as

dangerous animals, placing them in the same category as lions, tigers, bears, and sharks [4]. A novel way to address the issue is to treat chickens as a separate category of animal, giving homeowners, city inspectors, and animal control officers clear guidelines on how to approach and handle personal flocks [5]. In at least one instance, a city allowed a homeowner to keep her chickens because the owner herself considered them to be pets and the chickens did not create a nuisance [6].

Once the HOA/neighborhood association hurdle is cleared, the next step is to review city codes and ordinances. Internet access to city records is now almost universal even in small towns, and although this has simplified access, it can be bewildering to find the appropriate and applicable ordinances. Interestingly, most large American cities have at least some provision that allows for backyard poultry, and smaller jurisdictions seem to be the most restrictive [7].

In one report, the United States Department of Agriculture (USDA) Animal and Plant Health Inspection Service (APHIS), while conducting a survey of backyard/small production flocks in the United States, defined a backyard flock as being less than 1000 birds and those with 1000 or more birds as being a commercial poultry operation [8].

Navigating City Charters and Ordinances

Zoning and the law of local government often are regarded as subjects that are arcane and parochial. It is best to avoid projecting what you expect to find (and where) and simply be open to acquiring local knowledge [9]. A simple Internet search for "City of . . . . . ." usually yields the entire charter, ordinances, zoning, permitting regulations, and health codes. Once the documentation is retrieved, the process of finding pertinent material can begin as regulations may be placed in different areas of a city's codified ordinances. The first and most logical place to look is under an Animals/Animal Control heading or subsection. If chickens are addressed under a city's animal control ordinances, then further regulations concerning lot size, setbacks, or coop requirements may be conveniently located here. As noted, it may be unclear as to whether backyard poultry are considered pets or livestock. If such a distinction is not clear, the opinion of the city clerk or the city's legal counsel may be sought. If an animal control department exists, then the advice of the department should be sought, as they are very likely the people who actually have policing authority. In many cities, this function is carried out by the police department (or sheriff if county laws are applicable).

Another place to investigate will be health codes. Features such as cleanliness, sanitation, and noise control can often be contained in the health code, although the latter may be codified under a "Nuisance" section. The problem of free roaming birds may also be addressed as a public health issue, and owners should be particularly concerned about containing their birds as this can be especially disturbing to neighbors and may spark complaints that could result in uninvited scrutiny. At least two cities consider escaped chickens to be illegal trespassers if they enter your neighbor's property [10]. Fly and rodent control may figure prominently in local health codes, with some cities mandating the use of insecticides [11] and others requiring fly-proof enclosures designed to "prevent the entry therein or the escape therefrom of any bee, moth or fly" [12]. The cities that mention rat control usually just mandate that the coop be free of rats, although others specify the methods used to control rodents such as placing food in rat-proof containers or specifying that coops be designed to be rat-proof. Coop hygiene is another area that pops up frequently, and codes may stipulate how often coops must be cleaned, while most expressly prohibit odors or offensive odors.

The issue of slaughter may also be contained in city charters and vary widely in restrictions.

Most often, the slaughter of individual birds will have no state or federal inspection requirements if the meat is consumed on premises by the immediate family. However, some cities have outright bans [12] on slaughter or restrict it to a building or other structure [13], presumably so that neighbors or their children are not damaged by witnessing such actions (one city seems to be concerned about the negative effects of chickens witnessing their brethren succumb to such an end and requires that slaughter occur in an entirely separate room than the one that fowl occupy) [14]. Owners should also be aware that if backyard chickens are regarded as pets, then slaughter may run afoul of local animal cruelty laws or draw the attention of animal rights groups even if the practice is completely legal. It should also be pointed out that some jurisdictions specifically prohibit the slaughter of chickens for religious purposes, "applicable to any cult that kills (sacrifices) animals for any type of ritual, regardless of whether or not the flesh or blood of the animal is to be consumed" [15], but exempting Kosher slaughter. At least one city expressly allows slaughter for both food and religious purposes [16], whereas another bans slaughter for food purposes but allows it for religious purposes [17].

There is another issue involving carcass disposal if a bird has not been slaughtered specifically for consumption. Many jurisdictions have rules pertaining to burial of dead animals and may not allow for burial within city limits. Cremations often have legal requirements and if present may not allow for simple burning (actually, many cities and counties specifically prohibit burning of waste, which would presumably include incineration of animal waste including bodies). Obviously, veterinarians will have arrangements for carcass disposal that chicken owners can use. Even submitting a whole bird for necropsy can have unforeseen consequences. Diagnostic laboratories have specific rules pertaining to reportable diseases that are diagnosed on necropsy or other diagnostic testing. This may trigger the involvement of state or federal authorities who may dictate disposal of subsequent poultry deaths from the client's flock, either by natural death, euthanasia, or depopulation.

Roosters can present legal issues on several fronts. First, their presence may be specifically prohibited in a jurisdiction or the number of roosters allowed may be regulated [18]. There is the obvious noise problem, and clients may not be aware that roosters can and do crow at any time of day or night and do not restrict their vocalizations to daybreak. Rooster crowing may trigger a noise violation, even if a city specifically allows for roosters to be kept. Some clients may also mistakenly believe that a rooster is necessary for egg production, and it may be helpful to point out that almost all commercial laying hens never encounter a rooster once they have left the hatchery. The other problem with roosters is their mere presence if an owner is only interested in egg production and has no interest in chickens for the grill or soup pot. If an owner is keeping a rooster to allow at least some fertilized eggs to replenish the flock, then half of the chicks will have no place in an egg-producing flock. While many owners are successful in finding "homes" for these birds, few farmers are interested in accepting rooster "pets" and, unfortunately, many of these birds will end up at the local shelter (if one exists). A veterinarian may be presented with healthy rooster culls for euthanasia. Another potential legal problem exists with "rescue organizations" that claim to provide a no-kill option for unwanted chickens. While many of these operations do precisely what they claim, others are fronts for people who are hoarding animals. While hoarding increasingly appears to have a deep psychological basis, many jurisdictions are beginning to address the problem through legal prohibitions and interventions.

Zoning

Perhaps one of the most difficult areas in a municipal charter for laymen to navigate is zoning laws, as zoning cases are considered legally idiosyncratic and thus not subject to generalization [19]. Cities that regulate chickens through their zoning laws are much more likely to substantially restrict raising hens [20]. Generally, zoning regulations are designed and written for experts in the areas of land development and building construction, and while the language contained therein may be perfectly understandable for someone in those businesses, it may seem impenetrable to an outsider. A client must determine what zone his/her property falls within and whether that zone allows for backyard chickens. To compound the problem, the municipal employees responsible for interpreting and enforcing these codes are working with developers and builders on a daily basis and may struggle to explain the process to laypeople.

Local zoning boards serve as the forum where conflicting preferences over land use are articulated, disputed, and sometimes accommodated [21]. After all, zoning is "the primary legal mechanism through which the community attempts to influence the evolution of its physical structure. The community as a whole attempts to preserve that which it values, plan for that which it desires, and discourage or eradicate that which it dislikes" [22]. If a city's zoning laws only allow for chickens on land zoned for agricultural use, then most urban/suburban dwellers will have no options other than requesting a zoning variance or attempt to change the law itself. Zoning laws change in response to changing community values, and the community's cultural values are affected by the structures that an earlier era first permitted and then discouraged [23]. Under the Standard Zoning Enabling Act, any community that engages in zoning must set up a zoning board that serves the function of granting variances. In its simplest form, the zoning board is authorized to grant variances from zoning regulations only when (i) the impact of the regulations constitutes an unnecessary hardship on the petitioner, (ii) granting the variance will not harm the public welfare, and (iii) the situation is unique [24].

Coop Construction

Many cities will regulate how a coop should be built and maintained, specifying the dimensions of the coop, how it must be built, and exactly how it must be cleaned. Although some city's building requirements are specific to chicken coops, many are not particular to chickens and cover any structure meant to house animals. Some HOAs and municipalities will have requirements and permits that must be obtained prior to the construction of ANY unattached structure on a property.

The most common requirement concerns the amount of space allotted to the chickens. Again, there is wide variability, but it is usually calculated on the amount of square footage available per bird: anywhere between $2\,\text{ft}^2$ per bird [25] to $15\,\text{ft}^2$ per bird [26]. Rather than set a particular amount of space per bird, one city requires that the space be twice as big as the bird [27]. A relatively recent shift in animal welfare measurement focuses on welfare outcomes rather than setting engineering standards. These requirements can be so vague as to require that the chickens not be cramped or overcrowded [28] or they may be more specific, requiring that birds have space to stand, turn around, and lie down [29] or that they must be able to move freely [30]. A few cities have requirements designed to ensure that birds are protected from the environment. These standards range from specific protection from the sun or extreme temperatures [31] to simply requiring that enclosures protect the animals from inclement weather [32]. Some ordinances are downright peculiar, requiring windows if possible [33] or prohibiting keeping chickens in cellars [34]. Some cities will also restrict how large the coop may be, capping either total square feet or a maximum height for the structure.

Lot Size

Many cities restrict raising chickens based on the lot size of the property. Some cities require a lot of an acre or more in size [35] before allowing the presence of any chickens at all. Such a requirement effectively bans backyard chickens for most people in an urban or suburban setting. Another twist is that while some cities will not have a specific requirement for the size of the lot, the lot size is used to determine the maximum number of chickens allowed. Like most local codes, the specific ordinances can vary greatly. Some cities allow for a maximum number of chickens for properties of a certain size (and under), then allow for more birds as the property size increases. This kind of step system can become somewhat intricate and be based on number of birds per square foot, per acre or division of acre, and may allow for a mixture of chickens and other animals. On the other hand, some cities appear to be very lenient in lot requirements, allowing up to 30 chickens per $240\,\text{ft}^2$ [36] (about the size of a modern bedroom). Yet one more way to regulate is to determine the number of chickens allowed based on zoning, for example, allowing a certain number of birds on property not zoned agricultural [37]. A simple, albeit arbitrary, way to limit flock size is to limit the number of chickens any household can keep, no matter the size of the property. Of the cities that use this simple method, the number of birds allowed varies from 2 [38] to 50 [39] chickens. Still other cities set a maximum number of chickens that can be owned before requiring the owner to apply for a permit [40].

Setbacks

Setbacks are an extremely common way for cities to regulate chickens, especially requirements that chickens and/or coops be kept a certain distance away from other residences or neighboring buildings. These setbacks can range from $10\,\text{ft}$ [41] to $500\,\text{ft}$ [42] and may be mixed with zoning requirements and/or lot size. Some cities will relax setback requirements if the client is granted permission from surrounding neighbors [43]. This can be especially useful in multifamily residences and densely constructed neighborhoods such as zero–lot-line houses in which the structure comes up to or very near to the edge of a property line (in other words, an exterior wall of one home is the lot line of the other person's property). Some cities may cite specific setbacks from the owner's own home, while others exclude any such restriction [44]. As an example of how variable such codes can be, at least two major cities frame the setback not from the structure itself, but specifically to a door or window of the structure [45]. Setbacks from structures may also not be confined to residences, but from schools, hospitals, or businesses. Grand Rapids, Michigan, places a 100-ft setback from any "dwelling unit, well, spring, stream, drainage ditch or drain" [46]. Very few clients would find themselves able to escape from such tight restrictions.

More restrictive may be setbacks from property lines, no matter if a dwelling is much further away. Property line setbacks may vary from just inches [47] to many hundreds of feet [48]. As in the case with other setbacks, the rule may be relaxed if permission is granted by neighbors. In an effort to prevent direct visualization of chicken coops or possibly contain escapees, a city may prohibit coops in front yards or corner lots [49] or have a setback from the street.

Permits

Many cities will require a permit or license to keep chickens. As is always the case with local laws, the permitting authority is highly variable. It may reside within a city's public health department, animal control office, inspections department, or even the city clerk. For what must truly be the ultimate in frustration, some cities do not even specify in their ordinances by what means a person actually procures a permit. Permitting fees will also vary widely as will the term of the permit; some will require annual renewals, others biennial, still others may only need to renew every 5 years. A few municipalities appear to have open-ended terms, either not specifying the term or being valid unless revoked. Some cities

will issue a permit only with the consent of all or a percentage of neighbors that either border on the property or within a prescribed radius [50]. The permitting process may only apply to flocks of a certain size or if roosters will be present. Many of the permitting/licensing requirements appear to address concerns over potential complaints from neighborhood residents.

It must be noted that municipal codes and ordinances sometimes conflict with each other, creating confusion and frustration for an owner trying to be fully compliant. Animal control codes may conflict with zoning laws or with health codes [51]. This kind of discordance may pit different city departments against each other or even put into question whether a city's board of health has precedence over the zoning board. These conflicts may need to be resolved by the full city council and obviously may not be a priority for a busy council. At best, it will likely not be resolved quickly. As an example of the kind of confusion that can drive a client to frustration, the animal section of one city's code allowed chickens if the zoning ordinance permitted it. The zoning ordinance allowed chickens if the animal code permitted it. The city clerk resolved this viscous loop by interpreting the provisions to ban chickens entirely [52]. The contradictions that occur in local government are simply more visible and by no means preclude their presence in statewide or national forums.

Perhaps in retaliation for clients to have to navigate such a labyrinth of local laws, some homeowners are simply refusing to cooperate, or more constructively, are organizing local and regional movements to create or amend local ordinances. Commonly referred to as the "Poultry Underground" or "Chicken Underground," the movement gained momentum and publicity after some citizens convinced the Madison, Wisconsin, City Council to legalize backyard coops and resulted in the production of a documentary, "Mad City Chickens" [52]. Another dispute in Augusta County, Virginia, began with a ban on backyard poultry and eventually culminated in the county board of supervisors approving to update the county code to keep small numbers of chickens in residentially zoned neighborhoods. Websites and T-shirts frequently display slogans such as "When Chickens Are Outlawed, Only Outlaws Will Have Chickens."

State and National Laws and Regulations

Once your client has cleared the local hurdles (HOA, municipal and county), then the next set of rules and regulations will come from state and federal authorities. It is important to realize that rules and regulations at this level are designed for commercial poultry operations and protection of public health, whereas local ordinances are also concerned with property values, odor, noise, and other "nuisance" factors. As far as the extent of involvement of state and federal authorities, if a backyard enthusiast obtains their starter chicks legally and consumes either the eggs or the meat themselves, within their own household, then it would be rare and unique for them to have any contact or problems. Even if they are breeding their own birds, as long as the chickens they produce essentially live and die on premises, there are really no state or federal entanglements to ensnare them. But if birds (live or dead) or eggs move off their property, then an entire series of hurdles must be cleared. The penalty for non-compliance can be severe- including fines and depopulation of the flock.

A backyard enthusiast must realize that the commercial poultry industry can take a very cautious view of small flocks of chickens. The problem is not a shrinking market share—at least in the United States, eggs and meat produced by a household for their own consumption has a negligible financial impact on industry, insofar as regards lost revenue from egg or meat sales at supermarkets and restaurants. The real problem is the danger of a commercial operation being quarantined or even being depopulated because a small group of

chickens has been diagnosed with a highly contagious disease a few miles down the road in someone's backyard. If faced with the choice of depopulating a dozen chickens in a backyard flock versus the loss of millions of dollars of revenue because eggs or poultry cannot be transported away from the commercial operation, state and federal regulators may show little hesitation in their decision. This kind of situation is not simply an economic decision; a few backyard layers could potentially threaten the health and lives of hundreds of thousands of chickens living in commercial housing. Commercial producers are highly protective of their very large and very expensive investment, and small flocks of chickens present a credible and ever-present danger to their livelihood and the lives of their birds.

Matters become even more fraught when public health is at stake. The state has a responsibility to protect its' citizens and the state takes this matter seriously. Even though there has not been a single human case of avian influenza within the United States, you would be hard pressed to find any American who has not heard of the disease. Many millions of dollars and thousands of hours of work are expended to prevent and control the entry of Avian Influenza into the United States. While these efforts understandably focus on large commercial operations, officials are acutely aware of the dangers that small backyard flocks present.

Movement of Live Poultry to a Backyard Flock

A client must obtain starter birds from somewhere, and that somewhere must be from a neighbor, another backyard enthusiast, a feed store, a farmers market, a local hatchery, or mail-order. It is recommended to purchase chicks from hatcheries or breeders that participate in the National Poultry Improvement Plan (NPIP), which will be described shortly. It is important for both the veterinarian and client to at least have some awareness of what the

NPIP is, what it does, and why. The danger of entry of contagious diseases such as *Salmonella pullorum*-Typhoid or avian influenza is a real threat, not just to your client's personal flock or their family's health but also to public health and the commercial poultry industry. Beyond satisfying legal requirements, it is the duty of a small flock owner and the veterinarian as an advisor to prevent the entry of disease into small flocks and spread of disease to other small flocks and commercial flocks as well as protecting human health.

National Poultry Improvement Program

The NPIP [53] was established in the early 1930s to provide a cooperative industry, state, and federal program through which new diagnostic technology could be effectively applied to the improvement of poultry and poultry products throughout the country. The development of the NPIP was initiated to eliminate Pullorum disease caused by *S. pullorum,* which was rampant in poultry and could cause upward of 80% mortality in baby poultry. The program was later extended and refined to include testing and monitoring for *Salmonella typhoid, Salmonella enteritidis, Mycoplasma gallisepticum, Mycoplasma synoviae, Mycoplasma meleagridis*, and low pathogenic avian influenza. In addition, the NPIP currently includes commercial poultry, turkeys, waterfowl, exhibition poultry, backyard poultry, and game birds.

The NPIP is a voluntary program, and although a particular focus is the registration of breeder flocks to ensure disease-free chicks, the guidelines set up by the NPIP are particularly important when birds are being transported. All states (with the exception of Hawaii) will require that poultry being imported across their state border come from flocks that either participate in the NPIP or follow the guidelines set forth for participation in the NPIP. Further, many states will require that birds being transported *within* a state originate from an NPIP-registered flock or follow the guidelines set forth for participation in the

NPIP. The practical consequences of the establishment of the NPIP are simply this: although it is *possible* for a backyard enthusiast to have poultry that have never been subject to NPIP guidelines, it is not advisable as this will be the safest source for starter or replacement birds. Perhaps even more importantly, if your client is going to be moving birds off their premises to be sold, traded, or exhibited, then it is highly likely that your client must either be a participant in, or follow the guidelines of, the NPIP. Although the NPIP program is voluntary, every state (except Hawaii) has chosen to use NPIP guidelines in some shape or form to regulate movement of poultry into and within their state.

The technical and management provisions of the NPIP have been developed jointly by Industry members and state and federal officials. These criteria have established standards for the evaluation of poultry with respect to freedom from NPIP diseases. Each state runs its own NPIP program; the federal government (USDA) only manages and coordinates state efforts. The NPIP website has direct links to the official state agencies [54] in each state (Hawaii is the only state that does not participate in the NPIP). All of the regulations for the NPIP are detailed in Title 9 of the Code of Federal Regulations (CFRs) [55]. Each official state agency that implements the NPIP must follow the Plan as stated in the CFR, but they may have their own rules and can adopt rules that are more stringent than those in the NPIP.

Sources of Starter or Replacement Birds

Neighbors, Friends, or Other Backyard Hobbyists
The supplier has the responsibility to ensure that all applicable laws have been followed before delivery of live birds. While a health certificate or similar documentation may be required for the purchaser to transport the birds to their home, these requirements are typically fulfilled by the seller. It is important to note that states have the authority to restrict not only import of animals into their state but

also transport of animals within the state. Therefore, it is conceivable that your state may have rules that restrict the movement of birds even within your own neighborhood. It would be prudent to contact your state's animal control office to be sure that there are no state requirements. Identifying the appropriate state agency is the difficult part, as jurisdiction varies widely and often falls across several different agencies or departments.

Feed Stores, Flea Markets, and Roadside Stands

These sources very often have legal requirements, although it is not uncommon for these vendors to be completely unaware of such and they can be in gross violation of existing rules. Again, it is the responsibility of the seller, not the purchaser, to be in compliance with all applicable laws and regulations, although it would be wise for the purchaser to know if health certificates or similar documentation is required while transporting the birds from the source to their home (this applies to both intra-state and interstate transport). Pragmatically and realistically, however, it is virtually impossible for state regulators to oversee and enforce rules with every possible outlet or source. These sellers have very small batches of birds, often from myriad sources, and almost always have transient supplies. Most of the year, these sources will have no animals available at all. An aspiring backyard enthusiast will have no luck acquiring birds from these sources in deep winter, only to see a glut in the spring. "Chick Days" at feed stores and flea markets are common throughout the country.

One final note must be made regarding acquiring birds from the above-mentioned local sources that has nothing to do with laws or regulations. First, your client may have no assurance that they are buying a specific breed of chicken. In fact, there is no assurance that the available chicks are even egg layers as opposed to meat-type birds (referred to as broilers within the poultry industry). Often, these chicks are hybrids. Second, except for some breeds with sex-linked traits, your client will also have no idea whether they are buying pullets or roosters. Finally, it must be pointed out that this is the simplest way of introducing severe disease into a starter flock or, more importantly, into an established flock. A much safer way to acquire new birds is from the following sources.

Commercial Hatcheries and Hobby Farm Breeders

Virtually all commercial hatcheries and the majority of hobby farm breeders will be participants in the NPIP. There are several advantages to this for the backyard enthusiast. First and foremost, these sources will be certified free from *S. pullorum*-Typhoid. Additionally, they may also be certified free from mycoplasma and avian influenza. It is absurdly easy to find out if these sources participate in the NPIP program—just ask. Most hatcheries and breeders prominently display their participation in the program; in fact, if they are transporting birds across state lines they will be required to do so. Even transportation within a state will probably have rules either requiring participation in NPIP or have rules modeled on NPIP guidelines.

There is another advantage for obtaining birds from NPIP participants regarding legal movement (transportation). Birds that are shipped from an NPIP hatchery or breeder may use a form (specifically called the VS Form 9-3) *in lieu of* a health certificate for transportation [56]. To the author's knowledge, poultry are the only species that have such an exemption from health certificates. The hatchery or breeder will typically include this form along with the chicks. As far as means of transportation for small numbers of chicks from these suppliers, the most common (and inexpensive) will be through the United States Postal Service (USPS). The USPS does not assume responsibility for ensuring that shipped birds have required documentation—that responsibility lies with the shipper. The USPS does, however, have very specific mailing and packaging requirements [57] that can be accessed from their website [58]. Of course, if a breeder or hatchery is within driving distance, your clients can simply pick up the birds themselves, although it would still be advisable to receive the VS Form 9-3. A client may be frustrated to learn that they may not be allowed to inspect the premises or meander within a commercial hatchery to observe first-hand the conditions under which chickens are raised. This has little to do with concealing practices and everything to do with biosecurity. All commercial operations are either private or corporate entities, and they have every reason and authority to restrict entry onto their premises.

One final note is to point out that fertilized eggs are treated legally in the same fashion as live birds.

Transportation of Poultry from a Backyard Flock

While discussing acquiring starter or replacement birds into your client's backyard flock, it becomes apparent that state and federal authorities highly regulate the movement of poultry, both when crossing a border into a state and during movement within a state. Again, these regulations are designed to protect both the public health (as in the case of avian influenza) and the health of commercial flocks (as in the case of virulent Newcastle disease). These laws and regulations may cover movement of live birds (including fertilized eggs), unfertilized eggs for consumption, and bird carcasses (meat) intended for consumption. In fact, a state may have entirely different agencies that control each separate kind of chicken or chicken product. For example, in the State of Texas, the Texas Animal Health Commission regulates the movement of live birds. At least two (possibly three depending on the venue and destination of the meat) different groups within the Texas Department of State Health Services are in charge of poultry meat. Both the Texas Department of Agriculture and the Department of State Health Services regulate eggs. Remember, these regulations are in addition to

any restrictions that are placed at the municipal or county level. Large cities especially will usually have their own requirements that often are in the jurisdiction of their respective health departments.

The transport of live birds falls squarely within most state regulations, and every state has rules and regulations governing such movement. It is not wise to assume that even giving a few birds to a neighbor for them to start a new backyard flock has no legal restrictions. In some states it will not matter whether a financial transaction has occurred; it is the movement itself that is regulated. Depending on the state, the rules may vary from non-existent to very stringently regulated. Often, it is the presence or absence of large commercial flocks within the state that dictate the degree of regulation and severity of penalties.

If your client is transporting live poultry on an airline, they must be aware that each individual airline will have requirements that may or may not coincide with federal and state requirements for transport. Often, these requirements will be in addition to whatever governmental regulations are applicable. In addition to their own paperwork, they will also have stringent rules on the types of containers that must be used, food and water instructions, the number and types of birds allowed, or other requirements. Individual airlines have their own set of rules that may not be applicable on another airline. Most commercial air carriers have a division that specifically handles live animals.

Health Certificates/Veterinary Accreditation

In 1921, the USDA established the veterinary accreditation program so that private practitioners could assist federal veterinarians in controlling animal diseases. In 1992, the APHIS of the USDA began managing the program nationally, but authorization of veterinarians continued on a state-by-state basis. Every state has an area office that can easily be obtained at the veterinary accreditation website [59]. Any veterinarian writing health certificates since this time has been familiar with the program.

In 2010, the program was enhanced due to threats of emerging disease; in the case of birds, this has included an epizootic of exotic Newcastle disease (END) and epizootics of West Nile virus. In the vast majority of these incursions, these epizootics have successfully been eliminated with the veterinary practitioner being the first line of defense against such catastrophic disease events [60]. The enhanced program strengthens the accredited veterinarians' understanding of the program and increases their knowledge on current animal health issues. It also allows for the administration of a consistent and uniform program.

The program now has two accreditation categories (Category I and Category II) in place of a single category. Category I accreditation is designed primarily for companion animal practitioners and includes such species as dogs, cats, laboratory animals (rats, mice, gerbils, hamsters), ferrets, reptiles, and even native nonruminant wildlife. Category II accreditation includes all animals including food and fiber species. Accredited veterinarians who wish to write health certificates for any type of bird must obtain a Category II accreditation. All birds within the Class Aves are included, whether they are poultry intended for food, parrots intended for human companionship, or wild birds. As many veterinarians who are seeing backyard poultry are primarily companion animal veterinarians, it is important to either apply, renew, or reinstate for the Category II classification if you wish to be able to write health certificates for your client's birds. USDA-APHIS has an easily navigable website [61] that details requirements for accredited veterinarians and first-time applicants, as well as general information for the public.

All veterinarians who were accredited before the enactment of the enhanced program have (or will have) chosen that category they wish to continue being accredited in and have (or will have) completed supplemental training. Initial training will be required for all newly accredited veterinarians or those previously accredited veterinarians who did not renew before the deadline. All accredited veterinarians within the new, enhanced program will be required to renew their accreditation every 3 years to maintain the program as the core of veterinary preparedness and response. Although provisions were also made for accreditation specializations, such specific rules do not exist at the time of publication.

As small backyard flocks increase in number, some clients may become interested in competing in shows and fairs. Transporting poultry to a destination where birds of differing origin are congregating compounds the possibility of dispersing disease. Therefore, almost every state will have stringent rules regarding such movement and clients should be advised as such. Mandatory testing of individual birds for avian influenza is extremely common. Once more, the rules and the enforcing agency will differ state by state, but the state veterinarian's office should be the first place to contact. The organizers of such exhibitions are generally experienced and many of these events (such as county fairs) have been held for decades; therefore, the requirements and rules for registering show animals are distributed to participants well in advance. Regarding shows, fairs, and other exhibitions, there is another consideration to keep in mind: the Animal Welfare Act (AWA).

The AWA was signed into law in 1966. It is the only federal law in the United States that regulates the care and housing of animals in research, exhibition, transport, and breeding for wholesale and by dealers. Other laws, policies, and guidelines may include additional species coverage or specifications for animal care and use, but all refer to the AWA as the minimum acceptable standard. The Act is enforced by the USDA-APHIS Animal Care Program. While animals intended for food are specifically excluded from the AWA, animals that are exhibited are covered and therefore chickens that are entered in fairs, shows, and exhibitions are covered by its provisions. The AWA was amended in 2002 to include birds not bred for use in research; however, the regulations have not yet been released at the time of publication, so facilities with birds used for purposes described in the AWA are not subject to enforcement action. An overview of the AWA and specific provisions are accessible on the USDA-APHIS Animal Care website [62].

Slaughter, Processing, and Distribution of Poultry

The overarching law that applies to poultry slaughter and processing is the Poultry Products Inspection Act (PPIA) [63], which is administered by the Food Safety and Inspection Service (FSIS) of the USDA. The PPIA was passed by Congress to ensure that only wholesome poultry that is not adulterated and not misbranded enters interstate or foreign commerce, but it has been amended to extend the mandate for federal inspection to all businesses or persons that slaughter or process poultry within a state, when the state does not enforce requirements at least equal to the inspection requirements of the PPIA. Therefore, any business in any state that slaughters or processes poultry for use as human food is required to do so under federal or state inspection, unless the slaughter or processing operations at the business meets certain exemption criteria in the Act.

Twenty-seven states have their own meat inspection program (for intrastate sales), which will meet or exceed standards set forth in the PPIA. Inspection programs in states that do not have their own program are managed by USDA, specifically the Office of Policy Evaluation and Enforcement Review [64]. Although a backyard flock may be exempt from inspection, it may be necessary for your client to apply for an exemption or follow specific criteria to satisfy the exemption.

Exemption requirements vary but will often require a minimum level of sanitation or other requirements. In any case, if an exemption is granted, then the rules that the owner must comply with will be clearly spelled out by the regulatory agency requiring it.

Although it was not the intent of Congress to mandate federal or state inspection of an owner's private holdings of poultry or to mandate inspections of small numbers of poultry, even owners who operate under an exemption are not exempt from all requirements of the Act. USDA-FSIS has developed a flowchart [65] to help owners determine if they qualify for an exemption, but please note that this guide only applies to poultry and not to other kinds of livestock (cattle, sheep, goats, etc.), as they fall under the requirements of the Federal Meat Inspection Act and not the PPIA. Generally, if the client is not engaged in selling poultry meat, there are no federal requirements under the PPIA. Importantly, if your client slaughters and processes less than 1000 birds a year or if they are for personal or private use, they may qualify for either a Personal Use or a Producer/ Grower-1000 Limit exemption.

If your client qualifies for an exemption, then they may slaughter and process poultry without the benefit of federal inspection. However, the Act does not exempt any person slaughtering or processing poultry from the provisions requiring the manufacturing of poultry products that are not adulterated and not misbranded. Therefore, poultry must be slaughtered and processed under sanitary conditions and using procedures that produce sound, clean poultry products fit for human consumption. Specific sanitary practices are described in FSIS's Sanitation Performance Standards Compliance Guide, dated October 13, 1999 [66]. The specific sanitary practices in the document are not requirements; however, establishments that follow the guidance can be fairly certain that they comply with the requirements in the Act.

The regulations in the PPIA require that poultry products transported or distributed in commerce bear specific information. Poultry products inspected and passed under USDA inspection at official USDA establishments must bear the official inspection legend and meet specific labeling requirements prescribed in the regulation. However, exempt poultry products cannot bear the official mark of inspection. In addition, there is specific labeling or identification requirements for exempt product to meet in lieu of bearing all required elements of a label. The information that packages of exempt poultry products must bear varies depending on the exemption and on each state's regulations. In addition to labeling and packaging, states usually also have storage requirements, particularly refrigeration standards.

But even clients who qualify for both federal and state exemptions cannot donate the meat for use as human food outside of their immediate household in many states without meeting explicit criteria. In other words, your client is often not legally allowed to give away unlabeled, uninspected poultry meat to their neighbors or food pantries, although it is permissible for the neighbors to consume poultry that the client has slaughtered and processed (under sanitary conditions) on their own premises, as long as the neighbors consume the meat on the client's premises and the client does not receive money or any other type of compensation for the meal. Even then, if a family member or guest becomes ill from the meal, the owner may soon find themselves under the scrutiny of health officials.

Eggs for Consumption

If selling or even giving away poultry meat seemed complicated, then the rules that may apply to eggs will seem even more so. Starting at the federal level, egg regulations will fall across several departments and agencies.

Food and Drug Administration
Egg wholesomeness and safety will fall under the authority of the Food and Drug Administration (FDA) (Department of Health and Human Services). The FDA obtains its authority through both the Food, Drug, and Cosmetic Act and the Public Health Service Act and regulations will be found in Title 21 of the CFRs. Safety requirements, particularly regarding *S. enteritidis*, are exempted at the federal level for backyard flocks of less than 3000 birds [67]. However, refrigeration requirements, specifically that stored eggs be kept below 45°F, are not exempted for any operation; not even for very small flocks or distribution from the owner's homestead [68]. It does not appear to matter whether commerce is involved in the transfer of eggs from the owner to another person—only that food is being provided for human consumption.

Likewise, there is a labeling requirement [69] under the authority of the FDA that seems to apply to all shell eggs, which is that all shell eggs bear the following statement: "*SAFE HANDLING INSTRUCTIONS: To prevent illness from bacteria: keep eggs refrigerated, cook eggs until yolks are firm, and cook foods containing eggs thoroughly.*" As with the refrigeration requirement, this rule appears to have no exemptions or exceptions.

Agricultural Marketing Services
Ensuring egg quality is the responsibility of this agency, which is in the USDA and derives its authority from the Egg Products Inspection Act and whose regulations can be found in Title 7 of the CFRs. USDA-Agricultural Marketing Services (AMS) surveys egg distribution to ensure that only eggs fit for human consumption (acceptable and unadulterated) are used for such purposes. This function is enforced under the AMS Shell Egg Surveillance Program, which involves quarterly inspections and sampling at egg-processing facilities. There are exemptions from these requirements, specifically for producers who sell directly to consumers from their own flock, sell less than 30 dozen eggs, and have fewer than 3000 hens. Such eggs to be sold must not contain any more loss or leakers than allowed in the official standards for Grade B shell

eggs [70]. These exemptions do not apply to restricted eggs when prohibited by state law.

Additionally, the AMS provides for uniform standards, grades, and weight classes for shell eggs through its Voluntary Grading Program [71]. This is familiar to consumers as weight classes (Jumbo, Extra Large, Large, Medium, Small, Peewee) and consumer grades (AA, A, and B). It is important to note that although this is a voluntary program of the federal government, it is a requirement in some shape or form in every state. It should not be surprising that state requirements vary wildly. For small, backyard flocks, some states will not allow for the sale of ungraded eggs under any circumstances, even when sold directly from the owner to the consumer from their own home. Other states have extremely lax requirements or no requirements for grading at all if sold directly from the owner to the consumer. Eggs must generally be graded for eggs to be used in restaurants and retail food establishments. Most states have a mixture of requirements such as allowing for ungraded eggs to be sold in certain circumstances as long as the eggs are prominently displayed and labeled as being ungraded.

Some states do not allow eggs to be resold in used egg crates or cartons collected from friends or neighbors. In states that do allow this, there are almost always requirements to obliterate markings such as USDA grade shields, expiration dates, distributer information, and any other certification logos.

Food Safety and Inspection Services

This is another division of the USDA, and it also derives its authority from the Egg Products Inspection Act. Its regulations can be found in Title 9 of the CFR. While the FSIS has broad authority over poultry meat (under the Poultry Products Inspection Act described earlier), the bulk of its regulatory capacity with eggs involves egg products. Egg products are those that contain dried, frozen, or liquid eggs—essentially eggs that are intended for human consumption that have been broken. While most backyard enthusiasts will not be engaged in this sort of

activity, it is noteworthy to realize that these types of egg products have their own set of regulatory requirements that are separate and distinct from whole shell eggs. Oddly enough, the FSIS also has refrigeration requirements for whole shell eggs [72], and although there is an exemption for personal use, the FDA requirement (which is the same, i.e., that eggs be maintained below 45°F) has no known exemptions.

Sanitation

Finally, there may be sanitation requirements for washing or otherwise cleaning or sanitizing the eggs and these requirements can be very specific, such as a three-compartment sink necessary to wash, rinse, and sanitize equipment and eggs (with a separate sink for hand washing). Wastewater must be disposed of properly. When using a municipal sewage system you may need the utility provider to sign off, certifying that the provider is approved by state and/or local authorities. Onsite sewage disposal systems (e.g. septic tanks) are usually regulated by the county health department, which is responsible for approving this step of the process. A residential septic system may not be suitable; your local department of health will determine if an additional tank is required for the processing facility. Be sure to communicate the small-scale size of the operation to the inspector.

Roadside Sales and Farmer's Markets

Anyone considering selling their eggs or poultry meat onsite (on the owners own premises), at a roadside stand, flea market or farmers market should consult with their state officials to determine whether there are any inspection, storage, or labeling requirements related to their sale. Typically, the state's department of agriculture is the best place to start asking questions although rules may also be found within a state's department of health, environmental safety, or consumer safety divisions. Unfortunately, jurisdictions often overlap. Some farmers markets are highly regulated by either the state or local authorities, and even sale from the home may require a roadside vendor's permit. Additional permitting may be required such as a retail food establishment or food manufacturer's license. Flock registration for small, backyard flocks is not yet universal, but more and more states are requiring this if birds (live or dead) or eggs will be leaving the owner's property, regardless of the size of the flock. If selling eggs, an additional egg license may be required by the state. Misleading advertising may be considered an offense at national and state levels. Owners should be extremely careful when using such words as "fresh," "selected," "cage-free," etc. Use of the word "organic" has very specific legal meanings and unfortunately the definition will vary depending on the state and the product.

Live bird markets and auctions are increasingly coming under the scrutiny of both state and local health officials and the trend is to require that the birds come from NPIP-certified flocks (or follow NPIP guidelines for *S. pullorum*-Typhoid testing), be avian influenza tested, be from a flock registered with the state, and have record-keeping requirements. Many states are conducting regular inspections at markets and other venues to conduct surveillance testing and to ensure compliance with all existing regulations.

Transitioning from Hobby to Commercial Operation

If a veterinarian has a client with a rapidly growing backyard flock and is becoming concerned that they are flirting with crossing the line from a hobbyist to a commercial (albeit specialty) producer, the 3000-bird threshold would appear to be at least an easily quantified red line. Engaging in commerce itself (i.e. exchanging money for birds, live or deceased, or eggs), does not in itself define a commercial producer, not even if the birds or eggs are specifically intended for consumption. Direct sales to customers, either privately or in a farmers market, is exempted from food safety

rules except as regulated locally through state, county, or local health codes.

Each state has its own department of agriculture that sets regulations regarding poultry, whether commercial or backyard, and a quick check on your state's website will generally yield state-specific laws and rules. In addition, each state will have a state veterinarian who should be considered as a primary reference when in doubt. The state veterinarian also often directs, manages, or is affiliated with a state animal health commission or board. The state veterinarian will be primarily involved in areas of both animal health and increasingly animal welfare.

Some states will require registration or permitting if a client is selling even small numbers of live birds, even at a roadside stand or feed store. These rules specifically target disease control, especially those diseases that could affect commercial poultry producers. Laws and regulations governing transportation of poultry are largely concerned with the same health issues—that is, the health not of humans but of the larger commercial chicken population. Following are the diseases that are of gravest concern to state and federal officials:

Salmonella-Associated Pullorum and Typhoid Diseases

These conditions are caused by two very closely related organisms that were once thought to be different species but have recently been classified as biovars of *Salmonella enterica* subsp. *enterica*. Pullorum disease is usually symptomatic only in young birds. The mortality rate varies, but it can be as high as 100%. Fowl typhoid resembles Pullorum disease in young birds, but it is also a serious concern in growing and adult poultry. The control of these diseases is complicated by vertical transmission: hens can become subclinically infected carriers and pass the infections to their embryos in the egg. Fowl typhoid and Pullorum disease have been eradicated from commercial poultry in many developed countries, including the United States and Canada, but they may persist in backyard poultry flocks and game birds.

Avian Influenza

State and federal officials closely monitor two types of avian influenza based on their ability to cause disease in poultry: low pathogenicity avian influenza (LPAI) and high pathogenicity avian influenza (HPAI). LPAI naturally occurs in wild birds and can spread to domestic poultry. These strains pose little threat to human health, but the mere potential to mutate into more highly pathogenic forms has led the USDA to closely monitor both LPAI H5 and H7 strains. Broad public concerns about highly pathogenic H5N1 virus has resulted in USDA efforts to very quickly respond to and eradicate HPAI. It is important to note that HPAI has been detected a handful of times in US poultry: in 1924, 1983, 2004, and 2014–2017. While more than 200 human cases have been reported since 2004, no strain of avian influenza that have been detected in US poultry, either HPAI or LPAI, have caused any human illness. (See Avian Influenza and Exotic Newcastle Disease Chapter and the Biosecurity Chapter for more detail.)

Virulent Newcastle Disease

END, also known as virulent Newcastle disease, is a contagious and fatal viral disease affecting all species of birds. END is so virulent that many birds die without having developed any clinical signs. END can infect and cause death even in vaccinated poultry. Mortality is up to 90% of exposed birds. The USDA APHIS is the federal agency that takes the lead in excluding END from the United States and responding to any END outbreaks that do occur. (See the Avian Influenza and Exotic Newcastle Disease chapter and the Biosecurity chapter for more details.)

Be Cautious, Not Afraid

It is difficult not to be so intimidated by the labyrinth of laws, regulations, restrictions, and exemptions discussed in this chapter that you want to throw up your hands in confusion and fear. And in fact it is possible for a well-meaning but uninformed client to find themselves in either serious trouble or face the tragedy of having their flock depopulated against their will. These rules were never intended primarily to quash backyard flocks; rather they are designed to accomplish some very simple goals:

- Be a good neighbor
- Protect our poultry industry
- Protect human health

These are worthy objectives even though it may be burdensome or even impossible for your clients to engage in their desire for a backyard flock and simultaneously fulfill their ethical and legal duties. At the very least, people should be aware and become at least minimally educated instead of pursuing such an endeavor on a whim. Stewardship of living creatures always carries responsibilities, and as veterinary professionals we should proudly carry that responsibility and pass it on to our clients.

References

1 Bouvier, J. (2012). Illegal Fowl: A Survey of Municipal Laws Relating to Backyard Poultry and a Model Ordinance for Regulating City Chickens. *Environmental Law Reporter*. 42, p. 10889.

2 Dallas, Tex., Code of Ordinances §7-1.1 (2011); Indianapolis, Ind., Rev. Code tit. III, ch. 531.101 (2011); Jacksonville, Fla., Ordinance; Code §656.1601 (2011); New Orleans, La., Code of Ordinances §18-2.1 (2011); Raleigh, N.C., Code of Ordinances §12-3001 (2011); Plano,Tex., Code of Ordinances §4-184 (2011); Spokane, Wash., Mun. Code §17C.310.100 (no date listed).

3 Phila. §10-100.

4 Lakewood Mun. Ordinance §505.18.

5 North Carolina State Bar Government and Public Sector Section. http://governmentandpublicsector.ncbar.org/newsletters/publicservantmarch2011/urbanhenfare (accessed 9 April 2019).

6 Bouvier, J. (2012). Illegal Fowl: A Survey of Municipal Laws Relating to Backyard Poultry and a Model Ordinance for Regulating City Chickens. *Environmental Law Reporter*. 42, p. 10904.

7 Ibid, p. 10901.

8 United States Department of Agriculture – Animal and Plant Health Inspection Service, Veterinary Services. (2004). National Animal Health Monitoring System (NAHMS). Part I: Reference of health and management of backyard/small production flocks in the United States. Poultry '04, 2005. https://www.nal.usda.gov/exhibits/ipd/frostonchickens/items/show/374 (accessed 4 April 2019).

9 VanderVelde, L.S. (1990). Local Knowledge, Legal Knowledge, and Zoning Law. *Iowa Law Review*. 75, p. 1057.

10 Richmond, Va., Code of Ordinances §10-88 (2011); Stockton, Cal., Mun. Code §6.04.130 (2011).

11 Kansas City, Mo., Code of Ordinances §14-15(d) (2011).

12 Glendale, Cal., Mun. Code §6.04.040 (2011). Chi., Ill., Code of Ordinances §17-12-300 (2011; Madison, Wis., Code of Ordinances §2809(9)(b)(6) (no date listed; Milwaukee, Wis., Code of Ordinances §78-6.5(3)(b) (2011); Sacramento, Cal., City Code §9.44.860 (2011); Wichita, Kan., Code of Ordinances §6.04.175(p) (2011)

13 Buffalo, N.Y., City Code §341-11.3(d) (2009); Charlotte, N.C., Code of Ordinances §3-102(c)(4) (2010); Pittsburgh, Pa., Code of Ordinances §911.04.A.2 (2011).

14 San Francisco, Cal., Health Code §37(d)(5) (2011).

15 Chi., Ill., Code of Ordinances §17-12-300 (2011)

16 L.A., Cal., Mun. Code §53.67 (2011).

17 Wichita, Kan., Code of Ordinances §6.04.175(p) (2011).

18 Bouvier, J (2012). Illegal Fowl: A Survey of Municipal Laws Relating to Backyard Poultry and a Model Ordinance for Regulating City Chickens. *Environmental Law Reporter*, 42, p. 10916.

19 VanderVelde, L.S. (1990). Local Knowledge, Legal Knowledge, and Zoning Law. *Iowa Law Review*. 75, p. 1058.

20 Anaheim §18.38.030; Birmingham §2.4.1; Jacksonville tit. XVIII, ch. 462, tit. XVII, ch. 656; Lubbock §4.07.001.

21 VanderVelde, L.S. (1990). Local Knowledge, Legal Knowledge, and Zoning Law. *Iowa Law Review*. 75, p. 1060.

22 Ibid, p. 1063.

23 Ibid, p. 1075.

24 Ibid, p. 1068.

25 Atlanta, Ga., Code of Ordinances §18-7(1)(d) (2011); Buffalo, N.Y., City Code §341-11.3(B)(3) (2009).

26 Mobile, Ala., Code of Ordinances §7-88 (2011).

27 Long Beach, Cal., Mun. Code §6.20.100 (2011).

28 Cincinnati, Ohio, Code of Ordinances §701-35 (2011).

29 Long Beach, Cal., Mun. Code §6.20.100 (2011); New Orleans, La., Code of Ordinances §18-2.1(a) (2)(2011); Plano, Tex., Code of Ordinances §4-1 Secure Enclosure & Shelter (2011); Tucson, Ariz., Code of Ordinances §4-3(2)(c) (2011).

30 Cleveland, Ohio, Codified Ordinances §347.02(b)(1)(D) (2011).

31 Irving, Tex., Code of Ordinances §6-1 Shelter (2011).

32 Norfolk, Va., Code of Ordinances §6.1-2 (2011); Plano, Tex., Code of Ordinances §4-1 (2011); Tulsa, Ok., Code of Ordinances §406 (2011).

33 Jersey City, N.J., Code of Ordinances §90-8(2011).

34 Rochester, N.Y., City Ordinances §30-19 (no date listed).

35 Nashville-Davidson, Tenn., Mun. Code §17-16-330(b) (2011); Pittsburgh, Pa., Code of Ordinances §§635.02, 911.04.A.2 (2011); Phila., Pa., Code §10-112 (2011); Oklahoma City, Okla., Mun. Code §59-9350 (2011); Richmond, Va., Code of Ordinances §10-88 (2011).

36 Rochester, N.Y., City Ordinances §§30-12, 30-19 (no date listed).

37 El Paso, Tex., Mun. Code §7.24.020(B) (2011).

38 Garland, Tx., Code of Ordinances §22.14 (2011); Honolulu, Haw., Rev. Ordinances §7-2.5(d) (1990).

39 Jersey City, N.J., Code of Ordinances §90-6 (2011).

40 Wichita, Kan., Code of Ordinances §6.04.157(a) (2011); Santa Ana, Cal., Code of Ordinances §5.6 (2011); San Jose, Cal., Code of Ordinances tit. 7 (2007); El Paso, Tex., Mun. Code §7.24.020 (2011).

41 Seattle, Wash., Mun. Code §23.42.052(C) (2011).

42 Richmond, Va., Code of Ordinances §10-88 (2011).

43 Las Vegas, Nev., Mun. Code §7.38.050 (2011); Phoenix, Ariz., City Code §8-10 (2011); St. Petersburg, Fla., Code of Ordinances §4-31(d) (2011); Tacoma, Wash., Mun. Code §§5.30.010 & 5.30.030 (2011).

44 Atlanta, Ga., Code of Ordinances §18-7 (2011). L.A., Cal., Mun. Code §§53.58 & 53.59 (2011).

45 Buffalo, N.Y., City Code §341-11 (2009); San Francisco, Cal., Health Code §37 (2011).

46 Grand Rapids, Mich., Code of Ordinances §8.582(2) (2010).

47 Cleveland, Ohio, Codified Ordinances Ohio, Codified Ordinances §347.02 (2011); Buffalo, N.Y., City Code §341-11.3 (2009).

48 Wash., D.C., Mun. Regulations for Animal Control §902.7 (no date listed).

49 Bakersfield, Cal., Mun. Code §17.12.010-RS (2011). Buffalo, N.Y., City Code §341-11.3 (2009); Cleveland, Ohio, Codified Ordinances §347.02(b)(1)(B) (2011); Des Moines, Iowa, Code of Ordinances §18-4 (2011); Milwaukee, Wis., Code of Ordinances §78-6.5(3)(i) (2011); Phoenix, Ariz., City

Code §8-7 (2011); Sacramento, Cal., City Code §9.44.860 (2011).

50 St. Paul, Minn., §198.04(b) (2011): Las Vegas, Nev., Mun. Code §7.38.050 (2011). Buffalo, N.Y., City Code §341-11.2 (2009).

51 Bouvier J. (2012). Illegal Fowl: A Survey of Municipal Laws Relating to Backyard Poultry and a Model Ordinance for Regulating City Chickens. *Environmental Law Reporter*. 42, p. 10902.

52 *Mad City Chickens*. Dir. Tashai Lovington and Robert Lughai (2008). Tarazod Films. Documentary.

53 North Carolina State Bar Government and Public Sector Section. http://www.aphis. usda.gov/animal_health/animal_dis_spec/ poultry (accessed 9 April 2019).

54 North Carolina State Bar Government and Public Sector Section. http://www.aphis.usda. gov/animal_health/animal_dis_spec/poultry/ downloads/osa-npip.pdf (accessed 9 April 2019).

55 9 CFR 56, 145, 146, 147, and 148.

56 9 CFR 145.52.

57 Mailing Standards of the United States Postal Service Publication 52- Hazardous, Restricted, and Perishable Mail, Dec 2012. Subchapters 526.31, 32, 33, 41, and 42.

58 US Postal Service. http://pe.usps.com/text/ pub52/welcome.htm (accessed 9 April 2019).

59 US Department of Agriculture, Animal and Plant Health Inspection Service. https:// www.aphis.usda.gov/aphis/ourfocus/ animalhealth/nvap/ct_areavet (accessed 10-23-20)

60 US Department of Agriculture, Animal and Plant Health Inspection Service. http://www. aphis.usda.gov/animal_health/vet_ accreditation/downloads/why-nvap.pdf (accessed 9 April 2019).

61 US Department of Agriculture, Animal and Plant Health Inspection Service. https:// www.aphis.usda.gov/aphis/ourfocus/ animalhealth/nvap (accessed 10-23-20)

62 US Department of Agriculture, Animal and Plant Health Inspection Service. https:// www.aphis.usda.gov/aphis/ourfocus/ animalwelfare/sa_awa (accessed 10-23-20)

63 US Department of Agriculture, Food Safety and Inspection Service. https://www.fsis.usda.gov/wps/portal/fsis/topics/rulemaking/poultry-products-inspection-acts (accessed 10-23-20)

64 US Department of Agriculture, Food Safety and Inspection Service. https://www.fsis.usda.gov/wps/portal/informational/contactus/phone/key-agency-contacts. (accessed 10-23-20)

65 US Department of Agriculture, Food Safety and Inspection Service. https://www.fsis.usda.gov/wps/portal/fsis/topics/regulatory-compliance/guidelines/2006-0001. (accessed 10-23-20)

66 US Department of Agriculture, Food Safety and Inspection Service. https://www.fsis.usda.gov/wps/portal/fsis/topics/regulatory-compliance/guidelines/2016-0003 (accessed 10-23-20)

67 21 CFR 118.

68 21 CFR 115.50.

69 21 CFR 101.17 (h).

70 7 CFR57.100.

71 7 CFR56.

72 9 CFR 590.50.

2

Common Breeds of Backyard Poultry

Lillian Gerhardt and Cheryl B. Greenacre

Avian and Zoological Medicine Service, Department of Small Animal Clinical Sciences, College of Veterinary Medicine, University of Tennessee, Knoxville, Knoxville, TN, USA

General Information

Chickens have coexisted with people for centuries. They have been a staple in farmyards around the world, providing nutritious eggs and meat. Today, chickens have reemerged as a companion animal. The modern chicken owner has discovered that their hens each have a distinct personality and readily interact with their humans, with the added bonus of delivering delicious fresh eggs. They are given names and live in fancy coops, and when not feeling well, veterinary care is sought.

All of today's many breeds of domestic chickens (*Gallus domesticus*) come from a single origin—the Red Jungle Fowl (*Gallus gallus*) of Southeast Asia that was domesticated about 10,000 years ago. There are hundreds of chicken breeds around the world, but exactly how many chicken breeds currently exist is not known because new varieties are continuously being developed.

Classification of Breeds

Chickens are kept for egg purposes (laying breeds), meat purposes (meat breeds), both egg and meat purposes (dual purpose), or show

purposes (ornamental breeds) [1–6]. The following descriptions are examples of some commonly kept breeds of chickens and are not meant to provide a complete list. There are several websites with complete descriptions of breeds, and one includes a program for identifying the right breed for your needs [5, 6].

According to the American Poultry Association (APA) Standard of Perfection, chicken breeds are classified first as to whether they are standard size or bantam (smaller) size. The standard size is further subdivided into six classes named after where the breed was first developed (Table 2.1). The bantam size is further subdivided into five classes based on the physical traits of that breed (Table 2.1).

Variety

Each breed is further subdivided into "varieties" based on physical characteristic such as color, comb type, leg feathering, or presence of a beard or muffs. For example, Plymouth Rocks have seven different color varieties, Leghorns have single comb or rose comb varieties as well as color varieties, and Polish have bearded or nonbearded varieties of varying colors. Each breed of chicken can come in many different APA-recognized colors, as well

Table 2.1 The American Poultry Association (APA) standard of perfection classifies breeds of chickens into six classes of standard size based on where the breed was first developed and five classes of Bantam size (smaller) based on physical traits of that breed.

A. Standard class
    a. American
    b. Asiatic
    c. Continental (Europe, not including England)
    d. English
    e. Mediterranean
    f. All other standard breeds
B. Bantam class
    a. Game
    b. Single comb, clean legged
    c. Rose comb, clean legged
    d. All other combs, clean legged
    e. Feather legged

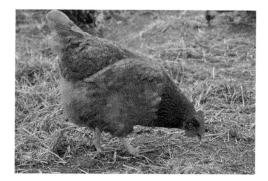

Figure 2.1 "Sexlink" chickens come in several varieties such as this Red Star hen.

as unrecognized colors; only one or a few examples are listed in the tables.

Strain

Each "variety" can then be further subdivided into "strains," a population of breeding birds (private or commercial) that exhibit a close common trait. An example would be the commercially popular chicken strain the Cobb500®.

Hybrids

Hybrids are a cross between two known breeds to acquire hybrid vigor. Sex-linked chickens produce a lot of eggs and are not broody. An example would be the Red Star (Figure 2.1), or Red Sex-Linked, chickens commonly sold at farm stores that are a cross between a New Hampshire or Rhode Island Red rooster and a Plymouth Rock, Rhode Island White, Silver Laced Wyandotte, or Delaware hen. A sex-linked chicken is one that at the time of hatch can be sexed by color. This helps to guarantee you have only pullets (females) for egg-laying purposes. With other breeds, the sexing of chicks is only about 90% accurate. Sex-linked chickens come in

several varieties such as Red Star, Black Star, and Golden Comets. The Rhode Island Red to Rhode Island White cross yields a female chick that is red with white undercolor, whereas the males are white [1]. The Black Star, or Black Sex-Linked, is a cross between a Rhode Island Red or a New Hampshire rooster and a Barred Plymouth Rock hen. The resulting offspring at hatching will be completely black females, and males will be black with a white spot on top of the head.

Laying Breeds

The main reason chickens are kept as backyard birds is for egg production. The physical traits and common characteristics of some commonly seen, or representative, laying breeds are listed (Tables 2.2 and 2.3). Some examples of laying breeds include Americauna (Figures 2.2 and 2.3), Hamburg (Figures 2.4 and 2.5), Lakenvelder (Figure 2.6), Leghorn (Figure 2.7), Maran (Figure 2.8), Plymouth Rock (Figure 2.9), and Welsummer (Figure 2.10). Some laying breeds may be considered dual purpose (for egg and meat), such as the Australorp, Barnvelder, Dominique, Maran, Plymouth Rock, and Rhode Island Red.

Egg Color

The Ameracauna breed is very popular because these hens are excellent layers of bluish-green tinted eggs (Figure 2.11). Technically, the "Easter eggers" that some hatcheries offer are

Table 2.2 Examples of some laying breeds of chickens and their physical traits.

Breed	S (class) M/F (kg)	B (class) M/F (kg)	Origin	Comb (points)	Wattles	Ear lobes	Legs	Example of color
Americauna (Figures 2.2, 2.3, and 2.11)	O 3.0/2.5	O 0.850/0.740	US	Pea	Red, small or absent	Red, small, round	C	Brown red, wheaten
Australorp	E 3.9/3.0	S 0.850–0.740	A	Single (5)	Red, small, round	Red, oblong	C	Black
Barnvelder	C 3.2/2.8	—	H	Single (5)	Red, medium	Red, medium	C	Double laced partridge
Dominique	A 2.0/1.6	—	US	Rose	Red, small to medium	Red, oblong	C	Barred
Hamburg (Figures 2.4 and 2.5)	C 2.3/1.8	R 0.740/0.625	T	Rose (with spike) (Figure 2.5)	Red, small to medium	White	C	Silver spangled
Lakenvelder (Figure 2.6)	C 2.3/1.8	S 0.680/0.570	G	Single (5)	Red, small	White, small, oblong	C	White body with black head/tail
Leghorn (Figure 2.7)	M 2.8/2.0	S 0.740/0.625	I	Single (5) or rose	Red, medium	White, oval	C	White
Maran (Figures 2.8 and 2.12)	a 3.9/3.2	a 1.1/0.910	F	Single (5+)	Red, long	Red, long	C	Black, silver cuckoo
Plymouth Rock (Figure 2.9)	A 4.3/3.4	S 1.0/0.910	US	Single (5)	Red, long	Red, long oval	C	Barred
Rhode Island Red	A 3.9/3.0	S 0.965/0.850	US	Single (5) or rose	Red, medium	Red, medium	C	Red
Rhode Island White	A 3.9/3.0	S 0.965/0.850	US	Rose	Red, medium	Red, oblong	C	White
Welsummer (Figure 2.10)	A 3.2–2.8	S 0.965/0.850	H	Single (6–7)	Red, medium	Red, long oval	C	Reddish brown with stippling

[S = Standard Class (Am = American, A = Asiatic, C = Continental, E = English, M = Mediterranean, O = All Other Standard Breeds) including average weights of males (M) versus females(F) in kilograms (kg)]; [B = Bantam Class (G = Game, R = Rose Comb – Clean Legged, S = Single Comb – Clean Legged, O = All Other Combs – Clean Legged, F = Feather Legged) including average weights of males (M) versus females(F) in kilograms (kg)]; [Origin = Country of origin, (US = United States, A = Australia, H = Holland, T = Turkey, G = Germany, I = Italy, F = France)]; R = rose comb; S = Single comb (number of points); [Legs; C = Clean, F = Feathered].
a Breed not yet recognized by the APA.

Table 2.3 Examples of some laying breeds of chicken and their common characteristics.

Breed	Eggs (#, size, color)	Laying period	Broodiness	Hardiness Cold/heat	Temperment	Bears confinement?	Other
Americauna	3/wk, large, light blue (Figure 2.11)	Very long	No, but will	Yes/not especially	Docile, fun	Yes	Differs from "Easter Egger" that lays blue and green eggs
Australorp	5/wk, large, brown	Long	Yes	Yes/not especially	Docile, sweet, shy, calm	Yes	Dual, Australia's National Breed
Barnvelder	3/wk, large, coppery/ chocolate brown	Long	No	Yes/no	Docile, lively, active, friendly	Yes	Dual
Dominique	3/wk, medium to large, brown	Long	Yes	Yes/not especially	Docile, calm nurturing	Yes	Dual, oldest US breed, excellent forager
Hamburg	4/wk, small, white	Long	No	Yes/yes	Active, alert, flighty	No, good fliers	Excellent forager
Lakenvelder	3/wk, small to medium, white to cream, or tinted	Long	No	No/yes	Flighty, active, alert, shy	Yes, good fliers	Ornamental layer, distinctive plumage appears after third molt
Leghorn	4/wk, extra large, white	Very long	No	Yes/yes	Active, intelligent, adaptable	Yes	Best feed: egg ratio
Maran	3/wk, large, dark brown (Figure 2.12)	Long	Yes	Yes/not especially	Varies, can be calm	Yes, do not fly	Dual, darkest eggs, "chocolate eggers"
Plymouth Rock	4/wk, large, brown	Long	Yes	Yes/yes	Docile, smart, plucky, adaptable	Yes	Dual
Rhode Island Red	5/wk, large to extra large brown	Very long	No	No/not especially	Easygoing, calm	Yes	Dual
Rhode Island White	5/wk, large to extra large brown	Very long	No	No/not especially	Easygoing, calm	Yes	Dual, used to cross with Rhode Island Reds to create "Red Sex-linked" hybrids
Welsummer	4/wk, large, chocolate brown	Long	Yes	Yes/yes	Intelligent, calm, friendly	Yes	Excellent forager, described as "what a farmyard chicken should look like"

H = Hardy in hotter temperatures; C = hardy in colder temperatures; FR = prefers free-range; Con = prefers confinement; US = United States; R = rose comb; S = Single comb (number of points).

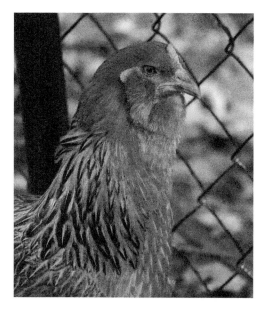

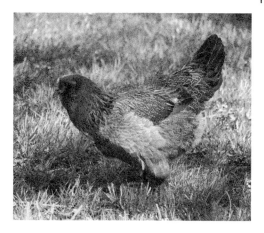

Figure 2.3 Ameraucana breed of chicken (hen). Source: Photograph courtesy of Dr. Katherine DeAnna.

Figure 2.2 Ameraucana breed of chicken (hen). Note the pea comb and "beard" or tuft on the cheek. Source: Photograph courtesy of Dr. Katherine DeAnna.

not Americaunas but a hybrid that lays blue-, green-, or pink-tinted eggs. The Americauna breed was developed from the Araucana, a tailless bird that lays colored eggs. Americaunas are easily identified by their beards and muffs on their cheeks. The Maran breed is known for

laying dark brown eggs that are the color of chocolate (Figure 2.12).

Egg Size

The United States Department of Agriculture (USDA) considers the minimum weight of a "jumbo" egg to be about 71 g, a "very large or extra-large" egg to be about 64 g, a "large" egg to be about 57 g, a "medium" egg to be about 50 g, a "small" egg to be about 43 g, and a tiny or "peewee" egg to be about 35 g (Figure 2.13).

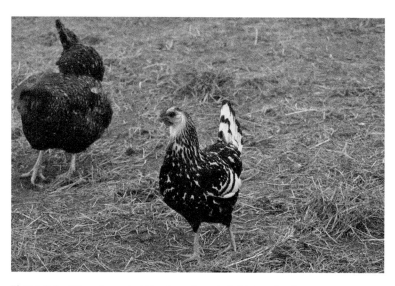

Figure 2.4 Silver Spangled Hamburg breed of chicken (hen).

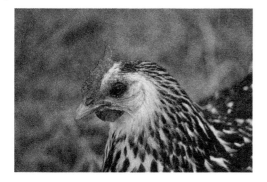

Figure 2.5 Rose comb of Silver Spangled Hamburg breed of chicken (hen).

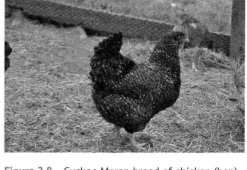

Figure 2.8 Cuckoo Maran breed of chicken (hen). They have a single comb.

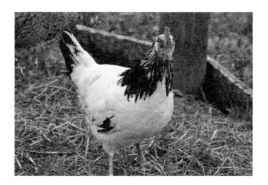

Figure 2.6 Lakenvender breed of chicken (hen). Note the single comb.

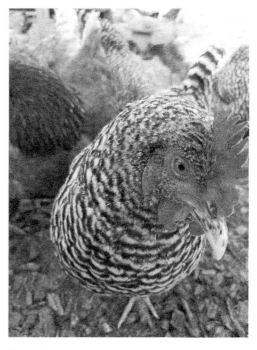

Figure 2.9 Barred variety of Plymouth Rock breed of hen.

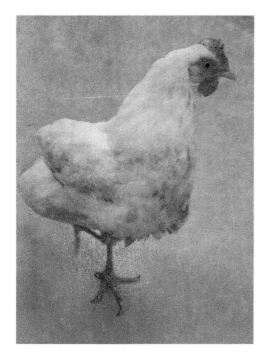

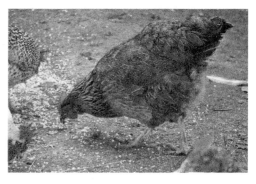

Figure 2.7 White leghorn breed of hen. Note the single comb.

Figure 2.10 Welsummer breed of chicken (hen). They have a single comb.

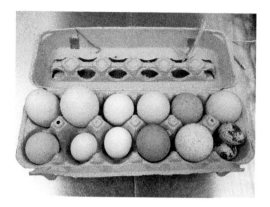

Figure 2.11 Variety of eggs from one farm. Top row from left to right: young duck, adult duck, Americauna chicken, barnyard mixed breed of chicken, "Olive Egger" chicken, Barnyard mixed breed of chicken; bottom row left to right: barnyard mixed breed of chicken, Old English Game Bantam chicken, Polish chicken, barnyard mixed breed of chicken, turkey, *Coturnix* sp. quail.

Egg Production

The White Leghorn breed is known for its excellent egg production (four per week, or 280 per year) of extra-large eggs and excellent feed-to-egg conversion ratio. The record number of eggs laid by a chicken is by a White Leghorn and was more than 365 large white eggs in a single year. Good egg production is considered to be about three eggs per week; fair, two eggs per week; and poor, one egg per week. Many of the hybrids, such as the Red Sex-Linked, are also excellent layers.

Broodiness

A broody hen is one that prefers to sit on the eggs, a trait that is desirable if one is trying to raise chicks but undesirable if one wants to collect the eggs. While brooding over eggs, the hen does not lay any additional eggs. Most laying breeds, like the Leghorn are not broody, but some are, such as the Welsummer.

Meat Breeds

Some backyard chickens are kept for free range meat production. The physical traits and common characteristics of some commonly seen, or representative meat breeds are listed (Tables 2.4 and 2.5). Some examples of meat breeds include Cornish (Figure 2.14), Delaware (Figure 2.15), Dorking, and Jersey Giant. Some meat breeds may be considered dual purpose (for meat and egg), such as the Brahma (Figures 2.16 and 2.17), Dominique, Maran, New Hampshire, Orpington (Figures 2.18–2.20), Sussex (Figure 2.21), and Wyandotte (Figures 2.22–2.26).

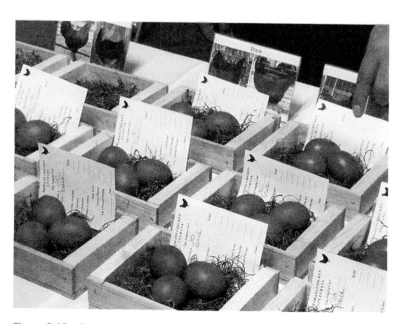

Figure 2.12 Eggs from Maran chickens showing their characteristic dark, chocolate brown color.

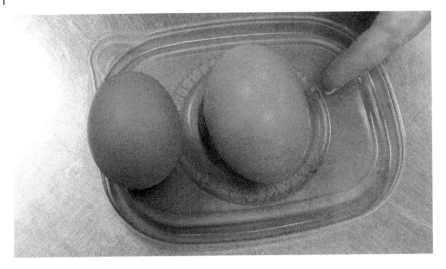

Figure 2.13 Examples of a "Large" (left), and "Extra-Large" (right) egg.

Skin Color

Some breeds are known for having yellow skin (preferred in North America), such as the Brahma and Wyandotte, whereas others have white skin, such as the Dorking and Orpington. Although the Silkie is an ornamental breed, it is prized in some countries for its black skin. They also have black periosteum on their bones and black peritoneal lining, as well as five toes (Figure 2.27).

Feed-to-Meat Conversion

The best feed-to-meat conversion occurs in commercial broilers that can reach market weight as young as 42 days of age. The Cornish breed is known for reaching a mature size quickly. They can reach 3 kg in 8 weeks and can get over 4 kg after that. The largest breed of chicken, the Jersey Giant, may take 6 months to reach mature size, and therefore does not have the best feed-to-meat conversion ratio.

Ornamental Breeds

Ornamental breeds are kept for show. The physical traits and common characteristics of some commonly seen, or representative ornamental breeds are listed (Tables 2.6 and 2.7) Some examples of ornamental breeds of chicken include American Game Bantam (Figure 2.28), Bearded d'Uccle (Figures 2.29 and 2.30), Cochin (Figures 2.31 and 2.32), La Fleche (Figure 2.33), Orloff (Figures 2.34 and 2.35), Polish (Figures 2.36 and 2.37), Seabright (Figure 2.38), Sicilian Buttercup (Figures 2.39 and 2.40), and Silkie (Figures 2.41 and 2.42). Some ornamental breeds can lay a respectable number of eggs, examples include Orloff, Sicialian Buttercup, Langshan (also a respectable meat chicken), La Fleche, and Cochin.

Many of the Game birds were originally bred for cock fighting, consequently the males of these breeds should not be housed together as some may even fight to the death. In contrast, the Silkie breed is one of the most docile chicken breeds and consequently they make good pets. Most Silkies in the United States are the bearded variety of bantam-sized Silkies. It is believed this breed originated in Asia, perhaps China, as far back as the thirteenth century. The feathers can be white, black, buff, blue, partridge, or gray. They are distinctive for their hair like feathers, the feather tuft on their head, their very dark, even black skin, and for having five toes instead of the usual four.

Table 2.4 Examples of some meat breeds of chicken and their physical traits.

Breed	S (class) M/F (kg)	B (class) M/F (kg)	Origin	Comb (points)	Wattles	Ear lobes	Legs	Example of color
Brahma (Figures 2.16 and 2.17)	A 5.5/4.3	F 1.1/0.965	US	Pea	Red, small	Red, large, long	F	Buff
Cornish (Figure 2.14)	E 4.8/3.6	A 1.3–1.0	E	Small pea	Red, small	Red, small	C	White
Delaware (Figure 2.15)	A 3.9/3.0	O 0.965/0.850	US	Single (5)	Red, medium to large	Red, elongated oval	C	White with neck and tail
Dorking	E 4.1/3.2	S,R 1.0/0.910	B	Single (6) or rose	Red, large	Red, medium	C, short, five toes	Silver gray
Jersey Giant	A 5.9/4.5	S 1.1/0.965	US	Single (6)	Red, medium	Red, medium	C	Black
New Hampshire	A 3.9/3.0	S 0.965/0.850	US	Single (5)	Red, medium	Red, long	C	Chestnut red
Orpington (Figures 2.18–2.20)	E 4.5/3.6	S 1.1/0.965	US	Single (5)	Red, medium	Red, medium	C	Buff
Sussex (Figure 2.21)	E 4.1/3.2	S 1.0/0.910	E	Single (5)	Red, small	Red, medium	C	Speckled
Wyandotte (Figures 2.22–2.26)	A 3.9/3.0	R 0.850/0.740	US	Rose (Figure 2.22)	Red, medium	Red, oblong	C	Silver or golden laced

[S = Standard Class (Am = American, A = Asiatic, C = Continental, E = English, M = Mediterranean, O = All Other Standard Breeds) including average weights of males (M) versus females(F) in kilograms (kg)]; [B = Bantam Class (G = Game, R = Rose Comb – Clean Legged, S = Single Comb – Clean Legged, O = All Other Combs – Clean Legged, F = Feather Legged) including average weights of males (M) versus females(F) in kilograms (kg)]; [Origin = Country of origin, (US = United States, A = Australia, H = Holland, T = Turkey, G = Germany, I = Italy, F = France, B = Britain, E = England)]; R = rose comb; S = Single comb (number of points); [Legs; C = Clean, F = Feathered].

Table 2.5 Examples of some meat breeds of chicken and their common characteristics.

Breed	Eggs (#, size, color)	Laying period	Broodiness	Hardiness Cold/heat	Temperment	Bears confinement?	Other
Brahma	3/wk, medium to large, brown	Long	Yes	Yes/not especially	Quiet, tame	Yes, but prefers outdoors	Dual, one of the largest breeds
Cornish	1/wk, small, light brown	Long	Yes	Yes/not especially	Loud, active, not docile	Well, does not do well with free range	Eats a lot of food, crosses used to develop commercial broilers, stocky build, skeletal, and heart disease
Delaware	4/wk, large, brown	—	Yes	Yes/not especially	Quiet, docile, friendly	Well, do not fly	Once popular, now quite rare
Dorking	3/wk, medium, cream, or tinted	Long	Yes	Yes/not especially	Docile, gentle, shy, calm	Well	Old breed, only breed with solid red ear lobe to lay a white egg
Jersey Giant	3/wk, large to extra-large, brown	Long	Can	Yes/not especially	Docile, easy going	Well	Largest chicken breed, 6 mo to grow to full size, dual
New Hampshire	3/wk, large, brown	Long	Yes	Yes/not especially	Usually calm, but some can be aggressive	Well	Dual
Orpington	3/wk, large, brown	Long	Yes	Yes/not especially	Calm, quiet, affectionate, patient, docile	Well, do not fly	Dual, big round fluffy feathered body shape
Sussex	4/wk, large, light brown	Long	Yes	Yes/not especially	Confident, curious, mellow, calm	Well, do not fly	Dual
Wyandotte	4/wk	Long	Yes	Yes/not especially	Easygoing, calm, tendency to dominate others	Well, do not fly	Dual

H = Hardy in hotter temperatures; C = hardy in colder temperatures; FR = prefers free-range; Con = prefers confinement; US = United States; R = rose comb; S = Single comb (number of points).

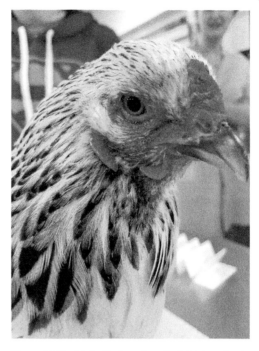

Figure 2.14 Cornish Game chicken (rooster).

Figure 2.17 Light Brahma breed of chicken (hen). Note the pea comb.

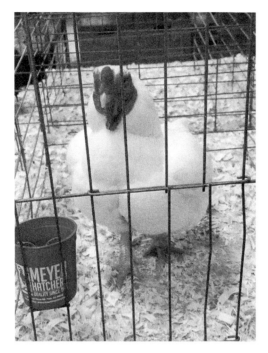

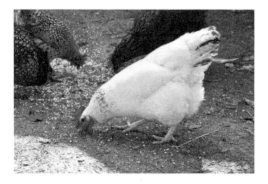

Figure 2.15 Delaware breed of chicken (hen).

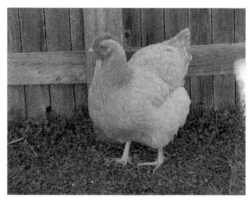

Figure 2.18 Buff Orpington breed of chicken (hen). Source: Photograph courtesy of Phil Snow.

Acknowledgments

Thank you to Phil Snow for taking some of the photographs for this chapter, and the "girls" (hens) at Happy Hen Farm, Rutledge, TN, who have given me (Gerhardt) great insight to the vast personalities of these charming creatures.

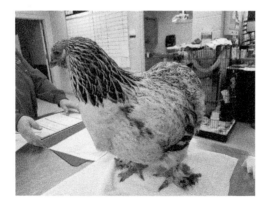

Figure 2.16 Light Brahma breed of chicken (hen).

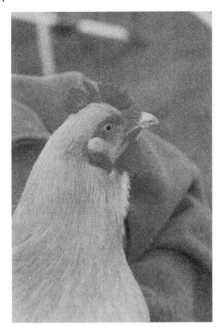

Figure 2.19   Buff Orpington breed of chicken (hen). Note the single comb. Source: Photograph courtesy of Phil Snow.

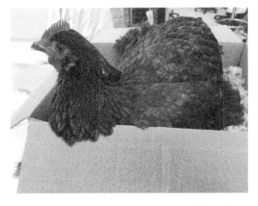

Figure 2.20   Black Orpington breed of chicken (hen).

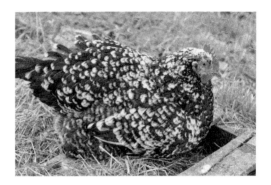

Figure 2.21   Speckled Sussex breed of chicken (hen). Note the single comb.

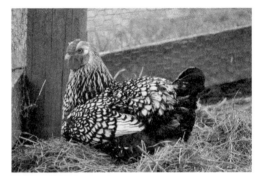

Figure 2.22   Silver-laced Wyandotte breed of chicken (hen).

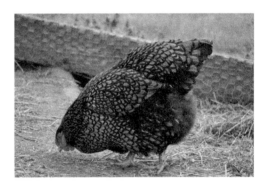

Figure 2.23   Golden-laced Wyandotte breed of chicken (hen).

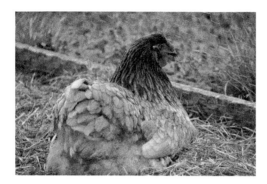

Figure 2.24   Black-laced Blue Wyandotte breed of chicken (hen).

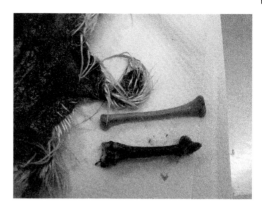

Figure 2.27   Photographs taken at necropsy showing the black (melanotic) skin and periosteum characteristic of all Silkie breeds of chicken. This occurs even if the feathers are white. The pink colored bone at the top of the picture has had its melanotic periosteum removed to show the melanotic color is in the periosteum.

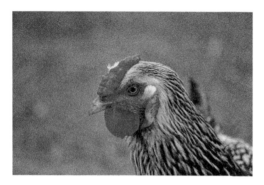

Figure 2.25   Silver-laced Wyandotte breed of chicken (hen) exhibiting a rose comb.

Figure 2.26   White Wyandotte breed of chicken (hen).

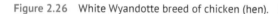

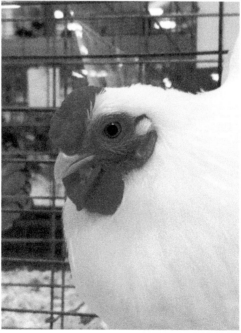

Table 2.6 Examples of some ornamental breeds of chicken and their physical traits.

Breed	S (class) M/F (kg)	B (class) M/F (kg)	Origin	Comb (points)	Wattles	Ear lobes	Legs	Example(s) of colors
American Game Bantam (Figure 2.28)	—	0.850/0.765	US	Single (5) or dubbed	Red, small	Red, small	C	Silver Duckwing
Bearded d'Anvers	—	R 0.740–0.625	B	Rose	Absent, bearded	Red, covered by muffs	C	Black
Bearded d'Uccle (Figure 2.29)	—	F 0.740/0.625	B	Single (5)	Red, small	Red, small	F	Mille Fleur
Cochin (Figures 2.31 and 2.32)	A 5.0/3.9	F 0.910/0.795	C	Single (5)	Red, long	Red, long	F	Buff
La Fleche (Figure 2.33)	C 3.6/3.0	O 0.850/0.740	F	"V" shape, large	Red, long	White, long	C	Black
Langshan	A 4.3/3.4	F 1.0/0.910	C	Single (5)	Red, medium	Red, medium	F	Black with black skin on legs
Modern Game	O 2.8/2.0	G 0.625/0.570	E	Single (5) or dubbed	Red, small	Red, small	C	Blue
Naked Neck	O 3.9/3.0	S 0.965/0.850	EE	Single (5)	Red, medium	Red, medium	C	White
Old English Game	O 2.3/1.8	G 0.680/0.625	B	Single (5) or dubbed	Red, small	Red, small	C	Splash
Orloff (Figures 2.34 and 2.35)	— 3.6/3.0	— 0.935/0.850	P	Walnut, small (Figure 2.13)	Red, small	Red, small	C	Spangled
Polish (Figures 2.36 and 2.37)	C 2.8/2.0	O 0.850/0.740	H	"V" shape, small	Red, small, +/−bearded	White, small, +/−muffs	C	White Crested Black

Breed								
Seabright (Figure 2.38)	—	S 0.625/0.570	B	Rose, medium	Red, small in hens	Purplish-red or blue, small	C	Reddish brown with stippling
Sicilian Buttercup (Figures 2.39 and 2.40)	M 3.0/2.5	O 0.740/0.625	I	Cup, susceptible to frost bite (Figure 2.10)	Red, small	White, almond shape	C	Golden buff, hens very colorful
Silkie (Figures 2.41 and 2.42)	—	F 1.0/0.910	Asia	Walnut, purplish	Purplish small	Blue, small	F, 5 toes	White with black skin, black periosteum, bony crest on skull (Figure 2.27)

[S = Standard Class (Am = American, A = Asiatic, C = Continental, E = English, M = Mediterranean, O = All Other Standard Breeds) including average weights of males (M) versus females(F) in kilograms (kg)]; [B = Bantam Class (G = Game, R = Rose Comb - Clean Legged, S = Single Comb - Clean Legged, O = All Other Combs - Clean Legged, F = Feather Legged) including average weights of males (M) versus females(F) in kilograms (Kg)]; [Origin = Country of origin, (US = United States, A = Australia, H = Holland, T = Turkey, G = Germany, I = Italy, F = France, C = China, EE = Eastern Europe, P = Persia)]; R = rose comb; S = Single comb (number of points); [Legs; C = Clean, F = Feathered]; —, denoting no information.

Table 2.7 Examples of some ornamental breeds of chicken and their common characteristics.

Breed	Eggs (#, size, color)	Laying period	Broodiness	Hardiness Cold/heat	Temperment	Bears confinement?	Other
American Game Bantam	3/wk	—	Yes	Yes/not especially	Docile, fun	Yes, but keep males separate	Easy show bird for beginners
Bearded d' Anvers	2–3/wk, small, cream, or tinted	—	Can	Yes/not especially	Can be aggressive to other chickens, friendly, easily handled	Yes	Good pets, AKA "Barbu or Belgian d' Anvers"
Bearded d' Uccle	2/wk, small (tiny), cream to tinted	—	Yes	No/yes	Sweet	Well	AKA "Barbu d' Uccle"
Cochin	2/wk, medium, light brown	—	Yes	Yes/not especially	Peaceful, friendly, easily handled	Well, do not fly	Dual, puffy tail feathers, slow to mature, yellow skin on leg
La Fleche	3/wk, large, white	Long	No	No/yes	Wild, untamed	Well	Dual, good flier, avoids human contact
Langshan	3/wk, medium, brown	—	Yes	Yes/not especially	Calm, self-possessed	Well	Dual, characteristic "U" shape to body on side view
Modern Game	1/wk, medium, white	—	Yes	No/yes	Noisy, alert, curious, active, friendly but can be aggressive	No	Combs dubbed for show, long-legged upright posture
Naked Neck AKA "Turken"	2/wk, medium, light brown	—	Yes	Yes/not especially	Calm, friendly, easy going	Well	Naked neck and vent area, 50% less feathering over rest of body
Old English Game	2/wk, medium, cream, or tinted (Figure 2.11)	—	Yes	Yes/not especially	Aggressive, self-sufficient, noisy	No	House males separately since will fight to death, don't house hens with docile breeds, great longevity

Breed	Eggs		H	C/—	Temperament	Confinement	Notes
Orloff	2/wk, medium, light brown	—	No	Yes (known for cold hardiness)/not especially	Calm, quiet, not especially friendly	Well, like to free roam	AKA "Russian Orloff" although originated in Persia, rare
Polish	2/wk, tiny, white (Figure 2.11)	—	No	No/yes	Calm, friendly, quiet, will be on low end of pecking order	Well	Known for bouffant crest of head feathers
Seabright	1/wk, tiny, cream, or tinted	—	No	Not especially/not especially	Cocky but not aggressive	Tolerates	Males and females have the exact same feathering, poor hatchability
Sicilian Buttercup	2/wk, small, white	—	No	No/yes	Very active	No	Rare breed in North America
Silkie	3/wk, small, cream, or tinted	—	Yes	Yes/yes	Sweet, tame, mothering	Well	Silky fluffy feathers, ideal pet chicken

H = Hardy in hotter temperatures; C = hardy in colder temperatures; FR = prefers free-range; Con = prefers confinement; US = United States; R = rose comb; S = Single comb (number of points).

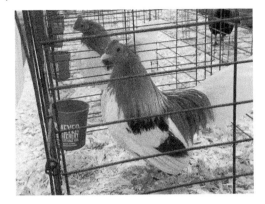

Figure 2.28 Red Pyle American Game Bantam breed of chicken (rooster).

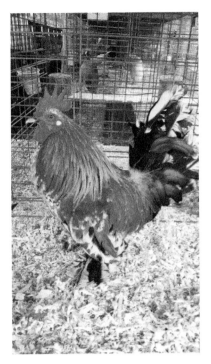

Figure 2.30 Mille Fleur Booted Bantam rooster, a close but non-bearded relative of the Bearded d'Uccle breed of chicken.

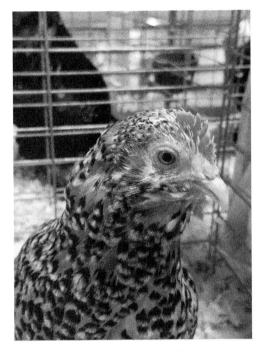

Figure 2.29 Mille Fleur Bearded d'Uccle breed of chicken (hen).

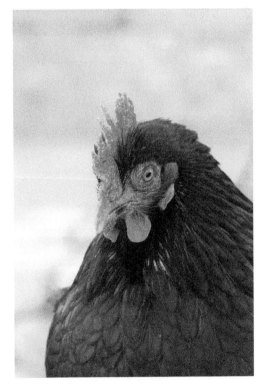

Figure 2.31 Cochin breed of chicken (hen). Note the single comb.

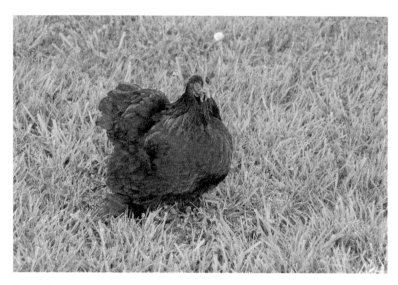

Figure 2.32 Cochin breed of chicken (hen). They are a large bird with a distinctive curve from the neck and shoulders to its short "fluffy" tail. Source: Photograph courtesy of Phil Snow.

Figure 2.33 The La Fleche breed of chicken is nicknamed the "devil bird" due to the large "V" shaped comb as seen in this rooster.

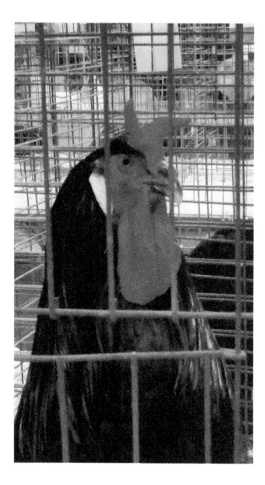

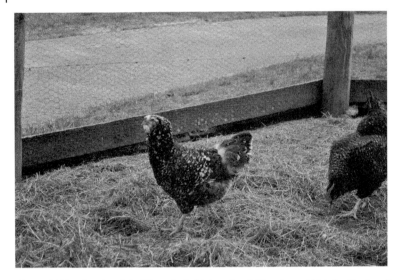

Figure 2.34   Russian Orloff breed of chicken (hen). They have thick feathering down the neck with a distinctive beard and muffs.

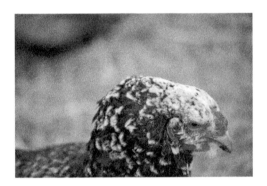

Figure 2.35   Russian Orloff breed of chicken (hen) exhibiting a walnut comb.

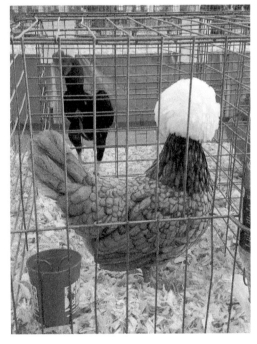

Figure 2.36   Non-bearded, non-muffed variety of White Crested Polish breed of chicken looking away from the camera.

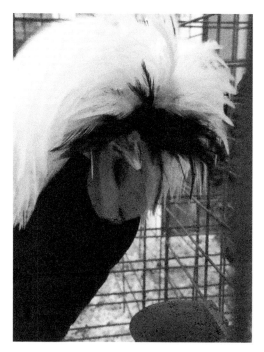

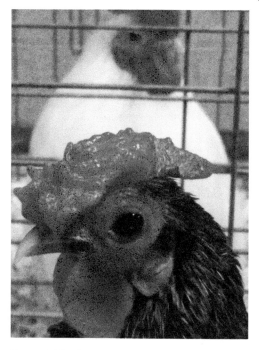

Figure 2.37 A White Crested Black Polish breed of chicken. The feathers of the crest sometimes interfere with sight.

Figure 2.38 Golden Seabright rooster. Note the well-developed rose comb.

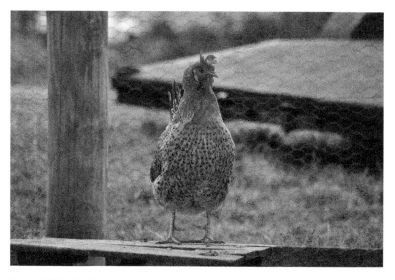

Figure 2.39 Sicilian Buttercup breed of chicken (hen).

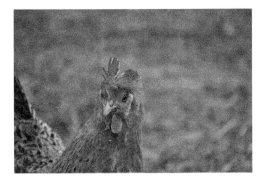

Figure 2.40 The Sicilian Buttercup breed of chicken has a unique cup-shaped comb, which appears as two single combs that have connected in the back and front to make a cup shape.

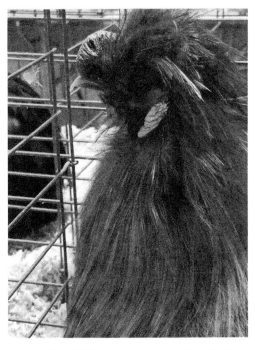

Figure 2.42 Silkie rooster showing the hair like glossy feathers, walnut comb and blue ear lobes characteristic for this breed.

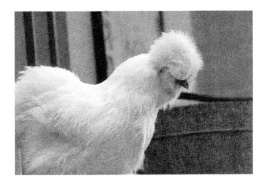

Figure 2.41 White Bearded Bantam Silkie hen presenting for examination. Note the distinctive blue ear lobes, hair-like feathers, and top knot of feathers on the head.

References

1 Ekarius, C. (2007). *Storeys' Illustrated Guide to Poultry Breeds* (ed. N. Adams). MA: Storey Publishing.

2 Head, H. (2012). *Backyard Duck Keeping Made Easy. Guide to Backyard Chickens*, Grit Country Skills Series. Ogden Publications, Inc.

3 Waller S. (2012). Breed profiles. chicken breeds. Popular Farming Series. *Hobby Farms Magazine*. Bowtie Inc.

4 Will, O. (2012). *Perfect Chickens. Guide to Backyard Chickens*, Grit Country Skills Series. Ogden Publications, Inc.

5 My pet chicken. www.mypetchicken.com (accessed 25 May 2019).

6 Poultry pages. http://www.poultrypages.com/chicken-breeds.html (accessed 25 May 2019).

3

Basic Housing and Management

Darrin Karcher

Department of Animal Sciences, Purdue University, West Lafayette, IN, USA

Introduction

Raising backyard poultry can be a very pleasant experience for those involved. However, the average person is not cognizant of the time, effort, and knowledge that are required for a successful experience. In this chapter, basic management will be covered including housing, chick purchasing, brooding, daily care, and predator control options.

Housing

Design

Housing design will affect bird care, comfort, welfare, and well-being. There are numerous aspects associated with housing that need to be considered. The backyard chicken coop may be elaborate and esthetically pleasing to the owner's eye, resembling a child's playhouse: windows, flower boxes, painted, and so on. The chicken coop might also be very simple, consisting of a cube made of treated lumber with chicken wire or composed of bits and pieces of metal, wire, and wood found around the home. There is no wrong way to create the chicken coop, but the design of the backyard chicken coop should be easy to clean, protect the birds from predators, and provide adequate space for the birds. The ideal structure would have a cement floor and be insulated with washable walls. This would allow the coop to be thoroughly cleaned and disinfected between each flock of birds. Typically, most chicken coops will have dirt floors, which can create problems if a disease outbreak occurs.

As mentioned, the housing can be constructed from numerous materials and appear very different. Egg-producing birds can be housed in cages where they might have access to nest area, feeders, waterers, and perches. Flocks might be housed on a floor where nest boxes are located along the wall and feeders and waterers are distributed throughout the floor area. Another type of floor system would provide a slatted floor, where the waterers and feeders might be located, which can help to reduce the amount of fecal matter in the litter as it is accumulated in an area below the slatted floor.

Perches and nest boxes are not needed for all types of poultry. For example, a nest box on the wall will not be used by waterfowl, but a nesting area on the floor will be. Perches can be used to various extents by turkeys, broilers, and other chickens. The turkeys and broilers will use them for a period of time, but eventually

Backyard Poultry Medicine and Surgery: A Guide for Veterinary Practitioners, Second Edition.
Edited by Cheryl B. Greenacre and Teresa Y. Morishita.
© 2021 John Wiley & Sons, Inc. Published 2021 by John Wiley & Sons, Inc.
Companion website: www.wiley.com/go/greenacre/medicine

the body weight may prohibit the use of the perch toward the end of the production cycle. Other chicken breeds will extensively use the perch. Six inches of perch per bird will be sufficient to allow all birds to perch at the same time and is the recommended minimum.

The perch and nest box should be introduced at the correct time, stage of life, or the birds will use them incorrectly. Perches should be provided to pullets at about 6 weeks of age. While the perches can be provided at any point, the early introduction allows the birds to develop the coordination and musculature to effectively use the perches throughout the life span. Nest boxes are only introduced around 17 weeks of age. As birds come into egg production, they will seek out a nesting area. Birds having access to the nest boxes prior to 17 weeks are not seeking a nest area and will identify the nest box as an area for feces. A nest box can accommodate four to six hens. However, nest use may be limited to a few nest boxes due to hen preference.

The backyard flock housing structures may be completely enclosed or have access to an outdoor run. Either method is acceptable, but the design of the house needs to attempt to limit the access of wild birds and predators. Further discussion on predator control can be found later in the chapter. Ideally, any openings in the chicken coop should be covered with hardware cloth and open doors should have a screen door. This will limit wild bird access because a constant supply of food and water will attract them. However, this may not be an option with an outdoor run and one must be comfortable with the liability of the increased biosecurity risk.

Stocking Density

Stocking density varies by species and performance outcomes. There is considerable debate and investigation into the impact of management decisions on bird welfare. The scientific community and animal welfare certification guidelines for U.S. commercial poultry production is moving

Table 3.1 Minimum stocking density for backyard poultry production.

Species	Live weight (lb)[a]	Number birds/ area (in.^{2})
Meat bird (chicken) [1]	<5.5	1.5/144
Meat bird (chicken) [1]	>5.5	1/144
Turkey [2, 3]	>30	1/288
Laying hen – cage [4]	NA	2/144
Laying hens – non-cage [4]	NA	1/144
All other chickens [5]	NA	1/144
Waterfowl [5]	NA	1/288

[a] Live weight is only applicable to meat production species. NA = not applicable.

toward outcome-based measures of welfare. Conversely, the current standards dictate the amount of the resource that should be provided to the birds. Table 3.1 provides guidance to the minimum area that should be provided to different poultry species. This is only a recommendation and as was published by Dawkins et al. [6], many other factors have more impact on the welfare of the bird beyond the stocking density. Backyard birds can easily be provided with additional space but limitations of housing structure, location (urban or country setting), or number of birds can have an impact. The general trend is to increase space provided as the birds age. The space requirements suggested in Table 3.1 do not include outdoor access and are derived from commercial strains.

Ventilation

A common misconception is that the exchange of oxygen is the main reason for ventilating the chicken house. Ventilation is important for moisture removal, excess heat removal, exchange of gases produced by the litter, and fresh air. Spring, summer, and fall tend to see the least amount of ventilation problems occurring. However, a very common issue arises as the weather changes from warm days to cool evenings, where the owner may increase the ventilation during the day and close the house at night. There may be times that temperature swings are not accounted for, resulting in a warm day with limited ventilation. This tends to result in increased respiratory problems as a result of too much humidity in the chicken coop.

The summer months may see high temperatures, and ventilation becomes important for circulating air to help remove excessive heat in the chicken coop. Ventilation is controlled by computer systems in the commercial poultry industry. The system will increase fan speeds and turn on additional fans to circulate the air as temperature increases. A backyard coop may open windows and doors, ideally screened, to increase the amount of air blowing into the chicken coop (natural ventilation). Another option is to use a small fan to circulate the air (mechanical ventilation). A fan purchased at a pet supply store would work sufficiently. The idea is not to provide enough fan for each bird to rest in front of the air flow but to circulate or exhaust the air within the coop.

The tradeoff between ventilation and temperature becomes apparent during the winter months. If you maximize the ventilation to remove all of the moisture within the coop, you will lose all of the warm air, resulting in an increase in input cost to maintain the temperature. On the other hand, if you maintain the temperature, then you will not remove the moisture in the coop, resulting in significant management issues. Therefore, minimum ventilation should be practiced meeting both objectives: removing moisture and maintaining temperature. Minimum ventilation describes the situation where a small amount of cold air enters the chicken coop, is warmed by the temperature in the house, absorbs moisture within the coop, and then is exhausted. This can be achieved with air inlets along the roof line of the coop or, depending on the house design, a slight cracking of a window could achieve the same objective. However, the incoming air must blow toward the roof. An opening where air enters and is not directed toward the roof will result in cold air descending downward and can create an unnecessary draft in the coop. As a result, the chickens can become chilled, resulting in health issues or a higher input cost as the owner tries to heat the coop.

A chicken coop designed with insulated sidewalls and roof can result in the house becoming too tight. This means that no external air can enter the chicken coop, resulting in no air exchange. This can lead to several problems. One issue is the accumulation of moisture causing condensation to form on the walls or ceiling and can result in "rain." This can lead to bedding issues that can affect bird health, as discussed later in the chapter. Additionally, the moist environment can provide opportunities for molds and other diseases to propagate. Second, excessive levels of ammonia can result from the damp litter and lack of airflow. When the ammonia levels become too high, >25 ppm, then birds can experience detrimental effects to their respiratory system and eyes.

Temperature

A chicken's body temperature falls within the range of 105–107 °F with males having a higher body temperature than females. Although their body temperature is high, birds have a thermal neutral zone, or an area where they do not need to actively regulate their body temperature. The extremes, hot or cold, can be detrimental to the birds and, depending on body size, age, and breed, these zones can vary. Baby birds are going to have a higher tolerance for hotter temperatures, while older birds are more forgiving of colder temperatures. A good rule of thumb is to aim for the temperature in the chicken coop to be between 50 and 75 °F. The largest consideration is whether the birds have the opportunity to get out of the weather to allow them to self-regulate their body temperature.

A ramification of extreme cold weather is frost bite. Poultry feet and head parts (combs, wattles, snoods, etc.) are most likely to become frostbitten. This can be a result of being outside for too long or having to stand, walk, or not being able to get out of snow for a long period of time. On the flipside, heat stress is a result of excessive hot weather. Birds will pant, spread their wings, increase water consumption, and decrease feed consumption in an effort to cool their bodies; proper ventilation can help reduce the chance of heat stress.

Lighting

Poultry can grow sufficiently with normal daylight and do not necessarily need any special lighting requirements. However, light intensity and duration can have an impact on birds. Light intensity can be as low as 5 lx to stimulate activity and can be as bright as desired. Very bright lights may lead to behavioral problems such as aggressiveness and bird picking. Therefore, lowering the light intensity will provide a remedy. A rule of thumb for intensity is whether you can read a newspaper at arm's length. If so, then there is sufficient light for the birds.

The other consideration is light duration. If the goal is to produce meat, the birds only need natural daylength to grow. Some individuals believe that providing 23–24 hours of light results in increased performance, but poultry are like humans and need a natural dark cycle. Therefore, 16 hours of light would be the maximum suggested for meat birds.

Poultry that are being reared for egg production, table eggs or fertile eggs, are more sensitive to daylight duration. Bird biology does not vary between songbirds and poultry. The increasing daylength in the spring results in songbirds laying eggs and hatching young. The decreasing daylength in the fall signals to songbirds that it is no longer a good idea to reproduce and egg cessation occurs. Poultry respond in the same way with increasing daylength triggering egg production and decreasing daylength stopping egg production.

A laying hen should reach a daylength of 16 hours light and 8 hours dark. Egg production will naturally occur in the spring with the increasing daylength, but artificial lighting will be needed to maintain egg production following the summer solstice. Similar to natural daylengths, a sudden jump from a short-daylength to a long daylength should be avoided. Therefore, a suggested lighting scheme is found in Table 3.2. The important thing to remember about egg laying is that once the daylength has increased and is established, any decrease in daylength will result in egg cessation. For example, an owner begins to artificially increase the light in the hen house but does not set the timer correctly. The daylength increases, but the birds receive 22 hours of day light for several weeks. The owner observes the mistake and wishes to decrease the length to 16 hours. Decreasing the light at this point will knock the hens out of production, so the only

Table 3.2 Suggested lighting programs for egg producing poultry.

Age (wk)	Light (h)	Dark (h)
0–18	8	16
19	9	15
20	9:30	14:30
21	10	14
22	10:30	13:30
23	11	13
24	11:30	12:30
25	12	12
26	12:30	11:30
27	13	11
28	13:30	10:30
29	14	10
30	14:30	9:30
31	15	9
32	15:30	8:30
33	16	8
34 to end of lay	16	8

option is to maintain the 22 hours of daylight if eggs are desired.

Litter Substrate

Many options exist when discussing litter substrate or bedding material. Ideally, the bedding material should be absorbent, loose, and fairly inexpensive. The most common substrate used is pine wood shavings (Figure 3.1). Straw, sand, shredded newspaper, crushed corn cobs, and soybean hulls are just some of the substrates that can be used. Table 3.3 summarizes the positives and negatives for some litter substrates. Poultry can be bedded with any of these materials, but management techniques may change depending on the litter substrate. Hard wood shavings should not be used with poultry due to the potential presence of fungus and molds. This can result in respiratory infections if the levels are high enough in the shavings; therefore, the safest recommendation is to not use hard wood shavings.

Managing Different Life Stages

Brooding

The management of chicks, ducklings, goslings, poults, and other baby poultry is similar with the largest difference attributed to dietary need. The brooder pen or area should be set-up

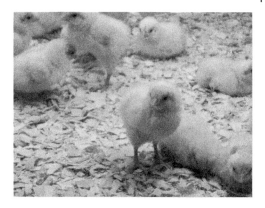

Figure 3.1 Example of pine shavings being used as a substrate for this chick's enclosure. *Source:* Photograph courtesy of Dr. Cheryl B. Greenacre.

48–72 hours prior to chick arrival to ensure all equipment is functioning correctly and allow time for all environmental variables to warm to the brooding temperature. The layout of the brooding area needs to provide feed, water, and heat to ensure a good start for the baby poultry. The ideal set-up is illustrated in Figure 3.2. The heat bulb is centrally located with feed and water alternating around the heat source, providing baby poultry access to feed and water in every direction. Smaller set-ups may use a box, cattle tank, or other similar area in which to brood.

The rule of thumb for brooding is to start with a 95 °F temperature for the first week and decrease by 5 °F each week until the outdoor temperature is met. This may indicate

Table 3.3 The positives and negatives of various litter substrates available for poultry.

Substrate	Positive	Negative
Wood shavings	Absorbent, fairly cheap	Depending on location availability may be challenging or very expensive
Straw	Cheap, abundant	Does not absorb moisture due to wax sheath on straw, but chopping into 1–2 in. pieces can help reduce this deficiency
Sand	Abundant, moisture easily drained, maintains coolness in hot weather	Hard to heat, can be costly
Newspaper	Abundant, cheap	Slippery when wet unless shredded, not very absorbent

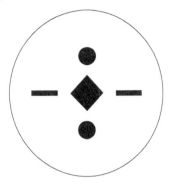

Figure 3.2 Brooding area layout. The brooder should have waterers (●), feeders (▬), and heat lamp (◆) arranged within the brooder ring.

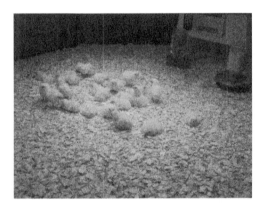

Figure 3.3 Chicks shown huddled together under a heat lamp, suggesting they are kept at too low a temperature. They should be scattered throughout the enclosure. Notice the food and waterer are placed away from the heat lamp. *Source:* Photograph courtesy of Dr. Cheryl B. Greenacre.

that during the day heat lamps will not be needed, but at night with cooler temperatures chicks still have access to heat lamps. The heat lamp can be purchased at a pet store or local agricultural food store and is different from a 100 W light bulb. The heat lamp can be purchased to illuminate with white or red light. White light can be used, but red light tends to be most common. Observation of the chicks around the brooder can provide lots of information to the poultry enthusiast. Chicks huddled under the heat bulb are an indication that they are cold (Figure 3.3); observing chicks on the perimeter of the brooding area indicates

that chicks are too hot; seeing chicks huddled together in one area of the brooder, not under the bulb, indicates there is a draft. The chicks will be most comfortable when they are evenly distributed throughout the brood area. Besides the physical location of the chicks in the brood area, the amount of noise produced by the birds will indicate whether they are cold or hot (excessive chirping by all) or comfortable (some chirping, but not all of the chicks).

Grow-Out

Poultry growing results in changes to body weight and the loss of down, which is replaced by feathers. Outdoor access should be limited to birds 6 weeks of age and older. The birds will be predominantly feathered by 6 weeks and can tolerate the environment better than chicks. The feed and water should be maintained within the chicken coop and, depending on location, additional water may be placed outside during the summer months. Outside water should be located in the shade, but preferably not under a tree or bush. Wild birds will be attracted to the water and you do not want to provide a drinking source under an area where wild birds can excrete into the water.

The young poultry can be trained to re-enter the house at night by keeping the lights on in the house for an additional 20–30 minutes past sunset. The first week or two might require additional help in catching and placing the birds back into the chicken coop, but the birds will learn to go in at night as sunset approaches.

Adulthood

Mature chickens are easy to care for and can provide a sense of self-worth to a young or aged person. All aspects of water, feed, and temperature have been discussed previously and no additional management changes are needed with adult birds. An important item to remember is that birds establish a social hierarchy and disrupting this by removal of hens or roosters will result in aggressive fighting behavior between the birds. This is common and will resolve quickly as the new hierarchy is established.

The length of time for which an individual has backyard chickens can vary depending on the end goal (meat, eggs, or pleasure). Chickens that are producing eggs or are kept for pleasure will go through a molt period. A molt indicates that the hen biologically needs to rest from egg production and results in the growth of new feathers and cessation of eggs. Individuals may be concerned about the excessive loss of feathers or loss of egg production. A molt period will usually last 6 weeks; if the proper lighting and feeding is in place the hens will again produce eggs.

General Management Practices

Litter

Litter substrate was discussed earlier, but litter management was not. There is no need to remove the litter from the brooding area unless there is a water spill that soaks the bedding. New substrate can be added as needed to keep the bedding cleaner but does not require removal of the existing material. Unless there is a disease issue or government regulations that require bedding material to be cleaned every so often, the material can be removed every 6–12 months. The recommendation would be to remove litter in April and October if litter is to be removed twice. If clean-out is going to occur once, then April would be the best time. The cleaning out following the winter months allows for removal of damp material, a spring cleaning, and in the fall would provide a time to disinfect for external parasites before confining the flock to the house for the winter months. A downside to a fall clean-out is that litter material that can provide additional insulation for the winter months will be eliminated.

Feed and Water

Consumption

Daily feed and water consumption should be monitored by recognizing the disappearance of the resources. This allows the backyard client to be cognizant of changes that are occurring due to life stage, production or potential health problems. Sudden fluctuations in water consumption are strong indicators that problems are occurring within the flock. Table 3.4 provides a suggested daily feed intake by species and age. Water consumption is more challenging to provide suggested intake, but water consumption should be approximately 0.3 gal to 1000 g of feed. Feed and water consumption will be impacted by numerous management and housing factors.

Height and Access to Waterers and Feeders

The commercial poultry industry has many auditing programs relating to feed and water access. Every person and backyard resource has different recommendations on the required access for poultry. Table 3.5 provides minimum requirements for feeders and waterers [6].

Feeder and waterer heights are important in the flock management to reduce spillage and wastage of the resources. The use of pin-metered drinkers, commonly called nipple drinkers, drinker cups, open sources of water, and drinkers could be used to provide water. The height can be variable for each of these different watering options; therefore, a recommendation needs to be followed that birds can freely access the water source at all times. If nipple drinkers are used, the nipple should be located just above eye level of the bird so the droplet of water can be visualized attracting them to the water droplet. The other waterers used should be positioned at the level of the "shoulder" on the bird. This will allow the bird to easily access the water and will minimize the amount of water wastage. Regardless of the type of feeder used, the height should be adjusted so birds reach over the lip of the feeder to access feed. This minimizes the feed wastage. Similar to the waterers,

Table 3.4 Feed intake ranges of poultry species at different weeks of age.

Species	Age (wk)	Feed intake (g/bird/d)
Chicken (meat) [7]	1	17–33
	2	37–63
	3	68–100
	4	106–140
	5	145–176
	6	180–204
	>7	207–230
Chicken (other) [8, 9]	1–4	15–30
	5–8	40–50
	9–12	50–60
	13–16	65–80
	17–20	75–95
	>20	85–100
Turkey [10]	1–4	20–100 (g/b/d)
	5–8	150–280
	9–12	325–470
	13–16	510–630
	17–20	657–760
	>20	800
Waterfowl [11]	1	225
	2	750
	3	1150
	4	1150
	5	1475
	6	1630
	>7	1770

Table 3.5 Resource space requirements for chickens.

Age (wk)	Feeder space (linear inch)	Waterer space (linear inch)
0–6	0.72	0.44
6–18	1.50	0.58
18 or older	3.00	0.75

Source: Hester, P. (2010) [5].

if needed, to help control bacteria and as a disinfectant, by making a stock solution (1 tbsp bleach: 0.5 gal water) and adding 2 tbsp stock solution to a gallon of water. The stock solution should be replaced weekly to ensure the effectiveness of the chlorine is not lost.

Feed Storage

Birds need to have fresh feed and water on a daily basis. The feed should be stored in a cool dry environment inside a rodent-proof container (Figure 3.4). Plastic or metal trash cans can provide the necessary protection against rodents and other animals (raccoons, opossum, etc.) that might try to access the feed. Animals that are not intended to eat the diet can introduce disease and other impurities into the diet that should not be presented to the flock. One should only purchase enough feed that can be consumed within 30 days to ensure nutritional content and reduce the chance of spoilage.

Rodent Control

Rodent control is vital to backyard flocks to reduce the chance of disease and financial cost to the flock owner. As discussed, preventing rodents from accessing the poultry feed is important. Periodic checking of the housing structure and location where feed is stored will provide insight into whether a rodent infestation is prevalent [12]. Rodent tracks, sightings, droppings, and burrows can provide insight into where they are active. Upon identification of the area, the owner can determine the best

the top of the feed pan should be located at the shoulder of the bird. This will require adjustment of height throughout the production cycle for both feeders and waterers.

Water Management

Water should be changed daily and, if needed, the waterer can be scrubbed with soapy water to remove any dirt or bacterial films that may develop. The drinking water can be chlorinated

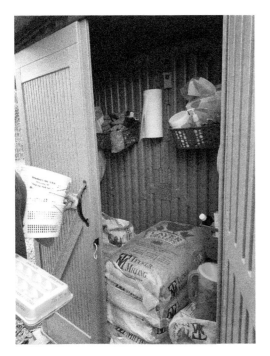

Figure 3.4 This prefabricated shed shows one method of storing food that provides a dry, rodent proof environment. *Source:* Photograph courtesy of Dr. Cheryl B. Greenacre.

way to trap and bait for the rodents. If rodenticides are used, a bait station should be used to keep the bait fresh, allow for monitoring of consumption and prevent accidental ingestion by other animals or the birds in the flock [12].

Cleaning and Disinfection

Cleaning and disinfecting the poultry house and equipment should be a part of the small flock experience. The poultry house should be cleaned at least once a year. Some backyard flock owners may choose to clean the house more often, but one should note that excessive cleaning (biweekly) has been documented to have severe implications on the health and welfare of chickens [13]. The cleaning provides the flock owner a chance to disinfect the house to reduce the presence of any ectoparasites, disease agents and removal of dirty litter. If there is a complete break in flocks, cleaning of the house and disinfection with a 2- to 3- week down period is ideal.

The recommended procedure would be to (i) remove all the birds and equipment from the house. (ii) Dry clean the house by sweeping or blowing down all dust and loose dirt starting at the ceiling and moving toward the floor. Remove the litter and dust from the floor. (iii) Wet clean the house by soaking heavily soiled areas to more easily remove softened material, wash the entire house with a neutral detergent followed by rinsing the house. (iv) Allow the house to completely dry before applying the disinfectant. (v) Disinfect the house following the manufacturer's directions.

This procedure can be used to clean and disinfect the equipment that was removed from the house. An important note: whenever used equipment or borrowed equipment comes back to the owner, this procedure should be used to ensure equipment is clean prior to introduction to the flock.

Behavior Disorders

Following are a few common behavioral issues that can occur associated with housing. For more information on chicken behavior, please refer to Chapter 22 on "Behavior" in this book.

Cannibalism

Birds are naturally aggressive and are omnivores. Chickens can become cannibalistic (peck at one another) if they are too densely populated or do not have enough resource space, that is, feeder, waterer, nestbox; incorrect lighting; abrasions or tears as a result of injury or mating; dietary deficiencies; prolapse; or meanness of a breed. As a result, the management of the flock needs to be adjusted to limit or reduce the behavior. Some potential remedies may include increasing space, dimming the lights to minimize activity, removing the wounded bird, applying an "anti-pick" compound to cover the affected area, or beak modification "trimming." Attempts can also be made to redirect the behavior by suspending hay slices to promote manipulation of the individual pieces of grass, broadcasting mixed grains into the litter to promote foraging behavior, or spreading grass clippings over the litter. While these are suggested remedies, each flock may react differently so several things may need to be tried until successful. Some suggest a red light may decrease pecking of others since blood or hemorrhagic areas may not induce curiosity and tempt them to peck.

Broodiness

Hens can go "broody," during which time the hen's hormones have changed her behavior, indicating time for nesting and hatching the young. A broody hen will cease egg laying, identify a nestbox or area within the coop that is her nest, and may increase aggressiveness as she attempts to protect her eggs. The best way to reduce the chances of having a broody hen is to remove eggs from the hen house on a daily basis. However, this may not always prove to be successful. A broody hen should be removed from the flock for a short period of time to break the hormonal cycle. This is achieved by eliminating her nest area and any eggs, even those laid by other hens, to prevent her from attempting to claim them as her own. Most backyard flock owners want their hens to lay eggs rather than nest and hatch them out.

Egg Eating

Chickens may occasionally develop a habit of eating their own or other hen's eggs. The behavior can develop as a result of overcrowding, uneven nest space, nutritional deficiency, too bright light intensity, or disposing of cracked or broken eggs in the chicken coop. Similar to other behaviors discussed above, the behavior can be broken or redirected at times. Solutions may include frequent gathering of eggs, increasing nest availability, darkening the nests, or beak modification. If the egg eating cannot be stopped, the best approach may be to induce a molt, causing the cessation of eggs to break the behavior and bringing the hens back into production several weeks later.

Predator Control

Predator control is a must for anyone who wishes to keep backyard poultry. As was previously mentioned, the design of the chicken coop can help reduce the number of wild birds, and in some instances predators, that enter the chicken coop. A small hole where a predator can gain access or pull a chicken body part through the hole can result in a grizzly scene the following day. The best approach is to ensure all holes or other access into the chicken coop is secured to eliminate the potential for predators. Raccoons, opossums, mink, skunks, foxes, coyotes, or weasels may find ways to enter the chicken coop or pull the chickens through wire and holes to consume them. If the birds have outdoor access, a sufficient wire enclosure may be needed to protect them (Figure 3.5). A wire fence can be used for the outdoor run, but should be buried 8 in. deep to ensure that predators are unable to dig under the fence to enter the chicken yard. Additionally, shrubs and bushes can provide cover from an aerial attack by raptors, or a mesh can cover the top of the chicken yard to prevent bird of prey attacks. Depending on state laws, consultation with animal control can provide information on how best to deal with a predator attack in the backyard flock. Dogs can be responsible for what appears to be

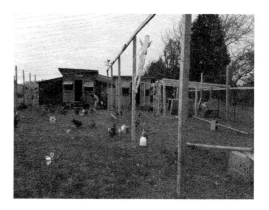

Figure 3.5 This outdoor enclosure had wire strung every 2 ft to discourage aerial predators. *Source:* Photograph courtesy of Dr. Cheryl B. Greenacre.

a predator attack as well. Dogs tend to kill the birds as a result of trying to play with them. The birds are typically not maimed as in a predator attack.

Conclusion

Backyard poultry can be an exciting endeavor as long as proper management practices are used. Chicken coop design can dramatically impact the effectiveness of ventilation, temperature, and predator control. Management practices tend to be more intense early in life (brooding), but as the birds age they are more forgiving to management errors. Paying attention to the bird behavior, their environment and provided resources will give you considerable information on the health and well-being of the flock. Finally, behaviors may develop that are detrimental to the birds or eggs and need to be addressed as quickly as possible.

References

1 National Chicken Council (2017). Animal welfare guidelines and audit checklist for broilers. https://www. nationalchickencouncil.org/wp-content/ uploads/2017/07/NCC-Welfare-Guidelines-Broilers.pdf (accessed 31 May 2019).

2 Erasmus, M.A. (2017). A review of the effects of stocking density on turkey behavior, welfare, and productivity. *Poult. Sci.* 96: 2540–2545.

3 Beaulac, K. and Schwean-Lardner, K. (2018). Assessing the effects of stocking density on turkey tom health and welfare to 16 weeks of age. *Front. Vet. Sci.* 5: 213.

4 United Egg Producers (2017). Animal husbandry guidelines for U.S. egg-laying flocks. https://uepcertified.com/wp-content/ uploads/2017/11/2017-UEP-Animal-Welfare-Guidelines-Cage-Housing-11.01.2017-FINAL.pdf; https://uepcertified.com/ wp-content/uploads/2017/11/2017-UEP-Animal-Welfare-Cage-Free-Guidelines-11.01.2017-FINAL.pdf. (accessed 31 May 2019).

5 Hester, P. (2010). Poultry In: *Guide for the care and use of agricultural animals in research and teaching*, 3e (eds. J. McGlone and J. Swanson), 103–128. Champaign: Federation of Animal Science Societies.

6 Dawkins, M.S., Donnelly, C.A., and Jones, T.A. (2004). Chicken welfare is influenced more by housing conditions than by stocking density. *Nature* 427: 342–344.

7 Aviagen (2019). Ross 708 performance objectives. http://en.aviagen.com/assets/ Tech_Center/Ross_Broiler/Ross-708-BroilerPO2019-EN.pdf (accessed 31 May 2019).

8 Hy-Line (2016). W-36 commercial layer management guide. https://www.hyline. com/UserDocs/Pages/36_COM_ENG.pdf (accessed 31 May 2019).

9 Hy-Line (2016) Commercial brown layer management guide. https://www.hyline. com/UserDocs/Pages/BRN_COM_ENG.pdf (accessed 31 May 2019).

10 Aviagen (2015). Nicholas select commercial performance objectives. http://www. aviagenturkeys.us/uploads/2015/11/13/ nicholas_comm_perf_obj_select_2015.pdf (accessed 31 May 2019).

11 Metzer Farms (2019). Daily feed consumption of pekin ducklings. https:// www.metzerfarms.com/ DailyFeedWaterDucklings.cfm (accessed 31 May 2019).

12 Loven, J. and Williams, R. (2010). Controlling rodents in commercial poultry facilities. AMD-3-W Purdue Extension Bulletin. https://extension.entm.purdue.edu/ publications/ADM-3.pdf.

13 Anderson, K.E., Mozdziak, P.E., and Petitte, J.N. (2010). The impact of scheduled cage cleaning on older hens (*Gallus gallus*). *Lab Anim.* 39: 210.

4

Anseriforme Husbandry and Management

M. Scott Echols

Mobile Avian Surgical Services, The Medical Center for Birds, Oakley, CA, USA

Introduction

Ducks have been called "the easiest domestic birds to raise" [1]. Combined with a tolerance to a variety of weather conditions, foraging and insect control abilities and resistance to numerous diseases that commonly plague chickens and other captive poultry, ducks are popular pets. Not far behind are pet geese and a distant third are captive swans. Collectively, waterfowl species are common in public and private collections as well as beloved pets. Ducks and geese are also raised for meat, eggs, and foie gras (although now outlawed in many countries), and this should be considered prior to the administration of any medications.

Particularly ducks can be used to reduce local pest insect and water plant populations. Holderread writes that 2–6 ducks per acre (0.4 ha) can be used to "control Japanese beetles, grasshoppers, snails, slugs, and fire ants" [1]. As a note, excessive fire ant populations can result in damage to ducks confined to land (Figure 4.1). Ducks may also be used to control livestock liver flukes by eating the snail intermediate host. Ducks are also used to clear out pest aquatic plants including duckweed (*Lemna* spp), pondweed (*Potamogeton* spp), green algae, skunkweed (*Chara* spp), widgeon grass (*Ruppia maritima*), wild celery (*Vallisneria americana*), arrowhead (*Sagittaria* spp) and more. Fifteen to thirty birds per water acre (0.4 ha) may be needed to remove heavy plant growths while 8–15 birds per acre can be used for maintenance control [1].

Waterfowl droppings are generally voluminous and can be both beneficial and detrimental. The obvious downside is that even a single bird can quickly contaminate a small area (land or water) and is one of many reasons that waterfowl should be provided adequate space and ideally outdoor housing. On a positive note, ducks can provide readily degradable fertilizer for gardens, (including geese) yards and (including swans) ponds and streams to feed fish and provide valuable nutrients to the water environment (provided water is adequately aerated, circulated, and replaced). To limit damage from ducks that forage through gardens, restrict access to tender crops (lettuce, spinach, cabbage, and young plants), low hanging ripe fruits and during irrigation [1]. See Chapter 10 (Zoonotic Diseases) regarding safe composting and use of poultry feces in gardens.

Pet waterfowl generally produce acceptable noise levels in urban environments. Small flocks of waterfowl are generally quiet except when disturbed. Single waterfowl (especially geese) may be quite noisy possibly as a result of being alone and more nervous. Of the duck

Backyard Poultry Medicine and Surgery: A Guide for Veterinary Practitioners, Second Edition.
Edited by Cheryl B. Greenacre and Teresa Y. Morishita.
© 2021 John Wiley & Sons, Inc. Published 2021 by John Wiley & Sons, Inc.
Companion website: www.wiley.com/go/greenacre/medicine

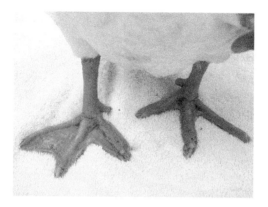

Figure 4.1 White Pekin duck (*Anas platyrhynchos*) with extensive damage to the foot webbing from fire ant bites. The lesions have healed leaving areas of missing interdigital webbing.

species, call ducks tend to be the noisiest with Pekin breeds in second place [1]. While not entirely mute, muscovy ducks (*Cairina moschata*) are the quietest of the domestic ducks.

General Groups and Features of Pet Waterfowl

While waterfowl are commonly classified via genetics or taxonomy, feeding, and movement styles are used here. The reason is that how a bird feeds and moves around helps one set up environments that best suit the animal. For example most domestic ducks are mallards (*Anas platyrhynchos*) and are dabblers that benefit from walking on land but also feed and spend time on water. Common backyard setups for pet ducks often lack clean accessible water and many birds spend most of their time standing or walking on hard surfaces and eat from a bowl on land (Figure 4.2). This scenario may contribute to inactivity, obesity, arthritis, poor hygiene, pododermatitis, and more.

Dabblers

Dabblers are those waterfowl that feed primarily on the surface of water or graze under shallow water. Traditionally this group is assigned to ducks from the subfamily Anatinae. These birds rarely dive and tend to have their legs placed more centrally on their body, walk well on land and even feed terrestrially (Table 4.1). Most swans are also dabblers. The mallard is the best known of all ducks and is the wild ancestor to all domestic ducks except the muscovy (Figure 4.3a,b).

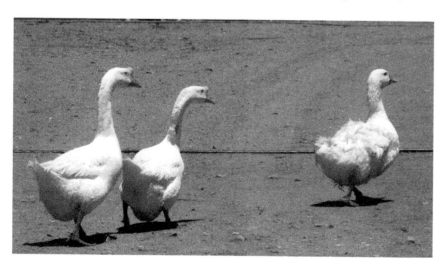

Figure 4.2 A gaggle consisting of two White Chinese (*Anser cygnoides*) and 1 Sebastopol (*Anser anser domesticus*) geese are walking on hard packed dirt. If no other substrate is available, this environment is conducive to foot and joint problems such as bumble foot and arthritis.

Table 4.1 Examples of types of waterfowl based on feeding and movement styles.

Type	Examples
Dabbling waterfowl	Teals, widgeons, mallards, shovelers, pintails, and gadwalls (all *Anas* genus)
Diving waterfowl	Bufflehead (*Bucephala albeola*), pochard, scaup, canvasback (*Aythya valisineria*), redhead (all *Aythya* genus), ruddy (*Oxyura jamaicensis*) and marbled (*Marmaronetta angustirostris*) ducks
Perching waterfowl	Mandarin (*Aix galericulata*), wood (*Aix sponsa*), torrent (*Merganetta armata*), maned (*Chenonetta jubata*), Hartlaub's (*Pteronetta hartlaubii*), muscovy and some whistling ducks (*Dendrocygna* genus) and the pygmy (*Nettapus* genus) and spur-winged geese (*Plectropterus gambensis*)
Grazing waterfowl	Canada geese (*Branta canadensis*)

Divers

Divers are those waterfowl that feed primarily under water. Ducks of this group belong to the subfamily Aythyinae. Compared to dabblers, divers have legs placed more caudally on their bodies to help propel them underwater. However, divers tend to walk poorly on land, if at all (Table 4.1, Figure 4.4a,b).

Perchers

Perchers tend to perch in trees, on top of logs or other raised surfaces (Table 4.1) Although not true of all, perchers tend to have longer legs and necks than dabblers and certainly divers (Figure 4.5a,b).

Grazers

Grazers are primarily limited to herbivorous geese that eat terrestrial grasses, grains, and other plants. These birds are good walkers and spend a significant amount of time foraging on land. The Canada goose (*Branta canadensis*) is a good example (Table 4.1, Figure 4.6a,b).

Important Physical Characteristics

Most domestic ducks and geese are poor or non-existent flyers- usually because they are simply too large and heavy for their wings. Domestic ducks the same size or smaller than mallards and all wild type waterfowl can be good flyers and precautions (pinioning, wing trims, appropriate housing) to prevent escape should be considered for captive populations.

The bill is a highly specialized organ and shows some degree of variation between different waterfowl species. Of note, female mallards and their breeds often develop dark spots

(a)   (b)

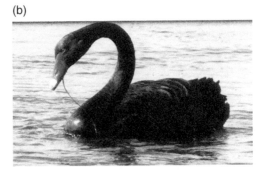

Figure 4.3 (a) This pintail drake (*Anas acuta*) is a dabbling duck. Notice the centrally placed legs which enable dabblers to walk well on land. (b) A black swan cob (*Cygnus atratus*) is dabbling on the surface of the water.

(a)

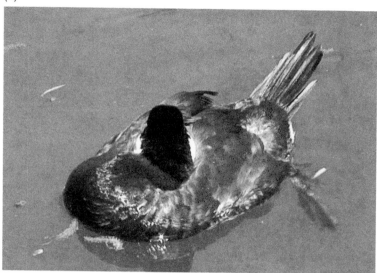

(b)

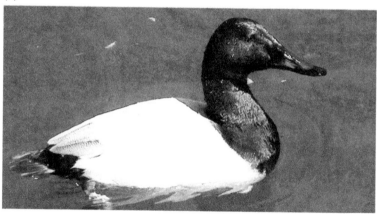

Figure 4.4 (a) A ruddy duck drake (*Oxyura jamaicensis*) is resting on the water. As is common with divers, ruddy ducks have caudally placed legs which aid in swimming but make them poor walkers on land. (b) Another diver, the canvasback (*Aythya valisineria*), will dive to retrieve tubers, insect larvae, seeds, snails, and more from the bottom substrate of waterways.

or streaks on their otherwise yellow to orange beak when they begin to lay. This is due to hormonal changes and is considered normal [1]. Mallards and other waterfowl have carotenoid pigmented beaks that may be used in mate selection [2]. The degree of coloration has also been linked to immune function [2].

Beak trimming is a practice sometimes used in commercial operations to reduce aggression and feather damage. If significant aggression

and cage mate feather damaging is present, this suggests crowded or otherwise inappropriate housing conditions. The author does not recommend beak trimming but rather environmental modification to reduce animal stress.

As mentioned above, the legs of waterfowl are quite variable and are best suited to their preferred environment. Divers reside primarily on water and occasionally rest on soft (grassy) land. Forcing divers to spend too much time

(a)

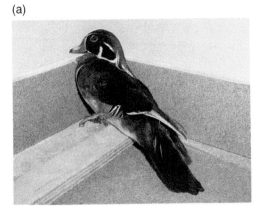

(b)

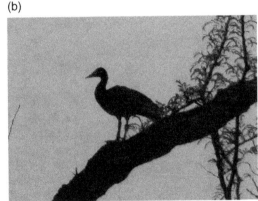

Figure 4.5 (a) A wood duck drake (*Aix sponsa*) is attempting to rest on a flat piece of wood in a holding pen. Ideally hospitalized perching ducks should be provided round surfaces (such as logs) to give the option to 'perch'. (b) The silhouette of a spur-winged goose (*Plectropterus gambensis*) is seen perched high in a tree.

walking on land can result in stress and leg and foot injuries. Most dabblers have legs designed for both agile swimming and walking and should be given access to both environments. Grazers and perchers generally have strong legs making them well suited to terrestrial life. Muscovy ducks in particular have sharp talon-like claws to aid in perching. All terrestrial waterfowl environments should include soft (grassy) areas (Figure 4.7). Perchers should also be provided with elevated rounded (logs or branches) surfaces. Chronically residing on hard substrates (packed earth, concrete, etc.), especially when combined with obesity, increases the risk of birds developing secondary pododermatitis (bumblefoot) and arthritis.

Only 3% of avian species, including waterfowl, possess a phallus. [3] Aside from external physical characteristics, most (adult) waterfowl can be sexed by identifying the phallus (or not as with females). With the bird standing or resting comfortably on its back, simply evert the cloaca and identify the phallus which is located on the ventral floor of the cloaca and within the phallic sac (*saccus phalli*) [4] (Figure 4.8a,b). Sometimes the phallus can be gently palpated by inserting a lubricated gloved finger into the cloaca. Females have a smooth cloacal floor. Juvenile birds may be difficult to sex until the phallus becomes better developed.

The phallus length in waterfowl varies from 1.5 to greater than 40 cm and may be smooth and simple or highly convoluted complete with grooves, spines, and a corkscrew shape. [3] Consequently, the female of the same species tends to have a vagina (simple to highly complex) that matches that of the male's phallus. The complexities of the phallus and vagina are positively correlated with the frequency of forced extra-pair copulations (FEPC) in that species. During FEPC, females generally struggle and do not show receptivity (prone position with tail up). [4] For example, the harlequin duck (*Histrionicus histrionicus*) and African goose (*Anser cygnoides*) (both of which do not engage in FEPC) have short simple phalli and vaginas. The opposite is true with the long-tailed duck (*Clangula hyemalis*) and mallard (both species engage in FECP) which have long phalli and elaborate vaginas. [3]

Basic Behavior

One of the best known characteristics of many waterfowl is their strong imprinting behavior. It has been noted that vocal imprinting (sounds encountered during incubation) predates visual imprinting – at least in ducks. [1] Young waterfowl tend to readily follow the first person

(a)

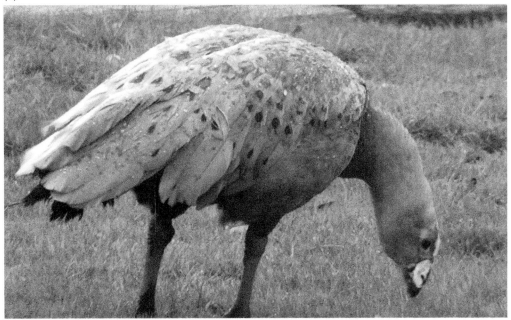

(b)

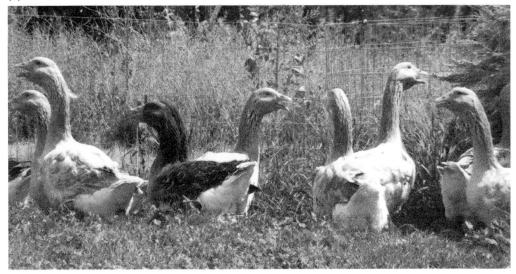

Figure 4.6 (a) Cape Barren Goose (*Cereopsis novaehollandiae*) is casually grazing on grass. The characteristic heavy body and strong legs are common among grazers. (b) Domestic geese are classic grazers. This gaggle of mixed breeds resides in a grassy field ideal for grazers.

or animal they see, and possibly hear, at hatch. Upon reaching maturity, most waterfowl will stop this tracking behavior and integrate with others of the same species (ideal) or other birds, animals or as a single animal (not ideal).

In general, waterfowl are gentle animals and tolerate the presence of humans and other non-predatory animals well. Intra-species aggression is most common with crowding, when food or other valuable resources are limited and

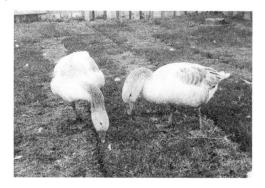

Figure 4.7 All captive waterfowl should be provided with soft grassy land. Grass sod strips can be seen in this backyard setting complete with 2 Buff geese (*Anser anser domesticus*). The grass provides forage and a soft substrate to walk upon for the geese.

during mating and rearing times. Waterfowl are most aggressive toward humans when young are present and can occasionally be territorial.

Waterfowl demonstrate a pecking order much like that of chickens with a top bird, then #2 and so on. Fighting may erupt especially when a new bird enters the flock. Generally, fights are limited in degree and intervention is only required if conflict results in serious injuries. As a means to reduce aggression among groups of drakes, Holderread suggests "light neutering" birds by placing them in totally dark enclosures for 14–18 hours a day. [1] If such "light neutering" is used, the author recommends doing this only for a short period until the source(s) of aggression (crowding, mating season, etc.) is (are) resolved. For information regarding behavior in poultry in general, see Chapter 22 (Behavior).

Common Species of Captive Ducks and Geese

Basic Terminology

Several poultry organizations have set standards that define class, breed and more for domestic ducks and geese. The American Poultry

(a)

(b)

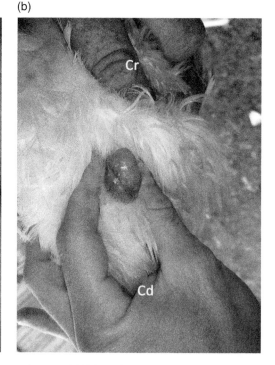

Figure 4.8 (a) When vent sexing waterfowl first expose the vent. (b) Using mild pressure slightly evert the cloaca. This Muscovy duck (*Cairina moschata*) is a hen. The phallus can be readily seen in species that engage in frequent forced extra pair copulations, such as with this Buff duck drake (*Anas platyrhynchos*), by everting the cloaca. Cr = cranial, Cd = caudal.

Association (APA, see www.amerpoultryassn.com) was founded in Buffalo, New York in 1873 is the oldest livestock organization in the United States. The American Bantam Association (ABA, see www.bantamclub.com) formed in 1914 and also sets standards for poultry including ducks. The APA and ABA recognize many, but not all, of the same breeds [5]. Additional organizations set waterfowl standards, provide basic education for owners, work to preserve breeds, and more.

The "class" of duck or goose is based on weight. The APA has defined four classes of domestic duck: Bantam Duck, Light Duck, Medium Duck, and Heavy Duck (Table 4.2, Figure 4.9a–h). Similarly, three classes of domestic goose are defined as follows: Light Goose, Medium Goose, and Heavy Goose [6] (Table 4.2, Figure 4.10a–f). As a note, the Egyptian goose (*Alopochen aegyptiacus*) is often placed in the shelduck family making it in-between a goose and a duck.

The "breed" of waterfowl (ducks and geese) is based on distinctive physical characteristics that were often developed over decades to millennia. As with dogs and other domestic animals, "breed type" and variation can be significant among domestic waterfowl. Breed and breed type may be distinguishable by size, body silhouette, plumage patterns and color, and more (Figure 4.11).

The "variety" of bird is usually distinguishable by the plumage color or pattern [1]. For example, White Aylesbury ducks are white and come in one variety. However, the Runner duck comes in eight recognized varieties: blue, black, chocolate, white, penciled, gray, fawn, and white and buff [1] (Figure 4.12a–c).

Finally, the "strain" of waterfowl refers to a particular breed that descends from one flock or breeding farm [1]. Birds within a strain are generally inbred to achieve specific traits, such as high egg production. These traits can actually be significantly different between strains and still be within the same breed. The strain is usually identified by the originator's name in the prefix. Examples of duck strains include;

Table 4.2 Examples of classes of ducks and geese based on weight according to the American Poultry Association (APA).

Class	Examples
Bantam duck	Call, mallard, East Indie
Light duck	Magpie, Campbell, runner, Welsh Harlequin
Medium duck	Buff, Cayuga, crested, Swedish (*Dendrocygna* genus) and the pygmy (*Nettapus* genus) and spur-winged geese (*Plectropterus gambensis*)
Heavy duck	Appleyard, Aylesbury, muscovy, Pekin, rouen, Saxony
Light goose	Canada, Chinese, Egyptian, Tufted Roman
Medium goose	American Buff, pilgrim, Pomeranian, Sebastapol, Steinbacher
Heavy goose	African, Embden, Toulouse

Legarth Pekins, Horton East Indies, Lundgren White Calls, and so on [1].

Basic terminology of names given to males, females, young, and groups of waterfowl is described in Table 4.3. A "mule duck" or "mule" is an infertile hybrid and most commonly refers to the offspring of a domestic mallard hen and Muscovy drake [7, 8]. A "hinny duck" or "hinny" is the offspring of a domestic mallard drake and Muscovy hen [8].

Ducks

Domestic ducks are either breeds of the mallard (*A. platyrhynchos*) or Muscovy duck (*Cairina moschata*). The Pekin, Khaki Campbell, Call, Runner, Rouen, Buff, Swedish, and Crested are examples of common duck breeds all believed to be descended from mallards while Muscovy ducks (and all of their color varieties) are distinctly different.

It is believed that duck domestication began in China during the Zhou Dynasty (514–495 BC) with the Pekin duck being one of the earlier breeds [9]. Pekin ducks are the

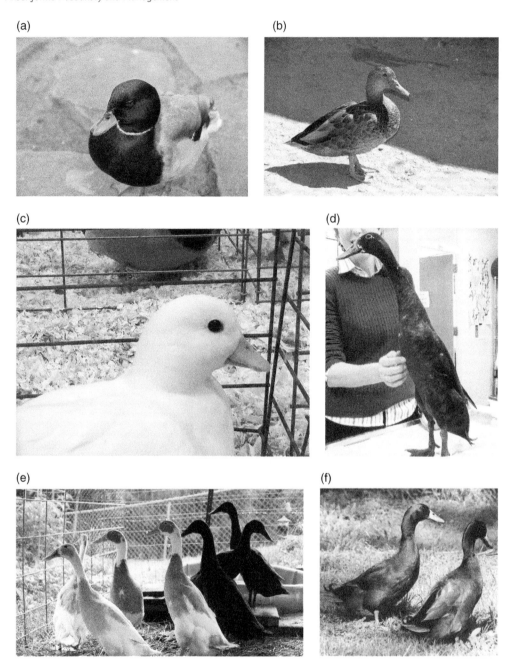

Figure 4.9 Domestic ducks can be divided into the following classes: Bantam Duck, Light Duck, Medium Duck and Heavy Duck. With the exception of the Muscovy duck (*Cairina moschata*) all other ducks are *Anas platyrhynchos*. This Gray Call drake (a), Mallard hen in molting plumage (b), and white Call hen (c) are all Bantam ducks. The Chocolate Runner (d), Fawn and White Runners (e), and Khaki Campbell (drakes) (f) are Light ducks. The Buff (g, foreground), and Crested (h, i) are Medium ducks. This Muscovy drake (j) and White Pekin (k) varieties are heavy ducks. *Source:* Figure 4.9c courtesy of Dr. Cheryl B. Greenacre. Figure 4.9e courtesy of Bridgette Napela, and Figure 4.9h courtesy of Dr. Abigail Duvall.

(g)

(h)

(i)

(j)

(k)

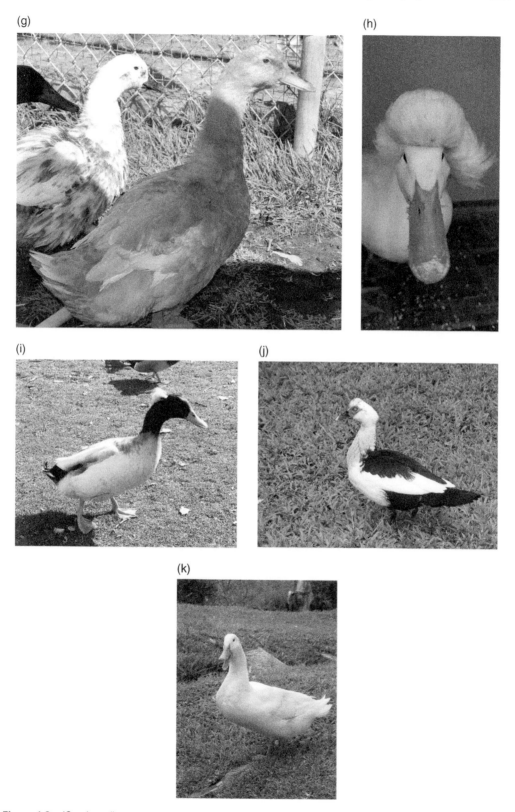

Figure 4.9 (Continued)

(a)

(b)

(c)

(d)

(e)

(f)

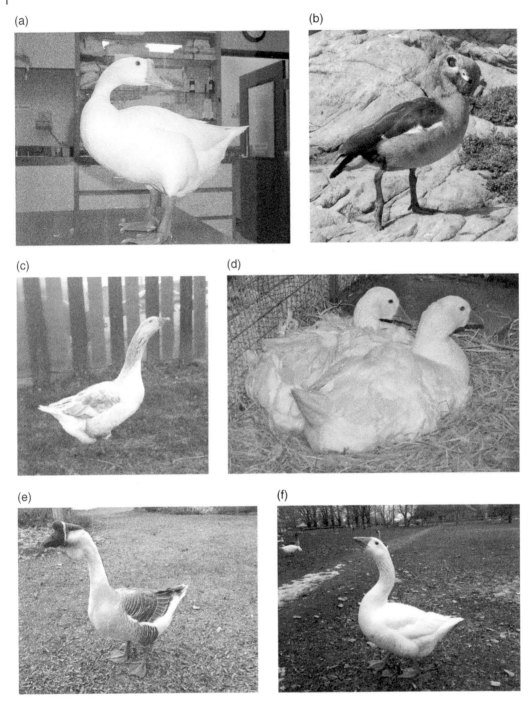

Figure 4.10 Domestic geese can be divided into the following classes: Light Goose, Medium Goose and Heavy Goose. African and Chinese geese are *Anser cygnoides*, the Egyptian goose is *Alopochen aegyptiacus* while the others are *Anser anser domesticus*. The White Chinese (a) and Egyptian (b) are Light geese. The American Buff (c) and Sebastopol (d), *Source:* Courtesy of Abby Perata are examples of Medium geese. The African (e) and Embden (f) are Heavy geese.

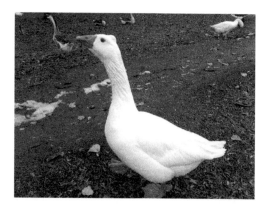

Figure 4.11 The Roman (*Anser anser domesticus*) is a breed of goose and is distinguished by the tuft of feathers on the top of its head, relatively small size with good meat to bone ratio. Contrast the Roman with another all white breed the Embden goose (Figure 4.10f) which is known as being heavy and the tallest of the domestic geese.

classic white-feathered, yellow billed ducks commonly kept as pets. Runner ducks are recognized by their vertical body posture and move with quick steps rather than waddle. Crested ducks have a unique crest on the back of their head sometimes associated with a malformed skull and brain, intracranial fat bodies and subsequent neurological disease [10, 11]. Khaki Campbell ducks are noted for their high egg production. Ducks are most often kept as companions, display (collection) animals and commercially for egg, meat, and foie gras production.

Several features can be used to distinguish males from females. Domestic female ducks "quack" while the males have a hoarse "wongh." [1]. Mature males tend to be larger, have a curled tail (although not while molting) and are more ornately colored (for non-white breeds). *Anas*, and other, genus males have an osseous syringeal bulla that is readily seen on radiographs (Figure 4.13a–c).

Muscovy ducks are best recognized by their warty features (caruncles) on the featherless portions of the face (mature birds), tendency to perch and roost like chickens, long claws on their feet and a hissing sound instead of a "quack" [12]. Drakes have a fleshy knob at the base of their upper bill, more pronounced facial caruncles and a short erectile crest of feathers on the top of the head. Muscovy ducks can breed with mallards, however their offspring are sterile (mule). Ducks commonly interbreed when kept with multiple species.

Geese

Domestic geese are derived from the graylag goose (*Anser anser*) or swan goose (*Anser cygnoides*). Although the exact origins can be argued, the eastern Asian (Chinese and African) geese are generally believed to come from the swan goose and the western Asian, North African, and European (European) geese are domesticated greylags. Domestic "Chinese" and "African" geese are distinguished by the large knob at the base of the upper bill which is not present in the "European" varieties.

Common goose breeds include the Toulouse, Embden, White Chinese and are either *Anser anser domesticus* or *Anser cygnoides* or hybrids. The Toulouse is well known for foie gras production and is dark gray (along back) to light gray edged (breast and ventrum) feathers. Embden is pure white with an orange bill. Chinese geese come in White and Brown varieties and have a characteristic knob at the base of the upper bill (Figure 4.14a,b)

Swans

Mute (*Cygnus olor*), trumpeter (*Cygnus buccinator*), black (*Cygnus atratus*), black neck (*Cygnus melancoryphus*), and Coscoroba (*Coscoroba coscoroba*) swans are most commonly kept as pets. As the name implies, mute swans are less noisy than others however they will hiss (usually defensively or aggressively), whistle or snort.

Zoos, aviaries and some specialized private collections may have a large number of different waterfowl species representing the approximately 150 members of the family Anseriformes. For more specific details, including breed characteristics, about common captive waterfowl, see Holderread and Ekarius [1, 5].

(a)

(b)

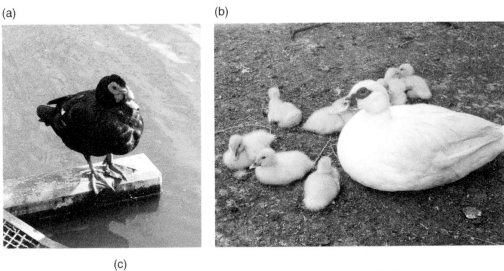

(c)

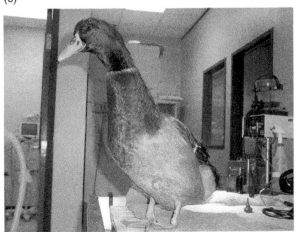

Figure 4.12 Domestic waterfowl breeds can come in many varieties. For example the Black Muscovy drake (a) and White Muscovy hen with brood of ducklings (b) are two varieties of the same breed (*Cairina moschata*). Some, such as this Rouen drake (*Anas platyrhynchos*) (c), only come in one variety.

Table 4.3 Names given to male, female, young, and groups of waterfowl.

	Males	Females	Young	Groups
Duck	Drake	Hen	Duckling	safe or badelynge (on land); brace (for a pair); flock (in flight); bunch, paddling, or raft (on water); brood (newly hatched with hen); team
Goose	Gander	Goose	Gosling	Gaggle (on land); flock; skein or wedge (in flight)
Swan	Cob	Pen	Cygnet	Bevy or wedge (in flight); lamentation, herd, game, team

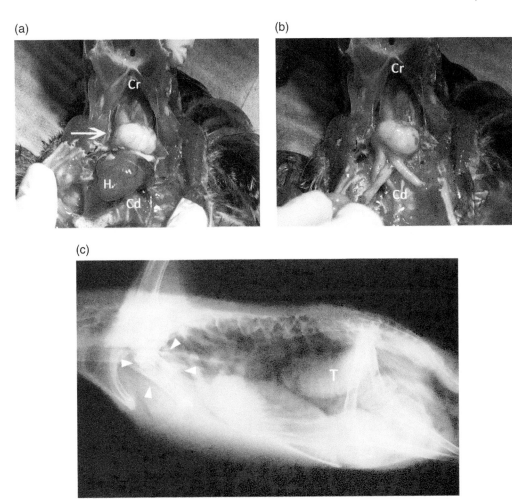

Figure 4.13 Some male ducks possess osseous syringeal bulla at the terminal end of the trachea and should be recognized as normal. (a) In this *Anas* genus duck, the sternum is reflected cranially exposing the heart (H) and osseous sryingeal bulla (arrow). (b) With the heart removed, the primary bronchi can be seen exiting the caudal aspect of the bullae. (c) This structure may be readily seen in drakes on radiographs (outlined by arrowheads). This domestic mallard drake (*Anas platyrhynchos*) was reproductively active and had enlarged testes (T). Cr = cranial, Cd = caudal.

Basic Reproduction

Swans and geese tend to form strong monogamous pair bonds whereas ducks (especially domestics) tend to be polygamous. Ducks will also breed, or at least attempt to breed, with different species of other ducks and small geese. Interestingly, the vagina of some waterfowl species has multiple blind pouches and spirals that may act as anatomical barriers to the phallus preventing conception resulting

from forced copulation [3, 4]. Interspecies breeding is especially common if the duck was raised in mixed species collections. Resulting mixed species ducklings are common but are often sterile (Figure 4.15a,b).

Waterfowl may breed on land or water. Few species such as the magpie goose (*Anseranas semipalmata*), Cape Barren goose (*Cereopsis novaehollandiae*), and Hawaiian goose (*Branta sandvicensis*) breed exclusively on land [3]. Most wild waterfowl tend to breed

(a) (b)

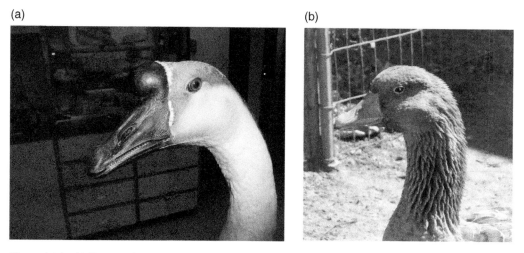

Figure 4.14 (a) Characteristic of the swan goose (*Anser cygnoides*) derived eastern Asian geese, a large knob is present at the base of the upper bill as with this Brown Chinese. (b) European breeds derived from the graylag goose (*Anser anser*) lack the knob such as with this Toulouse. *Source:* Photograph courtesy of Abby Perata.

(a) (b)

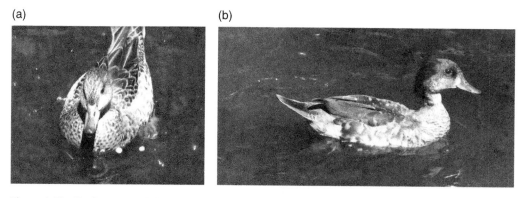

Figure 4.15 Ducks commonly interbred creating interesting offspring that are generally considered to be sterile mules. (a) American widgeon (*Anas americana*) X blue wing teal (*Anas discors*) hen. (b) marbled teal (*Marmaronetta angustirostris*) X wood duck (*Aix sponsa*) drake.

on water while domestic ducks commonly breed anywhere convenient.

Most waterfowl lay eggs on the ground and tend to make shallow nests composed of plant matter and feathers pulled from a "brood patch" (Figure 4.16). Wood ducks and buffleheads are examples of tree cavity nesters, but others such as the mallard will also opportunistically lay eggs in raised locations. Feather loss may or may not be evident over the ventral crop and breast regions. The mute (*Cygnus olor*) and other swans commonly build large raised nests from waterside vegetation (Figure 4.17).

It is common for hens to show behavior and physical changes just prior to lay that include apparent lethargy, anorexia, ventral coelomic swelling and a dilated vent that may easily be mistaken for illness. Males also sometimes display lethargy and anorexia during breeding season. Once breeding season is complete and eggs have all been laid, birds generally return to normal (excluding the sitting behavior of hens).

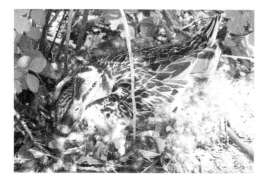

Figure 4.16 Nesting hens commonly pull feathers from their breast area creating a "brood patch." The feathers are often used in the nest construction as seen here with this wild mallard (*Anas platyrhynchos*).

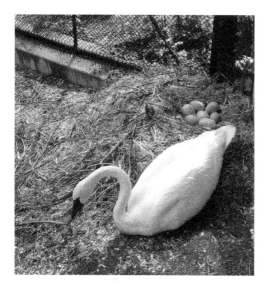

Figure 4.17 An exhibit trumpeter swan pen (*Cygnus buccinator*) sits next to her full nest. Items in the exhibit were used to create a large mound typical of many swan nests.

Handling

Because of the many species variations among waterfowl, handling techniques do vary. In general, waterfowl are easy to handle – especially domestic species. While most clinicians will be presented with individual birds, some may work with waterfowl flocks in private collections, zoos, aviaries, and through field work.

The discussions below will pertain to captive waterfowl. Wild animal capture techniques are discussed in more detail elsewhere.

Most waterfowl are presented as single or paired birds in boxes, dog carriers or simply unrestrained. Regardless, for the safety of the animal it is always best to transport birds in a sturdy enclosure such as a dog travel crate. While they may be nervous, most domestic waterfowl will permit an examination with minimal to no handling. Even some wild waterfowl are quite easy to handle when moved outside of their territory. Diving ducks generally require full handling for a complete examination simply because they don't stand or walk well and tend to rest on their breast when out of water. Of course handling is often required for fractious animals and those requiring more detailed examinations or collections of diagnostics.

The most common defenses waterfowl have when restrained are clawing (especially Muscovy ducks), wing flapping, and biting. The larger birds have the greatest potential to induce damage to handlers.

Most waterfowl can be restrained by simply placing a hand or arm over the back to keep the wings tucked against the body. The head is minimally restrained and only if needed as most don't bite once the body is secured (Figure 4.18a,b). If needed, the handler's hand or arm can be extended around the bird to the middle of the breast. From here, the bird can be turned on its side or back to facilitate necessary procedures. Some waterfowl will lay on their back in the crook of the handler's arm or on a flat surface (Figure 4.19a–c). Alternatively, the handler can use two hands with the palm on the back of the bird and each set of fingers extending to the bird's breast (Figure 4.20). If the bird is in respiratory or cardiac distress, laying it on its back may exacerbate the problem and the bird should be kept upright.

With the bird secured either standing, suspended or on its back or side, the legs may paddle freely. Small waterfowl rarely need their legs secured. Strong legs and prominent nails can

(a) (b)

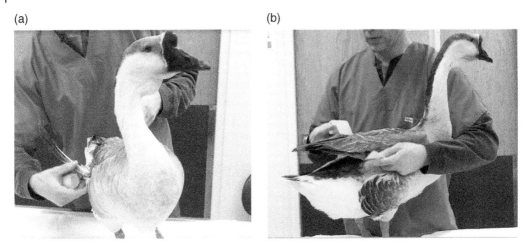

Figure 4.18 (a) Most domestic waterfowl can be examined with minimal restraint. This Brown African goose (*Anser cygnoides*) with angel wing deformity is standing with no restraint in preparation for a wing bandage. (b) If needed, the restrainer's arm can be placed around or over the bird.

(a) (b)

(c) (d)

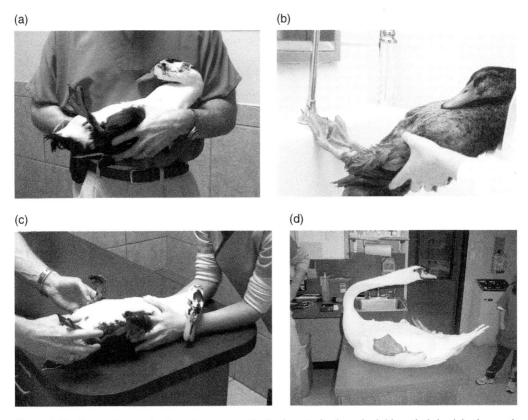

Figure 4.19 By gently securing the wings across the back, waterfowl can be laid on their back in the crook of the handler's arm (a), in the hands (b), or on a flat surface (c) as demonstrated on these mixed breed domestic ducks (*Anas platyrhynchos*). The same technique can be used with larger geese and swans such as the mute swan (*Cygnus olor*). (d) Birds should only be kept on their back long enough to complete necessary exams and sample collection. Unless absolutely necessary, do not place distressed animals or those with cardiac or pulmonary disease on their back. *Source:* Figure 4.19b courtesy of Dr. Cheryl B. Greenacre.

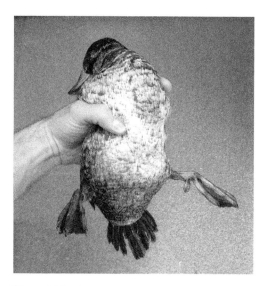

Figure 4.20 Small waterfowl, such as this Argentine ruddy duck drake (*Oxyura vittata*), can be handled by securing both wings using one (seen here) or two hands. The breast area is left unrestrained.

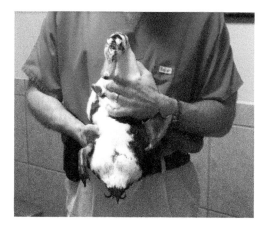

Figure 4.21 This mixed breed domestic duck (*Anas platyrhynchos*) is being held up against the handler's chest with the bird's body facing forward. If flailing legs pose a problem, gently secure the tibiotarsi being careful to not put pressure on arthritic joints.

result in scratch injuries to handlers. If needed, bring the restrained bird's back up against the handler's chest and use a free hand to hold the legs at the level of the tibiotarsii (Figure 4.21). Use caution when handling legs on waterfowl with arthritis (which is common) as it may cause pain and result in more struggling.

Herding

Domestic ducks of mallard descent and domestic geese tend to form tight groups when pressured to move by predators and humans [1]. This behavior allows caretakers to direct birds to certain areas such as night and holding pends using simple methods. For small groups, handlers (working singly or in groups) can "herd" birds with outstretched arms, flashlights, flags, or other small visual devices (Figure 4.22). For large flocks, consider working in (human) teams using bamboo poles, herding nets (seine, volleyball, etc.) or other devices to help span a larger area. Non-mallard ducks and wild waterfowl rarely follow these rules and swans are rarely encountered in groups making other forms of group handing necessary.

Catching Birds on Water

Occasionally birds need to be captured on open water in private collections and parks. Before attempting to capture wild waterfowl on open waterways, consult with local fish and game authorities as many waterfowl species are protected and capture may be considered illegal without appropriate authorization.

Assuming the animal is not trained and cannot be baited and captured at the water's edge or on land, the bird may need to be netted. Grazers and dabblers can be "herded" on water using poles and nets (sometimes spanning the water and with the help of multiple people) and brought close enough to easily capture with a hand held net. Divers pose a different problem and should be carefully netted. Hand held nets are the best but seine and other multiple person operated nets can be used as long as the netting is frequently checked to ensure the bird is not entangled unseen under water.

Swans

Swans are large birds and are generally docile unless threatened. The author finds swans easy to handle outside of their territory. In addition

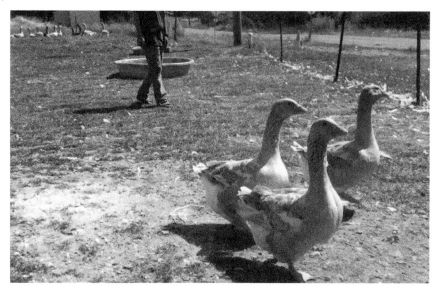

Figure 4.22 Mallard descent (*Anas platyrhynchos*) and domestic geese readily form tight groups when "herded" by people as shown with this small gaggle of Buff geese (*Anser anser domesticus*).

to biting and kicking; swans will often hit opponents using their wings which can potentially cause serious damage. If the swan is docile, minimal if any handling is needed as most will tolerate a full but gentle examination. If the swan is unruly or making threatening gestures, the wings should be secured first (the biting is minor in comparison). This is most safely accomplished by approaching swans from behind (usually with a second person in front of and in the line of sight of the bird). The wings are tucked into a normal resting position and secured while a second person performs a physical examination and any diagnostics if needed. The head is managed by simply moving the distal end of the neck away from the restrainer(s). Grabbing the neck may make the bird panic and

is generally avoided. Chemical restraint may be needed for select individuals and for performing some diagnostics such as radiographs.

Basic Housing

Waterfowl ideally need housing that protects them from inclement weather and predators while offering room to freely walk around and have access to natural sunlight, fresh water for swimming and drinking, soft substrate and, especially in the case of geese, fresh grass to graze (Figures 4.23a-g). Suddenly changing the substrate may lead to waterfowl eating the new substrate (if small enough) leading to gastrointestinal impactions. While some pet waterfowl

Figure 4.23 (a) Backyard ducks can be successfully provided swimming and comfort movement opportunities with a simple "kiddie" pool provided the water is kept clean as with this Khaki Campbell (*Anas platyrhynchos*). (b) Mute (*Cygnus olor*) and other swans ideally have access to water with naturally growing grasses to provide for swimming and natural forage. (c) Wood ducks (*Aix sponsa*- drake) and other perching waterfowl should be provided opportunities to perch on logs, branches or similar structures out of the water. (d) Grazers such as this Brown African goose (*Anser cygnoides*) spend most of their time on land and need grass as their primary substrate. (e) Dabblers like this cinnamon teal drake (*Anas cyanoptera*) need access to fresh water and comfortable places to rest on land. (f) Diving ducks such this redhead drake (*Aythya americana*) spend most of the their time on water and need enough depth to fully submerge their body and swim freely underwater. (g) Waterfowl ponds should have easy entrance/exit sites, some type of

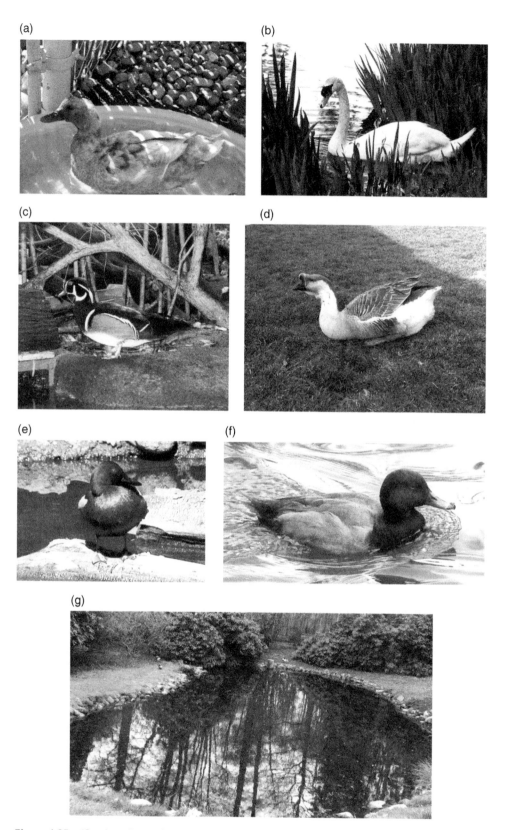

Figure 4.23 (Continued) aeration and fresh water flow, grassy soft banks and large enough to accommodate the number of animals present.

are pinioned to prevent flying, many simply don't fly and prefer to walk or swim.

Ponds can be natural or manmade ("kiddie" pool) and fresh cool drinking water that allows waterfowl to completely submerge their head (as is needed to clean their nostrils and preen feathers) should be available at all times [13]. Bodies of water should be designed such that birds can easily enter and exit as needed. This generally means ensuring there is a gentle slope (natural or manmade) between the land and water. Larger ponds that are at risk of stagnation (especially in summer months) should be aerated to reduce the risk of botulism and other disease outbreaks. Waterfowl produce voluminous droppings and tend to dirty small bodies of water very rapidly. Frequent water changes are often needed.

Waterfowl incidentally consume sediment as they feed in water. "Sediment" includes non-food items that are associated with foraging behavior and includes mud, grit, man-made objects, and more. The bird's feeding style generally dictates how much sediment is ingested. For example the piscivorous red-breasted merganser (*Mergus serrator*) feeds on fish within the water column and ingests less than 2% of its diet (dry matter) as sediment. In contrast, the benthos-feeding (feeds at the bottom of bodies of water) canvasback ingests 22% of its diet (dry matter) as sediment [14]. Dabblers and perchers, including the common mallard, generally ingest low amounts of sediment (less than 4% of its dry matter diet). Divers (ducks) and water grazers (geese and swans) generally ingest more sediment. To the best of the author's knowledge, sediment ingestion from land grazing has not been studied in waterfowl.

Heinz et al. showed that mallards experimentally fed diets containing up to 70% sediment (which was an estimated 46% consumed on a dry matter basis) had no adverse effects. When sediment reached 80–90% of the diet (representing 50–52% ingested on a dry matter basis), the birds lost a significant amount of weight [15]. While it is clear that some waterfowl (naturally and experimentally) safely ingest a large amount of sediment, the bigger

concern is when the sediment contains toxins and other contaminates.

This sediment can provide nutrition, pass through unprocessed or expose the bird to environmental toxins, foreign bodies and other dangers. Areas with slow moving water and fine textured sediment tend to be associated with elevated environmental toxins [14] Lead ingestion is an obvious concern, however waterfowl morbidity and mortality due to other toxins in ingested sediment is well documented [14, 16].

The foraging style of captive waterfowl should be considered when creating enclosures that include natural bodies of water such as streams, ponds, and lakes. Environmental sediment sampling should be considered prior to placing at risk waterfowl in natural settings. Man-made water bearing structures in exhibit and private collections have the benefit of reducing risk of toxin exposure as long as the construction and materials are well designed and safe.

The larger the birds, the more destructive they can be on the enclosure. Mute swans typically feed in water by uprooting or cropping vegetation [14]. This normal behavior can be quite destructive to a nice planted exhibit.

Basic Nutrition

General

Compared to commercial poultry, far fewer nutrition studies exist in relation to waterfowl. Commercial waterfowl diets are often formulated based on the National Research Council's (NRC) publication *Nutrient Requirements of Poultry,* 9th revised edition published in 1994. The NRC publication offers detailed information on specific chicken diets as well as recommendations for other poultry species. However, much of the duck information is extrapolated from other species or based on limited studies in waterfowl.

For example, energy values for formulating duck diets are generally adopted from chicken bioassay data [17]. Rush et al. found that white

Pekin duckling growth and toe ash weight were maximized with 0.95% and 0.85%, respectively, dietary calcium [18]. This is in contrast to the NRC recommendation of 0.6% dietary calcium and is just one example where published NRC guidelines may not be appropriate for all waterfowl. Rodehutscord and Dieckmann showed that young domestic ducks utilize plant and mineral phosphorous (in diets) very differently than that of same age turkeys, broilers, and quails [19]. These studies only serve to highlight nutritional differences between waterfowl (of which primarily domestic ducks have been evaluated) and chickens.

The NRC guidelines should only serve as a rough guide for waterfowl species. Some nutrients are even omitted for waterfowl. For example, there are no NRC guidelines for dietary zinc in waterfowl diets. Attia et al. evaluated several forms and levels of dietary zinc in white Pekin ducklings from 1 to 56 days old. [20] The authors concluded that 30 ppm was adequate for growth rate and zinc excretion in their studied birds. [20]

Most of the waterfowl nutrition studies are limited to production ducks. Marie-Etancilin et al. noted that duck breeding is primarily directed toward fatty liver production with fat meat being a co-product [7]. Basso et al. stated that the most important economic factor with duck production is feed efficiency during growth (which is represented as optimal growth in the studies later in this section) [21]. As a result, our nutrition data pertinent to waterfowl is generally optimized for short lived commercial duck production and not backyard, pet, or exhibit animals. Regardless, some of these studies provide insight into common nutrition based diseases and means to improve overall health that may affect non-production birds. Specific nutrients and their additives will be discussed below.

Total Energy and Body Scoring

Total energy requirements may be calculated by numerous means and are generally established for growth, maintenance, healing, etc. For adult animals, energy requirements are often described with the intent to maintain an animal at a constant live weight. Cherry and Morris established that maintenance requirements for 7 genotypes of domestic drakes were $583\,\text{kJ/kgW}^{0.75}$ per day at $10\,°\text{C}$ ($50\,°\text{F}$) and $523\,\text{kJ/kgW}^{0.75}$ per day at $26\,°\text{C}$ ($78.8\,°\text{F}$). [22]

There are many factors that go into energy needs for animals including, but not limited to, health status, reproductive activity, age, species, breed, strain, environmental conditions, activity level, stressors, and more. While calculating energy requirements for production animals can be important when determining feed rations and more, such calculations are not typically performed for non-production birds. The variables listed above make definitive energy requirements difficult to calculate for non-production birds.

Rather the author relies on individual animal evaluation to determine if the bird is in an energy positive or negative state. The author uses a combination of three methods to subjectively assess energy needs for birds (not just waterfowl); pectoral muscle score (PMS), body condition score (BCS) and health/environmental status. PMS and BCS have been described for many animals but have not been critically evaluated in birds (with the exception of budgerigars [*Melopsittacus undulatus*]). Using "yes" and "no" answers following an algorithm tree, a 1–7 physical scoring system correlated with total body fat has been reported in budgerigars [23].

The systems described below are used by the author and have also not been critically evaluated or correlated with any disease or health status. As a note, advanced diagnostics such as radiographs, ultrasound, computed tomography and magnetic resonance imaging can give a much more accurate account of muscle and fat content and can be used on conjunction with the scoring system below.

Pectoral Muscle Scoring

PMS is simply based on pectoral muscle mass and to a lesser degree strength (see Table 4.4).

Table 4.4 Pectoral muscle score (PMS) system.

	PMS 1	PMS 2	PMS 3	PMS 4	PMS 5
Physical findings	Minimal pectoral muscle mass and it is concave, keel is readily palpable	Pectoral muscle mass is either linear or slightly convex, keel is readily palpable on its anterior surface	Pectoral muscle fills the breast, is slightly convex and forms an arc over the keel making a smooth transition from the left to right pectorals	Pectoral muscles are convex enough to create a mild depression at the keel	Pectoral muscles form a significant convex arc and readily palpable depression at the keel commonly referred to as "cleavage"
Potential causes	Starvation, end-stage illness, chronic disease	Disuse atrophy, chronic disease, non-specific weight loss	Normal	Normal to overweight, strong flyer	Obese

Additionally, the breast muscle can be palpated to assess the softness or firmness of the pectorals. Pectoral muscles can be classified as soft (easily depressed when pressed with a finger), normal (minimally depressed when pressed with a finger) or firm (no depression with pressed with a finger). Soft pectoral muscles are most commonly associated with inactivity and obesity but may also be palpated with bruising and early localized inflammation. Firm muscles are most commonly associated with scar tissue, severe starvation and some infiltrative diseases such as sarcocystosis, granulomatous infections and neoplasia.

Scoring systems vary, however the author uses a 1–5 system with 3 being average or "normal." A PMS of 1 means the pectoral muscle mass is minimal, concave, and the keel is easily palpable. A PMS of 2 indicates the keel is slightly palpable (in addition to the leading edge) and the pectoral muscle mass is either linear or slightly convex. A PMS of 3 indicates that the pectoral muscle fills the breast, is convex and forms an arc over the keel making a smooth transition from the left to right pectorals. A PMS of 4 indicates the pectoral muscles are convex enough to create a mild depression at the keel. A PMS of 5 indicates the pectoral muscles form a significant convex arc and readily palpable depression at the keel commonly referred to as "cleavage." The pectoral muscles may also be classified as soft (easily depressed when pressed with a finger), normal (minimally depressed when pressed with a finger) or firm (no depression with pressed with a finger).

Body Condition Scoring

BCS refers to the amount of fat detected in the skin, subcutaneous, and coelomic tissues (see Table 4.5). Scoring systems vary, however the author uses a 1–5 system with 3 being average or "normal." A BCS of 1 is only assessed during celiotomy and/or with advanced diagnostics and generally means that no dermal or subcutaneous and minimal to no intraceolomic fat is found. A BCS of 2 is also assessed during celiotomy and/or with advanced diagnostics and indicates that no dermal or subcutaneous but a mild amount diffuse intraceolomic fat (usually mesenteric) is present. A BCS of 3 can be assessed subjectively with physical examination and indicates that no dermal and minimal subcutaneous fat is present (usually along the caudal ventral coelom). A BCS of 4 indicates that no to minimal dermal and significant subcutaneous fat is present in one or more parts of the body (commonly along the caudal ventral coelom, breast, inner thighs, caudal dorsum [near base of tail], and neck). A BCS of 5 indicates dermal and significant diffuse subcutaneous fat is present.

The obvious disadvantage of this BCS system is the need for advanced diagnostics to assess scores of 1 and 2. However, the system

Table 4.5 Body condition score (BCS) system.

	BCS 1	BCS 2	BCS 3	BCS 4	BCS 5
Physical findings	No dermal or subcutaneous and minimal to no intraceolomic fat is found[a]	No dermal or subcutaneous but a mild amount diffuse intraceolomic fat (usually mesenteric) is present[a]	No dermal and minimal subcutaneous fat is present (usually along the caudal ventral coelom)	No to minimal dermal and significant subcutaneous fat is present in one or more parts of the body (commonly along the caudal ventral coelom, breast, inner thighs and neck)	Dermal and significant diffuse subcutaneous fat is present
Potential causes	Starvation, end-stage illness, chronic disease	Normal, chronic disease, non-specific weight loss	Normal	Overweight, "well-conditioned"	Obese, metabolic derangement

[a] Can only be determined via celiotomy and/or by using advanced diagnostics such as computed tomography, magnetic resonance imaging or ultrasonography. Other findings are based on physical examination.

presented herein is designed to be used with PMS and health and environmental status considerations. At a minimum, BCS's of 3–5 can be accurately determined with physical exam and scores of 1 and 2 can deduced based on other findings.

While a PMS and BCS of 1 often indicate severe catabolism and scores of 5 indicate significant energy excess, values of 2–4 can represent some variations of normal. For example, a non-flighted and inactive bird can have a PMS of 2 with soft muscle and a BCS of 4 with excess subcutaneous fat. So the bird in this example is overweight with decreased pectoral muscle mass due to inactivity and is very common with pet ducks. Conversely, a strong flighted duck may have a PMS of 4 with normal muscle and BCS of 2. This is common with healthy wild birds, especially toward the end of migration, or those in aviaries with large flight areas.

Last, health and environmental status are used when considering energy needs. For example a clinically obese Pekin duck kept indoors will generally have lower energy requirements than a similarly obese bird kept outdoors with access to swim. Additionally disease states can alter PMS and BCS values.

For example, a bird with a wing injury will often have overall decreased PMS with more significant ipsilateral pectoral loss. Some birds with metabolic derangements (especially associated with liver and reproductive tract disorders) may have unusual fat deposits in areas not commonly seen. Because of the significant variables present, adjusting for health and environmental status are obviously the most subjective aspects of calculating energy needs for birds.

Aside from more accurate measurements using advanced diagnostics, the physical examination and daily weights often give clinicians the best assessment of a bird's energy needs. Accounting for the food in the gastrointestinal tract, weights typically fluctuate faster than PMS and BCS. PMS and BCS give clinicians better assessment of long term trends (over days to weeks).

Using PMS, BCS and by understanding the health and environmental conditions present, clinicians can better assess total energy needs for waterfowl. Caloric needs are adjusted based on the above findings. Underweight birds are provided more calorie dense and frequent feedings. Overweight birds are given fewer total calories and encouraged to exercise.

Total energy plans can be set for hospitalized birds and those in their normal environment. This may include using tube feeding products (usually ill individuals) and measured bowl (or other container) fed foods. As a note, calorie restriction in flocks may result in aggression and stress (see Foraging Enrichment) and should be considered prior to implementation.

Carbohydrates

Many breeds of domesticated ducks and geese have been developed for foie gras production and are predisposed to liver steatosis [24–26]. Studied mule ducks (Muscovy X Pekin) and specific breeds of domestic geese are highly susceptible to liver steatosis. Liver weight may increase 7–10-fold after just two weeks of overfeeding [26, 27]. In a separate study, 70-day old mule ducks were fed a carbohydrate rich diet (corn) for 12.5 days and developed severe fatty livers. Liver weights (8% of body weight) were nearly 10-fold that of controls (1% of body weight) primarily as a result of lipid accumulation (60% of total weight). The study showed that by simply overfeeding a carbohydrate rich diet (corn), de novo hepatic lipogenesis in mule ducks predominated over dietary lipid intake to significantly alter lipid composition in hepatocytes. Liver steatosis is likely common in certain waterfowl species (primarily domestics) because overfeeding results in intense lipogenesis that almost exclusively occurs in the liver of these birds [24, 26]. Saez et al. noted that even with basal dietary conditions (non-overfed), Muscovy ducks "have a tendency for hepatic steatosis" [25].

Fatty liver disease and fat accumulation in general may result with excessive carbohydrate ingestion in ducks and geese [24, 26–28]. Hepatic steatosis is strongly correlated with metabolic syndromes and is associated with liver injury, blood lipid metabolism, and peroxidation [28]. Species and breed determine the degree of hepatic steatosis development. As an example, liver lipids increased 85-fold and 50-fold in carbohydrate overfed Muscovy and common ducks, respectively [26]. Maize (corn) is the main component of foods used in overfeeding diets needed to achieve hepatic steatosis [8, 25, 26]. Ground corn, a simple carbohydrate source, is often the main ingredient in commercial waterfowl diets.

The author has noted significant obesity in geese and especially captive ducks fed diets high in simple carbohydrates. Just as domestic ducks and geese are predisposed to hepatic steatosis resulting from overfeeding, fatty liver is (generally) considered reversible when overfeeding is discontinued [26]. Strategies to reduce excessive body and (presumably) liver fat are to reduce dietary simple carbohydrates (corn, and flour based food, many pellet products), limit total food availability (except natural forage), encourage foraging, feed higher fiber leafy greens, increase physical enclosure space and encourage swimming opportunities.

Reducing total pellet consumption is best accomplished in adult birds. Young waterfowl have specific dietary requirements for growth and inappropriate rations (as with reduced commercial pellets and increased other foods without the total diet being balanced) may result in serious nutritional diseases. As a result, the author recommends either feeding specific waterfowl grower pellets or using published and proven alternate diets for growing birds (at least until fully grown). The author does encourage young birds to forage on vegetation and insects (which does supplement the diet) but use pellets as the base food.

Protein

Amino acids have multiple roles in both protein and non-protein metabolism. While the many different amino acids have important roles, only methionine and arginine will be discussed in any detail here. Recommended total protein amounts will also be covered.

Methionine is especially important because it is considered the first limiting amino acid of poultry diets [29–31]. Common diets offered to waterfowl are often composed of cereal grains and soybean meal which have limited methionine content [29]. As a result these diets are usually supplemented.

Unfortunately, nutrition information in young waterfowl is scarce [32]. The methionine research is limited to production ducks and geese but does offer useful information as to growth and other factors which are important in young animals. This understanding becomes important when homemade or other non-commercial foods are fed to captive young waterfowl and should be a consideration if stunting or other problems are noted.

The NRC (1994) requirement for dietary methionine for ducks two to seven weeks old is 0.3% and is based on research in Muscovy ducks [30]. Jamroz et al., found that a diet containing a total of 0.40% methionine resulted in the best body weight (productive output) and ileal digestibility of cysteine and methionine for 1–21 day old Pekin ducks [29]. Similar methionine supplementation resulted in improved body weight gain after four days of a duckling's life [32]. Xie et al., found that diets containing 0.377–0.379% methionine resulted in maximum weight gain and breast meat yield, respectively, in 21–49 day old Pekin ducks [30]. During the same study, the authors found that the proposed methionine levels also resulted in decreased "abdominal" fat deposition as a possible result of this amino acid's effect on key enzymes of lipogenesis and lipolysis.

Wang et al. studied the effects of methionine on growing Yangzhou geese (common domestic goose in China) [31]. The authors reported that 28–42 day old and 28–56 day old goslings needed 4.07 g/kg and 4.14 g/kg feed, respectively, of methionine for optimal growth (maximum daily weight gain). These values are slightly higher than the dietary methionine (3.77 g/kg feed) level shown to result in maximum weight gain in 21–49 day old white Pekin ducklings. "Abdominal" fat in the geese decreased linearly with increased methionine (as also shown in ducks). Although specific adverse effects were not elaborated upon, the authors noted that an excess of methionine resulted in an imbalanced dietary amino acid profile and altered metabolism [31].

In common with other uricotelic species, waterfowl cannot produce endogenous arginine and this amino acid must be available in the diet. The 1994 NRC arginine requirements for 0–2 and 2–seven week old White Pekin ducks are 1.1% and 1.0% of the diet respectively [33]. Wang et al. concluded that for optimal weight gain, feed/gain, and breast meat yield of 1–21 day old White Pekin ducklings, dietary arginine requirements should be 0.95% (9.5 g/kg), 1.16% (11.6 g/kg), and 0.99% (9.9 g/kg) of the diet respectively [33].

Wu et al. found that by adding 10 g/kg of L-arginine to a basal diet meeting NRC requirements for ducks, white Pekin ducklings gained significant weight and increased breast muscle size relative to total body weight by 5.2% and 9.9% respectively [34]. Arginine supplementation also resulted in significantly decreased skin fat and "abdominal" fat pad contents by 7.6% and 4.9% respectively. Twenty one day old male and female ducks were given either a control or L-arginine supplemented diet for three weeks total. The basal diet contained 11.6 g/kg of arginine. [34]

Other research has shown that lysine and valine requirements in starter and duck grower rations are higher than published NRC (1994) values [30]. The above findings and future research may reshape methionine, arginine, and other amino acid recommendations for young (and potentially adult) waterfowl.

By evaluating jejunal fluid contents, Zhao showed that dietary protein consumption significantly and directly altered intestinal amylase, trypsin, and chymotrypsin activity in 18-week old Pekin ducks [35]. As protein consumption increased, so did intestinal enzyme activity. While this finding may be intuitive it does support the concept that adequate dietary protein is required for optimal digestive enzyme activity and nutrient digestion.

Protein requirements are known to be variable between different young and aged ducks and likely between different species of water-fowl. The studies above were generally completed to determine methionine and arginine levels that result in maximum growth which may not be an appropriate goal for display or pet birds. Also, methionine and other amino acid requirements can change based on total available protein and other nutrients in the diet. Because waterfowl (at least domestic ducks and geese) may have specific amino acid requirements (such as methionine) unique from other poultry, the author advises working with a nutritionist prior to creating a formulated diet for captive birds.

General Dietary Protein Levels

Protein recommendations for waterfowl are more generalizations than critically studied rules. In general, commercial starter and grower diets contain 18–20% protein. Maintenance diets commonly contain 13–14% protein. Breeder and layer diets are typically between 16% and 20% protein. The higher the dietary protein content, the larger the eggs for laying birds. These general recommendations are in line with some popular literature such as with Holderread [1].

While protein malnutrition often results in poor growth rates, excess can commonly be associated with "angel wing deformity" in young waterfowl (especially geese) (Figure 4.24). Angel wing is pronation of the carpus. If left untreated, the wing is permanently deformed. Overfeeding and high protein diets are commonly blamed and result in rapid distal pin feather growth that outweighs the strength of the wing bones and muscles. Carpal rotation results and the affected distal wing has a "flipped up" appearance. If caught within a few days, the wing is simply taped or lightly bandaged (figure of 8 wing bandage, or Braille bandage) into correct position and diet modified as needed (lower protein, more access to natural forage). The bandage is removed in 5–7 days or when the wing remains in normal position. Acute malformations and treatment carry an excellent prognosis. Geese are likely

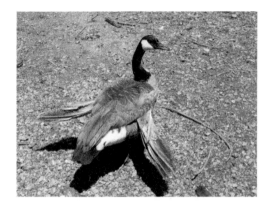

Figure 4.24 A wild Canada goose (*Branta canadensis*) with bilateral angel wing deformity. The bird was raised on a private park, developed angel wing when young, was not treated and is now a permanent resident as he can not fly.

more prone to excessive protein supplementation as their natural diet is generally poor quality grasses and forage.

Fats and Omega-3 Fatty Acids

Most commercial waterfowl diets are minimally supplemented with fat. Soybean oil (SBO) and other plant based oils (typically significantly higher in omega-6 than omega-3 fatty acids) are added bringing the total fat content between 2% and 4% of the diet. The discussion below will focus on the addition of omega-3 fatty acids (O-3 FA) to supplement waterfowl diets for captive birds.

O-3 FA have been shown to have increasing roles in a variety of health and disease processes in multiple birds and mammals. Omega-3 research is limited in respect to waterfowl. However, the research completed so far in waterfowl and other avian species supports consideration of omega-3 fatty acid supplementation.

Omega-3 fatty acids have gained popularity for their anti-inflammatory, lipid-stabilizing and anti-neoplastic effects, renal protective properties and other qualities. O-3 FA are polyunsaturated and are designated by their first carbon-carbon double bond occurring at the third carbon from the methyl group. O-3 FA are those rich in eicosapentaenoic (EPA), docosohexaenoic (DHA) and/or linolenic acid (α–linolenic acid or ALA). DHA and EPA are considered the functional O-3 FA as they exert the most beneficial biologic effects on body tissues [36].

Flax seed (and limited other plant sources) and menhaden (and other select fish and shellfish) oils contain predominately linolenic acid and EPA and DHA, respectively and therefore have different O-3 FA compositions. DHA and EPA are more readily incorporated into biological tissues, but also carry greater potential to create metabolic oxidative stress than linolenic acid. As a general rule, the more herbivorous the animal, the better that species is at converting ALA to DHA and EPA. Conversely, the more carnivorous the animal the poorer its ability to convert DHA and EPA from ALA.

The clinical impact of supplementation with various sources of O-3 FA has not been clearly defined although more attention has been given to the fish oils (FOs) in recent research. Regardless, various studies support that adding either fish oil and/or ALA to bird diets (multiple species) increases plasma levels of EPA, DHA and (with ALA supplementation) linolenic acid and reduces arachidonic acid. These findings indicate that supplemental O-3 FA result in incorporation into the body and doing so exerts biologic effects. Specifically, fish oil supplementation (2% herring oil, O-3 FA source) has been shown to be relevant in Muscovy ducks [36]. Schiavone et al.'s work showed that supplementing Muscovy ducks with fish oil significantly altered breast muscle fatty acid composition by increasing the O-3 FA content and decreasing omega-6 fatty acid (O-6 FA) content [36].

Similarly, Liu at al supplemented growing 17-week old Shaoxing laying duck diets with one of 4 fat sources for 70 days total: 3 g/kg fish oil (FO), 25 g/kg sunflower oil (SO), 30 g/kg palm oil or 20 g/kg beef tallow. [28] Serum triglycerides (FO group) and total cholesterol (FO and SO groups) were significantly decreased. Polyunsaturated fatty acids in the eggs and meat were significantly higher with birds fed FO and SO. Meat and egg O-3 FA levels were significantly higher in the FO group [28]. These findings in ducks are similar to those shown in other animals supplemented with dietary omega-3 fatty acids.

Birds cannot manufacture linoleic acid (an O-6 FA) or ALA and must get these from their diet [37]. Depending on the species of waterfowl, ALA or EPA/DHA are likely the main sources of O-3 FA in free-living birds. Based on research in other animals, herbivorous waterfowl (such as most geese) likely naturally consume more ALA (over DHA/EPA) in their diet as this would be the predominate source of O-3 FA in plants. However, omnivorous and more carnivorous birds likely naturally consume a mix of O-3 FA.

As most commercial bird foods are made from corn and soybean components, these diets are typically high in O-6 FA. Fish oils are highly unstable when manufactured in foods. Flax seeds provide a more stable source of O-3 in manufactured diets. Flax seed oil provides a more concentrated source (than flax seeds) of O-3 FA and can be added to the diet. Finally, fish oil (EPA and DHA) provides the most biologically potent form of O-3 FA and must be supplemented fresh due to its instability to heat, oxygen, and physical mixing. Based on research in multiple animals, fish oil supplementation is likely the best means to increase body EPA and DHA levels- even for herbivorous species that would naturally consume more ALA.

Bone Health

While it may seem an unlikely connection, O-3 FA contribute to several factors involving bone health. Studied four-week old quail fed identical diets for seven months except for fat content (SBO, hydrogenated soybean oil [HSBO], chicken fat [CF] or menhaden fish oil [FO] all at 50 g/kg of feed) had notable differences in bone parameters. [38] The ratio of O-6 FA:O-3 FA in the diets were as follows: SBO 12.55, HSBO 17.85, CF 18.47 and FO 0.66.

As O-3 FA's reduce the concentration of arachidonic acid and subsequent production of PGE$_2$ (the opposite is true with O-6 FA), bone formation is increased. PGE$_2$'s long term goal is to stimulate bone resorption. As expected, quail fed FO (and HSBO) had markedly improved cortical bone thickness and density compared to the other groups. Also, quail fed FO had higher percentages of tibial ash, Ca, and P. Last, quail fed FO or HSBO had increased bone shear force over the other groups. All of the findings indicated bones from FO and HSBO groups were stronger. As a potential negative, HSBO quail had more trans-fatty acids in studied tissues [38].

A similar study used 16-week old chickens fed diets of varying O-6 FA:O-3 FA (ranging from 48.7:1 to 4.7:1) for 42 weeks. While the study did find increasing cortical bone thickness as the O-3 FA concentration increased (up to the highest O-3 FA level), other parameters such as bone strength and mineral content were similar between the different diets [39]. One of many differences is that this second study used a much lower O-3 FA content diet than in the quail study above. These findings support a role of supplemental O-3 FA in improving bone quality in young Galliformes and may similarly affect waterfowl species.

Brain Development

O-3 FA, especially DHA, has been given special attention in terms of neurologic development. Studies in humans, rats, and dogs support that when young are supplemented with O-3 FA and specifically DHA, they perform better on a variety of intelligence and agility tests compared to age-matched peers given placebo. Precocial avian species, such as chickens, are known to have better developed brains and higher brain-DHA concentration than atricial species (such as swallows) at hatch [40]. These findings suggest that higher DHA brain content is correlated with a greater need for neuromuscular coordination and nerve synaptic connection in precocial species whereas altricial species

reserve DHA-brain accumulation for later as their development is slower.

Domestic duck (*A. platyrhynchos*) and captive partridge (*Alectoris rufa*) chicks have been noted to have significantly lower brain-DHA compared to wild counterparts. The difference has been attributed to the low O-3 FA diet with the domestic species. [37] Studied one-day old partridge chicks showed decreased learning ability when their parents were fed low amounts of O-3 FA (fish oil) compared to chicks whose parents were fed higher amounts [41]. Although studies are limited, the findings seem to correlate well with those from other species- that O-3 FA appear to be important for neonatal brain development.

Cancer

It can easily be said that it is better to prevent cancer than work to treat cancer. The research on supplementing diets with O-3 FA and their effects on laboratory animals, dog, and human cancer prevention and treatment is extensive. In general, diets high in O-3 FA (usually through additional supplementation) are associated with a lower risk of a variety of cancers. For those patients (humans, dogs, and some laboratory animals) with cancer, O-3 FA supplementation has been shown to reduce lipolysis and muscle degeneration ("cancer cachexia"), increase survival time and disease free interval and improve overall quality of life (although the cancer is not "cured").

At least one study has evaluated the effects of O-3 FA supplementation in chickens with ovarian cancer. Two and a half year old white leghorn hens were fed a standard or 10% flaxseed enriched diet for one-year [42]. While the overall incidence of cancer was the same in both groups, the flaxseed supplemented hens had fewer late stage tumors with ascites and metastasis. Additionally, the flax seed supplemented group maintained weight (as opposed to lost weight in the control group), had significantly lower overall mortality (from all natural causes of death) and better overall health. The authors noted that the study began after the hens had already ovulated approximately 500 times (the equivalent of a woman entering menopause) and the damage (cancer formation) may have already been done prior to starting the study. The authors are next studying the effects of O-3 FA supplementation starting in 22-week-old chicks over four years [42].

Kidney Disease

O-3 FA are frequently studied in mammal kidney disease models. The major renal benefits of O-3 FA supplementation appear to be centered on decreasing intra-renal inflammation, decreasing thrombosis and improving overall renal blood flow and single nephron glomerular filtration rate. No such studies currently exist in avian models.

Regardless, the overwhelming literature does support the idea that O-3 FA supplementation can have renal benefits across species and should be a consideration with kidney health in waterfowl.

Obesity

Supplemental O-3 FA have been shown to substantially affect fat deposition in many animals including birds. The effects of dietary fats and body fat were highlighted in a study of three-week old chickens fed identical diets for five weeks except for fat content (tallow, fish oil or sunflower oil all at 80 g/kg of feed) [43]. The fats represented saturated fat (tallow), O-3 FA (fish oil- FO), and O-6 FA (sunflower oil, linoleic acid- SO). FO chicks had significantly lower plasma triacylglycerol and total plasma cholesterol levels than the other groups. The SO group also had lower triacylglycerol levels compared to tallow, but not as significant as with the FO group. Abdominal fat pad mass was significantly lower in the SO and FO groups (0.8% and 1.1%, respectively) than those receiving tallow (2.7%). The SO and FO also had significantly increased breast muscle and subsequently breast muscle: abdominal fat than the tallow fed group. Similar findings have also been reported in humans that FO can reduce overall body fat mass [43]. This study helps support the use of O-3 FA supplementation in birds that are overweight and has been used by the author for this purpose specifically in waterfowl.

One study involved feeding perilla seed oil (65% ALA, 14% linoleic acid, and 14% oleic acid [omega-9 fatty acid]) to 28 day old laying Shaoxing laying ducks for a total of 50 days [44]. Compared to controls, the fatty acid supplemented ducks had improved egg laying (without altering egg weight or feed to egg conversion ratio), altered lipid profiles (reduced serum cholesterol and triglycerides and elevated high density lipoprotein cholesterol) and down regulation of lipogenic enzymes and up regulation of fatty acid catabolism enzymes in the liver [44]. All of the findings were considered positive and suggest that diets high in O-3 FA may improve hepatic fat metabolism and serum lipids in ducks as has been shown in numerous other studied animals.

Omega-3 Fatty Acid Dosing

Specific dosing for O-3 FA have not been established for waterfowl. A dietary O-6 FA: O-3 FA ranging from 1:5 to 15:1 has been proposed as desirable for dogs and cats with renal disease. This guideline has also been challenged and ratios of 1:1 have been proposed as more ideal. Based on plasma conversion of lower O-6 FA ratios post-supplementation with O-3 FA in multiple species, it appears that at least three to four weeks is needed to reach "optimal" levels. Long-term supplementation (three to six months or more) is likely appropriate if O-3 FA are to be effectively used.

The author uses fish oil capsules (better stability than pumps or pour-on versions) to supplement waterfowl. Capsules can be fed whole or cut and squirted over fresh food daily. In general, the author supplements 300 mg (combined EPA/DHA) to small waterfowl (less than 9.0 kg) and 600 mg (combined EPA/DHA) to larger birds daily.

Vitamins

Unlike the Galliforme poultry literature, relatively few studies in ducks explore the role of micronutrients such as vitamins.

Niacin

Popular literature commonly mentions that ducks in particular have niacin (Vitamin B_3) needs above and beyond those in more commonly kept poultry [1]. Holderread states that "young waterfowl require two or three times more niacin in their diet than chicks other than broilers." Classic signs of niacin deficiency in ducklings include bowed bones, stunted growth and enlarged hocks. Holderread further notes that chick broiler feed has sufficient niacin for ducklings. Providing 100 to 150 mg niacin per gallon (3.75 l) drinking water to ducklings until 8–10 weeks old can "cure" niacin deficiency in affected birds. Alternatively 2–3 cups of brewer's yeast added to 10 # (4.5 kg) chicken feed will prevent niacin deficiency [1].

Wu et al. reported that day-old mule ducklings when fed for three weeks required 45 mg/kg niacin in the feed [45]. Also niacin deficiency was compensated for by excess tryptophan but the opposite was not true. Ducklings fed basal diets had poorer growth rates and bowed legs compared to those with higher levels of niacin. Maximum growth rate and absence of bowed legs was noted when ducks were fed rations containing 48 mg/kg niacin. While maximum body weight and feed efficiency was noted when 0–3 week old ducklings were fed 48 mg/kg niacin in the feed, regression analysis predicted the minimum requirement of 45 mg/kg niacin [45].

Niacin is synthesized from tryptophan, which requires dietary pyridoxine, and much of the niacin in food stuffs is unavailable due to its form [45, 46]. For example, only 30% of the niacin in corn is available to chicks. Wu consequently also found that optimal growth rate and feed efficiency in 0–3 week old ducklings was obtained by feeding 0.23% tryptophan in the diet. Wu et al. concluded that niacin supplementation was needed when tryptophan levels were suboptimal but not when tryptophan was given in excess [45].

Serafin studied the dietary requirements of nicotinic acid (niacin), riboflavin (vitamin B_2), choline, and pantothenic acid (vitmain B_5) in Embden goslings [46]. Previous reports had shown than goslings and ducklings require 22–55 mg/kg feed of available niacin for optimal growth. After 2–3 week trials, the author determined the goslings required no more than 3.84 and 31.2 mg/kg dietary riboflavin and nicotinic acid, respectively, for rapid growth and development. Dietary pantothenic acid requirement did not exceed 12.6 and 1530 mg/kg of dietary choline was adequate to allow rapid growth and prevent perosis. Bowed legs were noted in diets with suboptimal levels of riboflavin. Choline deficient birds developed perosis. However, no goslings developed bowed legs or perosis on nicotinic acid deficient (as low as 16.2 mg/kg feed) diets. Deficiencies in all of the nutrients resulted in slow growth. [46]

These studies highlight the complexity of the relationships between niacin, tryptophan, and naturally available niacin in the food and likely other nutrients. Niacin supplementation appears to be very safe. However, it should be noted that the limited research above shows that bowed legs and stunting in young waterfowl is not limited to niacin deficiency. If such developmental abnormalities are found, several nutrient deficiencies should be considered.

Vitamin C

Vitamin C has many roles in the body, primarily as an antioxidant, and has been heavily studied in many animals including poultry. Specific to Jin-ding female layers ducklings, Wang et al. found that supplementing vitamin C at 400 mg/kg feed resulted in maximum weight gain; reduced malondialdehyde and increased superoxide dismutase and glutathione peroxidase in serum and liver; and increased serum IgA, IgG, and IgM concentrations [47]. While vitamin C was supplemented at 150, 300, 400, 800, and 1400 mg/kg feed, the 400 mg amount appeared optimal. Ducklings were 1 day old at the start of the study and supplemented until 28 days of age. The base diet was formulated as per NRC (1994) guidelines and had no vitamin C.

While it is reported that adult poultry (assumption extended to ducks) are able to synthesize vitamin C, requirements are higher during stress [47]. This provocative study demonstrates how a single added nutrient can affect growth, oxidative status and immune system function.

Enzymes

Enzyme supplements have been shown to be beneficial diet additives as a means to degrade non-starch polysaccharides (NSP) and increase energy and nitrogen retention in chickens (with multi-enzyme blends more effective than single enzymes) and other animals. [48, 49] Limited such work has been performed in waterfowl.

Young poultry, including ducks, seem to be sensitive to the anti-nutritional effects of NSP [50]. These carbohydrates are not digested by endogenous enzymes and increase the viscosity of the gastrointestinal contents. This in turn may decrease excretion of endogenous enzymes and bile acids and have other effects that ultimately reduce digestibility of nutrients. Conventional poultry diets containing corn and/or wheat are low in NSP. However when foods like oats, rye, triticale and barley replace corn and wheat, the concentration of NSP can significantly increase. [50] The theoretical application of enzyme supplements would be in degrading dietary NSP and improving the bird's ability to digest and utilize nutrients.

Adeola et al. evaluated an enzyme supplement containing 7500 units protease, 44 units cellulase and side activities of pentosanase, amylase, and α-galactosidase all per gram (0 or 1 g/kg feed additive) [48]. The supplement was added to the diet of eight or nine week old white Pekin drakes and feed and excreta evaluated for nitrogen, dry matter, amino acids, and energy contents. The enzyme supplementation had no effect on nitrogen, dry matter or energy utilization but did improve limited amino acid digestibility (particularly methionine) in the ducks fed starter or grower diets [48].

Hong et al. added enzyme supplements (4000 units amylase, 12 000 units protease and 1600 units xylanase all per gram) at 0.375 and 0.5 g/kg feed to White Pekin duckling diets for 42 days (starting at 3 days of age) [49]. Compared to controls, enzyme supplemented ducklings showed a 6–8% gain in body weight and had improved nitrogen and amino acid retention. This all correlates to improved feed efficiency with enzyme supplementation under the conditions of the study [49].

Based on limited research, it appears that enzyme supplementation can be used to improve amino acid digestibility and weight gain when added to starter and grower diets in (at least) white Pekin ducklings. It should be emphasized that the efficacy of enzyme supplementation is based on the type and dose of enzymes used, the diet fed and likely the animals. However, commercially available enzyme supplements are generally considered safe.

Grit

While naturally consumed by wild waterfowl, the need for grit supplementation depends on how the birds are being kept and what they are fed. Birds kept on lakes, ponds, waterways, and large open spaces will likely naturally accumulate grit in their diet. Birds that consume fibrous foods (natural forage, grasses, grains, etc.) are more likely to need grit than those eating processed commercial pellets (which are easily digestible). Some authors, such as Holderread, do recommend adding variably sized granite grit to duckling and adult duck diets [1]. However, the "need" for supplemental grit in captive waterfowl diets has not been critically evaluated.

Grit supplementation in waterfowl has been studied for non-nutrition related purposes. Grit may be used as a drug delivery system and has been specifically used to successfully provide the wildlife contraceptive nicarbazin to mallards [51]. Grit supplementation next to waterways may reduce lead shot ingestion in wild birds. It is believed that the shot particles are specifically selected by waterfowl as "grit" and not mistaken as a food item [52].

Grit type can be variably digested in birds. Mateo and Guitart found the half-life of ingested calcareous grit was 1.4 days in mallard gizzards. This is compared to siliceous grit which has a half-life of 3.1 days in mallard gizzards [52]. The implication is that calcareous grit would need to be replaced more frequently than siliceous versions to maintain functional levels in the ventriculus.

Natural Zeolite and Vermiculite

As the production poultry industry works to move away from drugs to improve health and animal growth, newer natural products are being used. Zeolite is "crystalline, hydrated alumino-silicate of alkali and alkaline earth cations, able to absorb water and exchange nitrogen molecules" and has experimentally been shown to reduce toxicity associated with litter ammonia and aflatoxins in chicks [53]. Vermiculite is a "clay mineral, magnesium alumino-silicate which has a high cation exchanging capacity" [53].

Khambualai et al. found that by supplementing a mixture of zeolite (70%), vermiculite (10%) and extracted plant enzymes (pineapple and papaya 20%) to 14-day old farmed Aigamo ducks for 9 weeks, the experimental group birds gained significant weight over controls [53]. The experimental additive produced significant body weight gain at 0.1 g, 0.5 g, and 1.0 g/kg feed. Based on electron microscopy observations, the authors hypothesized the experimental mixture resulted in intestinal villi hypertrophy and activated cell proliferation which subsequently increased nutrition absorption. The authors concluded that the experimental mixture could be added at a rate of 1 g/kg feed as a natural means to improve weight gain in (Agaimo) production ducks [53].

Ducks

In general, ducks are omnivorous and captive birds can eat commercial pellets, live worms and other insects, fresh leafy vegetables, and some fruit. Obesity is common in waterfowl, especially ducks. Domestic ducks may be predisposed genetically to fat storage resulting in hepatic lipidosis, coelomic fat accumulation, and elevated plasma glucose, triglycerides, and cholesterol that is especially evident when overfed diets high in corn and corn flour (simple carbohydrates) [7]. Limiting high energy foods and total food quantity, increasing exercise, and providing either natural or artificial foraging opportunities help to reduce the incidence of obesity. As such, the author typically offers about 50% of the diet as commercial pellets and the remainder as chopped dark leafy greens, free access to forage outside, worms as treats and supplemental fish oil.

Geese

Geese are predominantly herbivorous and feed on young tender grasses, aquatic plants and some roots, rhizomes, and cultivated grains. The author typically offers about 25–50% of the diet as commercial pellets and the remainder as chopped dark leafy greens, free access to forage outside (especially grass), and supplemental fish oil.

Swans

Swans naturally primarily eat vegetation supplemented with animal matter. The author typically offers about 50% of the diet as commercial pellets and the remainder as chopped dark leafy greens, (ideally) free access to forage on water plants and supplemental fish oil.

General Comments on Feeding Waterfowl

Beyer et al. estimated the average digestibility of natural swan diets at 50% [14]. The result is a large amount of fecal matter. This is common with all waterfowl. However, the fecal matter increases in volume as pellets are decreased and fibrous foods increased.

The amount of food needed depends on multiple factors already discussed. The author uses BCS and PMS (which can be taught to owners) and regular weighing (if practical) to assess caloric needs. If the bird's weight is deemed too heavy, then pellets are generally reduced until an acceptable PMS and BCS are achieved. Food quantity and caloric density generally needs to be increased with inclement weather, increased activity, reproductive seasons and illness.

Female birds often have increased nutrient (especially total calories, protein, and calcium) demands when reproductively active. Commercial waterfowl breeding diets are available and are substituted for maintenance diets during reproductive seasons. Emptied, cleaned, and dried crushed (chicken) egg shells offer a good source of calcium and are readily eaten by many waterfowl. Crushed oyster shell also works but is less commonly accepted by some birds. Special "breeder" supplements are readily available and popular with many waterfowl owners. However, no peer reviewed research has been published evaluating these supplements.

Young waterfowl are precocial and grow rapidly. They will generally eat most food items offered but are at risk of developmental nutritional disease with unbalanced diets. The author recommends feeding commercial waterfowl starter diets as the main food from 0 to 21 days of age. Commercial waterfowl grower diets are then fed starting at day 22 until 90% grown (which may be several weeks to months depending on the species). Once young waterfowl have reached most of the adult size, they can be switched over to a lower protein maintenance diet during this slower last growth phase. As a note, avoid feeding layer rations (which typically have a significantly higher calcium level) to developing waterfowl. Doing so may result in boney abnormalities, organ failure, and death.

When with their mother, young waterfowl will start foraging on a large variety of food items (in addition to pellets) within a few days of hatch. When single or otherwise without an adult role model, the author recommends supervised foraging at 1–2 weeks old to supplement their regular diet. As the young bird matures, foraging progressively makes up more and more of the diet.

Avoid medicated feed if possible. Medicated feeds for poultry are commonly used to treat parasites and are usually not necessary for waterfowl. Coccidiosis and other parasitic diseases can occasionally be seen in waterfowl and should be carefully evaluated before considering feed-based treatment.

Waterfowl Pest Control

Resident populations of waterfowl (especially mallards, duck hybrids, domestic geese, and Canada geese) may be found in many urban environments (Figure 4.25). Whether availability of food, shelter, bodies of water, and/or appropriate breeding grounds are present, these birds can sometimes overbreed and overstay their welcome. The end result is often significant fecal accumulation and the potential for disease transmission to other animals (especially commercial poultry operations) and even people [51].

Several methods of pest waterfowl control have been used and will only be briefly discussed here. These methods include capturing and relocating birds, euthanasia, and use of chemical contraceptives (such as nicarbazin) [51]. Additionally as pest waterfowl nests are clearly identified, the eggs may be oiled shortly after the clutch is laid. This simple procedure requires one to paint the egg with safe consumable oils such as canola, corn or olive oil. To ensure the eggs don't mature and hatch, first shake the egg vigorously. Then apply the oil to the addled egg and repeat two more times over one week.

Each method of waterfowl control has its pros and cons. In the United States, waterfowl are protected species and unauthorized population control may be illegal. Prior to considering any waterfowl control measures,

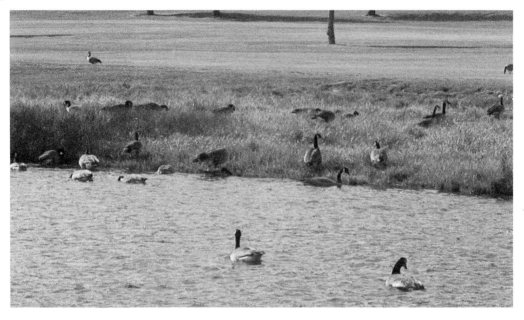

Figure 4.25   Domestic and wild waterfowl may overrun local ponds and urban environments and become pests. These wild Canada geese (*Branta canadensis*) are walking on to a golf course.

especially euthanasia or contraceptive use, work with local and state officials.

Enrichment for Captive Waterfowl

Enrichment Basics

In addition to plenty of room to walk around and a water source to swim in, waterfowl thrive with various forms of enrichment. Waterfowl are generally social and benefit when two or more of the same species are present. Overcrowding and lack of resources (food, water, etc.) can lead to aggression and should always be considered prior to adding new birds to a flock. Additionally closed aviary principles apply to waterfowl as with all other birds. Foraging is another means to improve enrichment. Geese will generally graze on new grass. However, ducks tend to be more sedentary when allowed to simply feed from a bowl. Small amounts of pellets can either be placed in multiple feeding stations or

foraging devices (such as "duck safe" foraging boxes) to increase the bird's effort and energy expenditure to find food. Also, leafy greens can be floated on water and worms can be placed in loose dirt or shallow water. If parasite transmission is a concern, then worms can be placed within foraging devices to prevent parasitic ova or larva contamination.

Enrichment is simply adding something to an animal's environment to improve its life and allow for species typical behaviors. The real challenge with enrichment is finding biological relevance that is practical. As its name suggests, biologically relevant enrichment is "effective" in that the animal actually uses the introduced enrichment to better its captive life. This is done in part by controlling stressors in its environment and allowing for species typical behaviors. Enrichment is only as successful as it is practical for caretakers to introduce and maintain.

What may be enriching for a mallard may not apply to a Canada goose. Because of physical, behavioral, developmental, natural history and other differences, items that are "enriching" can vary significantly between, and even within, species. While some enrichment may be readily accepted by most of a species, such as swimming areas for ducks, others may not be regularly used necessitating a trial and error approach.

Sometimes recognition for the need for enrichment can be challenging, especially if the waterfowl appear physically normal. Feather damaging is obvious to see. Cannibalism and feather "pecking" are serious problems recognized in captive production Muscovy ducks *(Cairina moschata)* and has resulted in the highly criticized practice of beak and claw trimming as a preventative measure [54]. Crowding and lack of access to adequate water troughs are just two of the proposed causes for these destructive behaviors.

Per the author's observations, one of the most common abnormalities with waterfowl is physical inactivity. This may lead to obesity, arthritis, and other complications or excessive reproductive activities (leading to coelomic reproductive disease in females and masturbation, phallus disorders, and aggression in males) and all are common with pet ducks. Lack of appropriate "comfort movements" as described by McKinney may be another means to assess whether or not captive waterfowl are performing normal behaviors [55]. Johnsgard gives detailed accounts of normal waterfowl behavior that may also be used to help recognize abnormal activities of captive birds [56]. Once explained, clients may recognize abnormal behaviors with their pets and be more willing to make appropriate changes (Figure 4.26a–e).

The benefits of environmental enrichment in numerous captive animal species are well documented. However similar research is rarely conducted in captive waterfowl.

Some biologically relevant enrichment can have unintended negative consequences. Introduced items may incite fear, especially in those animals poorly socialized to experience new items in the environment. Others may result in frustration, such as when enrichment holds prized items (food) that cannot be obtained because of physical limitations by the animal. Highly valued items, such as high protein food treats for ducks, may result in aggression with group housed animals (while the same enrichment can be very beneficial to a singly housed bird). Others may result in trauma or danger to the animal such as beak lesions caused by improperly made foraging devices. As with any item introduced into an animal's environment, complications should be considered and clients prepared accordingly.

Social Enrichment

Social interaction is the most effective and dynamic form of enrichment for the majority of captive animals. Due to the complexities of social enrichment, only generalizations will be made.

Recent attention has been given to the environment and conditions surrounding the development of young animals of many species as well as the long term consequences when raised under unnatural or stressful situations. In general, waterfowl are precocial and rapidly recognize movement, follow it and become socially attached (imprinted) during a short period of time after hatch (Figure 4.27). Usually the moving object is the bird's mother. However, many waterfowl are raised by people and their pets (dogs) for various reasons. Waterfowl recognize and associate with future mates in part based on their exposure to conspecifics when young.

Possibly the biggest concern with abnormal imprinting is that the bird may not be able to form pair bonds with its own species or attempt to, and successfully, mate/bond with a different species altogether. This is seen when ducks are raised in relatively crowded exhibits with multiple species. Once adults, the ducks of different species tend to fairly readily bred resulting in interesting offspring. However, this does not appear to be a problem for redhead ducks *(Aythya americana)* that often lay their eggs in and are raised by canvasback ducks *(Aythya valisineria)*. Canvasback reared redheads later appropriately pair with their own species.

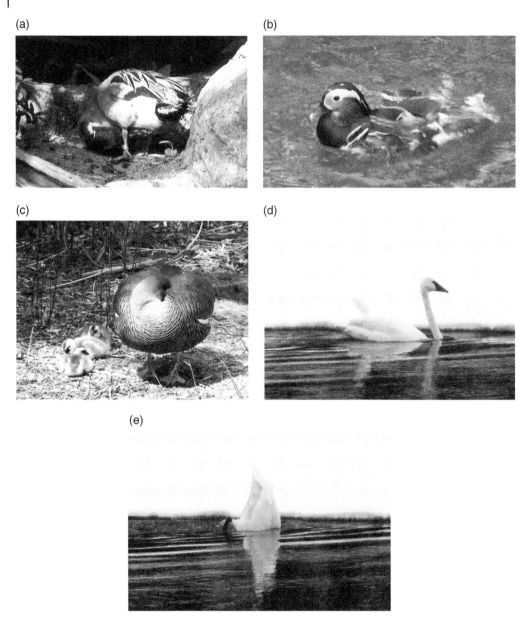

Figure 4.26 Evaluation of the presence of normal behaviors and comfort movements can be used to help assess the general well-being of captive waterfowl. Preening, as with this green-winged teal (*Anas carolinensis*) (a), and bathing, shown here with this Mandarin duck (*Aix galericulata*) (b), are examples of normal comfort movements. (c) Waterfowl should also feel secure enough to rest comfortably without disturbance as shown with this lesser Magellan goose and her goslings (*Chloephaga picta picta*). (d,e) This trumpeter swan (*Cygnus buccinator*) has enough room and water depth to dabble and completely submerge its head.

Light Enrichment

As waterfowl are primarily diurnal, they would naturally be expected to receive partial or full sunlight. While most zoos and aviaries have enclosures that allow their birds to receive unfiltered sunlight, some pet waterfowl (especially ducks) are kept in areas that receive little or no sun.

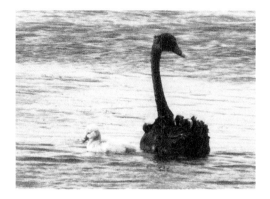

Figure 4.27 Hatchling waterfowl readily imprint. For proper social development, it is best to let hatchings imprint with conspecifics. As is normal, this black swan cygnet (*Cygnus atratus*) and pen are together.

The author does recommend regular exposure to partial and full sunlight for captive waterfowl. The reason is subjective and based on poor general (radiographic and surgical) bone density noted in captive waterfowl. One potential cause is low natural sunlight exposure (and subsequent inadequate vitamin D production). Also, birds kept outdoors are more likely

to engage in physical activity which helps build and maintain muscle strength and mass and bone density. The author recommends owners allow waterfowl to go outside. Be sure that there are plenty of hide spots or shelters should the bird choose not to "sunbathe" (Figure 4.28). Ideally, waterfowl should be left outside during the day but can be brought inside at night and during inclement weather.

Substrate Enrichment and Enclosure Design

Proper substrate is important for healthy feet and leg joints in waterfowl. It is also important to have an enclosure that gives waterfowl appropriate space security and adequate water.

In general waterfowl are either naturally on water, on soft (usually grassy) ground on perched on a rounded log or branch. Bumblefoot is commonly seen in waterfowl under one or more of the following conditions; obesity, hard substrate, lack of access of water to swim in, malnutrition and underlying disease, arthritis (resulting in placing extra weight on one leg)

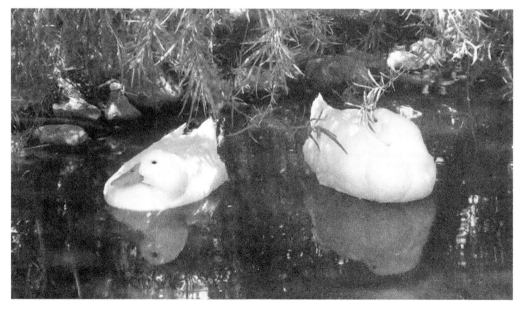

Figure 4.28 Natural unfiltered sunlight is extremely important for captive waterfowl. However protection from predators and the elements should be considered. This shaded pond housing a pair of White Pekin ducks (*Anas platyrhynchos*) provides relief from heat at an private aviary in a hot desert environment.

and foot trauma (fire ant bites, burns, etc.). Access to clean water seems obvious for waterfowl. However, research is just now showing how important various types of water enrichments (shallow water troughs, showers, etc.) are for production ducks [54]. Even without prior experience, ducks show clear preferences for open water and use the water for drinking, foraging and feeding, locomotion, preening and general exploration [57].

Proper space and enclosure set up can help reduce predation, aggression, sleeping/inactivity and possibly inappropriate interspecies breeding. Space requirements can be highly variable and can significantly affect social dynamics depending on how many birds and what species are present in a given enclosure. Aviaries with bird aggression and predation issues may need fewer animals, more hide spots, predator control measures, visual barriers and vertical rest spots or a combination to relieve tensions. In studied mallards, common teals (*Anas crecca*) and tufted ducks (*Aythya fuligula*), increased predation risk resulted in increased sleeping and decreased preening and foraging activities [58].

Toy Enrichment

Most waterfowl do not readily play with toys. However, some ducks seem to like balls or other objects that they can push around.

Foraging Enrichment

Just as with most wild animals, a significant portion of a duck's waking time is spent foraging. While it has been reported that Brent geese (*Branta bernicla*) forage an average of three hours a day, data on the specific amount of time most waterfowl spend foraging is lacking [59]. Ducks may not use a foraging device if the food is too difficult to obtain. Popular foraging feeders in group housing may result in stress and aggression if no other acceptable enrichment or food options are available.

Foraging devices and setups may also be used to encourage exercise and limit total food consumption. If total caloric needs are known, they can be measured and spread between multiple feeding stations or foraging devices. This is most easily accomplished with single birds or small flocks (2–4 birds) and is especially useful as a means of weight loss. Large flocks also benefit from foraging devices but often need supplemental and more traditional bowl feeding sites to reduce aggression and stress.

There are several simple types of foraging enrichment for waterfowl. For geese and some dabblers (mallards, for example) a grassy field offers the opportunity to graze (geese) or find insects (dabblers). Some dabblers will also pick at insects climbing trees and in and around logs. Of course, all ducks need water but divers live on and in water. Specific foraging devices are listed below.

Waterfowl Foraging Devices

Dive-to Feeder

Dive-to feeders are used to feed diving waterfowl separately from dabblers and grazers. The feeding device is enclosed on top, floating on the water and close to shore. Access to the birds is gained by diving under the floating feeder which is open. Caretakers can access the food through a hatch in the top of the cage.

Dive-to feeders can also be fitted with elevated feeding stations on the outside of the structure. The feeding stations are placed high enough off the water to only allow large dabblers to feed. This can be an effective means to feed swans and some geese while preventing ducks (especially invasive species) from eating the food (Figure 4.29a–c).

Deer Feeder

Waterfowl "deer feeders" are based on old style deer feeders. They are inexpensive and relatively easy to make and maintain. Deer feeders are meant to be hung and used by tall ground feeding birds (ratites, larger gallinaceous birds, etc.). However, waterfowl (of any size) that

(a)

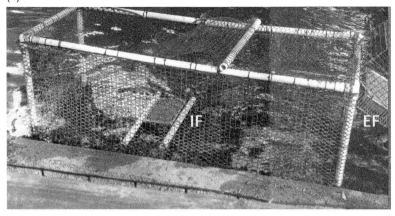

(b)

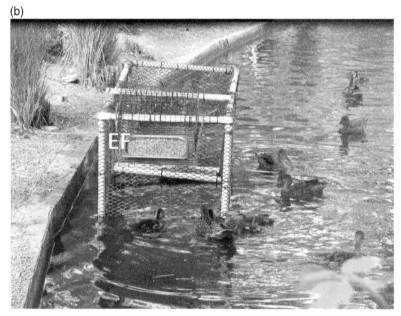

(c)

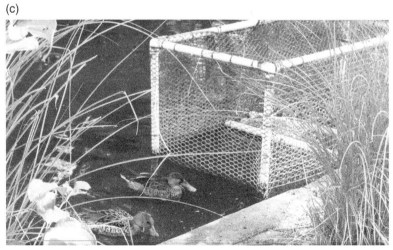

Figure 4.29 Dive-to feeders offer an excellent means to feed diving ducks separately from dabblers. (a) The floating rectangular box is next to shore allowing easy access to the internal feeder (IF) from a top hatch. The IF is suspended just above the water and can only be accessed by diving under the box (which has an open bottom). (b) An external feeder (EF) is elevated and placed on one side with a wire cage over the top. This allows tall birds such as swans to feed and prevents smaller birds from accessing the food from below or if on top of the box. (c) Dabblers generally do not swim under the box to gain access to the IF.

walk on land can also learn to use deer feeders. This is a good method to separately feed waterfowl that share time on land (such as dabbling ducks) from those that spend most of their time on water.

Use a standard 5 gal bucket (larger and smaller versions can be made too) with a lid and handle (optional). A hole slightly larger than 2–3 times the size of the food is drilled at the bottom of the bucket. For example, if the food is 1.0 cm in diameter, make the hole 2.5 cm. Next, get about 0.5 m of dowel rod that is the same diameter as the food. Use a 1.0 cm diameter dowel in this example. On one end of the dowel attach a washer that is significantly larger than the opening on the bottom of the bucket. Use a washer that is at least 5 cm in this example. The washer is either left flat or bent upwards (away from the dowel end) on both sides. Next place the dowel through the hole at the bottom of the bucket such that the washer end is inside the bucket and the dowel is left dangling below. The bucket is filled with food, covered with the lid and suspended via the handle, rope or both. Alternatively, the bottom of the bucket can be lined with a plastic cone such that all of the food is funneled to the central hole.

The bird then must learn to hit and move the end of the dowel to create an opening large enough for food to fall past the washer and dowel, through the bottom of the bucket and on the ground.

Alternatively, ornaments can be placed on the end of the dowel such as a bell or shinny object. Attach all items well enough that the bird cannot ingest the object (Figure 4.30a–e).

Foraging Logs

Foraging logs are good for birds that like to look into cavities for food. Many species of birds can learn to use foraging logs.

Use natural untreated logs or tree branches that are soft enough to drill holes with your existing equipment. The size of the logs can vary from a few inches (even using existing perches) to a few feet in diameter depending on the resources available. Logs can be oriented horizontally or vertically. These can further be rested on the ground or suspended (for perching waterfowl) (Figure 4.31).

Small (1–2 in.) to large (3–5 in.) holes can be drilled in the wood. Metal bowls can be placed within large holes and the logs oriented horizontally. Further, large holes can be covered (bark, leaves, etc.) to make it more challenging for the birds.

Note: If a large enough hole is drilled (on primarily vertically oriented logs), wild birds may try to enlarge the site to create a nest cavity.

Foraging Feed Troughs and Boxes

These devices are good for birds with poor "foraging dexterity" (especially those that do not handle food with their feet but can simply push things with their head and beak). Skilled birds can also use these devices.

Place feed troughs along the sides of the pen or along banks, trees or other structures within the enclosure. The troughs can vary in size but for ducks and geese should generally be about 2–4 in. deep, 4–6 in. wide, and 5–7 in. long. Foraging feed boxes are simply shorter versions of the troughs. Adjust size (bigger or smaller) based on the bird. Start with the troughs on the ground and leave open. Gradually raise the troughs off the ground by attaching them to the sides of the pens. Have 6–8 feed troughs scattered at different levels around the sides of (and/or within) the pen. Use dry foods in the troughs (pellets, grains, some veggies and some fruit- just as long as it can easily be cleaned).

Once the birds are accustomed to eating the food from the troughs, attach a flip top cover that the birds will have to flip up to find the food within. The flip tops can be wood, metal or durable plastic and attached via a hinge to the back side of the trough (Figure 4.32).

Long troughs (2–5 ft long) can have several flip tops along the length of the trough. So, one section of the trough may have a flip top up while the rest of the tops are down. The goal is that the

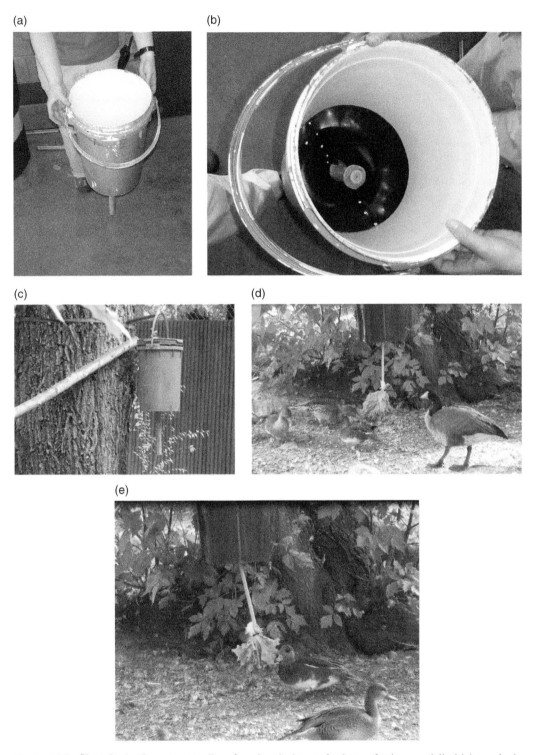

Figure 4.30 "Deer feeders" serve as excellent foraging devices to feed waterfowl terrestrially. (a) A standard 5 gal bucket is most commonly used. (b) A hole about 2–3 times the size of the food is drilled at the bottom of the bucket. A dowel rod with washer hangs suspended from the bottom of the bucket. In this example, a plastic lining was added to create a funnel leading to the central hole. (c) The finished product is filled with some food and then hung at the appropriate height such that the birds can easily grab the suspended dowel. This deer feeder was designed for southern ground hornbills (*Bucorvus leadbeateri*) and has a dowel too large for waterfowl. (d) A deer feeder being used in a mixed waterfowl species collection. Notice the lettuce tied to the end of the dowel being used to target the birds. (e) An American widgeon hen (*Anas americana*) grabs the lettuce, pulling the dowel which results in a small amount of food dropping on to the ground.

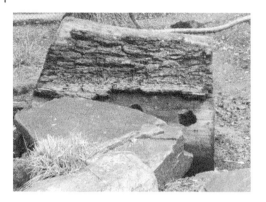

Figure 4.31 Foraging logs are simple and effective foraging devices for waterfowl. This horizontal log (partially covered by a rock in the foreground) has several large drilled holes each about 12–15 cm deep and 10 cm wide. Logs can be oriented vertically or horizontally and adjusted to the physical abilities of the bird.

birds don't know what is in each section (which should vary on a daily basis) and will have to open the flip top to check for food. Put small amounts of high energy food items in these feeding troughs. Troughs can be on the ground, suspended on the sides of cages or attached to trees. All suspended troughs or boxes should have an

adjacent branch to give the bird good solid footing when opening the boxes.

Note: Some birds risk getting their head stuck between the flip top and the box. Make sure to create a cut out area on the central section of the top edges of the box. If the flip top falls down and the bird panics, the cut out depressions will allow the bird to pull its head out unharmed.

Identification

Several methods of identification are available for waterfowl. The most common are leg bands, patagial bands, neck collars and/or microchips. Leg bands are best placed on birds a few days old. The band should be large enough to slip over the foot and rest over the tarsometatarsus. Bands need to be large enough to grow into without risk of constriction and small enough to prevent the foot from slipping through within a few days. Metal crimp, plastic, and spiral wire leg bands can be placed on adult birds.

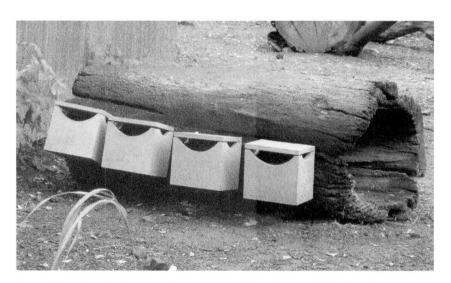

Figure 4.32 Foraging boxes and troughs are additional terrestrial feeding devices that work well with waterfowl. A series of 4 foraging boxes are attached to a log within an enclosure. Note the cut outs on each side of the box. These prevent injury to the bird if the lid of the box falls on the bird's head. While the boxes shown here are heavy duty, lighter construction materials work well for waterfowl.

Production birds will sometimes have notches or perforations in their webbing (using a poultry "toe punch") but is not recommended for pet birds [1]. Pet birds are most commonly fitted with leg bands and/or are microchipped.

Wild waterfowl may be banded by governmental agencies. The birds are banded to help track animal movement, disease monitoring and more. The most common bands used on wild waterfowl are leg, patagial, neck, nasal markers, web tags (for babies too young to place leg bands), and occasionally radiotelemetry devices. Each band generally contains information pertinent to the banding agency and may include contact information. Alternatively, one may call 1-800-327-BAND to report a bird band and get specifics on the animal. Hunters most commonly report bird band information back to the banding agency. This information is vital to understanding health and disease of wild waterfowl populations.

Pinioning and Wing Trims

Pinioning renders waterfowl flightless by removing the wing distal to the alula. Waterfowl are best pinioned between two and four days of age by simply amputating the proximal base of metacarpal III and IV on one wing leaving the alula intact. Typically, sterile clippers and no anesthesia are used. If the bird is sexed, pinion the right wing for males and left for females [60]. Adult birds can also be pinioned. However, the procedure requires full anesthesia, pain management, etc.

Alternatively wings may be trimmed in adult birds. The outer 5–10 primary feathers of both wings are trimmed just distal to the coverts. Avoid cutting new incoming or "blood" feathers. While wild waterfowl commonly molt twice a year, domestic birds may have more sporadic molts. Either way, the wing trim is temporary and feather regrowth should be periodically monitored.

Managing Excessive Egg Production

Domestic ducks and geese are well-known for their high egg production. Some breeds of domestic duck including Campbell, Harlequin, Magpie, Appleyard and, the most commonly kept pet, Pekin can produce 200–300 eggs per year [1]. In contrast, wild mallards lay approximately 5–16 eggs per clutch with 1–3 clutches per year depending on environmental conditions and the bird's health. With near year-round egg production, chronic nutritional and coelomic disease is common often requiring medical and sometimes surgical treatment (See Chapter 16: Soft Tissue Surgery-Female Reproductive Tract Surgery). The same problems are occasionally encountered in domestic geese and rarely in swans and non-domestic geese and ducks.

Factors contributing to excessive egg production include genetics, presence of mates (including stimulation by the owner), lengthened daylight (natural or artificial), adequate to excessive calories, restricted access to exercise, and natural behaviors such as foraging, gonadotropin releasing hormone (GnRH) agonists and possibly more. Understanding and identifying these factors helps to set a plan to reduce chronic egg laying and its negative effects on a bird's body.

Prior to lay, waterfowl often undergo physical changes. White plumaged ducks tend to lose color intensity in the beak which fades to pale yellow while the bills of colored ducks tend to darken during breeding season. Receptive ducks assume a prone position with tail up. For testing purposes only, this behavior can be induced in some by simply placing a hand on the bird's back. Also, the ventral coelom of many waterfowl noticeably distends as the reproductive tract enlarges in preparation for egg laying. The pubic bones on some ducks will also spread just prior to lay [1].

Associated risk factors and suggestions on how to reduce excessive egg laying in waterfowl are listed below. One or a combination of the described management changes may be needed to address egg over production. As a side note, some of the same management changes can be used to help reduce recurring phallus prolapses in drakes.

Genetics

Genetics is the least controllable factor. Many domestic duck and goose breeds have been inbred for decades, centuries, and in some cases millenniums. Combined with a propensity for development of fatty liver disease when fed simple carbohydrate rich diets, persistent egg laying has been selected to meet the needs of the foie gras, meat, and egg industries. Owners should understand that while such high egg production is unnatural compared to wild counterparts, it is very common in domestic ducks and geese. The management changes proposed below are essentially working to counteract the bird's genetic drive to lay.

Stimulation from Other Birds and Owners

Ducks and geese seem to be stimulated by other reproductively active birds and, especially ducks, by inappropriate human interaction. While placing the bird in isolation with no nest often will stop egg production the author recommends other measures. If a flock is present, place the over productive hen or goose with non-reproductively active birds (including non-waterfowl species) or other non-predatory animals. If the bird is paired and over production is a problem, consider splitting the pair and placing both birds with other animals as above. If the bird is single and is being stimulated by the owner (frequent petting, holding, close contact), have the owner discontinue the behavior and focus more on positive reinforcement training (clicker, trick, etc.) as the means of interaction (Figure 4.33a–d). All of these techniques can be stressful to the bird (and sometimes owner) and may need to be modified based on the response(s).

Light Exposure

Manipulating light (day length) in poultry is a well-known means to modify egg production. The same appears to be true in production waterfowl. Holderread notes ducks are more sensitive to light changes than chickens and a reduction in as little as 15–30 minutes of light per day can result in diminished rate of lay [1]. Typically lay will start toward the end of winter and early spring as day length increases.

A simple strategy is to reduce light exposure (including indoor lights) to mimic the shortened winter days. This strategy often requires that the bird be brought inside in a dark room. Using public weather charts, determine the sunrise and sunset times and total day length (in terms of hours of light) one month prior to the (approximate) day or week when the reproductive behavior was first noticed or suspected. Bring the bird into a lighted room with no external light visible starting at the calculated sunset time. Start by keeping lights on to match outdoor lighting. Over a period of one to two weeks, gradually decrease the artificial light time until no additional light is in the room. Each morning, take the bird out at the calculated sunrise time. This same pattern can be created with automatic lights for indoor birds. It is best to keep the bird with a companion(s).

The above strategy works best to prevent egg laying for female waterfowl with a known history of reproductive problems. If needed, birds can be kept in reduced light throughout the entire breeding season (which may be six to nine months for some birds). However, once the physical and behavioral signs of reproductive activity have ceased, the bird can be returned to a full light schedule and simply monitored. If needed, the light reducing procedure above can be repeated until day length is shortening significantly in the fall.

Dietary Management

With excess calories comes the energy to produce eggs. The first step is to assure the diet is appropriate and correct dietary inadequacies

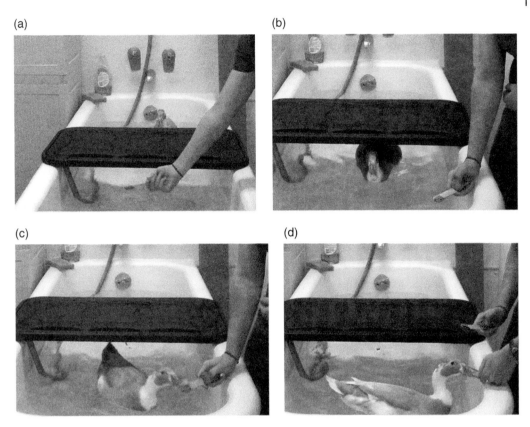

Figure 4.33 A mixed breed domestic duck (*Anas platyrhynchos*) is being used to demonstrate clicker training. (a) The owner holds a clicker attached to a tongue depressor with a target. While being prompted with clicks, the duck follows the target under an obstacle (b), then touches the target (c) and finally receives a food reward (d).

as needed. Next, reduce the amount of simple carbohydrates in the diet as this energy source will be the primary driver for hepatic lipogenesis and lipoprotein production of which some is used for the eggs. Holderread notes that egg production is lowest for ducks fed whole or cracked grains, with free access to pasture and pond and normal day length compared to the same breeds fed pellets with no pond time and either natural or increased day length [1].

Significant calorie restriction, especially when combined with diminished light, can result in cessation of reproductive activity and a "forced" molt. This often involves restricting all food (but free choice water) for three to four days. Food is then reintroduced on the fifth day.

Intermittent fasting is described in wild waterfowl and is often needed during migration [61]. In common with some other migrating species, hepatic steatosis is a main mechanism of energy storage in waterfowl and easily occurs with excessive carbohydrate ingestion (hence the development of the foie gras industry) [26]. However, long term steatosis is not expected under natural conditions as fasting (during migration) reverses this physiologic change. Unfortunately captive waterfowl often experience long term energy excess.

Black ducks (*Anas rubripes*) have been studied after four day fasts (no food) and shown to have lost weight and delayed egg production but otherwise underwent no significant adverse health effects [61]. Even young (10 and 20 day old)

Pekin ducklings have been studied with five days of calorie restriction (just enough to maintain relatively stable body mass). The study showed that ducklings adapted to calorie restriction by decreasing resting and peak metabolic rates and returned to normal growth when free feeding resumed [62]. Collectively these studies highlight a natural adaptive response in ducks that is common in other migratory animals and those with intermittent food supplies.

If such a fast is considered, the duck should be otherwise healthy and the owner instructed on a clear plan as to providing plenty of water, possible light restriction (outlined above) and monitoring for any problems.

Exercise and Natural Behaviors (Foraging)

Providing access to exercise and foraging opportunities serves many purposes. First, it fulfills the need to perform natural behaviors. Doing so may also reduce or prevent abnormal behaviors such as feather damaging, inactivity, and more. Restricting access to perform normal behavior is also considered poor welfare and goes beyond the scope of this chapter. Second, exercise is needed to utilize excess fat and maintain good muscle strength and tone. The obvious end results are better weight control and reduced side-effects of a sedentary lifestyle. Additionally, strengthening legs may help stabilize and decrease pain of arthritic joints. Last, by giving birds something to do beyond eating and minimal activity the drive for reproductive behaviors is sometimes decreased. Ideas for foraging activities are listed above. Providing access to outdoor space and water to swim in helps increase activity.

GnRH Agonists

Drugs such as leuprolide acetate (Lupron Depot, TAP Pharmaceuticals, Inc., Deerfield, IL, USA) and deslorelin (Suprelorin˚, Peptech Animal Health/Virbac, Australia) have recently become popular among veterinary and lay discussions. While these products have not been critically

studied in waterfowl, they are being used clinically. GnRH agonists are discussed in more detail in Chapter 21: Soft Tissue Surgery-Female Reproductive Tract Surgery. Editor's note: The Food and Drug Administration (FDA) may consider ducks a food animal species and therefore GnRH agonists would be a prohibited drug. In addition, deslorelin is a scheduled drug labeled for use in ferrets only.

In the author's experience, leuprolide acetate and deslorelin induce a very short term cessation in egg laying in domestic ducks with both reducing egg production for as little as a few days to weeks in some animals. Without other concurrent management changes listed above, currently available GnRH agonists alone are a poor means of managing excessive egg production in over-productive ducks. This is especially true when instituted after lay has begun.

It is not clear if the dosages being used are inappropriate, the drugs themselves have little biologic effect or if other intrinsic mechanisms easily override the effects of currently available GnRH agonists in ducks. Regardless, the author discourages use of these drugs as a sole means to manage egg overproduction in ducks, and other waterfowl.

Surgery

Unless a medical emergency is present, surgery should be one of the last means to control excessive egg laying in waterfowl. Surgery usually consists of salpingohysterectomy and coelomic cleanup with or without partial ovariectomy. See Chapter 16: Soft Tissue Surgery for more details of surgical correction of diseases of the female reproductive tract. The author generally reserves surgery for oviductal obstructions, ectopic eggs, advanced yolk coelomitis, neoplasia or other non-medically manageable reproductive tract diseases. Surgery should be performed in addition to some of the other management changes listed above.

Pre-emptive salpingohystectomy in young at-risk domestic ducks and geese has not been studied and reported at the time of writing.

References

1 Holderread, D. (2011). *Storey's Guide to Raising Ducks*, 2e. North Adams, MA: Storey Publishing.

2 Butler, M.W. and McGraw, K.J. (2012). Differential effects of early- and late-life access to carotenoids on adult immune function and ornamentation in mallard ducks (*Anas platyryhnchos*). *PLoS One* 7: e38043.

3 Brennan, P.L.R., Prum, R.O., McCraken, K.G. et al. (2007). Coevolution of male and female genitalia in waterfowl. *PLoS One* 2: e418.

4 Brennan, P.L.R., Clark, C.J., and Prum, R.O. (2010). Explosive eversion and functional morphology of the duck penis supports sexual conflict in waterfowl genitalia. *Proc. R. Soc. B* 277: 1309–1314.

5 Ekarius, C. (2007). *Storey's Illustrated Guide to Poultry Breeds*. North Adams, MA: Storey Publishing.

6 http://www.amerpoultryassn.com/PDF%20Forms/APA%20Recognized%20Breeds%20and%20Varieties%20Sept2012.pdf (accessed May 27 2013).

7 Marie-Etancelin, C., Basso, B., Davail, S. et al. (2011). Genetic parameters of product quality and hepatic metabolism in fattened mule ducks. *J. Anim. Sci.* 89: 669–679.

8 Chartrin, P., Schiavone, A., Bernadet, M.D. et al. (2005). The effect of genotype and overfeeding on lipid deposition on myofibres and intramuscular adipocytes on breast and thigh muscles of ducks. *Reprod. Nutr. Dev.* 45: 87–99.

9 LuJiang, Q., Wei, L., FangXi, Y. et al. (2009). Origin and domestication history of Peking ducks determined through microsatellite and mitochondrial marker analysis. *Sci. China Ser. C-Life Sci.* 52: 1030–1035.

10 Bartels, T., Krautwald-Junghanns, M.E., Portmann, S. et al. (2002). Ataxia and disequilibrium in domestic ducks (*Anas platyrhynchos* f. dom.) with intracranial lipomas. *Vet. Pathol.* 39: 396–399.

11 Frahm, H.D. and Rehkämper, G. (2004). Brain size, brain composition and intracranial fat bodies in a population of free-living crested ducks ('Hochbrutflugenten'). *Br. Poult. Sci.* 45: 590–597.

12 Morishita, T.Y. (1999). Clinical assessment of gallinaceous birds and waterfowl in backyard flocks. *Vet. Clin. N. Am. Exot. Anim. Pract.* 2: 383–404.

13 O'Driscoll, K.K.M. and Broom, D.M. (2011). Does access to open water affect the health of Pekin ducks (*Anas platyrhynchos*). *Poult. Sci.* 90: 299–307.

14 Beyer, W.N., Perry, M.C., and Osenton, P.C. (2008). Sediment ingestion rates in waterfowl (Anatidae) and their use in environmental risk assessment. *Integr. Environ. Assess. Manage.* 4: 246–251.

15 Heinz, G.H., Beyer, W.N., Hoffman, D.J., and Audet, D.J. (2010). Relating the ability of mallards to ingest high levels of sediment to potential contaminant exposure in waterfowl. *Environ. Toxicol Chem.* 29: 1621–1624.

16 Beyer, W.N., Spann, J., and Day, D. (1999). Metal and sediment ingestion by dabbling ducks. *Sci. Total Environ.* 231: 235–239.

17 Farhat, A., Normand, L., Chavez, E.R., and Touchburn, S.P. (1998). Nutrient digestibility in food wastes ingredients for Pekin and Muscovy ducks. *Poult. Sci.* 77: 1371–1376.

18 Rush, J.K., Angel, C.R., Banks, K.M. et al. (2005). Effect of dietary calcium and vitamin D3 on calcium and phosphorous retention in white Pekin ducklings. *Poult. Sci.* 84: 561–570.

19 Rodehutscord, M. and Dieckmann, A. (2005). Comparative studies with 3-week old chickens, turkeys, ducks and quails on the response in phosphorous utilization to a supplementation of monobasic calcium phosphate. *Poult. Sci.* 84: 1252–1260.

20 Attia, Y.A., Al-Hamid, A.E.A., Zeweil, H.S. et al. (2013). Effects of dietary amounts of inorganic and organic zinc on productive and physiologic traits of white Pekin ducks. *Animal* 7: 895–900.

21 Basso, B., Bordas, A., Dubos, F. et al. (2012). Feed efficiency in the laying duck: appropriate measurements and genetic parameters. *Poult. Sci.* 91: 1065–1073.

22 Cherry, P. and Morris, T.R. (2005). The maintenance requirement of domestic drakes. *Br. Poult. Sci.* 46: 725–727.

23 Burton, E.J., Newnham, R., Bailey, S.J., and Alexander, L.G. (2013). Evaluation of a fast, objective tool for assessing body condition of budgerigars (*Melopsittacus undulatus*). *J. Anim. Physiol. Anim. Nutr.* [Epub ahead of print].

24 Davail, S., Rideau, N., Guy, G. et al. (2003). Pancreatic hormonal and metabolic responses in overfed ducks. *Horm. Metab. Res.* 35: 439–443.

25 Saez, G., Baéza, E., Davail, S. et al. (2009). Hepatic metabolism of glucose and linoleic acid varies in relation to susceptibility to fatty liver in *ad-libitum* fed Muscovy and Pekin ducks. *Br. J. Nutr.* 101: 510–517.

26 Hermier, D., Guy, G., Guillaumin, S. et al. (2003). Differential channeling of liver lipids in relation to susceptibility to hepatic steatosis in two species of ducks. *Comp. Biochem. Physiol. Part B* 135: 663–675.

27 Molee, W., Bouillier-Oudut, M., Auvergne, A., and Babilé, R. (2005). Changes in lipid composition of hepatocyte plasma membrane induced by overfeeding in duck. *Comp. Biochem. Physiol. Part B* 141: 437–444.

28 Wei-Ming, L., Shu-Jing, L., Linzhi, L. et al. (2011). Effects of dietary fatty acids on serum parameters, fatty acid compositions, and liver histology in Shaoxing laying ducks. *J. Zhejiang Univ. Sci. B (Biomed & Biotechnol)* 12: 736–743.

29 Jamroz, D., Wiliczkiewicz, A., Lemme, A. et al. (2009). Effect of increased methionine level on performance and apparent ileal digestibility of amino acids in ducks. *Anim. Physiol. Anim. Nutr.* 93: 622–630.

30 Xie, M., Hou, S.S., and Huang, W. (2006). Methionine requirements of male white Pekin ducks from twenty-one to forty-nine days of age. *Poult. Sci.* 85: 743–746.

31 Wang, Z.Y., Shi, S.R., Zhou, Q.Y. et al. (2010). Response of growing goslings to dietary methionine from 28 to 70 days of age. *Br. Poult. Sci.* 51: 118–121.

32 Jamroz, D., Wertelecki, T., Lemme, A. et al. (2009). Dynamics of yolk sac content absorption and intestine development in ducklings fed mixtures with increasing dietary methionine levels. *J. Anim. Physio. Anim. Nutr.* 93: 381–390.

33 Wang, C., Xie, M., Huang, W. et al. (2013). Arginine requirements of white Pekin ducks from 1 to 21 days of age. *Poult. Sci.* 92: 1007–1010.

34 Wu, L.Y., Fang, Y.J., and Guo, X.Y. (2011). Dietary L-arginine supplementation beneficially regulates body fat deposition of meat type ducks. *Br. Poult. Sci.* 52: 221–226.

35 Zhao, F., Hou, S.S., Zhang, H.F., and Zhang, Z.Y. (2007). Effects of dietary metabolizable energy and crude protein content on the activities of digestive enzymes in jejunal fluid of Pekin ducks. *Poult. Sci.* 86: 1690–1695.

36 Schiavone, B.A., Romboli, I., Chiarini, R., and Marzoni, M. (2004). Influence of dietary lipid source and strain on fatty acid composition of Muscovy duck meat. *J. Anim. Physiol. Anim. Nutr.* 88: 88–93.

37 Petzinger, C., Heatley, J.J., Cornejo, J. et al. (2010). Dietary modification of omega-3 fatty acids for birds with atherosclerosis. *J. Am. Vet. Med. Assoc.* 236: 523–528.

38 Liu, D., Veit, H.P., Wilson, J.H. et al. (2003). Long-term supplementation of various dietary lipids alters bone mineral content, mechanical properties and histologic characteristics of Japanese quail. *Poult. Sci.* 82: 831–839.

39 Baird, H.T., Eggett, D.L., and Fullmer, S. (2008). Varying ratios of omega-6:omega-3 fatty acids on the pre- and postmortem bone mineral density, bone ash, and bone breaking strength of laying chickens. *Poult. Sci.* 87: 323–328.

40 Speake, B.K. and NAR, W. (2005). Timing of incorporation of docosahexaenoic acid into brain and muscle phospholipids during precocial and altricial modes of avian development. *Comp. Biochem. Physiol. Part B* 141: 147–158.

41 Fronte, B., Paci, B., Montanari, G. et al. (2008). Learning ability of 1-d-old partridges (*Alectoris rufa*) from eggs laid by hens fed with different n-3 fatty acid concentrations. *Br. Poult. Sci.* 49: 776–780.

42 Ansenberger, K., Richards, C., Zhuge, Y. et al. (2010). Decreased severity of ovarian cancer and increased survival in hens fed a flaxseed-enriched diet for 1 year. *Gynec. Oncol.* 117: 341–347.

43 Newman, R.E., Bryden, W.L., Fleck, E. et al. (2002). Dietary n-3 and n-6 fatty acids alter avian metabolism: metabolism and abdominal fat deposition. *Br. J. Nutr.* 88: 11–18.

44 Liu, W.M., Jhang, J., Lu, L.Z. et al. (2011). Effects of perilla extract on productive performance, serum values and hepatic expression of lipid-related genes in Shaoxing ducks. *Br. Poult. Sci.* 52: 381–387.

45 Wu, L.-S., Wu, C.-L., and Shen, T.-F. (1984). Niacin and tryptophan requirements of mule ducklings fed corn and soy-based diets. *Poult. Sci.* 63: 153–158.

46 Serafin, J.A. (1981). Studies on the riboflavin, pantothenic acid, nicotinic acid and choline requirements of young Embden geese. *Poult. Sci.* 60: 1910–1915.

47 Wang, A., Xie, F., Wang, Y.H., and Wu, J.L. (2011). Effects of vitamin C supplementation on growth performance and antioxidant status of layer ducklings. *J. Anim. Phys. Anim. Nutr.* 95: 533–539.

48 Adeola, O., Shafer, D.J., and Nyachoti, C.M. (2008). Nutrient and energy utilization in enzyme-supplemented starter and grower diets for white Pekin ducks. *Poult. Sci.* 87: 255–263.

49 Hong, D., Burrows, H., and Adeola, O. (2002). Addition to enzyme to starter and grower diets for ducks. *Poult. Sci.* 82: 1842–1849.

50 Jamroz, D., Jakobsen, K., Knudsen, K.E.B. et al. (2002). Digestibility and energy value of non-starch polysaccharides in young chickens, ducks, and geese, fed diets containing high amounts of barley. *Comp. Biochem. Physiol. Part B* 131: 657–668.

51 Hurley, J.C. and Johnston, J.J. (2002). Poly (methyl methacrylate) synthetic grit formulations sustain delivery of nicarbazin, a contraceptive agent, in pest waterfowl. *J. Controlled Release* 85: 135–143.

52 Mateo, R. and Guitart, R. (2000). The effects of grit supplementation and feed type of steel shot ingestion in mallards. *Prevent. Vet. Med.* 44: 221–229.

53 Khambualai, O., Ruttanavut, J., Kitabatake, M. et al. (2009). Effects of dietary natural zeolite including plant extracts on growth performance and intestinal histology on Aigamo ducks. *Br. Poult. Sci.* 50: 123–130.

54 Briese, A., Hänsch, F., and Hartung, J. (2009). Water provisions for Muscovy ducks–behaviour at duck showers and modified plasson drinkers. *Berl. Münch. Tieräz. Wochen* 122: 302–313.

55 McKinney, F. (1965). The comfort movements of Anatidae. *Behavior* 25: 120–220.

56 Johnsgard, P.A. (1965). *Handbook of Waterfowl Behavior*. University of Nebraska http://digitalcommons.unl.edu/bioscihandwaterfowl/7.

57 Knierim, U., Bulheller, M.A., Briese, A., and Hartung, J. (2004). Water provision for domestic ducks kept indoors–a review on the basis of the literature and our own experiences. *Dtsch. Tierarztl. Wochenschr.* 111: 115–118.

58 Zimmer, C., Boos, M., Bertrand, F. et al. (2011). Behavioral adjustment in response to increased predation risk: a study in three duck species. *PLoS One* 6: e18977.

59 Oppel, S., Powell, A.N., and O'Brien, D.M. (2010). King eiders use an income strategy for egg production: a case study for incorporating individual dietary variation into nutrient allocation research. *Oecologia* 164: 1–12.

60 Flinchum, G.B. (2006). Management of Waterfowl. In: *Clinical Avian Medicine Volume II* (eds. G.J. Harrison and T.L. Lightfoot), 831–847. Spix Publishing.

61 Barboza, P.S. and Jorde, D.G. (2001). Intermittent feeding in a migratory omnivore: digestion and body composition of the American black duck during autumn. *Physiol. Biochem. Zool.* 74: 307–317.

62 Moe, B., StØlevik, E., and Beck, C. (2005). Ducklings exhibited substantial energy-saving mechanisms as a response to short-term food shortage. *Physiol. Biochem. Zool.* 78: 90–104.

5

Biosecurity

Teresa Y. Morishita and Theodore Derksen

College of Veterinary Medicine, Western University of Health Sciences, Pomona, CA, USA

Biosecurity

Biosecurity is an important part of any avian health management program. "Bio" means "life" and "security" implies "protection," so such a program is designed to protect life. In its simplest terms, it means keeping the infectious agents away from the poultry and keeping the poultry away from infectious agents and other hazards to health [1]. To minimize the occurrence and spread of disease, the following steps can be taken to reduce the interaction of poultry and infectious agents: (i) a conscious examination of how infectious agents can be introduced to birds through humans; other poultry; food; water; infected equipment; and other animals such as pets and pests; and (ii) implementation of a routine cleaning and disinfection program [1–3]. Minimizing the contact between poultry and infectious agents such as bacteria, viruses, fungi, and parasites can reduce the likelihood of a disease outbreak. Steps can also be taken to reduce the risk of disease and other health risks to humans and other animals, such as pets, that may have contact with poultry and/ or their environment.

Informational resources are readily available for both poultry owners and veterinarians from a variety of sources. The United States Department of Agriculture Animal and Plant Health Inspection Service (USDA-APHIS) publishes a "Backyard Biosecurity 6 Ways to Prevent Poultry Diseases" poster and a "Backyard Biosecurity: Practices to Keep Your Birds Healthy" video and provides a toll-free help line (866-536-7593) [4, 5] (Figure 5.1). Many agricultural college extension websites offer information on biosecurity and many aspects of care for the backyard flock [6–13].

Besides U.S. government websites, other countries offer exceptional government websites with on-line manuals for poultry producers, backyard flock owners, and other domestic bird keepers [14, 15]. Clear advantages of practicing biosecurity include having healthy bird; minimizing the potential for significant costs and loss of revenue; protecting human health; protecting future ability to move birds without restriction; protecting other allied industries such as feed suppliers; and protecting export markets. It has been found that backyard poultry owners are typically lackadaisical when it comes to practicing good biosecurity protocols, but backyard poultry owners are eager to learn and implement good biosecurity protocols to ensure the health of their flocks [16]. Table 5.1 provides an overview of the personal protective equipment used in commercial poultry facilities

Backyard Poultry Medicine and Surgery: A Guide for Veterinary Practitioners, Second Edition.
Edited by Cheryl B. Greenacre and Teresa Y. Morishita.
© 2021 John Wiley & Sons, Inc. Published 2021 by John Wiley & Sons, Inc.
Companion website: www.wiley.com/go/greenacre/medicine

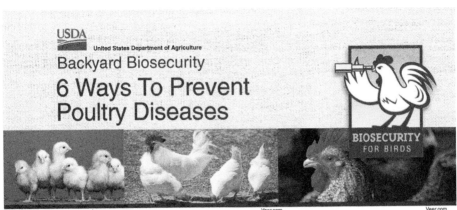

USDA
United States Department of Agriculture

Backyard Biosecurity

6 Ways To Prevent Poultry Diseases

BIOSECURITY FOR BIRDS

imagesource.com   Veer.com   Veer.com

1. Keep Your Distance.

Restrict access to your property and your birds. Consider fencing off the area where you keep your birds to form a barrier between "clean" and "dirty" areas. Allow only people who take care of your birds to come into contact with them. If visitors have birds of their own, **do not** let them enter your bird area or have access to your birds. Game birds and migratory water-fowl should not have contact with your flock because they can carry germs and diseases.

2. Keep It Clean.

Wear clean clothes and scrub your shoes with disinfectant. Wash your hands thoroughly with soap and water before entering your bird area. Keep cages clean and change food and water daily. Clean and disinfect equipment that comes in contact with your birds or their droppings, including cages and tools. Remove manure before disinfecting. Properly dispose of dead birds.

3. Don't Haul Disease Home.

Car and truck tires, poultry cages, and equipment can all harbor germs. If you travel to a location where other birds are present, or even to the feed store, be sure to clean and disinfect these items before returning to your property. Have your birds been to a fair or exhibition? Keep them separated from the rest of your flock for at least 2 weeks after the event. New birds should be kept separate from your flock for at least 30 days.

4. Don't Borrow Disease From Your Neighbor.

Do not share lawn and garden equipment, tools, or poultry supplies with your neighbors or other bird owners. If you do bring these items home, clean and disinfect them before they reach your property.

5. Know the Warning Signs of Infectious Bird Diseases.

Early detection is important to prevent the spread of disease. Here's what to look for:

- Sudden increase in bird deaths in your flock
- Sneezing, gasping for air, coughing, and nasal discharge
- Watery and green diarrhea
- Lack of energy and poor appetite
- Drop in egg production or thin- or soft-shelled, misshapen eggs
- Swelling around the eyes, neck, and head
- Purple discoloration of the wattles, comb, and legs (avian influenza)
- Tremors, drooping wings, circling, twisting of the head and neck, or lack of movement (exotic Newcastle disease)

6. Report Sick Birds.

Don't wait. If your birds are sick or dying, contact your agricultural extension office/agent, local veterinarian, local animal health diagnostic laboratory, or the State veterinarian. Or, call the U.S. Department of Agriculture (USDA) toll free at **1-866-536-7593**, and we'll put you in touch with a local contact.

You are the best protection your birds have.
For more information, go to http://healthybirds.aphis.usda.gov.

Animal and Plant Health Inspection Service
Program Aid No. 1764 • Revised March 2015
USDA is an equal opportunity provider and employer.
(Spanish on reverse side.)

Figure 5.1 The United States Department of Agriculture Animal and Plant Health Inspection Service (USDA-APHIS) publishes this poster titled "Backyard Biosecurity 6 Ways to Prevent Poultry Diseases" which members of the public can download for free from https://www.aphis.usda.gov/publications/animal_health/2015/pos_backyard_bio_six_ways.pdf. *Source:* United States Department of Agriculture. Public domain.

Table 5.1 Personal protective equipment for biosecurity measures utilized in the commercial poultry industry and recommendations for adaptations for backyard poultry owners.

Body area needing protection	Industry	Backyard
Feet	Rubber boots that are only worn on the farm. A footbath is used when entering and exiting barns and farm premise. Disposable plastic boots have been used with caution as rocks and other sharp flooring substrate can cause small tears on the sole of these boots.	A dedicated pair of shoes that only get worn around the flock is recommended.
Clothing	Coveralls that are worn only at the farm and are put-on in a dedicated dressing room. If cloth coveralls are used, company lauders the coveralls after use. Tyvek disposable coveralls can be used as an alternative.	Regular clothes can be worn but should be washed after contact with the flock
Head	Hairnets are commonly worn to reduce the risk of the spread of infectious agents that may be carried in the dust or debris.	If the owner is only handling their flock, no hairnet needed.

compared with suggested personal protective equipment for backyard flock owners. Table 5.2 provides some disease prevention tips that can be provided to backyard flock owners.

Methods Used to Reduce Interactions Between Poultry and Infectious Agents

The following procedures can be used to reduce interactions between poultry and infectious agents: minimizing human contact, establishing a visitor's policy, reducing exposure from contaminated food and water, reducing exposure from pests, and reducing exposure from new poultry introductions.

Minimizing Human Contact and Establishing a Visitor Policy

In the commercial poultry industry, a visitor policy is necessary to restrict human access to poultry. Disease agents can be transmitted to poultry through fomites such as the soiled soles of shoes, contaminated clothing and equipment, and even vehicles [1, 14]. The rationale for this biosecurity measure is that visitors to commercial poultry farms have probably come in contact with other birds, and contaminated soil is a primary mode of transmission of many infectious agents. For backyard poultry flocks, people may be visiting a farm to purchase eggs or poultry for their own flocks, or simply visiting the flock. If these visitors have exposure/contact with other poultry and/or bird species, they should wear coveralls or alternative protective clothing, and plastic disposable boots [1, 17]. Additionally, a footbath containing disinfectant that visitors step into prior to visiting the birds should be available. Recommended classes of disinfectants used in footbaths include phenols, iodophores, hypochlorites, quaternary ammonium compounds, and oxidizing agents. It should be noted that the footbath is only effective if it is kept fresh. If it is not routinely maintained, it can be a source of infection [2]. A typical footbath is changed every 2–3 days but should be changed more frequently if used often so that it remain effective. The footbath should include a long-handled scrub brush, a tray with short sides with plastic turf or some other synthetic bristled mat in the bottom, and sufficient disinfectant to cover the entire sole of the shoe [18, 19]. If there are no visitors who will have contact with the backyard flock other than the owner, there is a reduced need for protective clothing, disposable boots, and footbaths.

Table 5.2 Tips for the backyard flock owner to prevent diseases.

Recommendations	Recommendation rationale
1. Thorough cleaning and disinfection of the poultry house is an important factor in disease prevention.	This action keeps bacteria, viruses, fungi, and parasites from building up to levels that may cause disease outbreaks
2. It is not recommended that chickens, either young or old, be raised on old litter used by a previous flock of birds. Always add a new layer of bedding to the old litter if an entirely new bedding substrate is not possible. This top dressing should be 5–7 in. in depth.	Exposing birds to old litter is not recommended as the litter may have a build-up of disease agents to which the new flock has not been exposed. This can result in a disease outbreak.
3. Do not bring new chickens, especially adult birds from other flocks, and mix them immediately with your flock.	Chickens need a minimum 2-week quarantine period in a separate house in order to be monitored for any diseases.
4. Do not permit visitors in your poultry house if they have had contact with other poultry. If you do have visitors, they should not be wearing clothes and shoes that have come into contact with other birds and/or their feces.	Visitors can transfer diseases through their clothing, shoes, and unwashed hands. If you have frequent visitors that have exposure to poultry, provide footbaths and/or boot covering at minimum.
5. Prevent other birds (e.g. sparrows, pigeons) from direct contacting with your chickens.	These free-living birds can carry diseases and parasites to the chickens. Do not place bird feeders in areas where your poultry can congregate. One common backyard situation is having a bird feeder and chickens will often congregate under the feeder to eat the fallen bird food.
6. Purchase feed from a reliable source; do not use old moldy feed.	For health and productivity, chickens require a nutritionally balanced feed. Ensure that the feed is stored properly in a rodent proof container and in a cool dry area so that there is not heat degradation of nutrients and there is no mold growth.
7. Vaccinations are important in disease prevention, if needed.	Backyard chickens should only be vaccinated if there is a confirmed disease on your site. Marek's disease is common, so purchase chicks that were vaccinated in ovo or at 1 day of age.
8. Provide a well-ventilated but draft-free building with appropriate space available for the number of chickens housed.	This reduces ammonia build-up, stress, and pen-mate fighting.
9. Properly dispose of all dead birds and old litter.	This prevents flies and odor and reduces potential transmission of diseases. Flies can be carriers of disease from infected birds. Properly disposing of birds will reduce a potential source of odor and reduce a potential fly breeding source.
10. Keep all sick chickens separated from the rest of the flock.	Diseases can be spread through direct contact with infected birds. Isolate any sick chicken from the rest of the flock.
11. In the event of a disease outbreak in your flock, get an accurate diagnosis as soon as possible.	Since many diseases show similar clinical signs, it is advisable to get an accurate diagnosis before beginning treatment. Your veterinarian can help you with diagnostic procedures.
12. If the hobbyist also has pet birds of different species (e.g. parrots), extreme care must be exercised when undertaking routines between the different bird species.	Pet birds, like parrots, can pose a serious threat to chickens because they can harbor diseases that can be very devastating to a chicken flock, or vise versa.

Source: Adapted from Ebako and Morishita [14].

For veterinarians making field calls to multiple backyard flocks, it is imperative that clean coveralls be used when visiting each site and to have rubber boots that can be scrubbed and disinfected before and after each farm visit [18]. Additionally, vehicles should be parked at the edge of the property to reduce the likelihood of obtaining contaminated soil or feces in tires and wheel wells. Because Marek's disease, a common disease in chickens, can be spread from the feather dander of infected birds, wearing a hairnet is necessary to minimize this risk if visiting multiple flocks on the same day [18].

Backyard flock owners should have a separate set of shoes or boots to wear while working with the flock. This reduces the likelihood of bringing contaminated feces or soil into the house. Wearing a dedicated pair of shoes only when working around the flock also reduces the risk of bringing any contaminated feces or soil home from a feed store. Many people may have visited the feed store and may have brought in contaminated feces or soil from their flock. Appropriate hand washing after handling poultry is also advised [16].

Reducing Exposure from Contaminated Feed and Water

In the process used in commercial pelleted feed production, the temperature is elevated and the majority of infectious agents will be destroyed from the heat. However, feed can become contaminated during storage, often by rodent feces. Therefore, feed should be kept in rodent-proof containers and stored in a cool, out of direct sunlight, moisture-free environment to reduce nutrient degradation and mycotoxin production [1, 14, 16]. Additionally, appropriate containers should keep other animals, including pets such as dogs, from accessing feed.

A clean water source is necessary and daily cleaning of water containers will prevent build-up of organic debris and infectious agents [1, 18]. Periodic disinfection of the water containers will also ensure that the flock's exposure to disease agents is minimized. While the water supply for many backyard flocks is city municipal sources and generally clean, some farms may use well water, which should be tested annually as run-off after heavy rains may contaminate nearby wells [18]. Local public health agencies, land-grant state universities, state diagnostic laboratories, local extension offices, or water municipalities can be contacted for information on how and where well water can be tested.

Reducing Exposure from Pests

Rodents, specifically rats and mice, can serve as a reservoir for several poultry diseases including *Salmonella*, and rodent control measures should be in place for any backyard flock. The presence of readily available feed can attract rodents. Hence, appropriate containers for feed, minimizing feed spills and rapidly cleaning feed spills is of utmost importance to controlling rodents on the premises [18]. If you can see signs of rodents, including feces, then this usually indicates a rodent problem [1].

Free-living birds can serve as reservoirs for many diseases that can be shared among avian species, including, but not limited to, avian influenza, Newcastle disease, avian cholera, salmonellosis, chlamydiosis, campylobacteriosis, and avian tuberculosis [19–21]. Internal parasites tend to be host specific so they may not be readily spread to poultry, but external parasites like mites have a wider host range and can be spread through contact [22–25]. Like rodents, free-living birds are attracted to accessible feed, and exposure to free-living birds can vary per flock situation [26]. Feeding the poultry at night and before they are released from the coop in the morning could reduce contact with free-living birds and their feces [18]. The poultry could still have free access during the day to graze. In addition, bird feeders (for free-living birds) should not be hung near poultry areas as this will likely increase contact between free-living birds and poultry. Poultry may congregate under the feeders where they can become exposed to free-living bird feces or discarded food [18].

Predators, such as raptors and raccoons, can also serve as a source of disease or trauma for backyard poultry. Poultry should be housed in predator-proof housing at night [18, 27].

Reducing Exposure from New Poultry Introductions

For many backyard flocks, the addition of new poultry to the existing flock is one of the most common ways infectious agents are introduced. Obtaining background information such as vaccination history; previous diseases experienced in the birds being introduced or their parents; and causes of previous morbidity and mortality is important for the prevention of introducing infectious agent to the flock. New birds should have a minimum two week, preferably four week, quarantine period with no direct or indirect contact with the rest of the flock before being introduced to the rest of the flock [1]. This allows time for underlying diseases to manifest clinical signs because many disease agents have an approximately 2-week incubation period; it also allows for enough time to perform and receive serological testing and fecal examination results [1].

During quarantine, birds should have a physical examination performed to determine health status and appropriate vaccinations should be administered [28, 29]. A prominent keel bone indicates a thin bird, as a result of either chronic disease and/or a poor nutritional state (see Chapter 7) [30]. A poor nutritional state can also make a bird more prone to disease. Examine the ventral abdomen and the vent region of the bird as most lice and mite infestations can occur in these areas [24]. Clumps of lice eggs (nits) are found at the base of the feather shaft [24, 25]. Brownish black debris along feathers are often indicative of mite infestation [24, 25]. As a prevention, birds can be treated for external parasites at the start and end of the quarantine period

before they are added to the existing flock (see Chapter 12).

Also, during quarantine, blood should be collected to perform serological tests to determine exposure to certain disease agents, such as *Mycoplasma gallisepticum* [28, 29]. Fecal samples should be collected at the start of quarantine and 2 weeks later to ensure that birds are negative of parasites. If parasites are detected, the birds should be treated and retested during the quarantine period to evaluate the effectiveness of the treatment. The quarantine period will help prevent seeding of facilities with internal parasites that survive for prolonged periods in the soil [23].

Keeping Poultry Away from Infectious Agents

The following procedures can be used to minimize the introduction of poultry to areas where infectious agents are present: management of sick birds, carcass management, and vaccination.

Management of Sick Birds

Despite the best management practices, sometimes birds will become sick. It is important that poultry owners know what is considered normal behavior for their flock, including appetite. If any signs of clinical disease, such as diarrhea or respiratory signs, are noted, the affected bird should be removed from the flock to minimize the exposure to the other birds. Owners must also recognize that poultry are flock animals and an individual bird may get stressed if housed away from the rest of the flock [18]. While the sick bird is in isolation, provide extra warmth and ensure access to feed and water while collecting specimens for diagnosis [18].

Carcass Management

Proper management of a carcass can provide answers as to disease etiology and prevent further spread to other birds. Carcasses should be submitted for necropsy as soon as possible, or immediately disposed of in an area where other poultry, predators, and pets will not have access [18]. Do not allow flies to lay eggs on a carcass that develop into maggots because under certain circumstances other flock members could acquire botulism through ingestion of the maggots [18].

Vaccination Program

An appropriate vaccination program is necessary for all backyard poultry flocks [20, 29]. Vaccination protocols should be based on what diseases are present in the geographic region and what diseases have previously been diagnosed in the flock [20]. Diagnostic laboratories, extension veterinarians, and National Poultry Improvement Plan (NPIP) personnel can often provide information on which diseases are present in a region. It is also important to know if the birds will be taken off the farm and exposed to other birds, including at poultry shows or state fairs [26]. Owners must be made aware of potential disease exposure that might occur when birds are exposed to other birds of mixed or unknown vaccination history. Owners must also be willing to weigh this risk with the value of the birds [2, 20].

Typically, backyard flocks are only vaccinated against Marek's disease, and this is performed at the hatchery on day 1 of age or in ovo (vaccination while the chick is still in the egg), but vaccines for other diseases can be given if there is risk of exposure (see Chapter 30). Other vaccines that are available include a combination Newcastle disease and infectious bronchitis vaccine, laryngotracheitis vaccine, avian encephalomyelitis vaccine, fowl pox vaccine, and a fowl cholera bacterin [31].

Maintaining Adequate Records

Maintaining adequate records of bird transactions and movements, such as the name and address of who sold or purchased the bird, and bird mortality records, is crucial if there is a disease outbreak and an epidemiological investigation takes place. If a pet parrot, canary, or others birds are on the premises of a disease outbreak, having good records documenting biosecurity measures could save your pets from culling.

Cleaning and Disinfecting

"Cleaning" and "disinfecting" are two words that are commonly used interchangeably but have different meanings. Cleaning refers to the removal of organic matter such as bedding or feces from the coop, whereas disinfection involves the use of a disinfectant to kill or neutralize potential pathogens [32]. There is commonly much debate surrounding what can be considered a "clean" chicken coop. Some people believe that if the coop is visibly clean it can be considered clean, whereas others believe that there needs to be some sort of disinfectant applied [33].

To adequately clean a coop, all the dry organic matter should be removed and then ideally hot water with a detergent such as dish soap should be used on all surfaces to ensure that all organic material is removed and finally surfaces should be rinsed. The removal of organic matter is vital to do prior to disinfecting since most disinfectants cannot penetrate organic matter to reach potential pathogens [33]. For disinfection, there are a variety of different chemicals that can be used depending on major needs of the flock owner and include phenol compounds, iodine, chlorine compounds, quaternary ammonium compounds, and oxidizing compounds [32]. Regardless of the disinfectant that is chosen, all manufacturer instructions should be followed to ensure no harm is done to the flock or to people. Table 5.3 lists common diseases of poultry and the effectiveness of various disinfectants on the disease agents.

Table 5.3 Common disease of poultry and the effectiveness of selected disinfectants [3].

Disease name	Chlorhexadine	Chlorine-releasing agent	Iodophor	Phenol and bis phenols	Single ammonium compound	4-way (quaternary ammonium compound)
Salmonellosis	+++	+++	+++	+++	+	+++
Pullorum disease	+++	+++	+++	+++	+	+++
Fowl typhoid	+++	+++	+++	+++	+	+++
Paratyphoid infection	+++	+++	+++	+++	+	+++
Colibacillosis	+++	+++	+++	+++	+	+++
Pasteurellosis	++	+++	+++	++	+	+++
Tuberculosis	–	+	+	+++	–	+++
Infectious coryza	++	+++	+++	+++	+	+++
Mycoplasmosis	++	++	++	++	++	++
Campylobacteriosis	+	+++	+++	+++	+	+++
Botulism	–	++	++	–	–	–
Staphylococcosis	–	+++	+++	+++	+++	+++
Streptococcosis	–	+++	+++	+++	+++	+++
Aspergillosis	+	+++	+++	++	+/–	+++
Thrush (Candidiasis)	+	+++	+++	++	+/–	++
Marek's disease	+/–	+++	+++	–	–	++
Infectious bronchitis	++	+++	+++	–	–	+++
Laryngotracheitis	+/–	+++	+++	–	–	+++
Newcastle disease	+/–	+++	+++	+	–	+++
Pox	+/–	+++	+++	+	–	+++
Adenovirus infection	–	+++	+++	–	–	+++
Duck virus enteritis	+/–	+++	+++	–	–	+++
Reovirus infection	–	+++	+++	–	–	+++
Infectious bursal disease	–	+++	+++	–	–	+++
Chicken anemia	–	+++	+++	–	–	+++

– Not an effective agent; +/– May or may not be effective; + Weakly effective; ++ Effective; +++ Very Effective.

References

1 Morishita, T.Y. (2001). Biosecurity for poultry. Extension Factsheet, Veterinary Preventive Medicine, Factsheet #VME-9-2001. The Ohio State University Extension.

2 Morishita, T.Y. (1990). A word about . . . disinfectants. In: *California Poultry Letter, Cooperative Extension*. Davis, California: University of California-Davis.

3 Morishita, T.Y. and Gordon, J.C. (2002). Cleaning and disinfection of poultry facilities. Extension Factsheet, Veterinary Preventive Medicine, Factsheet #VME-013-02. The Ohio State University Extension.

4 United States Department of Agriculture Animal and Plant Health Inspection Service. http://www.aphis.usda.gov/publications/animal_health/content/printable_version/6-StepPoster-English_Araboc.pdf (accessed 14 September 2013).

5 United States Department of Agriculture Animal and Plant Health Inspection Service. http://www.aphis.usda.gov/animal_health/birdbiosecurity (accessed 14 September 2013).

6 http://www.healthybirds.umn.edu/Biosecurity (accessed 14 September 2013).

7 http://www.extension.org/poultry (accessed 14 September 2013).

8 http://edis.ifas.ufl.edu/an239 (accessed 14 September 2013).

9 http://www1.extension.umn.edu/food/small-farms/livestock/poultry/backyard-chicken-basics/, (accessed 14 September 2013).

10 http://www.caes.uga.edu/publications (accessed 14 September 2013).

11 http://web.uconn.edu/poultry (accessed 14 September 2013).

12 http://ag.ansc.purdue.edu/poultry/extension.htm (accessed 14 September 2013).

13 a http://www.ces.ncsu.edu/depts/poulsci/tech_manuals/small_flock_resources.html (accessed 14 September 2013); b Australian Government Department of Agriculture, Fisheries and Forestry, National Farm Biosecurity Manual-Poultry Producers. www daff.gov.au/animal-plant-health/pests-diseases-weeds/biosecurity/animal_biosecurity/bird-owners/poultry_biosecurity_manual (ISBN 978-1-921575-01-3, 1st edn., June 2009) (accessed 7 October 2013); c National Avian on Farm Biosecurity Standard, Canadian Food Inspection Agency, http://www.inspection.gc.ca/animals/terres-trial-animals/biosecurity/standards-and-principles/avain-on-farm/eng/1375193894256/1375193980266, (accessed 7 October 2013).

14 Ebako, G.M. and Morishita, T.Y. (2001) Preventive medicine for backyard chickens. Extension Factsheet, Veterinary Preventive Medicine, Factsheet #VME-12-2001. The Ohio State University Extension.

15 https://extension.umn.edu/poultry/poultry-biosecurity

16 Derksen, T.J., Lampron, R., Hauck, R. et al. (2018). Biosecurity assessment and seroprevalence of respiratory diseases in backyard poultry flocks located close to and far from commercial premises. *Avian Dis.* 62: 1–5.

17 Morishita, T.Y. (1995). Poultry management 101: Poultry management topics for avian veterinarian. In: *Section 7: Practice Management. Main Conference Proceedings, Association of Avian Veterinarians Annual Conference, Philadelphia, Pennsylvania*, 327–331.

18 Aye, P.P., Morishita, T.Y., and Bills, B. (1998). Conjunctivitis in Ohio's free-living passerines. *Wildl. Rehabil.* 15: 165–168.

19 Hauck, R., Crossley, B., Rejmanek, D. et al. (2017). Persistence of highly pathogenic and low pathogenic avian influenza viruses in footbaths and poultry manure. *Avian Dis.* 61 (1): 64–69.

20 Morishita, T.Y. (1999). Backyard poultry medicine: vaccination strategies and serological monitoring. In: *115th Annual Convention, Ohio Veterinary Medical Association Annual Conference (Midwest Veterinary Conference) Proceedings, Columbus, Ohio* (February 18–21), vol. 3 (Session 374), 467–469.

21 Keller, J.I., Shriver, G., Waldenstrom, J. et al. (2011). Prevalence of Campylobacter in wild birds of the mid-Atlantic region, USA. *J. Wildl. Dis.* 47 (3): 750–754.

22 Morishita, T.Y., Johnson, G., Thilstead, J. et al. (2005). Scaly-leg mite infestation associated with digit necrosis in bantam chickens. *J. Avian Med. Surg.* 19: 230–233.

23 Morishita, T.Y. and Schaul, J.C. (2007). Parasites of birds. In: *Flynn's Parasites of Laboratory Animals*, 2e (ed. D.G. Baker), 217–302. Ames, IA: Blackwell Publishing Professional.

24 Pickworth, C.L. and Morishita, T.Y. (2003) Common external parasites in poultry: lice and mites. Extension Factsheet, Veterinary Preventive Medicine, Factsheet #VME-18-03. The Ohio State University Extension.

25 Pickworth, C.L. and Morishita, T.Y. (2003) Less common external parasites in poultry. Extension Factsheet, Veterinary Preventive Medicine, Factsheet #VME-19-03.The Ohio State University Extension.

26 Morishita, T.Y. (2011) Backyard Poultry Medicine: Working with Fowl Patients. Proceedings of the 26th Annual Avian and Exotic Medicine Symposium, Avian and Exotic Medicine Club, School of Veterinary Medicine, University of California – Davis, Davis, California (April 30–May 1), 3 pp.

27 Ison, A.J., Spiegle, S.J., and Morishita, T.Y. (2005) Predators of poultry. Extension Factsheet, Veterinary Preventive Medicine, Factsheet #VME-22-05. The Ohio State University Extension.

28 Morishita, T.Y., Aye, P.P., Ley, E.C. et al. (1999). Survey of pathogens and blood parasites in free-living passerines. *Avian Dis.* 43: 549–552.

29 Morishita, T.Y. (1992). Vaccines and their implications to poultry health. In: *California Poultry Letter, Cooperative Extension*. Davis, California: University of California-Davis.

30 Spiegle, S.J., Ison, A.J. and Morishita, T.Y. Performing a physical exam on a chicken. Extension Factsheet, Veterinary Preventive Medicine, Factsheet #VME-20-04. The Ohio State University Extension.

31 http://www.amerpoultryassn.com/vaccination_guide.htm (accessed 26 Augest 2020)

32 Darre, M. J. (2014) Cleaning and Disinfecting Your Poultry House, Cornell Small Farms Program.

33 Bolder, N.M. and Ledoux, L. (2002). General protocol for cleaning and disinfecting poultry house and equipment. *World Poult.* 18 (12): 26–29.

6

Backyard Poultry Nutrition

Todd J. Applegate and Justin Fowler

Department of Poultry Science, The University of Georgia, Athens, GA, USA

Introduction

All of the processes a living thing undergoes to take in and use food for growth and reproduction is what we term "nutrition." For any animal to maintain its health, as well as grow and be productive, there are specific chemical compounds that must be in their diet in the right amounts. This is because no animal is capable of producing every one of the necessary components on its own. The study of nutrition is about understanding that there is no one ingredient that contains every nutrient an animal needs in the exact concentrations that it needs. Providing the right nutrition for poultry means ensuring that what they eat supplies all of the essential amino acids, fatty acids, carbohydrates, vitamins, minerals, and water that they will need to produce the meat or eggs we hope to collect.

Sufficient supply of nutrients is essential to drive the long-term health and well-being of any poultry flock. Nutritional insufficiencies/deficiencies are more likely to occur in smaller-scale, backyard poultry flocks than in commercial poultry production. There is a lack of nutritional knowledge and dogma of the backyard poultry owner, as well as a limited specificity of information on the nutritional needs of noncommercial poultry strains/breeds. Not surprisingly, the genetic "gap" between commercial poultry strains and that of backyard breeds has greatly increased. Current commercial livestock and poultry strains are more efficient in using nutrients and the commercial feeds are better formulated to meet the requirements of the rapidly growing animal [1, 2]. For example, nitrogen (N) and phosphorus (P) excretion per unit of live weight were 55 and 69% less, respectively, from a 1991 commercial broiler strain versus a 1957 commercial broiler strain fed the same diet. Also, modern broiler strains have been selected for an increased muscle mass, which has meant that broilers have had to decrease other supporting organs in proportion. Collins et al. [3] found that both external parts (feathers, head, neck, preen gland, and wings) and internal organs (heart, liver, lungs, gizzard [ventriculus], and viscera) have decreased in relative size among modern breeds.

Common Nutritional Issues in Backyard Poultry

While nutritional issues in any flock can be numerous, the most common issues seen in backyard flocks that will be discussed herein include:

1) Insufficient water quality or amount
2) Prolonged feed storage and degradation of vitamin efficacy

Backyard Poultry Medicine and Surgery: A Guide for Veterinary Practitioners, Second Edition.
Edited by Cheryl B. Greenacre and Teresa Y. Morishita.
© 2021 John Wiley & Sons, Inc. Published 2021 by John Wiley & Sons, Inc.
Companion website: www.wiley.com/go/greenacre/medicine

3) Dilution of dietary nutrients with a "cheaper" and less nutrient dense ingredient(s)
4) Feeding a diet for the wrong life-stage of the bird

Insufficient Water Quality or Amount

Water comprises 85% of young birds, 67–70% of adult birds, and 65% of the egg, whereas poultry feed is typically only 10% moisture. Thus, water is the nutrient that is required in greatest quantity by the bird. However, quantity and quality of water is often forgotten about and overlooked. Water intake is tied directly to feed intake. In fact, poultry require 1.5–3.5 parts water for every 1 part of feed consumed (up to 5–6 times for waterfowl), and birds will reduce feed consumption if they do not have access to water. Water is also critical for the regulation of body temperature in hot weather via evaporative cooling during panting. Several factors can influence water consumption, including (but not limited to):

A) Salts
B) Dietary fiber content
C) Ambient temperature
D) Medications
E) Disease status

Generally, monitoring water consumption can be an initial gauge of flock health, as deviations from "normal" consumption patterns often occur with initial onset of disease. Monitoring water quality is also important. The crop of a chicken is a holding reservoir for food, and adding poor quality water to a crop of nutritious feed makes for a perfect bacterial environment. Poor water quality can increase the risk of disease, decrease bird performance, and reduce the effectiveness of medications. Drinking water guidelines (namely maximum acceptable levels) can be found in Table 6.1.

Vitamin and Mineral Deficiencies

All of the chemical reactions that are needed for an animal to take carbohydrates, fats, and protein and use them to sustain its life require a group of chemicals called vitamins. Typical vitamin and mineral deficiencies observed in poultry are elaborated further in Tables 6.2 and 6.3. Vitamin deficiencies are typically seen when either not enough of a vitamin premix has been included into the diet or when using a vitamin premix that is well beyond its shelf-life (and thus efficacy). In either case, the fat soluble vitamin deficiencies will present themselves prior to the water-soluble vitamin deficiencies, particularly vitamin D_3. Thus, skeletal abnormalities that would be observe would include beading of the ribs, scoliosis, soft and pliable bones, keel, and beak, and rickets due to lack of hydroxyapatite crystallization at the growth plate in long bones such as the tibia, femur, or humerus (Figure 6.1).

Backyard producers may try to produce their own feed in some cases with the thought they could either do it better or more affordably than what could be bought commercially. One of the biggest limitations for doing this is the availability of a vitamin and micro-mineral premix. There are some readily available that they could purchase, likely from a toll-mill that mixes poultry rations, but usually in 50-lb quantities. For most of vitamin/mineral premixes, the range of inclusion typically would be between 3 and 10 lb of vitamin/mineral premix per ton of feed. Usually a laying hen would eat no more than 0.25 lb of feed per day. Thus as an example, if a backyard producer would have 25 hens, it would take 320 days to use 1 ton of feed. If the inclusion of vitamin/mineral premix were 5 lb per ton, it would take 8.75 years for them to get through a 50-lb bag of premix. With a maximum shelf-life of 3–6 months, it is easy to see why the birds in a smaller producer's flock may have vitamin deficiencies.

Proper and thorough mixing of all ingredients is essential to ensure the bird is able to ingest proper proportions of nutrients on a daily basis. For example, a newly hatched chick will eat enough feed in its first meal that can fit on the surface of a U.S. quarter. Thus, it is easy to see that adequate mixing (particularly of the vitamin/mineral premix)

Table 6.1 Suggested maximums for drinking water for poultry.

Contaminant	Average concentration	Maximum acceptable concentration	Remarks
Total bacteria		Less than 100 cfu/mL	
Total coliforms		Less than 50 cfu/mL	
Total hardness	60–180 ppm	110 ppm	< 60 is unusually soft; > 180 is very hard
pH	6.8–7.5	6.8–8.0	< 6. is undesirable; < 6.3 may degrade performance
Arsenic		0.2 ppm	
Calcium	60 mg/L	—	—
Cl$^-$		250 ppm	
Copper	0.002 mg/L	250 mg/L	Even 14 mg/L may be detrimental if sodium level is higher than 50 mg/L
Fluorine		2.0 ppm	
Iron		500 ppm	
Lead		0.02 mg/L	Higher levels are toxic
Magnesium	14 mg/L	125 mg/L	Higher levels may have laxative effect
Mercury		0.01 ppm	
Nitrates		50 ppm	
Nitrites		10 ppm	
Sodium	32 mg/L	50 mg/L	> 50 mg/L may affect performance if sulfate or chloride are high
SO$_4$		250 ppm	
Zinc		1.5 mg/L	Higher conc. are toxic

Source: Adapted in part from [4].

may be of particular difficulty by the small flock owner. Variation within the feed caused by inadequate mixing leads to variation within the flock, with some birds obtaining more or less of certain nutrients in others.

When considering minerals, poultry have specific requirements for calcium, phosphorus, sodium, chloride, potassium, sulfur, magnesium, iron, copper, zinc, manganese, iodine, and selenium. Grains are generally low in essential minerals, so supplementing the diet with a micro-mineral premix is needed for optimal health. The three from this list that are not routinely supplemented within a mineral premix are potassium, sulfur, and magnesium

as it is presumed that the feed ingredients in the rest of the diet would contain sufficient amounts to meet the bird's needs for these.

Also, much of the phosphorous in plants comes in a form that poultry cannot use (called phytate or phytic acid). Phosphorus is a major constituent of the hydroxyapatite crystals that make up bone. It is important for a poultry diet to contain an inorganic source of phosphorus such as dicalcium phosphate, deflourinated phosphorus, or meat and bone meal. When analyzing a feed for nutrient content, it is important to remember that in a predominately plant-based formulation, much of the total phosphorus there is not considered

Table 6.2   Vitamin requirements, deficiencies, and sources for poultry.

Vitamins	Major deficiency signs (in addition to growth reduction)	National Research Council [5] requirements (per kg feed)	Good sources
Vit. A	Drowsiness, incoordination, emaciation, ataxia, reduced vision, urate deposits in soft tissues, reduced hatchability, more susceptible to disease	C – 1500 I.U. H – 4000 I.U. P – 4000 I.U.	Fish oils, synthetics, and carotene from yellow corn and alfalfa meal
Vit. D$_3$ (cholecalciferol)	Rickets, thin egg shells, poor reproduction	C – 200 I.C.U. H – 500 I.C.U. P – 900 I.C.U.	Fish oils, some animal products and synthetics
Vit. K	Hemorrhagic disease (poor blood clotting)	C – 0.5 mg H – 0.5 mg P – 1.0 mg	Synthetics and low levels in plants
Vit. E	Encephalomalacia, exudative diathesis and poor reproduction	C – 10 mg H – 5 mg P – 12 mg	α-tocopherols in plants and synthetics
Thiamine (vit. B$_1$)	Polyneuritis and anorexia	C – 1.8 mg H – 0.8 mg P – 2 mg	Many natural feedstuffs
Riboflavin (vit. B$_2$)	Curled-toe paralysis, enlargement of sciatic nerve, poor protein utilization	C – 3.6 mg H – 2.2 mg P – 3.6 mg	Pure substance, milk products, alfalfa meal, Brewer's yeast
Pyridoxine (vit. B$_6$)	Reduced nitrogen retention, dermatitis, convulsions, anemia	C – 3.5 mg H – 2.5 mg P – 4.5 mg	Pyridoxal & pryidoxamine in animal products Pyridoxine – whole grains Up to 40% loss w/ processing & storage
Pantothenic acid	Dermatitis on top of feet and corners of mouth, poor hatchability	C – 10 mg H – 2+ mg P – 11 mg	Many feedstuffs, yeasts and milk products, synthetics
Nicotinic acid (niacin)	Pellagra-like syndrome, scaly dermatitis, hock disorders in poults	C – 27 mg H – 10 mg P – 70 mg	Wheat products, synthetics
Choline	Perosis-like condition, fatty liver	C – 1300 mg H – 500 mg P – 1900 mg	Soybean meal, wheat products, synthetics
Biotin	Dermatitis on bottom of feet, around vent and eyes and beak	C – 150 μg H – 150 μg P – 200 μg	Liver meals, yeast, and alfalfa meal, synthetics
Vit. B$_{12}$ (cobalamine)	Poor livability, poor hatchability, perosis-like condition	C – 9 μg H – 3 μg P – 3 μg	Meat and other animal products, fermentation products, synthetics
Folic acid	Anemia, poor feathering, hock disorders in poults	C – 550 μg H – 350 μg P – 1000 μg	Widely distributed in feedstuffs but may be limited in availability

C = growing chicks; H = laying hens; P = growing turkey poults.

Table 6.3 Mineral requirements and deficiency symptoms in poultry.

Mineral	Major deficiency signs	National Research Council–recommended minimum dietary concentrations	
Calcium	Rickets, decreased activity and sensitivity, tetany, thin egg shells, poor embryonic development	Chicks (C)	0.8%
		Hens (H)	3.40%
		Poults (P)	0.55–1.2%
Phosphorus (available)	Rickets, depraved appetite, weakness, thin egg shells	C	0.4%
		H	0.32%
		P	0.28–0.60%
Sodium	Softening of bones, gonadal inactivity, corneal keratinization, decreased plasma volume, decreased cardiac output	C	0.15%
		H	0.15%
		P	0.12–0.17%
Potassium	Overall muscular weakness; intestines, heart and respiratory muscles	C	0.4%
		H	0.15
		P	0.4–0.7%
Chlorine	Dehydration, hemoconcentration, low blood chloride, tetany-like syndrome	C, H, & P	0.15%
Magnesium	Anorexia, low blood Mg, disorientation, hyperirritability, tetany, reduced hatchability	C	600 ppm
		H	500 ppm
		P	600 ppm
Iron	Anemia (microcytichypochromic), inadequate respiration	C	80 ppm
		H	50 ppm
		P	50–80 ppm
Copper	Anemia, bone disorders, depigmentation of hair and feathers, cardiovascular defects	C	8 ppm
		H	6 ppm
		P	6–8 ppm
Zinc	Poor feather development, skeletal malformations, poor wound healing, impaired function of reproductive organs	C	40 ppm
		H	50 ppm
		P	40–75 ppm
Manganese	Skeletal abnormalities, decreased reproductive performance	C	60 ppm
		H	30 ppm
		P	60 ppm
Iodine	Goiter and consequences of thyroid hormone inadequacy	C	0.35 ppm
		H	0.30 ppm
		P	0.40 ppm
Selenium	Muscular dystrophy (White muscle disease), degeneration of myocardium, liver necroisis, pancreatic fibrosis	C	0.15 ppm
		H	0.1 ppm
		P	0.2 ppm

"available phosphorous" (meaning it will be phosphorus tied up in the phytate molecule). In commercial poultry diets, a phytate-degrading enzyme (called phytase) would be supplemented to break down this molecule and make the phosphorous more available.

Laying hens may also experience periods of thin-shelled eggs for numerous reasons. In many cases, the hen will sacrifice bone resorption to readily supply the calcium needed in the egg if it is not sufficiently available in the blood during shell formation. Long-term consequences of

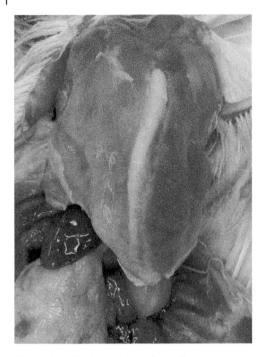

Figure 6.1 Keel angulation due to long-term consequences of cortical bone resorption from insufficient calcium in the diet.

cortical bone resorption can affect skeletal integrity, including keel angulation, long bone fractures, beading of ribs, and rib collapse. Supplementing additional calcium or phosphorus to the diet when the hen reaches these extremes will not alleviate long-term osteoporosis that has occurred. Any additional hydroxyapatite crystallization that occurs while the hen is laying eggs and circulating estrogen content is high will occur in the medullary portion of the bone. Rather, if a molt were induced through daylight length reduction to no more than 8 hours per day, a period of cortical bone remodeling could occur. Once adequate cortical bone regeneration has occurred, daylight length could be increased and another reproductive cycle could occur (albeit for a shortened duration).

Consequences of Diet Dilution

Small scale producers may also try to stretch their feed budget by purchasing a commercial diet, but diluting it directly or indirectly with other grains (often referred to as scratch grains), increasing the calories while reducing the protein, vitamin, and mineral content. General symptoms that usually occur when too low of nutrient density is fed are slow growth, slow, or cessation of egg production, and plausibly feather loss if the amino acid needs of the bird are not adequately met. Thus, while foraging behavior of hens can be desirable, the provision of scratch grains or diet dilution may compromise optimal performance. The total nutritional needs should be met by supplying supplemental feed formulated for the appropriate life stage of the birds.

Consequences of Feeding of the Wrong Life-Stage Diet (Hen Diet to a Nonlaying Bird)

A common mistake in feeding poultry can be as simple as feeding the wrong feed. For example, calcium levels in a layer feed will be upward of 4–5%, which can cause significant health problems in young birds that are not in lay. Also, growing broilers require as much as 23% protein, whereas laying hens and finishing broilers may need only 17–18%.

One of the common problems experienced with mixed age flocks, is avian urolithiasis and/or gout (Figure 6.2). Gout can occur as a result of numerous factors, but the commonality is demands for egg shell production

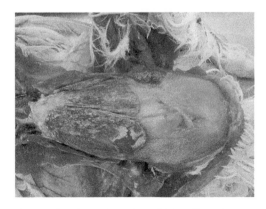

Figure 6.2 Visceral gout in a chicken. Note the urate deposits on the surface of the liver at necropsy.

along with prior renal damage. Predisposing factors could include infectious bronchitis, feeding of excessive levels of sodium bicarbonate (producing alkaline urine and an ideal medium for kidney stone formation), or, more commonly, a high-calcium (i.e., laying hen) diet to an immature bird. Even in commercial production, transition from birds not laying (i.e., the pullet phase) to laying is difficult to manage. Poultry species are photosensitive, and with increasing daylight lengths from 12 to 16 hours of daylight will induce egg production if the bird is old enough and proper body conditioning. Without housing where lighting is controlled, it can be difficult to match calcium needs of the bird coming into lay with proper, and not excessive, amounts of dietary calcium. Thus, the high (3.5–6%) calcium content of a laying hen diet can adversely affect the kidney in the proportion of the flock not in lay.

Changes to Nutrient Needs with Life Stages

Examples of changing nutrient and energy needs for egg-laying hens and broiler-type meat chicken strains are listed in Tables 6.4 and 6.5, respectively. Specific requirements for nutrient and energy can be found in the last National Research Council publication on the nutrient requirements for poultry published in 1994. Also, there are nutritional recommendations provided by the major commercial breeders for their strains. While there are recommended minimums for meeting bird's needs, realize that these may not be the concentrations needed for optimal or maximal productivity. Additionally, different strains of birds will also vary their intake due to factors such as environmental changes, disease state, and energy density of the diet. General nutrient needs for changing life phases are exemplified in Tables 6.4 (egg-laying strains) and 6.5 (broiler strains).

A general trend to notice for any type of poultry is that at the younger stages, birds require a greater nutrient density and diets will have slightly less energy than at the older stages. This reflects the changes going on in both the rate of growth and the maintenance energy requirement of the growing bird. A day-old broiler will not require very many calories to maintain its body condition, but it will quadruple its body weight in the first week of life, eating about 10–12% of its body weight per day. Then, as the bird ages and gets bigger, its growth rate slows down and the formulation will need less nutrient density but will need more energy to maintain the larger body size.

Table 6.4 Examples of changing nutrient needs for egg-laying chicken strains.

	Pullet starter	Pullet grower	Pre-lay	Hen	Rooster
Crude protein, %	20.00	18.62	18.40	18.30	11.54
Metabolizable energy, kcal/kg	3010	3005	2920	2890	3140
Calcium %	1.00	1.00	2.50	4.20	0.75
Phosphorus %	0.71	0.65	0.59	0.53	0.51
Available phosphorus, %	0.45	0.40	0.35	0.30	0.30
Methionine %	0.51	0.45	0.45	0.48	0.24
Methionine + cystine, %	0.85	0.77	0.77	0.79	0.47
Lysine, %	1.16	1.00	1.00	1.01	0.51
Threonine, %	0.77	0.72	0.71	0.71	0.44
Sodium, %	0.18	0.18	0.18	0.18	0.18

Table 6.5 Examples of changing nutrient and energy needs for broiler-meat type chicken strains.

	Broiler starter	Broiler grower	Broiler finisher
Crude protein %	22.50	18.25	17.50
Metabolizable energy, kcal/kg	3050	3175	3225
Calcium %	0.95	0.90	0.85
Available phosphorus, %	0.42	0.40	0.37
Methionine %	0.45	0.41	0.38
Methionine + cystine, %	0.88	0.83	0.75
Lysine, %	1.15	1.1	1.0
Sodium, %	0.18	0.15	0.15

Diet Formulation

Feed Ingredients and Feed Additives

While the nutrient needs of the bird for different life stages is fairly well defined (more so for commercial poultry strains), meeting them through the provision of combinations of ingredients into a diet can be accomplished with a range of ingredients and combinations thereof. Several ingredients, however, may contain antinutritional factors, toxic factors, and/or nutrient imbalances, which should be limited as a proportion of the diet. Considerations of maximal inclusions of certain feed ingredients are illustrated in Table 6.6.

All feedstuffs have the potential to be contaminated with mycotoxins in the field or during storage, and thus always should be monitored. For the backyard owner, it is also important to maintain proper storage of feed, as well as feeder hygiene. To prevent mycotoxin ingestion, make sure producers allow birds to clean up their feeders at least once a week, as well as never allow a bird to consume a visually moldy feed/feedstuff. Particular mycotoxins of concern and prevalence for poultry include that of aflatoxin, ochratoxin, T-2, and deoxynivalenol. All of these are of particular concern for young birds as they are more sensitive to their effects, but even older birds can be affected if there is long-term,

Table 6.6 Suggested ingredient maximums for feed ingredients for poultry for specific life stages.

Ingredient	Young birds <3 wk	>3 wk	Pullets	Laying hens
	(maximum, %)			
Corn bran	30	30	30	30
Barley	10	20	20	20
Rice bran	15	20	20	15
Wheat bran	10	15	15	15
Peanut meal	8	10	15	10
Fish meal	5	5	8	3
Blood meal	2	2	2	2
Palm oil	2	5	12	15

chronic ingestion. Some of these toxins have readily identifiable lesions while others do not. They are, in order of prevalence:

a) Aflatoxin – hepatic necrosis caused by free radical production, lipid peroxidation, and inhibition of RNA and protein synthesis. The liver will be enlarged and have a yellow/brown jaundice appearance. Aflatoxin is the only mycotoxin that can be readily adsorbed by certain feed additives (hydrated sodium/calcium alumninosilicates, bentonites, zeolites, and clinoptilotie).

b) T-2 toxin – causes contact dermatitis and can cause oral and dermal lesions within the mouth's palate, tongue, and/or corners of the mouth.

c) Ochratoxin – binds to plasma proteins and causes renal damage. Ochratoxin (of all the mycotoxins) causes the most body weight loss. In chronic cases, birds will have urate deposits in their joints and abdominal cavity. An increase in water consumption may occur, and polyurea is a common observation in the excreta.

d) Deoxynivalenol – does not have readily observable lesions but rather causes damage through inhibition of protein synthesis, thus making tissues with high protein turnover more susceptible (including the small intestine, bone marrow, lymph, spleen, and thymus). Of particular concern is damage to both the innate and acquired immune system, as well as the integrity of the gut lining.

Cereal Grains

Cereal grains are the primary energy source of the diet. These include ingredients such as corn, milo (grain sorghum), wheat, barley, oats, or triticale. Fiber content of the diet should be limited to 10–15% at a maximum. Higher amounts of fiber can be used, but litter wetness may become an issue, and lower-energy diets will have an impact on optimal performance. Several cereal grains also contain higher amounts of nonstarch polysaccharides (NSP) within the soluble fiber fraction. NSP increase the viscosity of the digesta, making digestion and absorption more difficult. For example, wheat-based diets will contain higher quantities of xylan sugars, which are not digestible by the bird. Also barley is high in an NSP known as β-glucans that can cause pasting of the beak and vent. In commercial poultry diets, NSP-degrading enzymes (e.g., a xylanase or a β-glucanase) would be supplemented to improve energy utilization if such ingredients were to be used. In addition to increasing intestinal digesta viscosity, higher content of NSP in a diet also increases mucin production. In many cases, this increased viscosity can predispose the bird to *Clostridium*

perfringens proliferation, and if prior intestinal damage has occurred (e.g., coccidial infection or mycotoxin contamination), *C. perfringens* can gain a foothold to cause a condition known as necrotic enteritis. Additional issues with cereals include that of rice bran, which can be high in trypsin inhibitors, and reduces the digestibility of protein and can result in feed passage (the presence of undigested feed in the feces).

Quality of feed ingredients should always be a concern. Particularly for grain ingredients, one needs to consider weed seed contamination, as certain weeds can be high in thiaminase activity. Grain byproducts are also readily available and, in the United States, include products of the dry and wet corn milling industries (gluten feed and hominy), from the brewing and distilling industries (wet or dry distiller's grains plus solubles), and wheat byproducts (wheat bran, wheat middlings, and screenings). Notably, many of these byproducts have mainly used the starch portion of the whole grain and thus, the fiber content may be higher, as well as the protein and fat fraction being more concentrated. While the protein content may be higher, typically it is of similar profile to that of the cereal grain itself and will still need a complement of amino acids from a legume and/or an animal byproduct meal to meet the amino acid needs of the bird.

Protein Sources

These are the primary amino acid source of the diet. Plant protein sources typically are from leguminous plant seeds, and are higher in protein than that of the cereal grains. The plant proteins' amino acid profiles complement the profile of cereal grains to help meet the amino acid needs of the bird. Specifically, corn has a much lower quantity of lysine and arginine relative to the requirement of poultry. However, an ingredient such as soybean meal has a much higher quantity of those amino acids, and so when mixed, the two ingredients provide an amino acid profile that better matches the needs of the bird. Often times, however, these needs cannot be fully met through the combination of the two types of ingredients and, therefore, supplemental amino acids must be added to the diet through addition of DL-methionine (or methyl hydroxyl analog), L-lysine HCl, and L-threonine. Typical protein meals from plant sources include soybean meal (without hulls containing 48% protein), canola meal (low glucosinalate varieties of rapeseed meal), corn gluten meal, peanut meal, peas, safflower meal, sunflower meal, sesame meal, and/or cottonseed meal.

Full-fat soybeans can also be fed (in addition to soybean meal), and provides additional energy compared with that of the meal. However, in both cases, raw soybeans contain a trypsin inhibitor that can be partially inactivated by heat. However, proper heating is essential as overheating will cause a Maillard reaction thus reducing lysine digestibility. Peanut meal is low in methionine, lysine, and threonine, high in tannins, and the trypsin inhibitors can only partially inactivated with heat. Cottonseed meal contains gossypol, an alkaloid, which if present in high enough levels in hens' diets can cause a discoloration to egg yolks, as well as cyclic fatty acids which may cause pink egg whites. Additional supplemental iron can be fed to partially alleviate these toxicities.

Animal byproducts can be used as protein sources, and include meat and bone meal, poultry byproduct meal, hydrolyzed feathermeal, fishmeal, and blood meal. Sources can be somewhat variable due to differing amounts of collagen, feathers, and hair, all of which have relatively low amino acid digestibility. Feathermeal, if processed properly by autoclaving to 145 °C for 30 minutes, can have improved digestibility but still has a relatively poor amino acid balance for poultry. Fish meal should be limited to only 2–3% to laying hens to prevent "fishy" tasting eggs. Fishmeal can also contain a thiaminase enzyme if not properly processed. It can also contain a biogenic amine (gizzerosine) known to cause gizzard (ventriculus) erosion and a condition called "black vomit." Blood meal can be a good source of lysine but is deficient in isoleucine and it can contain a high amount of sodium, which limits the amount of dietary inclusion. Proper processing is key for bloodmeal, as it has a greatly reduced amino acid availability if overheated (blackish in appearance).

Fats and Oils

These can supply a higher caloric density to the diet as well as reduce the dustiness of the diet and improve palatability. Typical sources include that of animal fats, vegetable oils, animal/vegetable oil blends, and restaurant grease. In poultry during their first 2 weeks of life, the digestibility of saturated fats is much less than that at older ages and thus accounted for in dietary formulation. Fats and oils need to be monitored routinely for quality control through the amount of free fatty acids, moisture content, unsaponifiable material, insoluble matter, and fatty acid stability. While unsaturated fats are more easily prone to oxidation, all fats are subject. Oxidation is catalyzed by any combination of trace metals, oxidative enzymes, light, and/or heat. Consequences of feeding oxidized fats to birds include degradation of the fat-soluble vitamins, increase in cellular membrane damage and friability, increase in intestinal enterocyte turnover rates, and reduction in xanthophyll content (and skin "bleaching"). Much of this damage occurs due to susceptibility to intracellular, extracellular, and membrane damage with reduced levels of antioxidants, especially vitamin E and glutathione peroxidase. Thus, often synthetic antioxidants such as ethyoxyquin, butylated hydroxytolulene, or butylated hydroxyanisole are included with the fat/oil source to suppress lipid oxidation.

Mineral Sources

Various mined sources are utilized primarily to provide needed macro- and micro-minerals to the diet. Calcium, phosphorus, and the electrolytes are macro-minerals usually provided separate from a trace mineral premix. Laying hens in particular can have a calcium-specific appetite, and thus many backyard poultry producers will provide a certain amount of oystershell or limestone for the birds to consume at will. A larger particle size of either of these two feedstuffs is also important to increase the amount of retention time in the gizzard (ventriculus). Ideally, two-thirds of calcium supplementation (in the mixed diet or otherwise) would come from a larger particle limestone or oystershell between 0.5 and 1.0 mm. This becomes important as the egg shell is being deposited onto the shell for 15–16 hours of the approximately 24 hours it takes to make an egg after ovulation of the follicle into the oviduct. Much of this occurs during the nighttime when the bird is not eating. Thus, having a slower release of calcium from the gizzard (ventriculus) helps supply some of the calcium need of the bird and can reduce the long-term resorption of medullary and cortical bone.

Phosphorus is typically supplied from dicalcium phosphate (18% phosphorus), mono- and di-calcium phosphate blends (21% phosphorus), and through the least bioavailable source, deflourinated rock phosphates (16% phosphorus) are also available.

Electrolytes supplemented into the diet include sodium chloride (salt), sodium bicarbonate, and potassium chloride. Imbalances in the electrolyte content can alter water intake, the regulation of blood pH, and certain enzyme reactions in the body. Micro-mineral sources in the mineral premix are supplemented either as sulfates, oxides, or as chelated forms with amino acids or proteins/peptides. Additional copper sulfate may be included in the diet (up to 1 pound per ton) to aide in prevention of mold growth and as an antimicrobial.

Other Feed Additives

Removal of sub-therapeutic antibiotics from poultry diets in Europe and the FDA's regulation of antibiotic use through Veterinary Feed Directives has led to recent pressure to reduce the use of these compounds or to raise birds without the use of antibiotics altogether. This has amplified interest and research into maintaining what specific functions growth-promoting levels of antibiotics elicit, namely: improving intestinal health, improving nutrient utilization, and reducing endogenous nutrient loss due, in part, to innate immune responses.

However, the ascribed "antibiotic replacements" used as feed additives have never been able to elicit the full range of physiological, microbiological, and immunological responses to that of sub-therapeutic antibiotics. Thus, poultry nutritionists can be hesitant to incorporate these categories feed additives due in part to (i) unfamiliarity, (ii) overselling of plausible effects, (iii) documented physiological and microbiological effects in vivo, and (iv) documentation of persistence from the feed and within the intestinal tract. Where antibiotic alternatives have documented effects, they largely have shown more narrow biological effects than that of sub-therapeutic antibiotics, including:

a) Organic acids (e.g., fumeric and propionic acids) – antimicrobial against gram-negative bacteria. Also, short-chain fatty acids (e.g. sodium butyrate), which promote intestinal development and the integrity of the intestinal lining.
b) Plant extracts (e.g., essential oils from oregano, thyme, cinnaminaldehyde) – varied physiological functions, including antimicrobial, altered intestinal mucin production, reduction in intestinal "turnover," and antioxidant capacity.
c) Probiotics (direct-fed microbials) – specific pathogen(s) exclusion, immunological modulation, improved nutrient use, antimicrobial action through pH modification and bacteriocin production.
d) Prebiotics (e.g., hydrolyzed yeast cell wall) – promote the growth of commensal microbes in the gut and reduce the ability of certain bacteria from attaching to the intestinal lining.

Additional feed additives can include antibiotics, coccidiostats (chemical or ionophore), mold inhibitors, mycotoxin binders, antioxidants, pigmenting agents, and pellet binders.

Interpreting a Feed Tag

Commercial feed that can be purchased will not have an exhaustive list of nutrient composition as was provided in Tables 6.4 or 6.5. Rather, it will likely contain a list of feedstuffs along with guaranteed minimums and maximums as illustrated in Table 6.7. Notably, the two most "limiting" amino acids for poultry in corn/soybean meal diets are that of methionine and lysine, and therefore are listed. As mentioned previously, a multitude of feedstuff combinations can be made to meet nutrient needs at various life stages. Example rations comprised primarily of corn and soybean meal are given in Table 6.8 (egg-type chicken strains) and Table 6.9 (broiler/meat chicken strains).

Table 6.7 Example of the nutrient minimums and maximum listings on a typical feed tag.

• Crude protein (CP)	min 26%
• Lysine	min 1.5%
• Methionine	min 0.5%
• Crude fat	min 6.0%
• Crude fiber	max 4.0%
• Calcium (Ca)	min 1.1%
• Calcium	max 1.5%
• Phosphorus (P)	min 0.8%
• Salt	min 0.4%
• Salt	max 0.7%

Summary

Nutrition is imperative to successful growth, reproductive performance, and health of the backyard flock. The fundamentals outlined in this chapter touch on the most common nutritional issues experienced by the small flock owner. More in-depth information is available in the following resources.

Table 6.8 Examples of diet formulation for egg-laying strains of chickens.

Ingredient	Pullet chick starter	Pullet grower	Laying hen	Rooster
		(%)		
Corn	66.8	66.8	54.35	85.93
Soybean meal (48% protein)	28.46	28.46	29.54	10.96
Soy oil	0.8	0.8	3.91	—
Sodium chloride (salt)	0.41	0.41	0.41	0.41
DL-Methionine	0.15	0.15	0.19	0.03
Limestone	1.8	1.8	10.42	1.42
Monocalcium phosphate	1.23	1.23	0.83	0.9
Vitamin/mineral premix	0.35	0.35	0.35	0.35

Table 6.9 Examples of diet formulation for broiler/meat strains of chickens.

Ingredient	Broiler starter	Broiler grower	Broiler finisher
	(%)		
Corn	57.66	63.76	66.9
Soybean meal (48% protein)	35.27	29.68	26.3
Soy oil	3.00	3.00	3.52
Sodium chloride (salt)	0.48	0.46	0.48
DL-Methionine	0.24	0.21	0.12
Lysine, HCl	0.11	0.10	0.02
L-Threonine	0.06	0.04	—
Limestone	1.41	1.38	1.49
Monocalcium phosphate	1.42	1.02	0.82
Vitamin/mineral premix	0.35	0.35	0.35

References

1 Havenstein, G.B., Ferket, P.R., Scheidler, S.E., and Larson, B.T. (1994). Growth, livability, and feed conversion of 1991 vs 1957 broilers when fed "typical" 1957 and 1991 broiler diets. *Poult. Sci.* 73: 1785–1794.

2 Havenstein, G.B., Ferket, P.R., and Qureshi, M.A. (2003). Growth, livability, and feed conversion of 1957 versus 2001 broilers when fed representative 1957 and 2001 broiler diets. *Poult. Sci.* 82: 1500–1508.

3 Collins, K.E., Kiepper, B.H., Ritz, C.W. et al. (2014). Growth, livability, feed consumption, and carcass composition of the Athens Canadian Random Bred 1955 meat-type chicken versus the 2012 high-yielding Cobb 500 broiler. *Poult. Sci.* 93: 2953–2962.

4 Carter, T.A. and Sneed, R.E. (1987). Drinking water quality for poultry. P&T Guide No. 42, Extension Poultry Science, North Carolina State University, Raleigh, N.C.

5 National Research Council (1994). *Nutrient Requirements of Poultry*, 9e. Washington, DC: National Academy Press.

Further Reading

Applegate, T.J. and Angel, R. (2008a). Phosphorus requirements for poultry. AS-583-W Purdue Univ. Coop. Ext. Publ. http://www.extension.purdue.edu/extmedia/AS/AS-583-W.pdf (accessed 10-3-18)

Applegate, T.J. and Angel, R. (2008b). Variation in nutrient utilization by poultry and ingredient composition. AS-585-W Purdue Univ. Coop. Ext. Publ. http://www.extension.purdue.edu/extmedia/AS/AS-585-W.pdf (accessed 10-3-18)

Applegate, T.J. and Angel, R. (2008c). Protein and amino acid requirements for poultry. AS-584-W Purdue Univ. Coop. Ext. Publ. http://www.extension.purdue.edu/extmedia/AS/AS-584-W.pdf (accessed 10-3-18)

Leeson, S. and Summers, J.D. (eds.) (2009). *Commercial Poultry Nutrition*, 3e. Sheffield, England: Notingham University Press.

Diaz, D. (2005). *The Mycotoxin Blue Book*. Sheffield, England: Notingham University Press.

Fairchild, B.D. and Ritz, C. (2012). Poultry drinking water primer. UGA Cooperative Extension Bulletin 1301. http://www.caes. uga.edu/applications/publications/files/ pdf/B%201301_3.pdf (accessed 10-3-18)

Leeson, S. and Summers, J.D. (2001). *Nutrition of the Chicken*, 4e. Guelph, Ontario, Canada: University Books.

National Research Council (1994). *Nutrient Requirements of Poultry*, 9e. Washington, DC: National Academy Press.

Pesti, G.M., Bakalli, R.I., Driver, J.P. et al. (2005). *Poultry Nutrition and Feeding*. Victoria, British Columbia, Canada: Traford Publishing.

Section 2

Initial Examinations

7

Anatomy and Physiology

Wael Khamas and Josep Rutllant-Labeaga

College of Veterinary Medicine, Western University of Health Sciences, Pomona, CA, USA

Anatomy and Physiology

Understanding the anatomy of chickens allows for recognition of normal versus abnormal findings and for an accurate description of abnormalities in the record. Only the relevant anatomical/physiological differences that differ from mammals will be included in the descriptions that follow.

Body Regions

The body regions divide the surface of the entire animal and can be subdivided into sub-regions with special clinical interest [1].

Head and Neck Regions

Several regions can be identified on the head including nasal, nasal arch, forehead, orbital, suborbital, crown, postorbital, anterior dorsal neck, posterior dorsal neck, lateral neck, and anterior ventral neck (Figure 7.1).

The natural orifices on the head (the eyes, external acoustic meatuses, nasal openings, and mouth) as well as the ornamental structures (comb, wattles, ear lobes) are frequently used to identify certain clinical signs in the diseased chicken. The ornamental structures differ in size between male and female chickens even at a young age, being more developed and much larger in size in the male (Figures 7.2).

External Trunk and Lower Extremities Regions

Major body regions that can be identified on a chicken include metatarsal, ankle, abdominal, knee, sternal, prolateral, wing, ventral abdomen, crop, ventral neck, lateral neck, and posterior dorsal neck regions (Figure 7.3).

Wing Regions (Ventral Aspect)

Wing regions may be used for blood collections or examination for external parasites and abnormal feather conditions. These regions include prolateral, shoulder, upper arm, forearm, prepatagium, wrist, hand, and alular patagium [1, 2] (Figure 7.4).

Backyard Poultry Medicine and Surgery: A Guide for Veterinary Practitioners, Second Edition.
Edited by Cheryl B. Greenacre and Teresa Y. Morishita.
© 2021 John Wiley & Sons, Inc. Published 2021 by John Wiley & Sons, Inc.
Companion website: www.wiley.com/go/greenacre/medicine

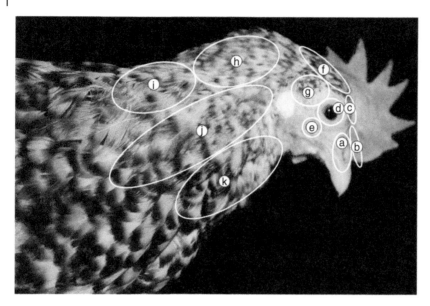

Figure 7.1 Regions of the head and neck of an adult female chicken. (a) Nasal; (b) nasal arch; (c) forehead; (d) orbital; (e) suborbital; (f) crown; (g) postorbital; (h) anterior dorsal neck; (i) posterior dorsal neck; (j) lateral neck; (k) anterior ventral neck.

(A)   (B)

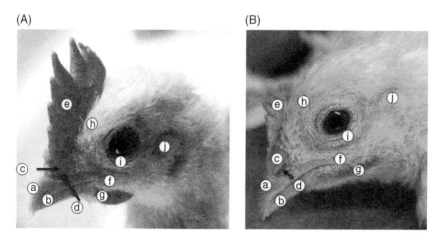

Figure 7.2 **A&B** External features of the head of a 5-week-old male (A) and female (B) chicks. (a) superior (maxillary) beak; (b) inferior (mandibular) beak; (c) operculum; (d) external nares; (e) comb (compare sizes between male and female of the same age); (f) maxillary rictus; (g) wattle; (h) frontal feathers, (i) eye feathers, (j) ear feathers.

Skeletal Anatomy

Only characteristic features of the chicken skeleton will be described here. Birds, in general, are noted for their exceptionally large eyes, which are accommodated by equivalently large orbits in the skull (Figure 7.5). The two bony orbits are separated from each other by an ossified partition, the interorbital septum. The quadrate bone is a very complex bone that articulates with the mandible to help in jaw suspension. It also forms the pivotal bone for the kinetic jaw mechanism.

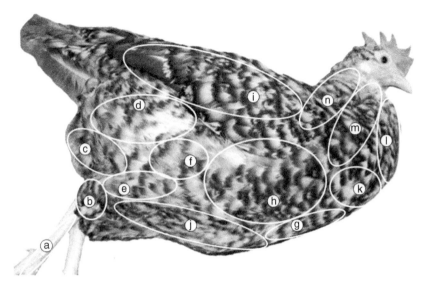

Figure 7.3 Body regions of adult female chicken. (a) metatarsal; (b) ankle; (hock) (c) abdominal; (d) prolateral; (e) shank; (f) knee; (g) sternal; (h) prolateral; (i) wing; (j) ventral abdomen; (k) crop; (l) ventral neck; (m) lateral neck; (n) posterior dorsal neck.

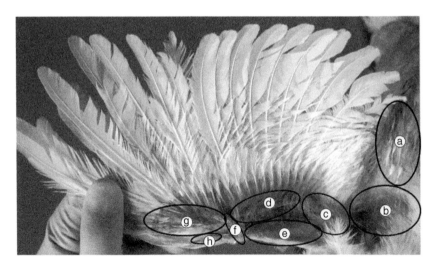

Figure 7.4 Regions of the ventral aspect of the wing of a 4-week-old chick. (a) prolateral; (b) shoulder; (c) upper arm; (d) forearm; (e) propatagium; wrist (carpus) (f) wrist; (g) hand region (area of major and minor metacarpal) (h) alular patagium.

The chicken has a single occipital condyle that articulates with a small ring-shaped atlas. The cervical vertebrae have characteristic saddle-shaped articular processes. In the last two cervical vertebrae, the vertebral segment of the ribs can be identified. The chicken has four to six thoracic vertebrae, and the lumbar and sacral vertebrae are fused into a structure called the synsacrum. The caudal vertebrae vary in number, and several of them fuse to form the pygostyle (plowshare, rump post) [3, 4].

There are seven pairs of true ribs. Except for the first and the last, the ribs have uncinate processes that overlap the succeeding rib, giving rigidity to the rib cage. In the sternum

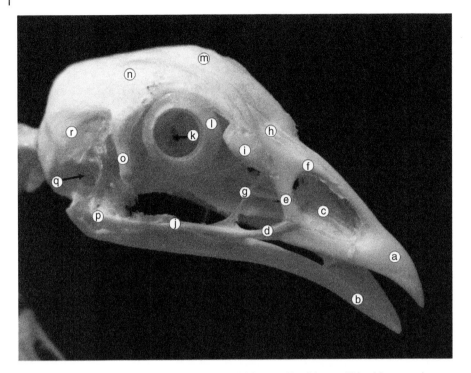

Figure 7.5 Bone of the skull of adult chicken. (a) Premaxilla; (b) mandible; (c) external nares opening (d) maxilla; (e) lateral ramus of the nasal; (f) nasal; (g) lacrimal process (h) nasal frontal suture; (i) lacrimal (prefrontal) (j) jugal bar (k) optic foramen; (l) scleral ring (bone); (m) frontal; (n) parietal; (o) postorbital process; (p) quadrojugal; (q) external acoustic meatus; (r) squamosal.

(breast bone), the keel (carina) can be identified and serves as the origin of major flight musculature (pectorals and supracoracoid). The pectoral girdle is comprised of three pairs of bones that support the wings: fused clavicle (furcula), coracoids, and scapulae (Figure 7.6). They come together dorsally leaving a triosseal canal (foramen triosseal) through which the tendon of the supracoracoid muscle passes to insert on the humerus. It acts to elevate the humerus and the wing.

The hyoid apparatus of the chicken is unique and is composed of several segments [5]:

1) Paraglossal (entoglossal), which extends into the free portion of the tongue
2) Two cornua extended laterally from the paraglossal bone forming the wide base of the tongue
3) Rostral basibranchial (basihyal) bone lies in the fixed portion of the tongue

4) Caudal basibranchial (urohyal) bone
5) Ceratobranchial bone
6) Epibranchial bone.

Myology

Because of the complexity of this system and the large number of muscles present on the chicken body, only those related to the wing and leg will be highlighted because they are anatomical landmarks for clinically relevant structures and procedures. The relevant muscles of the thoracic limb are latissimus dorsi, rhomboid, deltoid, coracoid, propatagial, scapulohumeral, trapezius, extensor carpi ulnaris, extensor carpi radialis, biceps brachii, triceps brachii, pronator, digital muscles, flexor carpi ulnaris, and alular muscles (Figures 7.7–7.9).

In the pelvic limb, to find the sciatic (ischiadic) nerve, the sartorius, quadriceps femoris,

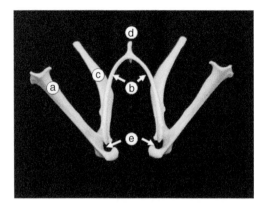

Figure 7.6 Thoracic limb girdle of the chicken. (a) coracoid; (b) clavicle; (c) scapula; (d) apophysis furculi (hypocleidum, lamina interclavicularis); (e) foramen triosseum (triosseal canal).

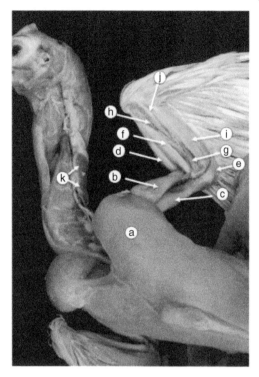

Figure 7.8 Ventral view of the muscles of the wing of an embalmed rooster. (a) thoracic pectoral (superficial); (b) biceps brachii; (c) triceps brachii (humeral head); (d) extensor carpi radialis; (e) expansor secondarum (dermoulnaris); (f) pronator superficialis (longus – deep et brevis – superficial); (g) deep pronator; (h) extensor indicis digital major (longus); (i) flexor carpi ulnais; (j) deep digital flexor (flexor digitorum sublimis); (k) thymus.

Skin and Appendages

Generally, the skin of poultry is thin and loosely attached to the body. Apterylae, non-feathered skin, is covered with extremely thin keratinized stratified squamous epithelium. In the areas where feathers are present on the skin (pterylae), a similar type of thin but highly keratinized stratified squamous epithelium is present. However, the amount of keratin increases as it approaches the feathers.

The spur (metatarsal spur) is a horny structure present on the caudal surface of the leg of domestic fowl (Figure 7.11). It is well developed in males and may reach several inches in length, while it is less developed in female fowl

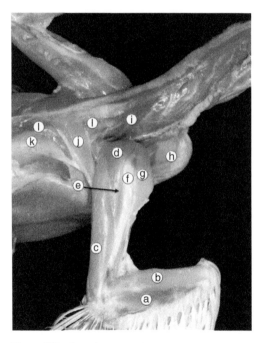

Figure 7.7 Dorsal aspect of the shoulder girdle of adult rooster. (a) extensor carpi (metacarpi) ulnaris; (b) extensor carpi (metacarpi) radialis; (c) triceps brachii; (d) deltoid major; (e) superficial coracoid; (f) humerus; (g) propatagial (deltoideus pars propatagialis; tensor propatagialis; pars longa/ brevis); (h) crop (ingluvies); (i) longissimus dorsi (cervical portion); (j) scapulohumeralis; (k) latissimus dorsi; (l) tapezius.

femrotibial, flexor crural medial, and lateral muscles should be identified (Figure 7.10) [6–8].

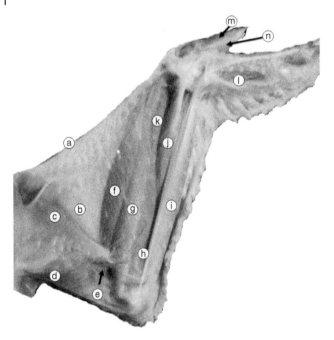

Figure 7.9 Ventral aspect of the left wing of adult rooster after complete removal of the feathers. (a) Skin of patagial fold and embedded within it is the propatagial ligament; (b) propatagium; (c) biceps brachii; (d) triceps brachii (humeral head); (e) basilic vein; (f) extensor carpi radialis (extensor metacarpi radialis); (g) superficial pronator; (h) deep pronator; (i) flexor carpi ulnaris; (j) deep digital flexor; (k) extensor indicis longus (extensor digiti longus majoris); (l) interosseous palmaris (ventralis); (m) abductor alulae (policis); (n) adductor alulae (policis).

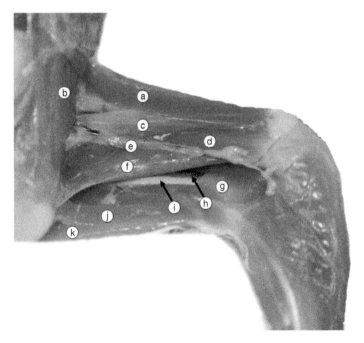

Figure 7.10 Medial aspect of the thigh of a chicken. (a) Cranial iliotibial (sartorius) m., (b) external abdominal oblique m., (c) quadriceps femoris/ambiens m., (d) internal femorotibial m., (e) circumflex femoral (femoral) artery, (f) adductor/puboischiofemoral m., (g), accessory head of puboischiofemoral m., (h) ischiatic (sciatic) artery and vein, (i) ischiatic nerve; (j) flexor crural medialis, (k) flexor crural lateralis.

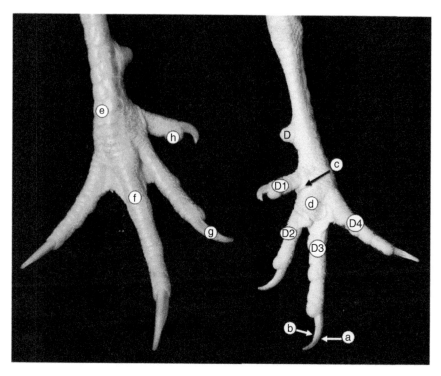

Figure 7.11 Right metatarsal and digits of adult chicken. (a) claw dorsal plate; (b) claw ventral plate; (c) metatarsal fold; (d) metatarsal pad; (e) metatarsal scutes; (f) carpal scutes; (g) claw; (h) digital pad; D. spur; D1–4 digits.

and could be very small. The spur may need to be trimmed, especially in larger breeds, as it results in injury of the back of the female during mating. This is more obvious in the heavy breeds [9, 10]. Chickens have four digits, or toes, numbering 1, 2, 3, and 4 medial to lateral, with 2, 3, 4, and 5 phalanges, respectively.

The comb and other ornamental structures differ among different breeds of poultry, and they are usually well developed in males (Figures 7.4 and 7.10). These structures are routinely used to detect the general health condition of chickens. The process of comb removal is called dubbing and if done is usually performed on day-old-chicks to avoid trauma from cannibalism or frostbite in cold climates. After caponization (castration), the comb shrinks in size, as its development is dependent on the androgen hormone level.

The ear lobes (ear flaps) are extensions of the skin with modified underlying tissues (Figure 7.4). The surface of the ear lobes is covered with a few cell layers of stratified squamous epithelium with little keratinization.

Double folds of skin extend downwards from the head region creating the wattles, which have two surfaces medial and lateral (see Figure 7.12). There are no feathers on the wattle in an adult chicken; however, with advancing age the folds will be drawn downwards carrying medially short feathers with it.

The uropygial gland, also known as the oil, preen, rump, caudal, or perunctum gland, is associated with the skin of the dorsal aspect of the caudal rump region. The gland has two lobes separated by an interlobular septum, which continues with the gland capsule. The gland duct from each primary cavity is carried through the papilla to its tip where it opens to the outside as the uropygial duct. The gland often elevates the dorsal skin of the tail to produce the uropygial eminence.

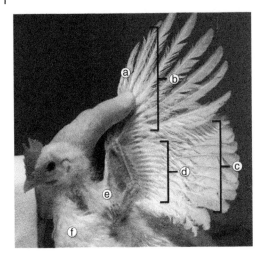

Figure 7.12 External features showing the wing feathers on a four-week-old male chick. (a) Alulae; (b) primary feathers (I-X); (c) secondary feathers (I-XVIII); (d) under cover for secondary feathers; (e) under wing feathers; (f) chest feathers.

The body of the chicken is covered with feathers apart from few regions, depending on the species and breed (Figure 7.12). The main type of feather covering the body are called contour feathers or pinnae. In general, the feathers can be described as consisting of a shaft (quill) and the vane [11, 12] (Figure 7.13). The shaft is composed of two portions, the calamus (proximal portion implanted in the skin) and the long solid segment above it called the rachis. On each side of the shaft, barbs and barbules are attached to form the vane (Figure 7.21).

Digestive System

The digestive system of the chicken consists of the beak, mouth, tongue, esophagus, crop, proventriculus, ventriculus, small intestine, and large intestine. The coprodeum is a portion of the cloaca that ultimately leads to the vent and is considered a continuation, or the end point, of the digestive system [13].

The *beak* is a highly keratinized structure covering the jaws (Figure 7.22). It is also known as the ramphotheca. It is pointed at its tip and composed of upper (superior, maxillary) and lower (inferior, mandibular) portions that meet at the angle of the mouth. The mandible forms the lower part of the beak. The base of the beak is sharply convex in the upper portion where it forms the operculum. The operculum covers the external nares in 1-day-old chicks. The keratinized region of the beak is supported caudally by the jawbones. The outer dorsal surface of the beak is keratinized, and the midline is called the culmen. The cutting edges of the

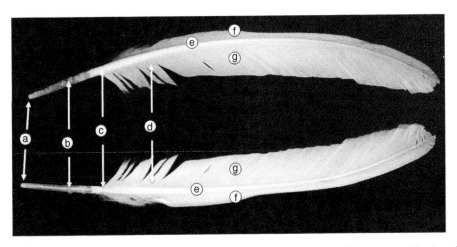

Figure 7.13 Adult male primary feather (remix). (a) Inferior umbilicus; (b) remnant of feather sheath; (c) calamus (quill); (d) barbs; (e) rachis; (f) anterior barbs; (g) posterior barbs.

beak are called tomia (singular tomium). When the mouth is closed, the two edges of the beak do not come together as the lower edge glides inside the edges of the upper beak.

A small protrusion (egg tooth) is found in 1-day-old chicks at the surface of the upper beak. It is used to break the shell of the egg during hatching and is usually shed soon after. The process of cutting the beak is called de-beaking, and if done, is preferably performed on 1-day-old chicks, as the beak is a highly innervated structure. One third of the distance from the tip of the beak is usually cut to prevent bleeding. De-beaking is routinely exercised in laying breeds to prevent cannibalism and picking of each other's feathers, especially under crowded conditions and if mineral deficiencies are present.

In the *mouth* (oral) cavity, the hard palate is incomplete and communication between oral and nasal cavities exists through a slit-like midline opening, the choana (Figure 7.14). The surface of the hard palate has several visible ridges with caudally oriented papillae. The cheeks are very much reduced, and the floor of

the mouth cavity has the median fold of the mucosal membrane connected to the free portion of the tongue and is called the lingual frenulum.

There are large numbers of salivary glands present in the roof and floor of the oral cavity, body of the tongue, and pharyngeal wall. They usually open by several ducts into the oral and pharyngeal cavities (Figure 7.14).

The *tongue* (glossa, lingua) is a pointed organ in the chicken and has a triangular shape in a cross section, adapting to the space of the lower beak where it lies. The tongue has a hyaline cartilage inside its rostral portion. This cartilage is an extension of the entoglossal portion of the hyoid apparatus that can be found in the caudal lingual segment or root. The tongue is covered by extremely thick stratified squamous epithelium on the dorsal surface and a much thinner and highly keratinized type of epithelium on the ventral surface.

The *pharynx* is a thickened muscular tube that connects the oral cavity to the digestive and respiratory systems. In the dorsal aspect of the pharynx, the opening of the infundibular

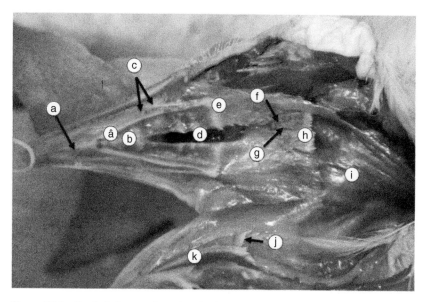

Figure 7.14   Roof of the mouth cavity of adult chicken. (a) median swelling; ā. Lateral palatine ridge; (b) palate; (c) opening of lateral palatine glands; (d) palatine (choanal) cleft; (e) papillae; (f) medial palatine glands; (g) infundibular cleft; (h) pharyngeal papillae; (i) pharynx; (j) lingual papillae; (k) tongue.

slit (Eustachian or auditory tubes openings) is present. There are rough caudally directed papillae similar to those described in the oral cavity. The caudal portion of the pharynx is connected to the esophagus. The floor of the pharynx is formed by the root of the tongue. The area of the junction between the pharynx and the esophagus is lined by a thick highly keratinized stratified squamous epithelium with papillae. Keratinization of the epithelium decreases, as well as the number of glands, as the esophagus is approached. A characteristic smooth muscle layer of the lamina muscularis mucosae starts to appear at this junction, where lymphoid follicles or tonsils are also present.

The *esophagus* is a muscular tube connecting the pharynx to the stomach. It has two distinct parts: the cervical and the thoracic part. The cervical part connects the pharynx to the crop, while the thoracic portion connects the crop to the proventriculus [14]. The crop is relatively large in diameter, and researchers consider it an embryonic dilation of the esophagus before it enters the thoracic cavity.

The cervical esophagus is shorter than the vertebral column of the neck. It starts dorsal to the larynx and trachea and, caudal to the fifth cervical vertebra, it lies on the right side of the neck. Close to the entrance into the thoracic cavity, the esophagus returns to the midline and enlarges ventrally to form the crop. The thoracic esophagus is much shorter than the cervical part and extends dorsal to the trachea along the base of the heart. The most caudal portion of the esophagus is reduced in diameter.

The crop (ingluvies) is a large thin-walled diverticulum, which can store food for a short period of time. It differs in shape and size among different breeds of poultry. In chicken, it is displaced toward the right side of the median plane, in front of the furcula, on the pectoral muscles. The crop is only covered by the skin and can be palpated easily when it is full [15]. On the dorsal wall surface of the crop, there is a cleft or a channel (crop channel) and easily digestible food may pass through it directly to the proventriculus.

The crop is lined by stratified squamous epithelium, which contains mucus glands at the crop channel only. The "crop milk" is produced by these glands.

The proventriculus (glandular stomach) is connected to the esophagus orally and to the muscular stomach (ventriculus, gizzard) aborally (Figure 7.15). It is a fusiform structure and has no separating point or clear sphincter

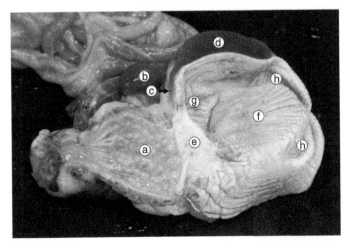

Figure 7.15 Chicken stomach interior structures. (a) proventriculus; (b) spleen; (c) thin muscle; (d) thick muscle; (e) intermediate zone (isthmus); (f) body (fundus); (g) cranial blind sac; (h) caudal blind sac.

with the esophagus. When the proventriculus is cut open, large numbers of papillae (openings of the glands) appear on the surface. The proventriculus has a typical tubular organ layers arrangement [14, 15]. The mucosa is represented by folds of simple columnar epithelium. Loose connective tissue with lymphatic cells is present in the lamina propria. In several areas, these cells form well-defined lymphatic nodules extending in a few places into the tunica submucosa. Thin scattered layers of well-defined lamina muscularis mucosae are present. Large compound tubular glands almost completely occupy the tunica mucosa [16, 17] (Figure 7.16).

The intermediate zone is the area of connection between the proventriculus and the ventriculus (gizzard). This segment is relatively short and has the characteristic features of the wall of the ventriculus in an unorganized way.

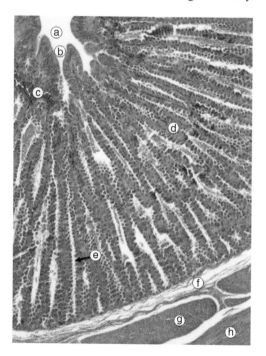

Figure 7.16 Cross section of proventriculus of an adult chicken. (a) Lumen of the gland; (b) simple columnar epithelium; (c) blood capillaries in the lamina propria; (d) body of the gland; (e) lumen of individual gland; (f) lamina propria; (g) muscularis mucosa; (h) inner muscular layer. Stained with H&E stain, magnification ×120.

The ventriculus (muscular stomach, gizzard) is a muscular flattened structure connecting the proventriculus to the duodenum. It is composed of four definitive muscular portions separated by constrictions and connected in the middle by a thick aponeurotic region (cranial dorsal, cranial ventral, caudal dorsal, and caudal ventral). The gizzard interior compartments are named anterior cul-de-sac and posterior cul-de-sac with a middle cavity connecting the two (body). The inner surface of the ventriculus is covered by a thick keratinized yellowish layer, which at necropsy or at butchering, can be stripped easily from the surface, as it is the secretion of the glands. The yellowish coloration results from the antiperistaltic movements of the small intestine, which brings contents from the initial portion of the duodenum. The epithelium has a thick layer on the surface called koilin that some authors call the horny layer of the stomach.

The *duodenum* is the first segment of the small intestine; it starts at the ventriculus and ends at the jejunum. It forms a long loop of descending and ascending portions. These two portions are connected by a fold of peritoneum (interduodenal ligament) (Figure 7.17). The pancreas is lodged between these two portions and extends the entire length of the duodenal loop. The site of termination of the descending duodenum and the beginning of the jejunum is considered the area of opening of the pancreatic and bile ducts.

The *jejunum* forms loose coils and has a long mesentery (Figure 7.18). The Meckel diverticulum (vitelline diverticulum) is a short blind remnant of the embryonic yolk sac and yolk stalk that is located on the surface of the jejunum (Figure 7.19).

The *ileum* is relatively short, and it is the last segment of the small intestine. It is lodged between the two ceca and attached by a fold of peritoneum called the ileocecal ligament/fold. The ileum has a relatively thicker wall when compared to the duodenum or jejunum.

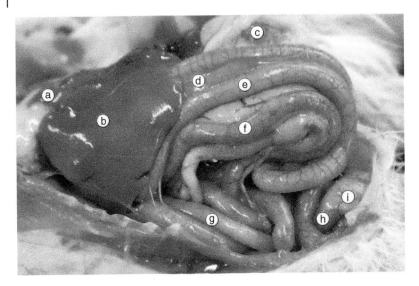

Figure 7.17 Visceral organs of adult chicken in situ. (a) heart; (b) liver; (c) gizzard (ventriculus); (d) pancreas; (e) duodenum; (f) cecum; (g) jejunum; (h) rectum (colorectum); (i) cloaca.

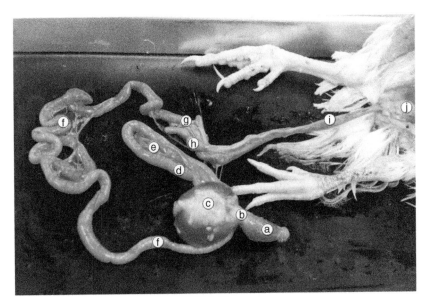

Figure 7.18 Digestive system of adult chicken removed from the body to show different segments starting at the proventriculus. (a) proventriculus; (b) intermediate zone; (c) gizzard (ventriculus); (d) duodenum; (e) pancreas; (f) jejunum; (g) ileum; (h) cecum; (i) colorectum; (j) cloaca.

The chicken has a pair of blind end sacs or ducts called ceca (Figure 7.17). They are smaller in diameter at their origin and wider as they ascend into the blind end. The ceca are lined by highly folded simple columnar villiated epithelium with relatively large numbers of goblet cells. Simple branched tubular glands extend down into the lamina propria.

The *colon* (colorectum) of the chicken is well delineated as it starts from the ileocecal junction and transitions to the *rectum*; therefore, it is also known as the colorectum (Figure 7.20). It is

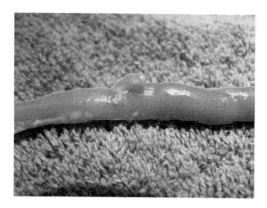

Figure 7.19 Meckel diverticulum (vitelline diverticulum) is a short blind remnant of the embryonic yolk sac and yolk stalk that is located on the surface of the jejunum. (Photograph courtesy of Dr. Cheryl B. Greenacre.)

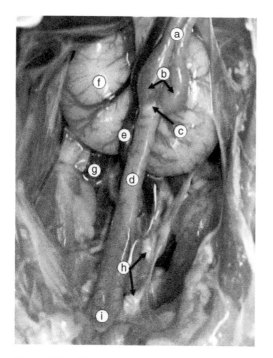

Figure 7.20 Dissected rooster showing testes and relationship to the distal segments of the intestinal tract. (a) Ceca; (b) cecal tonsils; (c) ileocecocolic junction; (d) colorectum; (e) common mesenteric vein; (f) testis; (g) kidney; (h) ductus deferens; (i) cloaca.

connected distally to the cloaca. Generally, it is a short and straight tubular structure. The internal surface of the colon appears folded with villi

and lined by simple columnar epithelium with large numbers of goblet cells.

The *cloaca* is the dilated end of the digestive and urogenital systems. It is composed of three compartments: The first (coprodeum) connects to the colorectum while the second (urodeum) is associated with the ureters and the genital system. The third compartment is the proctodeum, which opens to the outside through the vent. A well-developed fold of mucous membrane separating the coprodeum from the urodeum is usually seen (coprourodeal fold). An incomplete circular fold separating the proctodeum from the urodeum is called proctourodeal fold. The inner surface of the cloaca is thrown into folds and lined by simple columnar epithelium with goblet cells.

The external caudal opening of the cloaca is the vent, which has dorsal and ventral labii and a labial cleft between the two. An abrupt change in the type of epithelium is observed at the junction of the distal portion of the cloaca and the vent. The keratinization and the thickness of the stratified squamous epithelium decrease as it moves away from the vent to join the skin. In this area, it is composed of one or two cell layers with thin keratin covering. Herbst corpuscles are present in this area and close to the feather follicles [17, 18].

Liver (Hepar, Jecur)

The color of the liver is yellow in 1-day-old chick as it has pigments from the yolk lipids at the late stage of incubation. On the other hand, the liver in adult chickens varies in color depending on the nutritional status, general health condition, and method of sacrifice [7]. The normal color is reddish brown, light brown, to yellow. The liver can be easily seen when the abdominal wall is cut open (Figure 7.17). The liver is divided into two lobes with the right lobe larger than the left. The left lobe is clearly divided into two lobes (dorsal and ventral). The caudal vena cava passes through the cranial region of the right lobe close to its dorsal edge. The fusiform gall bladder lies on the visceral surface of the right lobe. Each liver lobe is drained by a bile duct. The so-called hepatocystic duct drains bile from the right lobe to the gallbladder, while the common hepatoenteric duct drains bile from both lobes to the duodenum [19, 20]. Histologically, the liver lobules are not well delineated, and each lobule is composed of hepatic cords arranged around a central vein. These cords are composed of double hepatocytes, while other histological characteristics are similar to those found in mammals [16, 17].

The hepatic portal vein is the functional circulation of the liver. It collects blood from the gastrointestinal tract except for the caudal portion of the cloaca, the pancreas, the spleen, and the air sacs. The hepatic portal vein divides to enter the right and left lobes of the liver.

Pancreas

The pancreas is situated inside the loop of the duodenum, inside a fold of peritoneum called the duodenopancreatic fold. Dorsal and ventral lobes, as well as a small segment rich in islets of Langerhans lying close to the spleen known as the splenic lobe, can be identified. This latter lobe is very thin and embedded in the adipose tissue and may be difficult to visualize but can be identified microscopically. The pancreas has three ducts: two from the ventral and one from the dorsal lobe, with the splenic lobe having no separate excretory duct. The pancreatic and bile ducts open into the ascending part of the duodenum opposite the cranial part of the muscular stomach. The exocrine portion is composed of compound tubuloalveolar glands. The lobulations of the gland are not as clear as in mammals because of the low quantity of connective tissue. However, the lobation is obvious externally.

The endocrine portion of the pancreas is composed of islets of Langerhans. These islets are scattered circular structures in between the exocrine portion of different lobes. They are usually surrounded by a thin layer of connective tissue. The cells inside the islets are arranged in the form of branching cords separated by sinusoidal capillaries. Researchers describe two types of islets, alpha and beta. Alpha islets are larger and usually present inside the splenic lobe and at the site of the junction of the ventral and dorsal lobes. These islets are also called the dark islets because they stain with argyntaffine (argyrophilic staining) and are associated with glucagon production. These islets have alpha and delta cells. Beta islets are scattered randomly in all pancreatic lobes. They are smaller than alpha islets and contain beta cells and a few delta cells. Beta islets are also called light islets because they do not take the argyrophilic stain and are associated with insulin production [21].

Respiratory System

The respiratory system consists of the nasal cavity, upper larynx (glottis), trachea, lower larynx (syrinx), lungs, and air sacs.

The nasal cavity has three conchae (rostral, middle, and caudal) and it opens posteriorly through the choanae to the pharynx. The choanae appear as a single slit in the roof of the mouth. The upper larynx (cranial larynx, glottis) is composed of cricoid and arytenoid cartilages only. It connects the pharynx to the trachea. The trachea is a long flexible tube made up of complete articulating cartilaginous rings (signet shape) connected cranially with the upper larynx and distally with the lower larynx (syrinx). These rings tend to become ossified with age, especially at the distal part close to the syrinx [22, 23]. They have narrow and wide portions to fit with adjacent rings to form a continuous tube of overlapping rings. No true trachealis muscle is present in the chicken, but two well-developed skeletal muscles ascend on both sides of the trachea. Each tracheal ring has a thickened segment at the periphery and is extremely thin at both the dorsal and the ventral sides. The syrinx is the organ of phonation in some species of birds and is considered a second larynx [22, 24]. It is situated at the distal end of the trachea and at the beginning of the lungs. The syrinx is composed of several modified tracheal cartilages fused with membranes and muscles. The wedge-shaped cartilage is covered by a semilunar membrane, which extends distally and is called the inner tympanic membrane. The external tympanic membrane connects the middle group of cartilages to the caudal group.

The lungs (pulmo) of birds are located in the uppermost dorsal part of the coelomic cavity. They are pink and relatively small [24]. The lung is not lobated like other species, with the ribs deeply embedded in it (Figure 7.21). The primary bronchi bifurcate into secondary bronchi, and then these will divide to become the tertiary bronchi (parabronchi) [24]. The smallest, terminal portion, known as air capillaries, are much smaller than mammalian alveoli.

The presence of air sacs in poultry is another unique characteristic feature that is not present in mammals [23]. Air sacs are connected with the lungs, where they develop at early stages of embryonic life. The air sacs are characterized by being easily expandable and having thin transparent walls. The outermost layer of the air sacs is covered by a serous membrane (simple squamous epithelium). The air sacs are poorly vascularized structures; therefore, they are not involved in gaseous exchange. They perform other functions like lessen the weight of the body to facilitate flying, body temperature regulation, distribution of weight and balancing during flying, in addition to their role in phonation and air storage. They include the clavicular (unpaired sac), cervical, cranial thoracic, caudal thoracic, and abdominal (paired sacs).

Urinary System

The urinary system is composed of paired kidneys and paired ureters. The kidneys are symmetrically positioned occupying the depression inside the synsacrum (renal fossae)

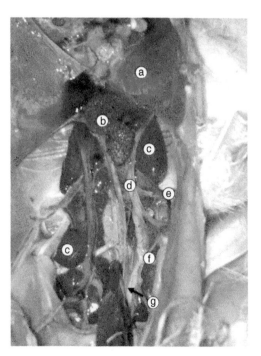

Figure 7.22 Dorsal view of the celomic cavity of young hen after removal of the gastrointestinal tract. (a) lung; (b) ovary; (c) cranial and middle lobes of the kidney; (d) left oviduct; (e) external iliac vein; (f) internal iliac artery; (g) uterus (left oviduct).

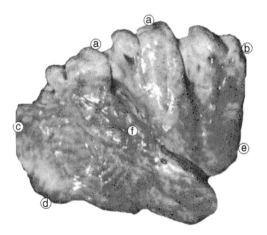

Figure 7.21 Lung left dorsal view. (a) Costovertebral border; (b) craniodorsal angle; (c) caudodorsal angle; (d) caudoventral angle; (e) cranioventral angle; (f) costal surface.

(Figure 7.22). Each kidney is divided into three distinct divisions: the cranial, middle, and caudal divisions, which are separated by the passage of the external iliac and the ischiatic arteries respectively [25].

On section, the kidney has a cortex and medulla. Three types of nephrons have been described, cortical with a relatively small glomerulus (mammalian type), medullary with large glomerulus (reptilian type), and intermediate (infrequently found). Microscopically, distinct lobulations inside the cortical region are seen following the branching of the duct system (Figure 7.23). The epithelial lining of the proximal tubule is simple cuboidal that can become pyramidal in shape. The lumen of the tubule is not always clear as a result of the presence of the brush border on the surface. The distal tubule is lined by lower simple cuboidal epithelium with larger lumen and darker cytoplasm (basophilic).

The collecting duct system starts at the periphery of the cortex and passes through it toward the medulla. These ducts increase in diameter progressively until they terminate collectively as a series of large ducts ending in the ureter [21].

Each kidney is drained by a ureter, which passes caudally to open at the urodeum of the cloaca. The ureter can be divided into two portions, intrarenal and extrarenal. The ureter is a well-developed muscular duct, which is described to receive about 13–17 large ducts from the kidney. Histologically, the ureter is lined by transitional or pseudostratified columnar epithelium, having variable thickness from one region to another [26].

Renal Portal System

Blood from the rectum, pelvis, and hindlimbs is carried to the kidney through the caudal mesenteric, ischiatic, and external iliac veins. The blood enters a venous ring lying on the ventral surface of the kidneys. The venous ring has connections with the common iliac vein to join the caudal vena cava. Branches of the vein enter the kidney and form the peripheral interlobular veins, which discharge into the capillary network surrounding the nephrons. The flow of blood inside the caudal mesenteric vein is usually toward the kidneys.

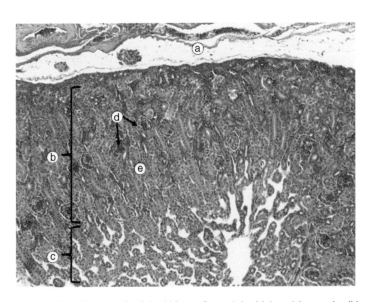

Figure 7.23 Micrograph of the kidney of an adult chicken. (a) capsule; (b) cortex; (c) medulla; (d) renal corpuscles; (e) renal tubules. H&E stain, magnification ×150.

Blood in the portal (renal) venous ring normally flows from the kidneys cranially into the caudal vena cava via the common iliac veins (under sympathetic influence). Alternatively, under parasympathetic influence, the flow can be diverted into the hepatic portal circulation via the caudal mesenteric vein. Within the lumen of the common iliac vein is the renal portal valve, which when open allows portal blood to enter the caudal vena cava (Figure 7.24). The renal portal system enhances renal tubular secretion and reabsorption and is

especially important in the secretion of urates. The renal lobules drain to the central intralobular veins, the branches of which eventually discharge into the caudal and cranial renal veins [18, 27].

Ideally parenteral medication administration should be confined to the cranial half of the body (pectoral muscles for intramuscular injections) just in case the renal portal system is causing blood to flow directly through the kidney to avoid potential renal damage from renal toxic medications.

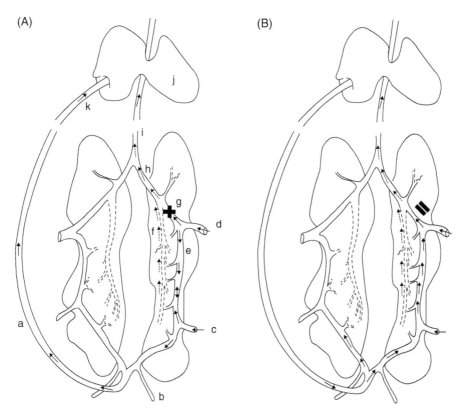

Figure 7.24 Drawing depicting the renal portal system blood flow under two different autonomic nervous system stimuli. A: under parasympathetic control, the valve (g) is closed (X) and the blood is diverted toward the kidneys as well as the caudal mesenteric vein to reach the hepatic portal vein. Branches of the caudal portal renal veins enter the kidney and form the peripheral interlobular veins, which discharge into the capillary network surrounding the nephrons. After being involved in renal tubular secretion and reabsorption, these vessels end up into the caudal renal veins that join the common iliac veins. B: under sympathetic control, the valve (g) is open (II) and the blood coming from the caudal mesenteric, ischiatic, and external iliac veins flow toward the caudal vena cava via the common iliac veins. A: blood flow under parasympathetic control; b: blood flow under sympathetic control; a: caudal mesenteric vein; b: internal iliac vein; c: ischiatic vein; d: external iliac vein; e: caudal portal renal vein; f: caudal renal vein; g: renal portal valve; h: common iliac vein; i: caudal vena cava; j: liver; k: hepatic portal vein.

Male Genital System

The male genital system consists of paired testes, epididymis, ductus deferens, and a phallus.

The two testes (testicle, orchis) are situated symmetrically in the dorsal portion of the coelomic cavity between the lungs and the cranial lobe of the kidneys [18, 27]. Each testis is bean-shaped and whitish yellow in color in the adult (Figure 7.25). The testes are covered by the abdominal air sacs, especially at their cranial portions. The seminiferous tubules are separated by extremely thin connective tissue, which contains some interstitial cells (Leydig, testosterone producing) and connective tissue.

The epididymis is much less convoluted compared to mammals. There are no clear demarcations between different segments of the epididymis as the efferent ductules open over all its length.

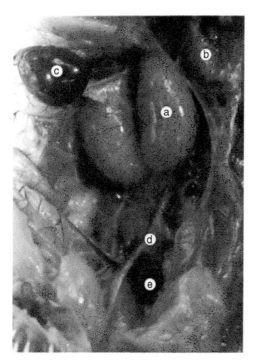

Figure 7.25 Exposed male genital system in a rooster after removal of the abdominal viscera. (a) testis; (b) lung; (c) spleen; (d) ductus deferens; (e) kidney.

The ductus deferens (vas deferens) has a small lumen, is white in color and relatively difficult to differentiate from the epididymis in its initial segment. Histologically it has a thick muscular wall. It courses toward the cloaca, lying next to the synsacrum and to the kidney. It ends at a small elevated papilla inside the urodeum. There are no accessory sex glands in chicken.

The phallus is the male copulatory organ and it is a non-protrusible intromittent structure. It has a spiral phallic sulcus where the ejaculate passes through. The phallus can be found on the ventral lip of the vent. It consists of a median white phallic body (few millimeters in diameter) and two lateral phallic bodies (2–4 mm) surrounded by two phallic folds.

Female Genital System

The female chicken has a single left ovary because the right ovary is not fully developed and regresses early during development. The remnant of the right genital organ in the adult hen is called the regressed right cystic oviduct (Figure 7.26 and Figure 7.27). The left ovary is found within the peritoneal (coelomic) cavity attached to the dorsal wall by the mesovarium. It can be described as active when it is composed of several follicles (yolks) at different stages of development and inactive when the follicles (yolks) are extremely small, white in color, and transparent. There is no corpus luteum described in the chicken ovary at any stage [18, 27].

The oviduct is a muscular tube that conveys the ovum from the ovary to the cloaca (urodeum). It is attached to the body wall by a mesentery called the mesotubarium. The oviduct is composed of five segments:

1) *Infundibulum* At the periphery of the free border of the infundibulum, the finger-like projection that extends toward the ovary are called fimbriae. The infundibulum length is close to nine centimeters in laying hens and is much shorter in non-laying

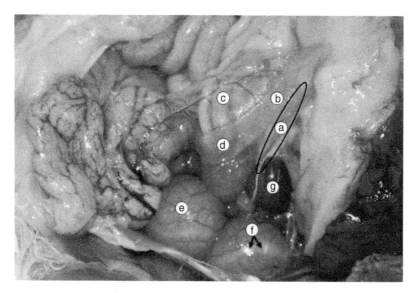

Figure 7.26 Female genital system of adult hen. (a) fimbria; (b) infundibulum; (c) mesotubarium; (d) ampulla; (e) developing ova; (f) stigma; (g) spleen.

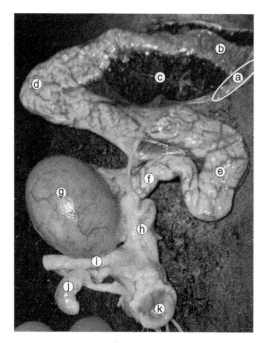

Figure 7.27 Female genital system of adult hen with an egg inside the uterus. (a) fimbria; (b) infundibulum; (c) mesotubarium; (d-e) ampulla; (f) isthmus; (g) uterus (egg shell gland); (h) vagina; (i) colorectum; (j) remnant of atretic (cystic)right oviduct; (k) cloaca.

hens. The wall is thin, and it has a funnel-shape which collects the ova after being released from the ovary. The infundibulum is lined by ciliated low columnar epithelium with few goblet cells.

2) **Magnum** The magnum participates in the formation of the thin and thick albumin on the developing egg. The ova descend spirally inside the magnum. The spiral chalaza is formed in this segment. The surface epithelium is ciliated simple columnar with large number of goblet cells. Well-developed branched tubular glands fill the propria-submucosa.

3) **Isthmus** The isthmus is a short segment of the oviduct (about 8 cm). The boundary between the isthmus and magnum is sharply distinguished by a narrow band of tissue called zona translucent. The membranous isthmus forms the internal and external shells of the egg.

4) **Uterus (egg shell gland)** The uterus functions in laying the shell on the outer shell membrane. It also works to deposit the pigment in certain species which produce colored shells. There is no distinct anatomical boundary between the isthmus and the uterus. The cranial part is short through which the egg passes rapidly. The major part is pouch-like and holds the egg during shell formation.

5) ***Vagina*** The vagina is a short muscular tube, which extends from the sphincter of the uterus to the cloaca. It has a thick wall as a result of the presence of a thick muscular layer. The mucosa is composed of primary and secondary folds.

Central Nervous System

The central nervous system is composed of brain and spinal cord surrounded by the meninges to protect and nourish. As in mammals, the meninges consist of the dura matter (outer), arachnoid and pia mater (inner) [28, 29].

The brain can be divided into cerebrum, cerebellum, and the brainstem. The cerebrum is composed of two cerebral hemispheres separated by a median (longitudinal) groove or fissure. A small pointed olfactory bulb projects from the rostral end of the cerebrum (Figure 7.28). Caudally, the hemispheres extend to contact the well-developed optic lobes in bird. The cerebrum has the lateral ventricles inside the hemispheres and the third ventricle around the thalamus. The fourth ventricle is found in the hindbrain. The choroid plexuses produce and regulate the amount of the cerebrospinal fluid. These ventricles are connected with the central canal of the spinal cord. The outer most portion of the cerebrum is the cortex. The cortex is composed of one or two layers of cells (neurons). Overall, the cortex is divided into three functional regions: the limbic, the general, and true olfactory cortices.

The paired optic lobes comprise a relatively large proportion of the mesencephalon, projecting laterally on either side of the brain from the posterior ventral aspect of the forebrain. Within each optic lobe the greater part of the structure consists of a well-developed optic tectum or rostral colliculus.

The cerebellum attaches to the dorsal aspect of the medulla oblongata by rostral and caudal peduncles. The cerebellum can be divided into three main lobes, rostral, middle, and caudal,

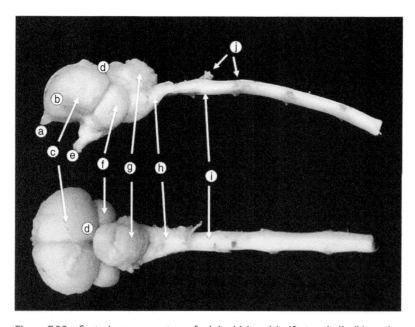

Figure 7.28 Central nervous system of adult chicken. (a) olfactory bulb; (b) cerebrum/frontal part; (c) cerebrum/parietal part; (d) occipital part (e) optic tract; (f) optic lobe (mesencephalon); (g) cerebellum; (h) medulla oblongata; (i) spinal cord; (j) cervical spinal nerves.

as a result of the presence of two fissures known as the fissura prima and fissura secunda (first and second fissures). Externally, the vermis can be observed with deep transverse sulci.

The pyramids and the decussation of the mammalian medulla are not seen in the chicken medulla oblongata. There is no obvious pons. Histologically, the arrangement of the nuclei of the cranial nerves inside the medulla shows similarity to the gray matter of the spinal cord.

The spinal cord extends along the spinal canal including the coccygeal (caudal) region; however, it decreases in diameter as it descends caudally. The conspicuous difference is the presence of the glycogen body, which is an elongated dilation at the lumbar region.

Endocrine System

The endocrine system includes glands and scattered glandular tissues [30]. These glands are:

1) Pituitary gland
2) Pineal gland
3) Thyroid glands
4) Parathyroid glands
5) Ultimobranchial gland (body)
6) Adrenal glands

Included within the endocrine system are the endocrine cells inside the pancreas (Islets of Langerhans), cells in the wall of the gastrointestinal tract, hypothalamus, testis (interstitial, Leydig cells), and ovary (thecal cells).

Pituitary Gland (Hypophysis Cerebri)

The pituitary is a small gland attached directly to ventral aspect of the brain stem, caudal to the optic chiasma. Histologically, there is no intermediate zone or region in the chicken pituitary gland. The glandular portion has two regions: distal and tuberal; while the nervous portion divides into infundibular, median eminence, and nervous parts. The glandular portion has six types of cells with different staining affinity. Their function or secretions are similar to those of mammals.

Pineal Gland (Epiphysis Cerebri)

The pineal gland is a small bean-shaped structure that arises from the roof of the diencephalon. It is situated in the mid-line between the two hemispheres of the brain at the junction of the cerebrum with the cerebellum. It consists of solid group of cells subdivided into lobules by connective tissue. It is the neuroendocrine gland that secretes melatonin.

Thyroid Gland

The thyroid gland is a paired gland, dark red in color, and situated at the vascular angle formed by the subclavian and common carotid arteries. The gland is oval shaped in the chicken, but the size may differ according to the season, sexual hormones, nutrition, and age. The thyroid gland is enclosed in a thin capsule of collagen bundles with numerous elastic fibers. The gland parenchyma consists of roughly spherical follicles with little interstitial connective tissue between them (Figure 7.29). Each follicle is lined by a single layer of cells with different heights depending on the gland activity. Follicles from very active glands, as in young growing chickens, are lined by low columnar to cuboidal cells. Active follicles contain small amounts of colloid. In relatively quiescent glands, as in the normal laying hen, the follicles are large as a result of accumulation of colloid and the lining epithelium is reduced in height, which may reach flattened or almost squamous in appearance. No parafollicular cells are seen within the thyroid gland of chickens.

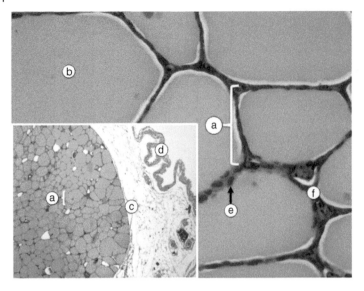

Figure 7.29 Thyroid gland of adult chicken. (a) thyroid follicle; (b) colloid; (c) thin connective tissue capsule; (d) lining epithelium of thoracic air sac; (e) follicular epithelium; (f) blood capillaries. H&E stain, magnification ×120, insert magnification ×80.

Parathyroid Glands

The parathyroid glands are normally found caudal to the thyroid glands inside the thoracic part of the coelomic cavity. Accessory parathyroid tissue is frequently encountered in different locations. Nodules of functioning parathyroid cells are found within nearly all ultimobranchial bodies. As many as three nodules have been described in the literature. Parathormone secreted by the gland regulates calcium and phosphate metabolism.

Ultimobranchial Glands (Bodies)

The ultimobranchial bodies (postbranchial) arise as an L-shaped sac from the caudoventral face of the fourth pharyngeal pouch [31]. These bodies migrated with the thyroid to the entrance of the coelomic cavity in birds. The ultimobranchial bodies frequently enclose parathyroid tissue within them and consist of strands of principal cells similar to mammalian C cells, as well as follicular structures formed by distinct endocrine cell types with larger granules. In mammals they become incorporated into the thyroid gland and differentiate into parafollicular cells (C cells) that secrete thyrocalcitonin hormone. This hormone acts to reduce concentrations of calcium in the blood.

Adrenal Glands

The adrenal glands are situated on both sides of the abdominal (caudal part) aorta, close to the cranial end of the kidney. In the hen, the left gland is normally embedded within the ovarian stalk, and in the cock, the adrenals are closely associated with the anterior end of the epididymis [30]. The gland is usually yellow in color with the weight varying considerably according to breed, age, health, and various environmental factors. There is no clear separation of cortex and medulla. The cortex is formed by columnar cells aligned in chords intermingled with the medullary cells which are arranged as clumps of irregular masses forming a meshwork. These cells are polygonal in shape and larger than the cortical cells. Cells have basophilic cytoplasm and a large, spherical, centrally located nucleus with diffuse chromatin. Secretions of both cortical and medullary tissues are similar to those in mammals.

Cardiovascular System (Heart, Cor)

The heart of chickens is composed of four typical chambers and is relatively large. It is dark red to bluish red in color and with a conical outline. It is surrounded by the pericardium [32]. The base of the heart is situated at the level of the second rib, while the apex is directed toward the sternum to reach the intercostal space between the fifth and the sixth ribs. The myocardium is relatively thick because of its high activity. The outermost layer of the pericardium is connected by a fibrous tissue to the hepatoperitoneal sac and the air sac in this region. It is further connected to the horizontal and oblique septa in addition to the sternum.

Lymphatic System

The normal lymphoid organs of the fowl are basically the spleen, thymus, bursa of Fabricius, and the mural lymphoid nodules. These small lymph nodules occur irregularly throughout the main lymphatic vessels of the neck, wing, and the hind limb. Apart from these organs, foci of lymphoid tissue of variable sizes are found in a large number of tissues and organs of the body.

Spleen

The spleen is spherical, dark red to reddish brown in color, and lies on the dorsal right side of the junction between the proventriculus and the gizzard (Figure 7.20). Small accessory spleens are reported in the literature close to the celiac artery.

Thymus

The thymus extends from the pharyngeal region to the distal part of the neck, in young chicks. The gland is embedded inside the connective tissue under the skin close to the jugular vein. During its development, the thymus is divided into 6–8 lobes separated by connective tissue (see Figure 7.8). The thymus eventually regresses almost completely in older bird.

Cloacal Bursa (Bursa of Fabricius)

The cloacal bursa is a unique structure to birds. It consists of a dorsal median diverticulum of the proctodeum. It is pear-shaped and it reaches its maximum size before the bird is fully mature [27, 33]. In domestic fowl, this size is attained at 4–12 weeks of age depending on the strain. The internal structure of the bursa consists of about 12 thick longitudinal folds and lymphoid tissues are found in each of these folds separated by collagen fibers (Figure 7.30). The internal lumen is lined by simple columnar epithelium. The cloacal bursa is the site of differentiation of immunologically competent bursal (B) lymphocytes. Involution of the bursa begins at about two to three months of age. However, remnants of the bursa persist for a relatively long time after involution.

Sensory Organs

Eye

The three main tunics of the eye (fibrous, vascular, and nervous) are present in the chicken. The main differences from the mammalian eye will be described here. Between the anterior-most part of the eye (cornea) and the large globular posterior component (sclera) is an intermediate region occupied by the bony scleral ring [33–35]. The avian retina is avascular and relatively thick compared to that of mammals. Another characteristic feature of

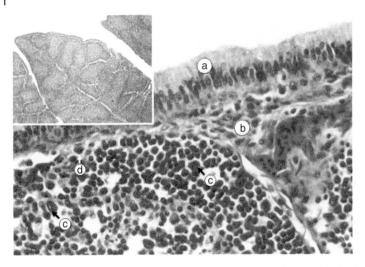

Figure 7.30 Cloacal bursa (bursa of Fabricius) of young chicken. (a) simple columnar epithelium; (b) lamina propria submucosa; (c) macrophage; (d) plasma cell; and darkly stained rounded nuclei represent lymphocytes predominate the bursa. H&E stain, magnification ×220, insert magnification ×100.

the chicken eye is the black trapezoid-shaped pecten oculi which projects from the linear optic disk into the vitreous body. For the purpose of lens and corneal accommodations the presence of striated ciliary muscles is described and sometimes they attach directly to the lens.

Ear

The pinna of the ear is absent and the entrance to the external acoustic meatus is 4–5 mm in diameter. It has glands and is covered externally by modified feathers.

References

1 Lucas, A.M. and Stettenheim, P.R. (1972). *Avian Anatomy Integument, Parts I, Chapter 1 Topographic Anatomy*, 39–48. Washington, DC: United States Government Printing Office.

2 Clarke, G.A. (1993). *Handbook of Avian Anatomy: Nomina Anatomica Avium*, 2e (eds. J.J. Baumel, A.S. King, J.E. Breazile, et al.), 1–45. United States of America: published by the Club.

3 Feduccia, A. (1975). Aves osteology. In: *The Anatomy of the Domestic Animals*, 5e, vol. II (ed. R. Getty), 1790–1801. Philadelphia, Chapter 60,: W.B. Saunders Company.

4 King, A.S. and McLelland, J. (1984). *Birds: Their Structure and Function, Volume 1*, 26–29. Eastbourne, UK: Bailliere Tindall.

5 McLelland, J. (1975). Aves Digestive System. In: *The Anatomy of the Domestic Animals*, 5e, vol. II (ed. R. Getty), 1857–1882. Philadelphia, Chapter 63,: W.B. Saunders Company.

6 Proctor, N.S. and Lynch, P.J. (1993). *Manual of Ornithology-Avian Structure and Function*, 166–168. New Haven, CT: Yale University Press.

7 Nickel, R., Schummer, A., and Seiferle, E., trans. W.G. Siller and P.A.L. Wight, (1977). *Anatomy of the Domestic Bird, Muscular System*, 34–38. Berlin, Germany: Paul Parey.

8 George, J.C. and Berger, A.J. (1966). *Avian Myology*, 370–384. New York: Academic Press.

9 Koch, T. and Rossa, E. (1973). *Anatomy of the Chicken and Domestic Birds*, edited and

translated from German manuscript by B.H. Skold and DeVries l., 145–151. Ames, Iowa: The Iowa State University Press.

10 McLelland, J. (1990). *A Color Atlas of Avian Anatomy*, 31–46. London, UK: Wolfe Publishing Ltd.

11 Lucas, A.M. and Stettenheim, P.R. (1972). *Avian Anatomy Integument*, part I, Chapter 3 and 5, 104–121. Washington, DC: United States Government Printing Office and 235–239.

12 Lucas, A.M. (1975). Integument. In: *The Anatomy of the Domestic Animals*, 5e, vol. II (ed. R. Getty), 2075–2083. Philadelphia, Chapter 70,: W.B. Saunders Company.

13 Nickel, R., Schummer, A., and Seiferle, E. (trans. W.G. Siller and P.A.L. Wight), (1977). Anatomy of the Domestic Bird. In: *Digestive System*, 40–56. Berlin, Germany: Paul Parey.

14 Poultry Anatomy (2008). USDA site. pp. 6–7. http://www.fsis.usda.gov/PDF/PSIT_ Anatomy.pdf (accessed 19 February 2013).

15 McLelland, J. (1990). *A Color Atlas of Avian Anatomy*, 51–57. London: Wolfe Publishing Ltd.

16 Eurell, J.A. and Frappier, B.L. (2006). *Dellmann's textbook of veterinary histology*, 208–211. Lippincott Wilkins and Williams.

17 Bacha, W.J. Jr. and Wood, L.M. (2012). *Color Atlas of Veterinary Histology*, 178–182. Philadelphia: Lea and Febiger.

18 King, A.S. (1975). Urogenital System. In: *The Anatomy of the Domestic Animals*, 5e, vol. II (ed. R. Getty), 1919–1961. Philadelphia, Chapter 65,: W.B. Saunders Company.

19 Lucas, A.M. and Denington, E.M. (1956). Morphology of the chicken liver. *Poultry Sci.* 35: 793–806.

20 Ritchie, B.W., Harrison, G.J., and Harrison, L. (1997). *Avian Medicine Principles and Application*, 274–275. Florida: Wingers Publishing Inc.

21 Machino, M., Sakuma, H., and Onoe, T. (1966). The fine structure of the D-cells of the pancreatic islets in the domestic fowl and their morphological evidence of secretion. *Arch. Histol. Jpn.* 27: 407–418.

22 White, S.S. (1975). The larynx. In: *The Anatomy of the Domestic Animals*, vol. II (ed. R. Getty), 1899–1902. Philadelphia, Chapter 64,: W.B. Saunders Co.

23 Nickel, R., Schummer, A., and Seiferle, E. (trans. W.G. Siller and P.A.L Wight), (1977). *Anatomy of the Domestic Bird, Respiratory System*, 62–69. Berlin, Germany: Paul Parey.

24 Whittow, G.C. (ed.) (2000). *Sturkie's Avian Physiology*, 5e, 234–236. San Diego, CA: Academic Press.

25 Siller, W.G. (1971). Structure of the kidney. In: *Physiology and Biochemistry of the Domestic Fowl* (eds. D.J. Bell and B.M. Freeman), 197–231. United Kingdom: Academic Press.

26 Liu, H.C. (1962). The comparative structure of the ureter. *Am. J. Anat.* 11: 1–15.

27 Nickel, R., Schummer, A., and Seiferle, E. (trans. W.G. Siller and P.A.L. Wight) (1977). *Anatomy of the Domestic Bird*, Urogenital System, 70–83. Berlin, Germany: Paul Parey.

28 Baumel, J.J. (1975). Aves Nervous System. In: *The Anatomy of the Domestic Animals*, vol. II (ed. R. Getty), 2019–2022. Philadelphia, Chapter 69,: W.B. Saunders Co.

29 Nickel, R., Schummer, A., and Seiferle, E. (trans. W.G. Siller and P.A.L. Wight) (1977). *Anatomy of the Domestic Bird*, Nervous System, 114–128. Berlin, Germany: Paul Parey.

30 Nickel, R., Schummer, A., and Seiferle, E. (trans. W.G. Siller and P.A.L. Wight) (1977). *Anatomy of the Domestic Bird*, Endocrine System, 108–113. Berlin, Germany: Paul Parey.

31 Hachmeister, U., Kracht, J., Kruse, H., and Lenke, M. (1967). Lokalishtion von C-Zellen in Ultimobrachialkörper des Haushuhnes. *Naturwissenschaften* 54: 619.

32 Nickel, R., Schummer, A., and Seiferle, E. (trans. W.G. Siller and P.A.L. Wight), (1977). *Anatomy of the Domestic Bird, Blood Vascular System*, 87–92. Berlin, Germany: Paul Parey.

33 McLelland, J. (1975). Aves sense organs and common integument. In: *The Anatomy of the*

Domestic Animals, 5e, vol. II (ed. R. Getty), 2063–2069. Philadelphia, Chapter 70,: W.B. Saunders Company.

34 Nickel, R., Schummer, A., and Seiferle, E., (trans. W.G. Siller and P.A.L. Wight), (1977). *Anatomy of the Domestic Bird*, Sensory Organ, 148–155. Berlin, Germany: Paul Parey.

35 Proctor, N.S. and Lynch, P.J. (1993). *Manual of Ornithology-Avian Structure and Function*, 250–252. New Haven, CT: Yale University Press.

8

Physical Examination

Cheryl B. Greenacre

Avian and Zoological Medicine Service, Department of Small Animal Clinical Sciences, College of Veterinary Medicine, University of Tennessee, Knoxville, Knoxville, TN, USA

Physical Examination

Introduction

A physical examination is important for identifying any abnormalities that may be occurring in the flock and in the individual bird. The following will focus on the chicken, but the information can be applied to physical examinations of most birds. It is important to understand normal, including behavior, before deeming a finding abnormal. Before restraining the bird for a physical examination, which can be stressful, obtain a thorough history, observe the bird and its droppings, and obtain a respiratory rate.

History

Signalment and Use
Obtain signalment of the bird (breed, age, and gender) and determine its use. Is it a pet, a pet that happens to lay eggs, is it kept for egg production, for meat production, for show, or for breeding? Are the meat or eggs sold? Determine how open or closed the flock is by asking how many chickens are owned, how long has the flock been owned, did they come from multiple sources at multiple times, when was the last addition to the flock, how long has this chicken been owned, where was it and the others obtained, any previous diseases or deaths, any previous treatments?

Housing
Determine how the chicken is housed by asking about housing, substrate, perch size and composition, and space of coop and range. Are they brought in at night? If a laying hen, how many nest boxes are set up and what is the laying history?

Diet
Determine diet by asking about diet including type, brand, amount, where purchased, how old is the food, is it medicated food, and if any treats or supplements are given. Are they offered greens and insects for enrichment?

Presenting Concern
Last, ask the presenting concern and how long has it been occurring, are multiple birds affected, and is it progressive?

Restraint

Prior to Restraint
Before restraining the bird, perform a visual examination of the bird and its surroundings

Backyard Poultry Medicine and Surgery: A Guide for Veterinary Practitioners, Second Edition.
Edited by Cheryl B. Greenacre and Teresa Y. Morishita.
© 2021 John Wiley & Sons, Inc. Published 2021 by John Wiley & Sons, Inc.
Companion website: www.wiley.com/go/greenacre/medicine

from a distance, preferably before the bird becomes aware of you. See if the bird brightens up after it is aware of your presence as this could be indicative of a bird trying to "put on a good show" or appear healthier than it is. Birds that look sick tend to be pecked by conspecifics or become a meal for a predator, so they tend to only look sick when they are very sick, decompensate, and cannot "put on a good show" anymore. Examine the alertness of the bird and if it is interacting with others in the flock or off in a corner by itself. Healthy birds are curious, active, and hold their head high with bright open round eyes, whereas sick birds hold their head down with the eyelids partially or completely closed (Figures 8.1a,b and 8.2). Observe stance and ability to walk normally. Examine the droppings for consistency, blood, or abnormal smell. Realize that chickens have two types of feces: the more common drier droppings and the wetter cecal droppings seen most often in the morning (Figure 8.3).

Restraint

The restraint of any bird begins with controlling the weapons of that bird—for example, with parrots the head is restrained first, and with raptors the talons are restrained first. Chickens do not bite or claw typically but they do flap their wings and may injure themselves or you, so first restrain their wings by gently holding them to the body in their normal folded position with your fingers spread wide apart to restrain as much of the wing as possible (Figure 8.4). Do not bend the wings backwards as the relatively flimsy wings of chickens can be easily luxated at the shoulder or elbow (Figure 8.5). Also remember to allow the normal up and down excursions of the keel so the chicken can breathe since birds lack a diaphragm. The bird can then be tucked under your arm either pointing forward or backward (Figure 8.6). Placing a towel on a table is a great way to evaluate a bird at your eye level and provide them with a nonslippery surface to stand on. Most chickens are very calm and usually the less restraint the better. If needed, drape a towel over the bird to calm it. Systematically evaluate the chicken from head to toe, but do save the oral examination for last as this is highly perturbing to the chicken. See Table 8.1 for a checklist when performing a physical examination. (See website for video of a complete physical examination in a duck.)

(a)

(b)

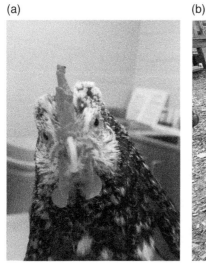
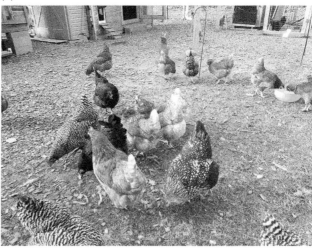

Figure 8.1 (a) Healthy, curious Speckled Sussex chicken with round, open, bright eyes, and head up. Note there is symmetry of the structures of the head (eyes, wattles, ear lobes, and sinuses) and a comb that is erect. (b) Flock of healthy chickens actively searching for and eating food and drinking water.

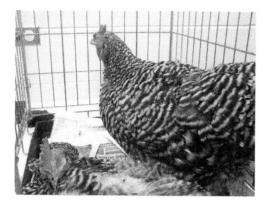

Figure 8.2 Two Plymouth Barred Rock chickens presenting with lethargy, feathers fluffed, dyspnea, and rales. Note that in strange environment of the examination room one is sleeping and the other has its head down with its eyes closed. Both were diagnosed later with Infectious Bronchitis virus.

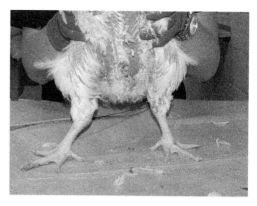

Figure 8.4 Restrain the wings of chickens by gently holding the wings to the body in their normal folded position with your fingers spread wide apart to restrain as much of the wing as possible. Note the abnormal stance in this white Leghorn chicken exhibiting a valgus deformity of the right leg.

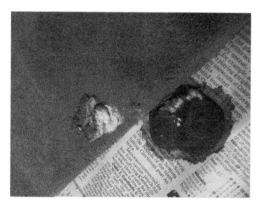

Figure 8.3 Normal chicken feces generally consists of semisolid green to brown excreta admixed with a cap of white urates (on red towel). Note the looser normal cecal dropping on the newspaper nearby.

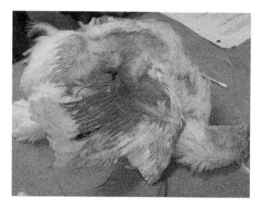

Figure 8.5 This 1.5 month old euthanized Cobb 500 broiler breeder chicken was improperly restrained by holding the wings over the back resulting in complete luxation of the elbow and puncture of the distal humerus through the skin.

Physical Examination

Head

Examine the head for symmetry of the beak, eyes, sinuses, nostrils, wattles, and ear lobes (Figure 8.7). Examine for ocular, nasal, or oral discharge, crusts, scratches, scabs, swellings, and discolorations (Figure 8.8a,b). The beak tips should come to a point. The iris should be the same color on both sides. A lighter color of one iris may be indicative of the ocular form of Marek's disease. Also, the eyes (anterior chamber or lens) should not be cloudy. Ocular discharge can appear as matted feathers along the cranial ventral lid margin (Figure 8.9). Flip the feathers cranially that cover the ear and examine the shallow ear of the chicken for discharge, blood or parasites.

The comb should be firm and red (Figure 8.10). There are many different shapes of comb (single, rose, walnut, buttercup), but the tissue should not invert as seen with a genetic condition known as ingrown comb/leader

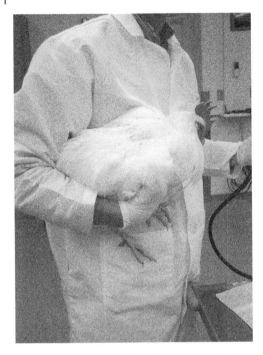

Figure 8.6 Demonstration of proper restraint in a chicken with the bird tucked under the arm with the head pointed forward. Alternatively, the head can be pointed backward.

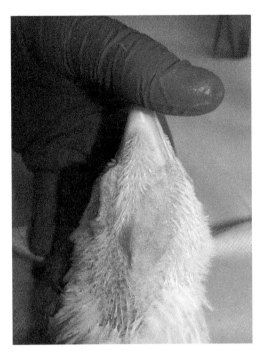

Figure 8.7 Note this 1.5-month-old Cobb 500 broiler breeder chicken has agenesis of the left wattle.

(Figure 8.11). A purple or darkened comb can suggest decreased oxygenation and the heart should be auscultated for murmurs (Figure 8.12a,b). A capillary refill time can be performed on the comb by digitally pressing and releasing (Figure 8.13). It should refill in about 2 seconds. The comb should not be pale, nor dark. Occasionally the comb is flopped

(a)

(b)

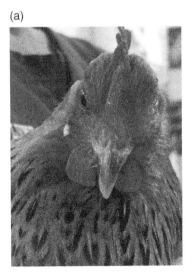
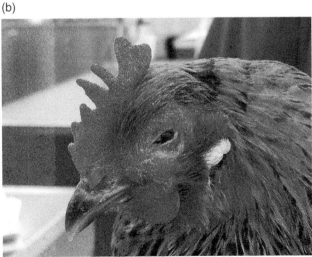

Figure 8.8 (a) Head on view of a chicken presenting with asymmetry of the head due to swollen left infraorbital sinus. (b) Side view of the same chicken. Note the beak tip comes to a normal point.

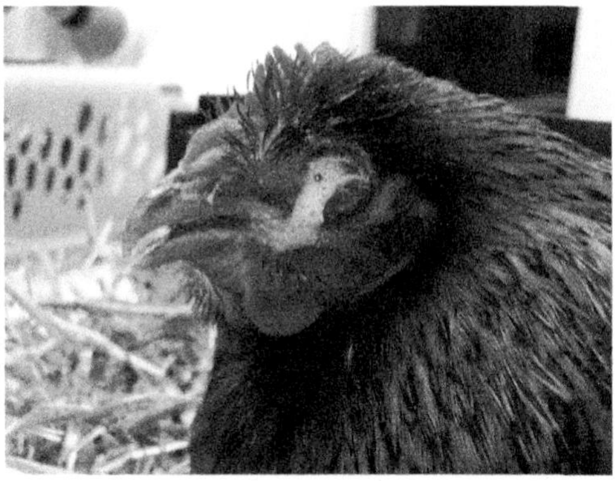

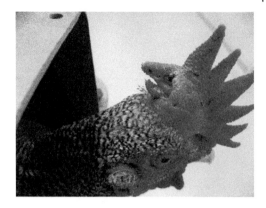

Figure 8.9 Chicken with closed eyes, head down, and copious oculonasal discharge. This chicken also had an abscess in the intermandibular area.

Figure 8.11 Plymouth barred rock rooster with a condition thought to be genetic in origin, known as ingrown comb/leader where the comb tissue inverts.

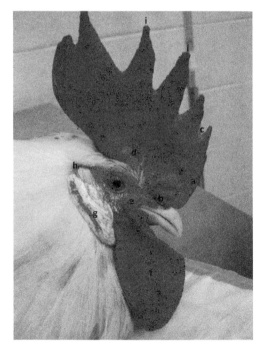

Figure 8.10 Healthy rooster with a firm, red comb. External features of the head are identified (a) blade of comb; (b) operculum; (c) crest of comb; (d) body of comb; (e) maxillary rectus; (f) wattle; (g) ear lobe; (h) external acoustic meatus; (i) points of comb.

Alternatively, the basilic vein (cutaneous ulnar vein) located just distal to the ventral surface of the elbow can be digitally pressed as in other birds to examine refill time (Figure 8.15). Normally when the finger is removed from the vein, refilling will be so fast that it cannot be witnessed visually, and if it can be witnessed visually then the birds is considered approximately 5% dehydrated, and if 1 second can be counted, then the bird is about 10% dehydrated or in shock. Decreased corneal moisture exhibited by a dull surface appearance to the eye, or in severe cases, recession of the globe is indicative of dehydration, as well as thick saliva in the oral cavity [1].

Body
Palpate the crop. It should feel soft and fluctuant, similar to a bean bag, and have crop movements about once per minute. Birds lack organized lymph nodes, so normally there should be no subcutaneous masses present. Birds possess only one gland, the bilobed uropygial gland (preen gland), on the dorsal caudal area just cranial to the base of the tail.

The keel should be straight with no deviations, and a slight "V" shape to the pectoral muscles on either side (Figure 8.16). In general backyard chickens normally feel thinner in the pectoral muscles and therefore normally have a more pronounced "V" shape than parrots.

over to one side, which can be normal as long as this did not occur suddenly (Figure 8.14). Sometimes the comb of roosters are "dubbed" or trimmed in show birds of the fighting bantam breeds.

(a)

(b)

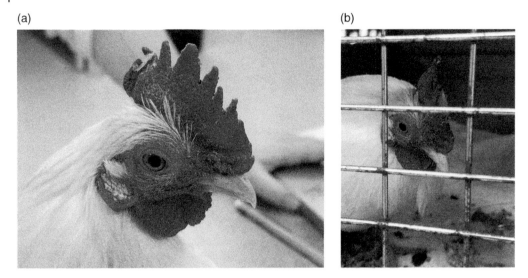

Figure 8.12 (a) Cornish rooster prior to restraint is exhibiting a darker than normal color to the comb. (b) During and immediately after restraint the comb turned purple and the rooster was visibly tachypnic. An echocardiogram confirmed heart disease.

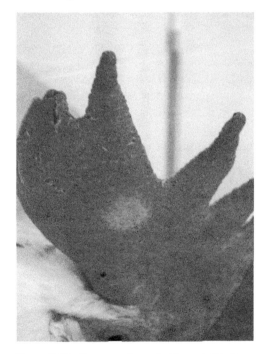

Figure 8.13 Same rooster as in Figure 8.10 after the comb has been digitally pressed and released. The normal "refill time" is approximately 2 seconds.

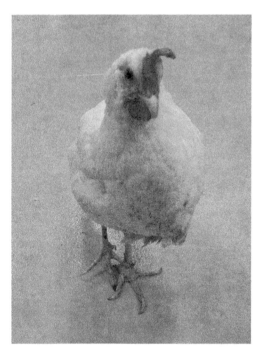

Figure 8.14 White Leghorn chicken showing a floppy comb and swollen left metatarsal area.

If "blisters," or any redness or swelling is seen on the keel, it may be indicative of a bird that has been in sternal recumbency and not walking for a period of time [2].

To auscultate the heart, place the stethoscope over the breast muscle on either side of the keel (Figure 8.17). Birds have a four-chambered heart and the sounds are similar to those of mammals

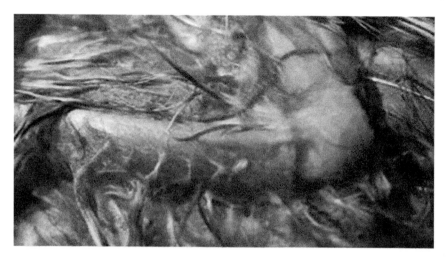

Figure 8.15 The basilic vein (cutaneous ulnar vein) that courses ventrally over the proximal ulna is an ideal location to digitally blanch the vein and observe refill time. Normally the vein refills almost instantaneously. If it can be seen refilling it is abnormal suggesting dehydration or shock.

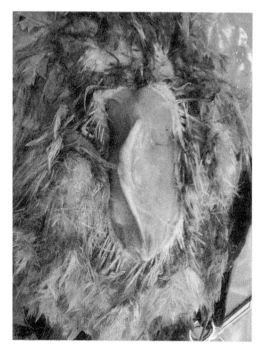

Figure 8.16 Note the deviated keel of this chicken at necropsy.

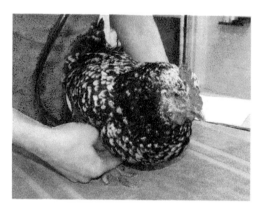

Figure 8.17 Physical examination of a chicken while it stands on a towel covered tabletop showing proper placement of stethoscope over breast muscle to auscultate the heart.

but faster at about 140–250 beats per minute. The heart rate can increase significantly with the stress of handling; therefore, if possible, it is recommended to obtain the heart rate while the bird is still in its carrier before restraint.

To auscultate the lungs, place the stethoscope over the craniodorsal body wall (Figure 8.18). Normal respiratory rate in the chicken is about 15–30 respirations per minute, but this too can increase with the stress of handling. Observe for a "tail bob" where the tail goes up and down with each breath indicating abnormal, increased respiratory effort (see video online). Try to obtain a respiratory rate prior to opening the door of the carrier and prior to handling the chicken if possible. Auscultate the lungs for abnormal sounds such as crackles, wheezes, or rales.

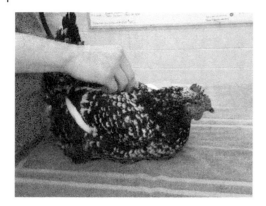

Figure 8.18 Physical examination of a chicken while it stands on a towel covered tabletop showing proper placement of stethoscope over the dorsum to auscultate the lungs and air sacs. (see Video 8.1 online "rales from Infectious Bronchitis Virus – IBV" and also Video 8.2 "tail bob in chicken with respiratory disease").

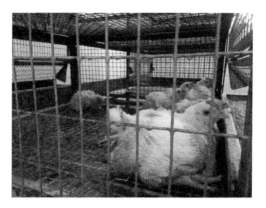

Figure 8.19 Note the bird in the foreground with visible coelomic distension. Also note the bird in the left background that is not with the others, stunted and is lethargic. This group of young birds was mistakenly given a diet with too much selenium resulting in coelomic effusion, stunting, and unthriftiness.

Palpate the coelomic cavity for firm masses (normal ventriculus, egg, or neoplasia), or fluctuant ascites [3,4]. The caudal coelomic cavity should be soft and doughy in an egg laying bird, but should not be distended or firm, fluid filled, or hanging down between the bird's legs. It would be abnormal to palpate multiple firm masses, or appreciate a fluid wave (Figure 8.19). The liver should not extend caudally past the caudal edge of the sternum. If gastrointestinal or reproductive disease is suspected a digital cloacal examination can be performed to better assess those structures.

Temperature is typically not taken in birds during routine physical examinations because it is generally higher than typical thermometers can read and there is debate over whether ill birds exhibit a fever like mammals. The normal core body temperature of a chicken is about 105.0–109.4 °F (40.6–43.0 °C) and can be measured with a thermistor thermometer with a small (2 mm wide) probe if needed. Temperatures are taken when birds are under anesthesia to determine degree of body heat loss during a procedure.

The feathers should lay down flat and smooth (Figure 8.20). Check for fluffed, dirty, or damaged feathers (Figure 8.21). Feathers that were

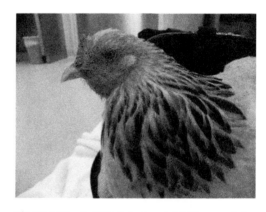

Figure 8.20 Buff Brahma hen exhibiting normal feathers laying flat and smooth.

damaged during the formation of the feather will show "stress bars," linear areas of barbule loss perpendicular to the shaft (Figure 8.22). Conspecific aggression may result in feather loss over the dorsal head and neck area (ducks), dorsum (chickens), or the vent area (Figure 8.23). Lift feathers up and look at the shafts especially under the tail near the vent and under the wings and base of primary feathers for evidence of lice and mites. Lice can be seen with the naked eye as beige oblong insects; their nit eggs look like clumps of white material at the base of feathers. Mites can cause abnormal

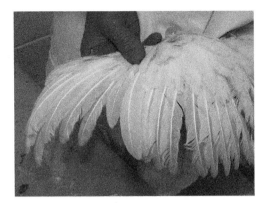

Figure 8.21 The left wing on this Cobb 500 chicken is gently extended at the carpus to examine the wing feathers, palpate the carpal joint, and extension of the elbow joint.

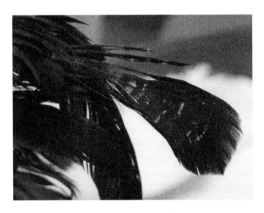

Figure 8.22 Feathers exhibiting "stress bars," linear areas of barbule loss perpendicular to the shaft, indicative of damage or stress during the formation of the feather.

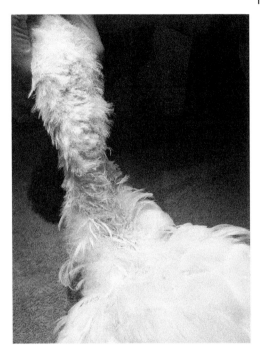

Figure 8.23 Duck exhibiting feather loss over the dorsal head and neck area suggestive of conspecific aggression. Feather loss from conspecific aggression in chickens is usually over the dorsum.

irritated, inflamed, or pitted looking skin. The skin is a light pink color in most chickens but can also be whitish, yellowish, or even black as in Silkies (Figure 8.24). Silkie chickens also have pigmented periosteum and peritoneum, as well as possessing six toes and a bony protuberance from the skull (see radiology chapter).

The vent should be clean and dry. There should not be a pasty vent (a vent with white urates stuck to it), nor should there be feces around the vent (Figure 8.25). The conformation of some egg laying birds requires the cutting of feathers around the vent to keep them clean.

Extremities

Examining the stance of the bird may give an indication as to the cause of the abnormal stance (Figure 8.26a–c). The "range paralysis" form of Marek disease often presents as a young bird in sternal recumbency with one leg forward and one leg back (Figure 8.27). Laying hens with the inflammation and pain of egg-related coelomitis commonly present with lameness (Figure 8.28).

All joints and limbs should be palpated and examined externally for range of motion, fractures, swelling, crackles, and clicks (Figure 8.29a,b).

The bird can then be lifted up to expose the smooth plantar surface of the feet and symmetrical appearance of the caudal surface of the hocks (tibiotarsal-tarsometatarsal joint) (Figure 8.30a,b). Scabs, callouses, swellings, keratin overgrowth, dark areas, or cuts are abnormal on the plantar surface of the feet.

(a)

(b)

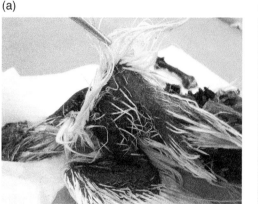 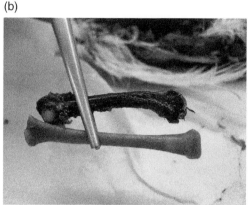

Figure 8.24   (a) Photograph taken at necropsy showing the normal black pigmented skin of a white feathered bantam Silkie hen, (b) as well as pigmented periosteum.

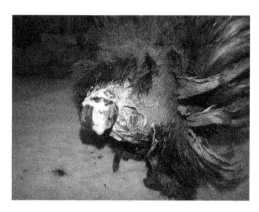

Figure 8.25   Chicken with cloacal prolapse and vent "pasty" with white urates.

The hocks should be of equal size and not swollen, and the tendon should be in the trochlear groove. The nails should be smooth, straight, and extend to just below the plantar surface when placed on a flat surface.

Oral Examination

Lastly, an oral examination is performed. Gently open the mouth by pressing the commissures to evaluate the oral cavity for white plaques, masses, abnormal smell, and evaluation of the choanal slit and choanal papillae on the roof of the mouth (Figure 8.31a–c). The beak should meet to a point and not be deviated (Figure 8.32a,b).

Remember to accurately weigh the bird on a gram scale in order to accurately calculate potential drug dosages or to compare to previous or later weights (Figure 8.33).

(a)

(b)

(c)

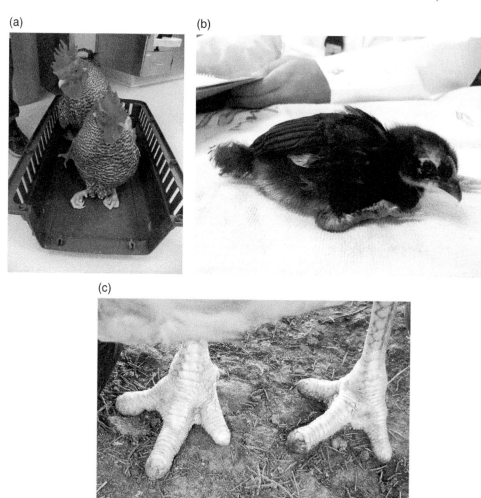

Figure 8.26 (a) Plymouth barred rock rooster presenting with lifelong curled toes. This condition was present in varying degrees in all birds in this clutch and was thought to be either genetic or congenital. (b) Young sex-linked chicken unable to stand due to perosis, also known as slipped gastrocnemius tendon (see Figure 8.30b). (c) A three-month-old broad breasted white turkey that was purchased with toes #2–4 "trimmed" at day of hatch, a common practice in commercial turkey flocks.

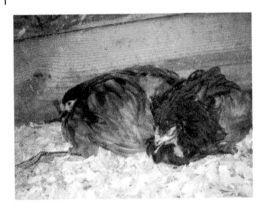

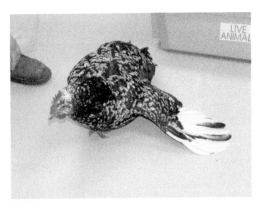

Figure 8.27 Two seven-week-old blue Orpington chicks with confirmed Marek disease exhibiting typical lameness and lethargy seen with this disease. Note sternal recumbency with one leg forward and one leg back (see Video 8.3 online "chicks with Marek's disease").

Figure 8.28 Adult speckled Sussex hen presenting for lameness due to egg related coelomitis. There were no palpable abnormalities of her legs. She was non-weight bearing lame in one or the other limb, could not be persuaded to walk, and when attempting to move put the wing out for balance (see Video 8.4 online "lameness due to egg related coelomitis").

(a)

(b)

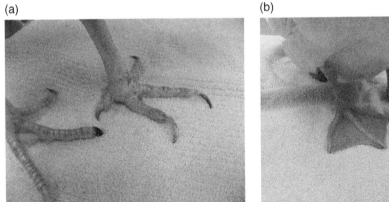

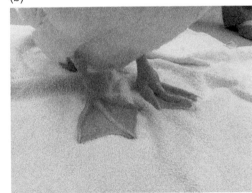

Figure 8.29 (a) Chicken with left metatarsal swelling. (b) Duck with left metatarsal swelling.

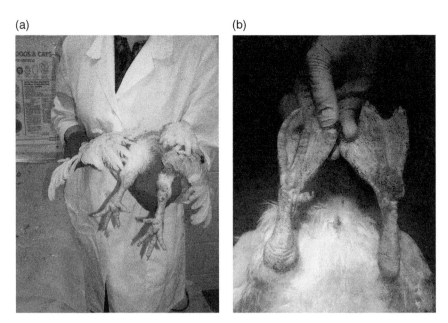

Figure 8.30 (a) The bird can be lifted up to examine the smooth plantar surface of the feet and symmetrical appearance of the caudal surface of the hocks (tibiotarsal-tarsometatarsal joint) such as what is being done in this normal chicken. (b) Alternatively, the bird can be flipped onto its back and the hocks evaluated in this direction. This white Pekin duck has a severe left metatarsal and phalangeal pododermatitis secondary to a swollen right hock joint from perosis/slipped gastrocnemius tendon.

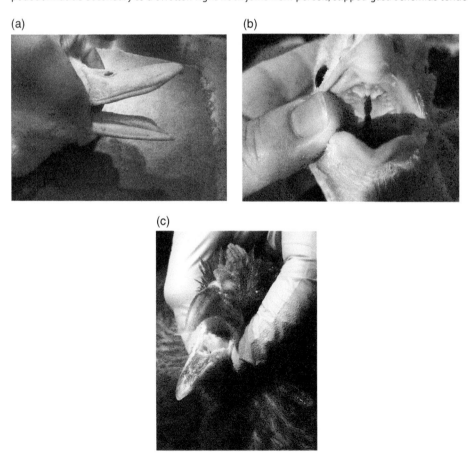

Figure 8.31 (a) Demonstration of how to open the mouth of this normal duck by gently pressing on the commissures. (b) Demonstrating normal choana in a healthy broad breasted turkey. (c) (Same chicken shown in Figure 8.9) demonstrating how to open the mouth to perform an oral examination. This chicken has a severe case of pox with white oropharyngeal plaques including the tongue and choana.

(a)

(b)

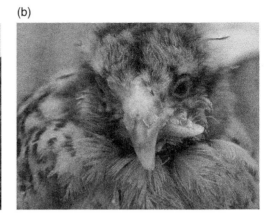

Figure 8.32 (a) A normal beak as in this chicken should meet to a point at the tip. (b) This chick has a severely deviated mandibular beak (gnathotheca).

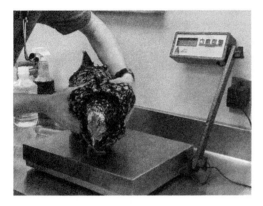

Figure 8.33 Accurately weighing the bird is part of a complete physical examination.

Table 8.1 Physical examination checklist.

From a distance:
- attitude, posture, gait, droppings, respiratory rate

Head:
- eyes, ears, comb, wattles, nares, sinuses, oral cavity, beak

Body:
- crop, keel, pectoral muscle mass, body condition score, auscult heart, auscult lungs, palpate coelomic cavity, preen gland

Feathers:
- general appearance, look under feathers at skin and feather base especially under wings and under tail

Extremities:
- joints and bones of wings and legs, hocks and feet

References

1 Tully, T.N. (2007). The avian physical examination. In: *NAVC Clinician's Brief: The Official Publication of the North American Veterinary Conference*, 74–78.

2 Spiegle, S.J. Ison, A.J., and Morishita, T.Y. Performing a physical examination on a chicken. In: *Poultry Health Resources* (ed. T.Y. Morishita), PHR Factsheet 2019–10. Pomona, CA: Western University of Heath Sciences.

3 Morishita, T.Y. (1999). Clinical Assessment of Gallinaceous Birds and Waterfowl in Backyard Flocks. In: *Veterinary Clinics of North America: Exotic Animal Practice*, 2(2); 383–404.

4 Lossle G., McDermott T. Performing a physical exam on a chicken. The Ohio State University Extension Fact Sheet. https://ohioline.osu.edu/factsheet/vme-20 (accessed 26 October, 2020).

9

Radiographic Evaluation of Normal and Common Diseases

Ashley L. Hanna[1], Marcie L. Logsdon[2] and John S. Mattoon[1]

[1] *Diagnostic Imaging, Department of Veterinary Clinical Sciences, College of Veterinary medicine, Washington State University, Pullman, WA, USA*
[2] *Exotics and Wildlife Services, Department of Veterinary Clinical Sciences, College of Veterinary medicine, Washington State University, Pullman, WA, USA*

Patient Positioning

Appropriate patient positioning and exposure techniques will maximize the information gained from each study. The patient is typically anesthetized and tape is frequently utilized for positioning, minimizing patient motion, and exposure to the handler (Figure 9.1a,b). Masking tape is superior to other types of tape as it causes less trauma to the feathers. A positioning device, known as a bird board, is also used in some practices to restrain birds for imaging. This device is usually composed of a board, with associated straps to the hold the patient in the correct position. In our practice, we have performed standing cross-table horizontal beam radiography in patients that were poor anesthetic candidates (Figure 9.2a,b).

Due to the small size of these patients, orthogonal, whole body projections are frequently obtained, allowing for a global assessment of the patient. A straight lateral radiograph and a ventrodorsal (VD) radiograph are often sufficient to complete the study (Figure 9.1). For the lateral projection, the wings should be pulled dorsal to the body and attached to the table with tape. Care must be taken not to overextend the "up" wing as that can cause rotation, or subluxation of the joint. Extending the legs away from the body will also minimize superimposition. On the VD projection, the patient is placed in dorsal recumbency, with the wings pulled out laterally and symmetrically from the body, and secured with tape. Full downward extension of the legs prevents superimposition of the stifles over the coelom. Inclusion of the contralateral wing or limb for comparison can be beneficial in cases where musculoskeletal pathology is suspected. Collimated images over a particular area of concern are useful for more detailed evaluation of the extremities (Figure 9.3).

If there is concern for injury to the shoulder girdle, a special projection, known as the "H view," can be included in addition to the standard views. This H view is a caudoventral-craniodorsal oblique projection that can be useful to evaluate the symmetry of the complicated pectoral girdle in birds [1]. This projection has

Backyard Poultry Medicine and Surgery: A Guide for Veterinary Practitioners, Second Edition.
Edited by Cheryl B. Greenacre and Teresa Y. Morishita.
© 2021 John Wiley & Sons, Inc. Published 2021 by John Wiley & Sons, Inc.
Companion website: www.wiley.com/go/greenacre/medicine

(a)　　　　　　　　　　　　　　　　　(b)

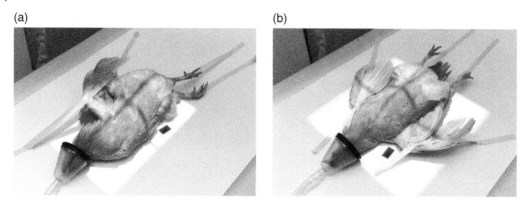

Figure 9.1 Positioning for lateral (a) and ventrodorsal (b) whole body radiographs. The appendages are pulled away from the body and secured with masking tape. The patient is under inhalant anesthesia.

(a)　　　　　　　　　　　　　　　　　(b)

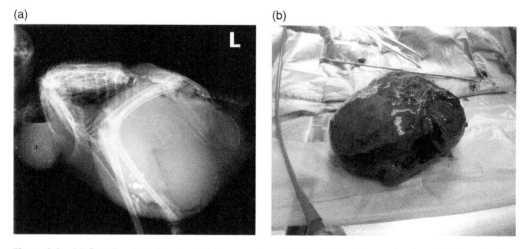

Figure 9.2 (a), Standing lateral horizontal beam radiograph of a chicken. The coelomic cavity is markedly distended with homogeneous soft tissue opaque material. The ventriculus is ventrally displaced and contains a metallic bolt as well as a small amount of mineral grit. Ventral displacement of the gas-filled intestines is present indicating a coelomic mass. The crop (denoted by an asterisk) is dilated, with a small amount of gas and a moderate volume of relatively homogeneous, soft tissue opaque material, indicating abnormal fluid retention; this is a common finding seen with diseases of the coelomic cavity. There is also a collapsed, thin shelled egg in the caudal coelom. (b) A very large ovarian tumor was removed at surgery (weighing 517 g).

been described specifically for use in raptors, with the projection made at 45° to the frontal plane. However, in our experience the specific angle of the beam often needs to be adjusted for poultry (Figure 9.4a,b).

Indications for Radiography

Indications for radiography include respiratory signs, coelomic distention, dystocia, lameness, trauma, and suspected metal ingestion/toxicity.

(a)   (b)

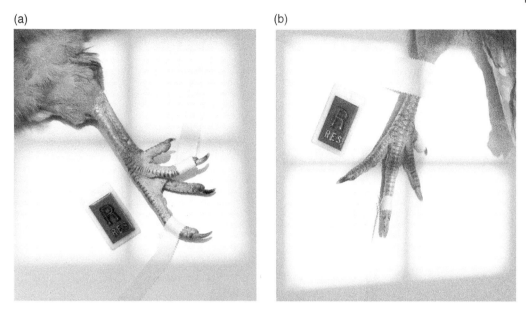

Figure 9.3   Positioning for collimated lateral (a) and dorsoplantar (b) images of the foot. The digits can be separated with tape to minimize superimposition.

(a)   (b)

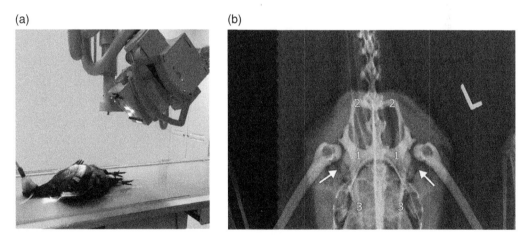

Figure 9.4   The "H view" for evaluation of the pectoral girdle. (a) The patient (chicken) is placed in dorsal recumbency and the beam is angled in a caudoventral to craniodorsal direction and centered on the shoulder region. (b) "H view" radiograph of a chicken, demonstrating the normal symmetry of the coracoid bones (1) and clavicles (2) of the pectoral girdle. The scapulae (3) can be seen coursing caudally from the region of the pectoral girdle and are partially superimposed over the coracoids. This view also nicely illustrates the location of the clavicular air sacs (arrows). In this patient the medullary cavities of all long bones (and bones of the pectoral girdle) are markedly increased in opacity, consistent with polyostotic hyperostosis.

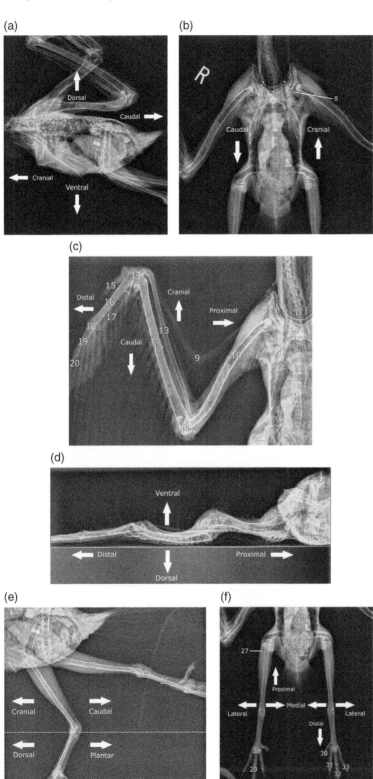

Directional Terms

Directional terms are described in Figure 9.5a–f.

Radiographic Anatomy and Common Abnormalities

Radiographic anatomy is represented in Figures 9.5a–c,e,f, 9.6a–c, 9.7a–d, 9.8a–e, and 9.9a,b.

Liver

In avian species, there is no distinct delineation between the heart and liver radiographically, and therefore the combination of these structures is referred to as the cardiohepatic silhouette. The shape of the cardiohepatic silhouette varies between species, but in a reproductively inactive bird, it usually has an hourglass appearance on the VD projection (Figure 9.10a,b). Enlargement of the cardiohepatic silhouette is usually a nonspecific finding and often is seen with caudal coelomic disease (not necessarily just the liver).

Alimentary Tract

The gastrointestinal (GI) tract can be evaluated with plain radiography, with the majority of structures best visualized on the lateral projection. Positive contrast medium administration can be used if a GI problem is suspected or to investigate a caudal coelomic mass effect. Typically, barium is used, unless GI perforation is suspected, in which case iodinated contrast is recommended. The reported avian barium dose is 25–50 mL/kg. A 60% weight/volume barium suspension is recommended [2]. A contrast study can be helpful to differentiate GI disease from a mass originating from a separate organ. Determining the direction of GI displacement can aid in identification of the affected organ.

The crop is typically located near the coelomic inlet, just to the right of midline on the VD projection and ventral to the cervical spine on the lateral projection. The crop normally contains heterogeneous, soft tissue opaque material, sometimes with small amounts of mineral opaque grit. The size of the crop is variable based on the time of the most recent meal. Fluid distention/stasis of the crop is often seen with coelomic disease (Figure 9.2a).

Figure 9.5 Radiographs of a turkey to demonstrate directional terminology. Whole body lateral (a) and ventrodorsal (b) radiographs. Cranial is toward the head and caudal is toward the tail. The terms dorsal and ventral are similar to those used in quadrupeds when referring to the trunk; however, these terms are also used to describe to the surfaces of the wings in avian species. Collimated lateral (c) and craniocaudal (d) projections of the right wing. As mentioned above, cranial is the surface of the wing toward the head and caudal is toward the tail. In this patient the elbow joint is luxated, with dorsal displacement of the distal wing relative to the humerus seen on the craniocaudal projection (d). This study demonstrates the importance of orthogonal views, as the extent of this injury is not as easily visualized on the lateral and VD projections (9.5a and 9.5c). Collimated lateral (e) and craniocaudal (f) projections of the limbs. Proximal to the intertarsal joint the terms cranial and caudal are used on a lateral projection, but distal to the intertarsal joint, the correct terminology is dorsal and plantar. In both the wings and limbs, proximal is toward the trunk and distal is away from the trunk. The inside surface of the limb is medial, and the outside surface is lateral, similar to in other veterinary species. Osseous structures: 1. Keel, 2. Notarium, 3. Synsacrum, 4. Pygostyle, 5. Cervical spine, 6. Coracoids, 7. Clavicles, 8. Left scapula (mostly superimposed over the coracoid) 9. Patagial tendon (pars propatagialis longus) 10. Humerus, 11. Elbow joint, 12. Ulna, 13. Radius, 14. Carpus, 15. Alula, 16. Major metacarpal bone, 17. Minor metacarpal bone, 18. Metacarpophalangeal joint 19. First phalanx, 20. Second phalanx, 21. Femur, 22. Stifle joint, 23. Tibiotarsus, 24. Intertarsal joint, 25. Tarsometatarsal bone, 26. Coxofemoral joint, 27. Fibula, 28. Tarsometatarsophalangeal joint, 29. Phalanges of the 3rd digit, 30. 1st digit, 31. 2nd digit, 32. 3rd digit, 33. 4th digit.

(a)

(b)

(c)

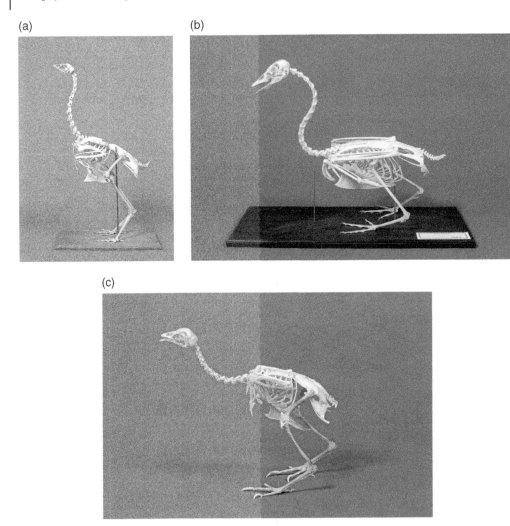

Figure 9.6 Skeletons of a turkey (a), goose (b), and chicken (c). The pectoral girdle is different between types of poultry; note the well-developed clavicles in the goose compared to the chicken and turkey.

The esophagus is seen as a soft tissue opaque tubular structure dorsal to the heart, that continues caudally into the proventriculus. The proventriculus blends into the ventriculus, which is located in the caudoventral coelomic cavity, just caudal to the liver and ventral to the coxofemoral joint. It is often easily identified, containing small mineral opaque foci (grit). This characteristic grit allows localization of the ventriculus (Figure 9.7). Metallic foreign material can also accumulate in the ventriculus, secondary to dietary indiscretion (Figure 9.11a,b; also see Figure 9.2a). This finding is of particular importance in patients with suspected zinc toxicity. The small intestines are usually filled with fluid and are identified in the mid to caudal coelomic cavity, with multiple segments superimposed over one another, making differentiation of individual loops of bowel difficult.

Spleen

The spleen is inconsistently seen on the lateral projection as a round soft tissue opaque structure, located dorsal to the proventriculus and ventriculus. The spleen should roughly be similar in diameter to the width of the femur. It is

(a)

(b)

(c)

(d)

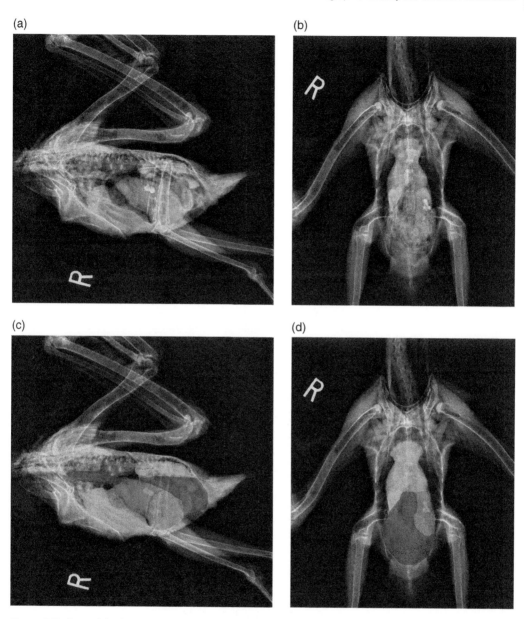

Figure 9.7 Lateral (a, c) and ventrodorsal (b, d) radiographs of a turkey to label normal coelomic anatomy. Cardiohepatic silhouette (yellow), esophagus (red), proventriculus (blue), ventriculus (orange), bowel (pink), gonads and kidneys (green). The renogonadal silhouette is not visible on the ventrodorsal projection due to the superimposition with the synsacrum and other coelomic viscera. Note the areas of air lucency within the humeri and femurs, indicative of normal pneumatic bone. The right humerus is abnormal, with the distal half being soft tissue opaque (this is the same patient as Figure 9.5 with the right elbow luxation).

not distinctly visible on the VD projection. Abnormalities associated with the spleen are uncommon, but generalized infiltrative disease processes (e.g., lymphoma) can result in splenomegaly. Additionally, juvenile birds tend to have larger spleens.

Respiratory System

The respiratory system of birds is composed of lungs and air sacs, both of which can be evaluated radiographically. Normal avian lungs have a honeycomb appearance, which is

(a)

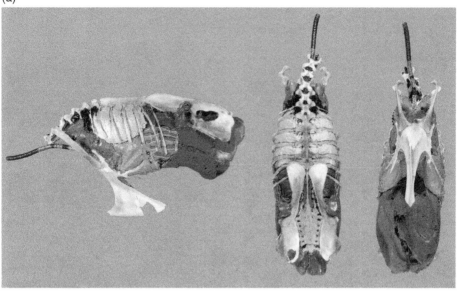

(b)

(c)

(d)

(e)

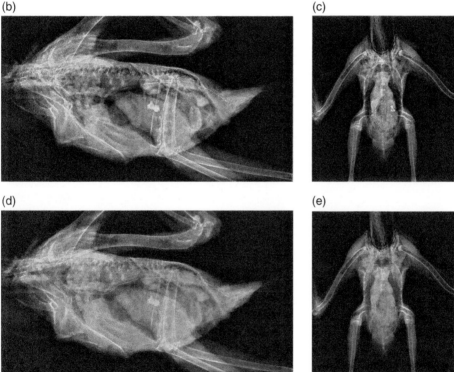

Figure 9.8 The avian respiratory system. (a) A cast of the lungs and air sacs in a chicken (lateral view on the left, dorsal view in the middle, ventral view on the right). In the lateral view, cranial is to the left; in the dorsal and ventral views, cranial is toward the top of the image. The trachea and surrounding osseous structures are left intact; however, there is a defect in the keel of this specimen. The lungs and thoracic air sacs are predominately located within the rib cage. Note the focal extension of the abdominal air sac that surrounds the acetabulum. Outlined are clavicular air sacs (green), cervical air sacs (dark purple), lungs (yellow), cranial, and caudal thoracic air sacs (Orange; caudal air sacs have green stripes), and abdominal air sacs (blue). Lateral (b, d) and ventrodorsal (c, e) radiographs of a turkey with the approximate positions of the lungs and air sacs highlighted (same colors as above). On the ventrodorsal projection, there is superimposition of the thoracic air sacs and lungs. There is variability in the relative volume of the air sacs between species. Note the pneumatic humerii and femurs.

(a)

(b)

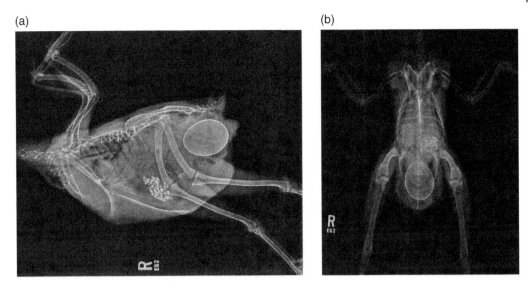

Figure 9.9 Lateral (a) and ventrodorsal (b) projections of a normal laying hen. There is a large, mineralized egg in the caudal coelomic cavity. The lungs, thoracic and abdominal air sacs are small in reproductively active hens. Note the large amount of mineral opaque material (grit) in the ventriculus, and to a lesser extent the crop, which is not fluid distended. The cardiohepatic silhouette is very wide, a result of cranial displacement of viscera by the enlarged reproductive tract.

(a)

(b)

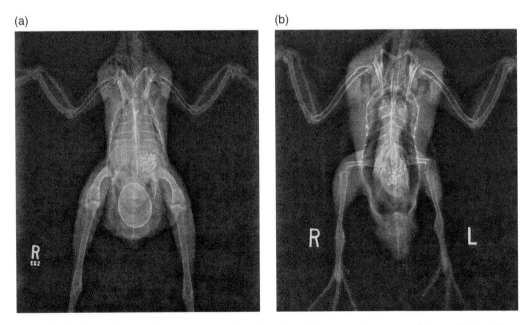

Figure 9.10 Cardiohepatic silhouette comparison. Note the difference in the shape of the cardiohepatic silhouette between a laying hen (a) and duck (b). The cardiohepatic silhouette in the laying hen is typically not an hourglass shape due to the large reproductive tract and cranial displacement of the viscera.

best seen on the lateral projection. Loss of this characteristic pattern indicates pulmonary disease. Healthy air sacs are gas filled and best visualized on the VD projection. The clavicular air sacs are seen just caudal to the shoulder joints. The thoracic air sacs are visualized caudal to the lungs and lateral to the cardiohepatic silhouette at the narrowest point ("waist").

(a)

(b)

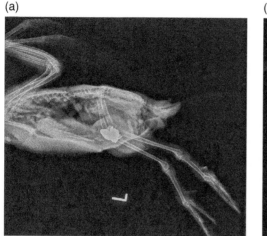
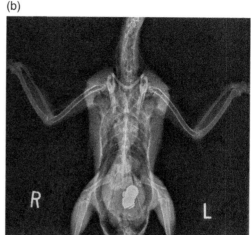

Figure 9.11 Orthogonal whole-body projections of a duck that presented for a 10-day history of lethargy and anorexia. Lateral (a) and ventrodorsal (b) radiographic images. There are multiple metal opaque structures in the ventriculus; the majority of these structures are disc shaped and thought to represent coins. Bloodwork confirmed zinc toxicity and a proventriculotomy was performed. Multiple foreign bodies were removed, including pieces of wire, washers, 2 dimes and 5 pennies. Note the very distinct hourglass shape of the cardiohepatic silhouette.

The abdominal air sacs are seen caudal and lateral to the majority of the coelomic organs (kidneys, gonads, GI tract) (Figure 9.8).

The easiest way to evaluate these structures radiographically is to look for symmetry. Decreased size or increased soft tissue opacity of an air sac could be an indicator of air sacculitis. The caudal abdominal air sacs are often decreased in size in reproductively active hens due to a space occupying effect. In cases of trauma to the shoulder region, increased opacity of the cervical and clavicular air sacs may be seen secondary to hemorrhage. Additionally, obese animals may have smaller air sacs that are more opaque than their normally conditioned counterparts. Respiratory signs in chickens are often secondary to a coelomic disease, resulting in decreased functional volume of the air sacs and lungs.

The syrinx is located at the level of the terminal trachea, similar to the carina is mammalian species. It should also be evaluated carefully for the presence of increased soft tissue opacity, which suggests focal infection such as a fungal granuloma (Figure 9.12a–c). It is important not to confuse major end-on blood vessels in this region for a diseased syrinx. An orthogonal projection is often necessary to differentiate vasculature from a fungal granuloma. Note that some species of male ducks, including mallards, have a normal bony structure called the syringeal bulla, arising from the left side of the syrinx (Figure 9.13a–d).

Urogenital Tract

The kidneys are best seen on the lateral projection, in the caudodorsal coelom, just ventral to the synsacrum. Radiographically detectable abnormalities associated with the kidneys are uncommon in poultry, as gout and renal tumors are rare.

The gonads are also visible in the caudodorsal coelom on the lateral projection, just cranial to the kidneys and caudal to the lungs. Differentiating renal from gonadal tissue is rarely possible radiographically. The ovary and testes demonstrate seasonal enlargement (Figure 9.13a). This change in size may not be evident in laying hens as they often are managed to be reproductively active year round. The salpinx is normally superimposed over the intestines, and when it does not contain an egg, it cannot be distinctly differentiated from bowel.

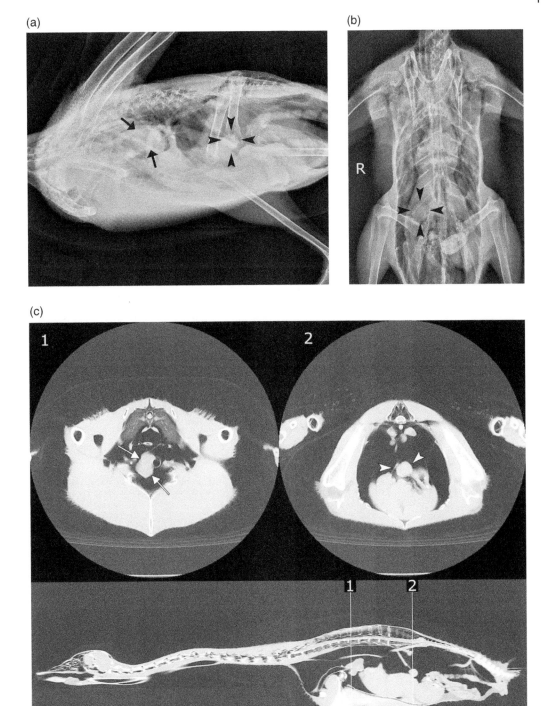

Figure 9.12 Orthogonal whole-body radiographs (a, lateral view and b, ventrodorsal view) and transverse CT images (c) of a Canada goose with a history of wheezing. (a and b) Two subtle soft tissue opaque masses are identified; one is located in the region of the syrinx (arrows) and the other is in the region of the right caudal thoracic air sac (arrowheads). These findings are most consistent with fungal granulomas.
(c) Transverse CT images showing the radiographically identified masses (sagittal slice is presented for transverse image location reference). This was confirmed to be aspergillosis. Follow-up CT examination (not shown) six weeks following antibiotic and antifungal therapy showed marked improvement.

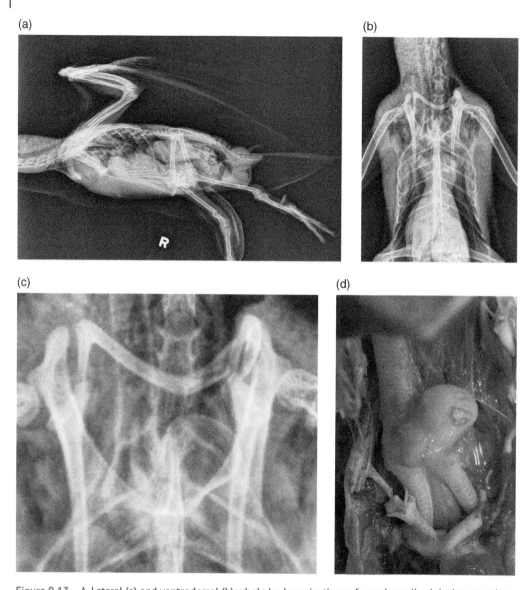

Figure 9.13 A, Lateral (a) and ventrodorsal (b) whole body projections of a male mallard duck presenting for a tibiotarsal fracture. Note on the lateral (a) view the normal large testicles of breeding season. Also note on both views the syringeal bulla, a normal bony structure arising from the left side of the syrinx. (c) A closeup view of this structure on the ventrodorsal view. (d) A photograph of a syringeal bulla, as seen at necropsy of another duck. Source: Photographs courtesy of Dr. Cheryl B. Greenacre.

Reproductive problems are a common indication for radiography in backyard poultry. In egg-bound birds, radiographs reveal a large mineralized egg in the caudal coelomic cavity and the egg can occasionally be malpositioned. This is more common in new laying hens, as the size of the egg often varies in young female birds. A history of straining in conjunction with an egg present in the caudal coelomic cavity is usually diagnostic for being egg-bound. However, it can be difficult to differentiate a normal egg from a retained egg on imaging alone. This can also occur secondary to pelvic or cloacal malformations, which are usually a developmental anomaly.

Radiographically, it is impossible to determine if an egg is located within the oviduct or free in the coelomic cavity. A free floating coelomic egg is usually a sequela of a ruptured oviduct secondary to dystocia. Reproductive disease resulting in retropulsion of an egg, shelled or unshelled, or repeated ovulation into the coelomic cavity can result in egg-related coelomitis. This typically results in coelomic distention and reduced serosal detail (Figure 9.14a–c).

In addition to egg-laying problems, the reproductive tract is a common location for neoplasia. There is such a high prevalence of ovarian cancer in chickens that they have been used as a model for human ovarian cancer [3]. See Figure 9.2 for an example of an ovarian tumor in a chicken.

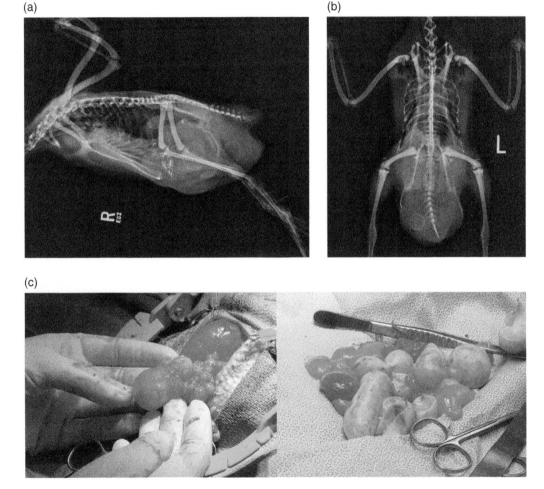

Figure 9.14 A, Lateral (a) and ventrodorsal (b) whole body projections of a duck presenting for coelomic distension and failure to start laying after the normal seasonal winter hiatus. There are multiple, variably sized eggs in the coelomic cavity, some of which are misshapen. The caudal coelomic cavity is pendulous and there is reduced serosal detail, concerning for egg yolk peritonitis. The medullary cavities of all long bones are markedly increased in opacity, consistent with polyostotic hyperostosis. (c) A salpingohysterectomy was performed. All yolk and undeveloped eggs were free floating in the coelomic cavity, with the exception of one that was in the distal oviduct/uterus.

Musculoskeletal System

Radiographs are extremely useful in evaluation of the musculoskeletal system, to determine a cause of lameness and evaluate the degree of osseous involvement in cases of soft tissue injury. The same basic principles of radiographic interpretation in mammalian species apply to avian species when evaluating the musculoskeletal system. The practitioner should look for areas of soft tissue swelling and underlying bony pathology such as a fracture or osteomyelitis. There are several anatomic variations between avian species, including nonpathologic tendon mineralization seen in chickens [4] (Figure 9.15), polydactyly seen in several Chinese and European chicken breeds

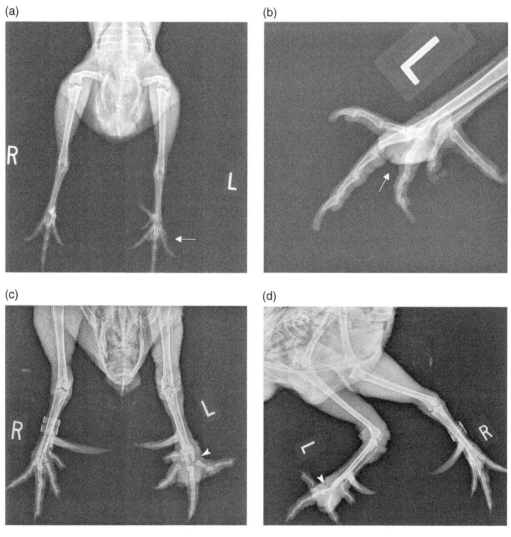

(a) (b) (c) (d)

Figure 9.15 Radiographic studies of two different chickens demonstrating variable severity of pododermatitis. Ventrodorsal projection (a) of the coelom and hindlimbs and a collimated lateral projection (b) of the left foot. There is focal soft tissue swelling surrounding the tarsometatarsophalangeal joints (arrows), with no involvement of the underlying bones. Ventrodorsal (c) and lateral (d) projections of the hindlimbs. There is marked widening of the left tarsometatarsophalangeal joints, with lysis of the distal tarsometatarsus and remodeling of the proximal phalanges (arrowheads), indicative of septic arthritis. Note the linear, striated mineralization of the plantar tarsometatarsal soft tissues, a variant of normal. Also note the radiographic appearance of normal spurs which consist of bone covered with keratin.

(a)　　　　　　　　　　　　　　　　(b)

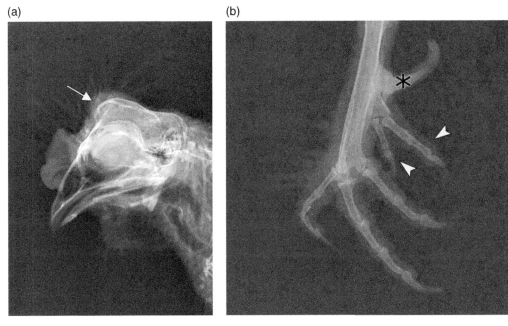

Figure 9.16　Lateral skull (a) and foot (b) radiographs showing unique bony features of the Silkie breed of chicken. (a) The skull has a "vaulted appearance" in this breed (arrow). (b) Polydactyly is a common finding in this breed. Note the extra toe compared to other chicken breeds (arrowheads). A tarsometatarsal bone spur in this rooster is seen as a mineralized, sharply pointed bony structure just proximal to the supernumerary digits (denoted with an asterisk).

(including the Silkie) [5] and the vaulted skull of the Silkie [6] (Figure 9.16a,b). The only notable gender difference in the chicken musculoskeletal system is the large tarsometatarsal spur in roosters (Figure 9.16b).

The radiographic appearance of a few notable, more common diseases are mentioned next.

- In cases of trauma, radiography allows identification of fractures and is often necessary for surgical planning (Figures 9.17 and 9.18). It is important to know that the humerus and femur are pneumatic bones, and subcutaneous emphysema surrounding a fracture in these regions is not necessarily indicative of an open fracture, nor is it indicative of the presence of a gas producing bacteria.
- Pododermatitis is a common cause of lameness in poultry. The infection can be limited

to the soft tissues; however, in more severe cases, osteomyelitis and septic arthritis can occur (Figure 9.15a–d).
- In lame birds, with muscle atrophy and no definitive underlying cause radiographically, Marek's disease should be considered as a cause for the clinical signs.
- Active laying hens often show regions of increased opacity in the medullary cavities of long bones. This appearance is termed polyostotic hyperostosis and typically has no clinical ramifications (see Figures 9.4b and 9.14a,b). However, it has been described in patients with oviductal tumors or cystic right oviduct.

Coelomic Cavity

Coelomic masses in birds are often difficult to localize to an organ of origin. As mentioned, oral administration of barium may help to

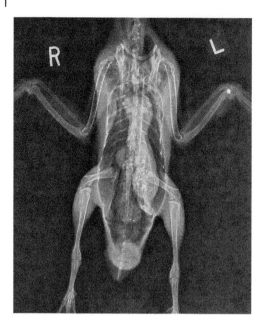

Figure 9.17 Ventrodorsal projection of a duck with an injured left wing. There is a mildly comminuted fracture of the left distal ulna. One large and several smaller metal opaque foci are identified just distal to the fracture, indicating gunshot trauma.

(a)

(b)

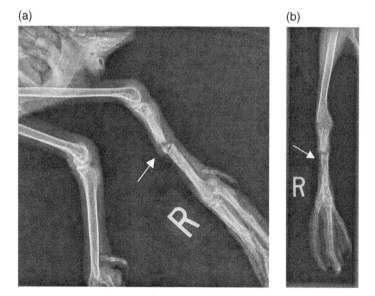

Figure 9.18 Open fracture and sequestrum of the tarsometatarsal bone of a goose. Lateral (a) and dorsoplantar (b) projections of the right limb. There is a fracture of the tarsometatarsal bone, with a large fragment between the proximal and distal portions of the bone. The proximal and distal segments are remodeled and smoothly marginated, indicative of chronicity. A small amount of periosteal reaction is seen on the proximal fracture segment; however, the fragment remains sharply marginated and demonstrates minimal new bone formation. These findings are consistent with sequestrum formation (arrow). There is surrounding soft tissue swelling and a defect in the skin at the level of the fracture, indicative of an open fracture.

differentiate the GI tract from the suspected mass (Figure 9.19a–c). Additionally, a focal ultrasound can also be helpful in some cases. A pendulous coelom with a convex ventral margin (normally concave to flat) and decreased serosal detail is usually indicative of effusion (Figure 9.20a,b).

Acknowledgments

We thank Henry Moore Jr., photographer II, Biomedical Communications Unit, Washington State University, College of Veterinary Medicine, for his outstanding positioning and specimen photography; and Darrel Nelson,

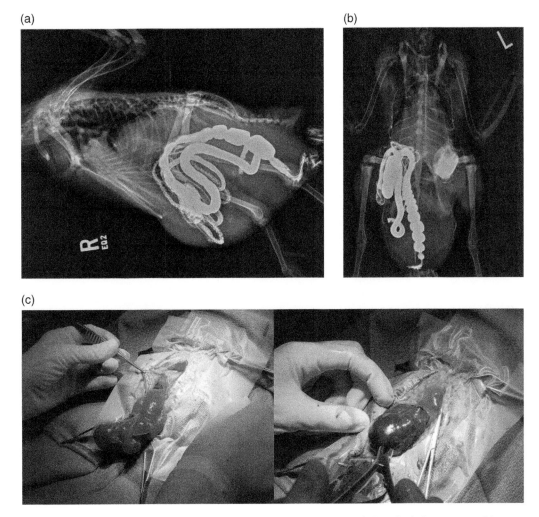

Figure 9.19 Lateral (a) and ventrodorsal (b) projections of a barium study in a duck that presented for marked, acute coelomic distension, and dyspnea. There is a mass effect in the left caudal coelom, resulting in displacement of the majority of the GI tract (outlined with barium) to the right side of the coelomic cavity. This is concerning for a mass originating from the reproductive tract. There is also increased soft tissue opaque material in the caudal coelomic cavity, seen both on the lateral and ventrodorsal projections; this could be associated with the mass or represent coelomic effusion. (c) Multiple large cystic structures (left), some of which were blood-filled (right), were found at surgery extending toward the region of the ovary. These abnormal structures correspond to the mass effect seen radiographically.

(a)

(b)

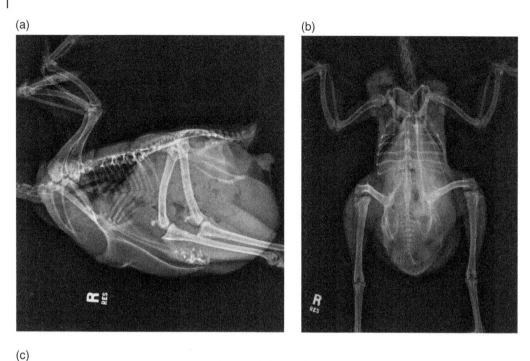

(c)

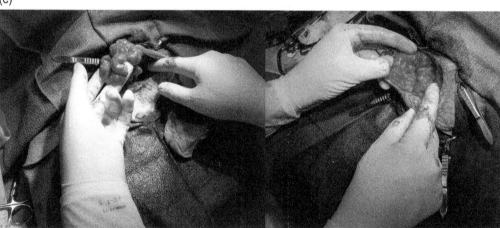

Figure 9.20 Lateral (a) and ventrodorsal (b) projection of a chicken with carcinomatosis confirmed at necropsy. The coelomic cavity is pendulous and distended with soft tissue opaque material, consistent with coelomic effusion. The ventriculus (filled with mineral opaque material) is ventrally positioned, with the remainder of the gas filled GI tract located centrally in the caudal coelom. The evenly distributed intestines are indicative of a diffuse coelomic disease process rather than a coelomic mass (compare with Figure 9.2a). (c) On necropsy, the small intestine was severely thickened (left) and there was abnormal tissue lining the entire serosal surface of the coelomic cavity (right).

instructional lab supervisor, Robert P. Worthman Anatomy Museum, Integrative Physiology and Neurosciences, Washington State University, College of Veterinary Medicine, for providing beautifully prepared anatomic specimens.

References

1 Visser, M., Hespel, A.M., De Swarte, M., and Bellah, J.R. (2015). Use of a caudoventral-craniodorsal oblique radiographic view made at 45 to the frontal plane to evaluate the pectoral girdle in raptors. *J. Am. Vet. Med. Assoc.* 247 (9): 1037–1041.

2 Wallack, S. (2003). The Handbook of Veterinary Contrast Radiography, 77. Solana Beach: San Diego Veterinary Imaging Inc.

3 Rodriquez, G.C. (2001). Characterization of the chicken ovarian cancer model. Defense Technical Information Center. https://doi.org/10.21236/ADA406141 (accessed 22 June 2019).

4 Abdalla, O. (1979). Ossification and mineralization in the tendons of the chicken (Gallus Domesticus). *J. Anatomy* 129 (Pt 2): 351–359.

5 Zhang, Z., Changsheng, N., Yaxiong, J. et al. (2016). Parallel evolution of polydactyly traits in Chinese and European chickens. *PLoS One* 11 (2): e0149010.

6 Rowshan, J. (2013). Study for Breeding of Japanese Silkie Fowl. ir.kagoshima-http://u. ac.jp. https://ir.kagoshima-u.ac. jp/?action=pages_view_main&active_ action=repository_action_common_ download&item_id=5390&item_ no=1&attribute_id=16&file_no= 2&page_id=13&block_id=21 (accessed 9/10/18).

Section 3

Diseases

10

Zoonotic Diseases

Marcy J. Souza

Department of Biomedical and Diagnostic Sciences, University of Tennessee, College of Veterinary Medicine, Knoxville, TN, USA

Zoonotic Diseases

Zoonotic diseases are infectious diseases that can be transmitted either directly or indirectly from animals to humans. An example of direct transmission would be *Salmonella* spreading via the fecal-oral route. An example of indirect transmission would be the transportation of infectious agents via fomites, such as shoes, clothing, equipment, and vehicles. Zoonotic diseases that can be spread by backyard poultry include but are not limited to salmonellosis, other enteric pathogens, chlamydiosis, influenza, Newcastle disease, eastern and Western equine encephalomyelitis, and West Nile virus [1–3]. The prevalence of most diseases in backyard poultry is unknown, but a recent publication examined causes of mortality in backyard poultry over a 5-year period [4]. The authors found a variety of infectious, including zoonotic diseases as well as non-infectious causes [4]. The risk of zoonoses to people exposed to backyard poultry is variable depending on many factors, such as immune status and biosecurity practices. However, veterinarians should be knowledgeable about these diseases and their implications to appropriately educate owners.

Seemingly healthy birds can be reservoirs and transmit disease. Owners of sick birds should be encouraged to consult a veterinarian. In most states, the following diseases and/or infectious agents are reportable: *Salmonella* Gallinarium, *Salmonella* Pullorum, eastern equine encephalomyelitis, West Nile virus, influenza, and *Chlamydia psittaci* (avian chlamydiosis). The National Poultry Improvement plan (NPIP) is a great resource and has been instrumental in controlling *S.* Pullorum and other diseases [5]. The Centers for Disease Control and Prevention (CDC) is also a good resource for salmonellosis and other diseases [3]. General hygiene practices, such as hand washing after handling birds or their excrement, not eating or drinking around the birds or their environment, and wearing personal protective equipment, helps to decrease exposure to zoonotic pathogens. Also, the CDC recommends that people who are immunosuppressed (elderly, children under 5 years of age, or those with HIV infection or receiving chemotherapy) avoid contact with chickens to prevent potential life-threatening disease, such as salmonellosis. The CDC goes on to say veterinarians should educate owners of these risks, and in some cases, education can be done with a handout that the owner signs after reading. Figure 10.1 shows a poster available from the CDC, outlining steps to keep both people and poultry healthy [6].

Backyard Poultry Medicine and Surgery: A Guide for Veterinary Practitioners, Second Edition.
Edited by Cheryl B. Greenacre and Teresa Y. Morishita.
© 2021 John Wiley & Sons, Inc. Published 2021 by John Wiley & Sons, Inc.
Companion website: www.wiley.com/go/greenacre/medicine

HEALTHY FAMILIES AND FLOCKS

Live poultry, such as chickens, ducks, geese, and turkeys, often carry harmful germs such as *Salmonella*. While it usually doesn't make the birds sick, *Salmonella* can cause serious illness when it is passed to people.

HANDWASHING PROTECTS YOU FROM GERMS

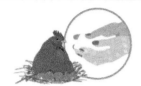

- Always wash your hands with soap and water right after touching live poultry or anything in the area where they live and roam.
- Adults should supervise handwashing for young children.
- Use hand sanitizer if soap and water are not readily available.

HANDLE BIRDS SAFELY

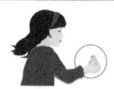

- Children younger than 5 years, adults older than 65 years, and people with weakened immune systems should not handle or touch chicks, ducklings, or other live poultry.
- Do not bring chicks, ducklings and other live poultry to schools, childcare centers, or nursing homes.
- Do not snuggle or kiss the birds, touch your mouth, or eat or drink around live poultry.

SAFELY CLEAN COOPS

- Clean any equipment used to care for live poultry outside, such as cages or feed or water containers.
- Set aside a pair of shoes to wear while taking care of poultry and keep those shoes outside of the house.

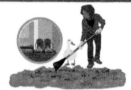

POULTRY BELONG OUTSIDE

- Do not let live poultry inside the house, especially in kitchens.
- Do not let live poultry in areas where food or drink is prepared, served, or stored.

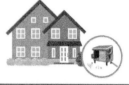

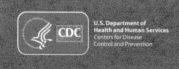

U.S. Department of
Health and Human Services
Centers for Disease
Control and Prevention

Have a Backyard Flock? Don't Wing it.
Visit www.cdc.gov/features/salmonellapoultry
for more information

Figure 10.1 This is a poster available from the CDC, outlining steps to keep both people and poultry healthy. *Source:* Available at https://www.cdc.gov/healthypets/resources/backyard-flock.pdf.

Salmonella

General Information

Most of the estimated 1.4 million annual cases of human salmonellosis in the United States are caused by ingesting contaminated food, including eggs, but recently, there has been an increase in cases resulting from direct exposure to live poultry [3].

Taxonomy

As a gram-negative bacterium in the Enterobacteriaceae family, *Salmonella* has a distribution worldwide, and most serotypes infect animals as well as people [7]. Due to the DNA analysis of bacteria in the *Salmonella* genus, two species have been designated: *S. enterica* and *S. bongori*. *S. enterica* is further subdivided into six subspecies, with the most frequent human pathogens being found within subspecies I, also known as subgroup 1, and designated, for example, as *S. enterica* subsp. *enterica*. Both the genus and species name are italicized and the serovar name begins with a capital letter. For example, instead of *Salmonella typhi*, the nomenclature is *Salmonella enterica* serovar Typhi, abbreviated S. Typhi or ST.

There are more than 60 serogroups (i.e., B and D) and more than 2400 serotypes, many of which are serologically classified by the geographic location where that serotype was first isolated. *Salmonella* from groups B and D account for approximately two-thirds of all reported *Salmonella* infections and include the two most common serotypes, *Salmonella enterica* serotype Enteritidis (S. Enteritidis) and *Salmonella enterica* serotype Typhimurium (S. Typhimurium), which together account for half of all human infections in the United States [8].

Great genetic variation exists within many *Salmonella* serotypes. Serotyping and phage-typing are now complemented by molecular subtyping techniques, such as pulse field gel electrophoresis and whole genome sequencing, for epidemiological disease surveillance and outbreak investigations. An overview of *Salmonella* and poultry can be found at the CDC's website at: https://www.cdc.gov/salmonella/ [3].

Reservoir and Incidental Hosts

Many species of wild and domestic animals, including poultry, can act as reservoirs for *Salmonella* bacteria. There are many reports of chicks and ducklings acting as a source of infection for humans, especially children. The CDC website has an informational page titled "Salmonella," which is available at: https://www.cdc.gov/salmonella [8].

Pathogenesis

Exposure to *Salmonella* usually occurs by ingesting the bacteria, which is shed in the feces of infected animals and found in feces-contaminated food or water. Relatively few bacteria can cause an infection; however, usually a quantity of more than 1000 is needed. The incubation period is generally from 6 to 72 hours but is usually between 12 and 36 hours. *Salmonella* naturally lives in the intestine of poultry and is considered normal flora in healthy, live poultry. Raw and undercooked foods, such as eggs, milk, and meat products; cooked foods not maintained at an appropriate temperature; and cross-contaminated foods are common sources of infection. Recently, it has become more common for live poultry to be a source of exposure to *Salmonella*. Anything that touches live poultry can also be contaminated with *Salmonella*, including food and water dishes, pens, coops, plants, and soil. To prevent exposure to *Salmonella*, wash hands with soap and warm water immediately after handling poultry or anything they touch, keep poultry and anything they touch outside the house, and follow other biosecurity recommendations discussed previously. The CDC further states: "Do not eat or drink where the birds live or roam, do not wash their bowls in the kitchen sink, and do not house poultry in bathrooms or keep where food is prepared, served, or stored" [8]. Those composting poultry feces to use as compost in gardens or elsewhere should consult the Environmental Protection Agency's website describing the various recommended safe composting methods known to kill bacteria available at https://www.epa.state.oh.us/portals/35/sludge/503_08_04_99.pdf [9].

Epidemiology

S. Enteritidis can survive several years in a favorable environment; the organism also accumulates and can survive for months in feed, fecal material, and soil [10]. Freezing will decrease its survival, but some bacteria can survive and replicate when thawed. *Salmonella* is susceptible to heating and drying and many common disinfectants, including phenolic compounds, chlorine, and iodine-based compounds, but organic material must be removed for disinfectants to be effective.

Since 2000, there have been 70 outbreaks of *Salmonella* linked to backyard poultry, with 2017 having the most cases. In 2017, there were 1120 cases of *Salmonella* in 48 states often due to contact with backyard poultry. There were 249 hospitalizations and 1 death associated with these multistate outbreaks. Ten different types of *Salmonella*, including *Salmonella* Enteriditis and *Salmonella* Typhimurium, were identified in the various outbreaks [11]. At the time of writing this text in July 2018, a new multistate outbreak has led to 124 cases of salmonellosis in 26 states with 21 hospitalizations and 0 deaths to date. Several different types of bacteria have been implicated in the current outbreak, including *Salmonella* Seftenberg, *Salmonella* Montevideo, *Salmonella* Infantis, *Salmonella* Enteriditis, *Salmonella* Indiana, and *Salmonella* Litchfield. Many of the affected people obtained chicks and ducklings from a variety of sources, including feed supply stores, websites, hatcheries, and relatives [12]. As backyard poultry continues to increase in popularity, the number of *Salmonella* outbreaks linked to live poultry will undoubtedly increase if appropriate preventive measures are not taken. If given the opportunity, veterinarians should educate poultry owners about the risks of all zoonoses, but particularly salmonellosis, as its prevalence continues to increase.

Additional Zoonoses from Oral Exposure

Campylobacteriosis

Campylobacteriosis is a commonly reported foodborne illness in humans and is estimated to affect 1.3 million people annually in the United States [13]. Transmission is usually through ingestion of contaminated food or water but can occur from live poultry as well [14]. *Campylobacter* bacteria are common in poultry but cause no clinical disease. Wild birds can be a source of infection for backyard poultry and humans. One study evaluating 333 wild birds in the mid-Atlantic region of the United States detected *Campylobacter jejuni*, *C. coli*, or *C. lari* via multiplex polymerase chain reaction (PCR) in six avian families, with an overall prevalence of 7.2% [15]. Crows (Corvidae) and gulls (Laridae) had the highest prevalence at 23% and 25%, respectively [15]. Another study evaluating 318 fecal samples from urban resident Canada geese in North Carolina detected six different strains of *C. jejuni*, including one strain (ST-4071) that has been associated with human illness [16]. The prevalence in the Canada geese was 5% in 2008 and 16% in 2009. Biosecurity measures described in Chapter 5, including exclusion of wild birds and proper hygiene around poultry, will reduce exposure to *Campylobacter* sp.

Colibacilosis

Colibacilosis is caused by many different types of *E. coli*, and the CDC estimates that approximately 400 000 human cases occur annually in the United States [17]. Similar to *Salmonella*, transmission of colibacilosis is typically through the ingestion of contaminated food or water. Human outbreaks are often associated with contaminated meat, fresh greens, or unpasteurized milk. Symptoms in people include stomach cramps, diarrhea, and vomiting. Most cases are self-limiting, but others can become severe and even fatal. Although *E. coli* is less commonly associated with poultry than *Salmonella*, a recent report found *E. coli* to be the most common bacterial cause of mortality or significant morbidity in backyard poultry [4]. Additionally, a study found colistin resistance genes in *E. coli* collected from backyard poultry in Vietnam; 12.8% of the samples collected from poultry were positive for the colistin resistance *mcr-1* gene [18]. Additionally, 4% of isolates from farmers were positive for *mcr-1* bacteria [18]. Although geographically distant from the United States, the spread of resistance genes is possible through global trade. Veterinarians must encourage prudent antibiotic use, including appropriate culture and sensitivity of ill animals, to ensure correct therapeutic applications.

Listeriosis

Sporadic outbreaks of listeriosis, caused by the gram-positive, non–spore-forming bacteria *Listeria monocytogenes*, have been described in chickens, turkeys, ducks, geese, pigeons, canaries, parrots, and other birds [19, 20]. A study found that backyard poultry's mortality due to the bacteria was rarely caused by *Listeria* sp. (3:305) [4]. Usually, affected birds are young and show signs of torticollis with the encephalitic form or emaciation and diarrhea with the septicemic form [20]. The usual route of human exposure is through consumption of contaminated poultry, resulting in neurological signs [20]. Presumptive diagnosis is based on gross and histopathological lesions, including inflammatory foci in the brain, splenomegaly, multifocal hepatic necrosis, myocardial necrosis, and pericarditis, but a definitive diagnosis is based on culture [20]. This organism is resistant to many commonly used antibiotics, and therefore, treatment is often unsuccessful in poultry.

Cryptosporidiosis

Currently, it is questionable whether contact with live poultry can be a source of human cryptosporidiosis infection, since *Cryptosporidium baileyi*, found in avian species, has not been found to infect animals other than birds. Further, *C. parvum*, found in mammals including humans, is not commonly seen in poultry [21]. Recent studies have suggested that because a *C. meleagridis* strain was shown to infect mice, it has the potential to be transmitted from birds to humans [22]. A recent study of 2579 fecal samples from 46 chicken farms and 8 Pekin duck farms in Henan Province, China, showed *C. baiylei* was present on many farms, but more importantly, *C. meleagridis*, which has the potential to be zoonotic, was isolated via PCR from 31 to 120 day old chickens from 3 of the 46 chicken layer farms [23]. Another study using PCR found the prevalence of *C. meleagridis* in turkeys from 16 farms and chickens from 23 farms in Algeria to be 44% and 29%, respectively [24].

Avian Chlamydiosis

General Information

Although human exposure to *Chlamydia psittaci* (formerly known as *Chlamydophila psittaci*) from poultry usually occurs at turkey slaughter plants, backyard chickens can carry the organism and potentially infect humans. A complete description of *C. psittaci* and the disease in humans and animals can be found in the periodically updated "Compendium of Measures to Control *Chlamydophila psittaci* Infections Among Humans (Psittacosis) and Pet Birds (Avian Chlamydiosis)," 2017, by the National Association of State Public Health Veterinarians [25].

Taxonomy and Nomenclature

The human disease psittacosis goes by the names parrot fever, ornithosis, and chlamydiosis. The term "psittacosis" refers to the human disease originating from a parrot (a psittacine bird), whereas the term "ornithosis" refers to the human disease originating from any species of bird. The term "chlamydiosis" is more generic, referring to an infective organism in any animal or person within in the *Chlamydia* genus. The term "avian chlamydiosis" is used to specify an infection with *C. psittaci* in birds.

Note that *C. psittaci* should not be confused with a related organism in humans, *Chlamydia trachomatis*, a sexually transmitted disease of people, or another related organism, *Chlamydia pneumoniae*, a common mild respiratory pathogen of humans.

Over the past two decades, the nomenclature of the family Chlamydiaceae has changed due to advances in DNA testing. When reading the literature, the same organism will be referred to as *Chlamydia psittaci* or *Chlamydophila psittaci* depending on the date and current genomic classification. The current term, *C. psittaci,* will be used throughout this document to refer to the organism formerly known as *Chlamydophila psittaci*.

Epidemiology

C. psittaci has been found in 130 species of birds worldwide and a variety of mammals, including humans. Birds are known to be a potential source of infection and include domestic or wild pigeons, passerines (soft-billed birds), or poultry, although poultry do not usually exhibit overt illness with this disease.

The general prevalence of chlamydial infection in captive and wild birds is thought to be low, but the prevalence may increase dramatically in birds stressed by shipping, crowding, chilling, and breeding [24]. Those who have an occupational risk for the disease include pet store employees, veterinarians, veterinary technicians, laboratory workers, workers in avian quarantine stations, farmers, wildlife rehabilitators, zoo workers, and employees of poultry slaughtering and processing plants (usually involving turkeys).

Pathogenesis

The *C. psittaci* organism is transmitted by either inhalation or ingestion of the spore-like elementary body phase of the organism. Shedding in birds can be activated by stress, such as shipping, crowding, chilling, and breeding. Individuals who are immunosuppressed are more susceptible to the disease and its effects.

The organism *C. psittaci* is relatively resistant, surviving in soil for 3 months or within bird droppings for up to 1 month. *C. psittaci* is a dimorphic organism, meaning it exists in two different forms called phases: the infectious phase and the replicating phase. In general, the *C. psittaci* organism enters the host via inhalation or ingestion and replicates in the host's cells. The infectious form is small (0.2–0.6 μm) and called an elementary body. After the elementary body is inhaled or ingested, it is endocytosed by a host cell, where it transforms into a reticulate body. The reticulate body is larger (1.5 μm) than the elementary body and is the replicating, or metabolically active, form of the organism inside the host's cell. The reticulate body uses nutrients from the host cell and undergoes multiple rounds of binary division before releasing multiple elementary bodies from the cell when it ruptures. Two or more days pass between the time the host cell is infected and the elementary bodies are released. These infectious elementary bodies then infect other host cells or are released into the environment via feces, nasal secretions, sputum, blood, or infected tissues. The elementary body is metabolically inactive and resistant to environmental forces, so it can survive long enough to be inhaled or ingested by another host.

Persons performing a necropsy of any bird suspected of having avian chlamydiosis should wear gloves and wet the carcass with soapy water to decrease aerosolization of organisms, as well as practice Animal Biosafety Level 2 practices, which includes containment equipment and facilities and respiratory protection.

Clinical Signs

Poultry, pigeons, and passerines seem to exhibit little if any clinical signs of disease while infected with the *C. psittaci* organism and, therefore, are sometimes referred to as asymptomatic carriers of the disease.

Diagnosis

There are many tests available for use in birds, including tests to detect antibodies in the serum (elementary body assay [EBA] and immunofluorescent antibody [IFA]) and tests to detect antigen in the feces or blood (enzyme-linked immunosorbent assay [ELISA], and PCR). It is best to perform a panel of tests, including PCR of blood, PCR of feces, and IFA of serum. Alternatively, a fluorescent antibody [FA] test can be performed on tissue, such as a liver, from a biopsy or necropsy and is available through most state diagnostic laboratories. For legal purposes, cell culture from the feces is the best test. However, the organism does not consistently grow in feces, and shedding of the organism in the feces is intermittent. There is also risk to personnel when the organism is grown in the laboratory. For backyard poultry, the most common situation resulting in a diagnosis of avian chlamydiosis is where PCR is performed on a necropsy specimen that died with a concurrent illness, such as mycoplasmosis.

Treatment

The treatment of birds should be supervised by a licensed veterinarian. The treatment of choice in birds is oral doxycycline, since it is absorbed better and eliminated slower than other tetracyclines (see chapter on drugs for further information regarding egg-laying or meat birds). During treatment, care should be taken to observe for signs of toxicosis, such as lethargy, anorexia, or biliverdinuria. If any of these occur, the doxycycline should be discontinued and the bird offered supportive care until recovered; afterward, a lower dose can be attempted.

Prevention and Control

People cleaning cages or handling infected birds should wear protective clothing, gloves, a disposable cap, and a respirator or appropriate mask. Accurate records should be maintained of all bird-related transactions to aid in identifying sources of infection and potentially exposed persons; records should include the date of purchase, species of bird, source of birds, leg band numbers, and describe any illness or deaths of birds. Avoid purchasing or selling sick birds and isolate newly acquired birds for at least 30 days. Test birds before they are to be boarded or sold on consignment.

Chlamydial organisms can be killed with most commonly used disinfectants, including freshly prepared 1:32 dilution of household bleach solution (1/2 cup per gallon), 1% phenol compounds, or 1:1000 dilution of quaternary ammonium compounds [25]. Gloves and a respirator should be worn in an avian outbreak in any areas exposed to the positive bird or its fecal matter. It is important to clean and remove all organic matter first and then disinfect. Chlamydiosis in humans is a Nationally Notifiable Disease. Avian chlamydiosis is reportable in most states, meaning if a veterinarian diagnoses chlamydiosis in a bird, the case must be reported to the state veterinarian or public health department. Usually the public health department becomes involved if humans are affected.

Mycobacteriosis

Mycobacteriosis has been diagnosed in many avian species, including Galliformes and Anseriformes.

Taxonomy

Mycobacteriosis in birds is generally caused by the acid-fast bacteria *Mycobacterium avium* or *M. genevense*. Other species have also been identified in infected birds. The bacteria can survive in soil for several months [26].

Epidemiology and Pathogenesis

Transmission of the bacteria is through inhalation or ingestion. Because of the long incubation period, it is sometimes difficult to determine the source of human or bird exposure. The reported prevalence of mycobacteriosis in wild bird populations varies from 4% to 40% [26]. It has been reported that poultry, pheasants, and sparrows are highly susceptible; guinea fowl and domestic turkeys are less susceptible; domestic geese and ducks are moderately resistant; and the domestic pigeon is highly resistant to *Mycobacteria* infection [26].

Clinical Signs

Avian mycobacteriosis generally causes chronic weight loss and unthriftiness. Unlike humans, infection of the respiratory tract is uncommon in birds; most birds develop granulomatous masses of the liver, spleen, and intestines.

Diagnosis

Radiographs of the granulomatous masses can be suggestive but are not definitive for diagnosis. Demonstration of acid-fast organisms in feces is also suggestive but not definitive, since other nonpathogenic acid-fast organisms can be in the feces. Demonstration of acid-fast organisms in tissues is highly suggestive. Usually *M. avian* is associated with large numbers of organisms in birds, whereas *M. tuberculosis* and *M. bovis* are not. The organism is difficult and dangerous to culture.

The intradermal tuberculin test used in many mammals is not reliable in most birds, but it has been used with some success in the wattle of chickens [26]. The standard purified protein derivative (PPD) is injected intradermally (0.05–0.1 mL, 2000 IU) into one wattle of the chicken [26]. Heat, swelling (>5 mm), and edema of the injection site 48 hours later are considered positive for infection with, or sensitization to, *M. avium* [26]. This tuberculin test is considered about 80% accurate in detecting infected birds compared to gross lesions, but birds in the advanced stages of disease may have no reaction [26]. If testing waterfowl, the whole blood agglutination test is considered better than the tuberculin test but may have false positives [26].

Treatment

Treatment of birds with mycobacteriosis should be discouraged and euthanasia should be the first option discussed for numerous reasons, including: the *M. avium* organism is often resistant to antimycobacterial drugs (e.g., isoniazid, ethambutol, rifampicin, and pyrazinamide); long-term (12–18 month) treatment can be excessively expensive; the organism has zoonotic potential; and there is a lack of pharmacokinetic or pharmacodynamic data of antimycobacterial drugs in birds.

Influenza A

Avian influenza is highly infectious and affects many species. The disease in birds is explained in detail in the chapter on avian influenza and exotic Newcastle disease in this book. The zoonotic capabilities of this virus are described next.

Taxonomy and Nomenclature

Influenza virus is in the Orthomyxoviridae family. There are three types of influenza, types A, B, and C, but only type A is found in birds. There are influenza A subtypes based on surface proteins: "H" for hemagglutinin and "N" for neuraminidase. There are 15 known H subtypes and 9 known N subtypes. All subtypes are found in birds, but only H1, H2, H3, N1, and N2 are typically found in humans. All avian virulent strains to date have been in the H5 or H7 subtype, but most H5 or H7 isolates are of low virulence.

History

In 1918–1919, there was an H1N1 influenza A pandemic in humans called the "Spanish flu." This outbreak may have killed 20–50 million people worldwide, and 50% were young, healthy adults. More than 500 000 deaths were attributed to the flu in the United States. In 1957–1958, the H2N2 "Asian flu" caused approximately 70 000 human deaths in the United States. In 1968–1969, the H3N2 "Hong Kong flu" caused 34 000 human deaths in the United States and still circulates today. In 1961, influenza A H5N1 was first isolated from terns in South Africa. In 1997, influenza A was shown to pass from birds to humans in an outbreak in Hong Kong, where 18 people became sick and 6 died after being in contact with infected birds. This outbreak was controlled by killing 1.5 million chickens. In 1999, in Hong Kong, China, H9N2 was confirmed in two children, both of whom recovered. Both children had previous contact with chickens.

In 2003, influenza A H5N1 was isolated from two human cases in Hong Kong, one of whom died. Then, the H5N1 subtype was confirmed in turkey poults in Cambodia, China (Hong Kong had a single positive peregrine falcon), Indonesia, Japan, Laos, South Korea, Thailand, and Vietnam. Human deaths of influenza A H5N1 were reported in Thailand and Vietnam after contact with infected birds or their excretions (nasal, saliva, or feces). This H5N1 subtype isolated from humans has been genetically sequenced and all genes were of bird origin; it was found to be resistant to two antiviral drugs, amantadine and rimantadine, but still sensitive to oseltamivir and zanamivir. To date, approximately 600 human cases have been reported with a 60% case-fatality rate. Also in 2003, influenza A H7N7 was isolated from poultry workers in the Netherlands. More than 80 cases were reported, and a veterinarian died from the infection. People in the Netherlands outbreak exhibited ocular symptoms, with some also having respiratory symptoms.

More recently in the spring of 2013, an H7N9 influenza virus emerged in China and has led to 1564 laboratory-confirmed human cases as of September 2017 [27]. This virus was particularly interesting because it did not lead to morbidity or mortality in poultry. Recent outbreaks of avian influenza in the United States have not led to any human morbidity or mortality [28, 29].

Epidemiology and Pathogenesis

Wild birds, especially waterfowl, are the natural hosts for influenza A and do not generally exhibit illness from infection. Domestic birds, particularly chickens, are very susceptible to high mortality with influenza A. Animal-to-human transmission has occurred but is unusual at the current time. The virus is currently not efficient at human-to-human transmission, but gene mutation is common and may lead to sustained human-to-human transmission in the future.

The World Health Organization (WHO), along with other organizations, is monitoring for human gene development in order to stop the virus before it spreads by killing birds infected or exposed to pathogenic strains (H5 or H7).

The Office International des Epizooties (OIE) is an international organization based in France. It was formed by 28 countries in 1928 and now comprises 165 countries. The OIE is a clearinghouse of reported cases of animal disease from each of the member countries and aids in the rapid response to multicountry outbreaks.

Diagnosis

Many tests are available to diagnose avian influenza, including the agar gel immunodiffusion (AGID) test, ELISA, and RT-PCR. Not all birds develop demonstrable antibodies on the ELISA. The hemagglutination and hemagglutination inhibition tests are also available. Birds with H5 or H7 are required to be depopulated.

Prevention and Control

People cleaning cages, handling infected birds, or slaughtering birds should wear protective equipment. Influenza is typically contracted through inhalation, so respiratory protection, such as a mask, is of utmost importance. Gloves and eye protection can also be beneficial. Areas where birds are housed or slaughtered should be regularly cleaned and disinfected. The virus can survive days to weeks in feces, depending on environmental conditions. The virus is typically susceptible to the most commonly used disinfectants.

Newcastle Disease

Newcastle disease is caused by a paramyxovirus and is classified as either velogenic (virulent) or lentogenic, depending on virulence [30]. Velogenic Newcastle disease is also known as virulent or exotic Newcastle disease and is a reportable foreign animal disease in the United States. In people, Newcastle disease causes a mild, acute granular conjunctivitis, general malaise, and sinusitis that resolves within 7–20 days. Exposure is usually from affected chickens but can also be from the live vaccine. In May 2018, an outbreak of virulent (exotic) Newcastle disease was identified in a small backyard flock in California and it has subsequently spread [31]. Please see Chapter 13 for further information on the disease in poultry.

Arboviruses

West Nile Virus

The causative organism of West Nile disease is a flavivirus. West Nile Virus was endemic in other countries, but in the late 1990s, it was identified in the eastern United States. The virus has since become endemic in the continental United States. Crows, jays, raptors, ducks, and horses are susceptible species, whereas most poultry species are considered resistant to clinical disease [32]. The WNV is spread by numerous species of mosquitos; there is no direct transmission from birds to people. If people are clinically affected, they are usually older or immunosuppressed. There is no vaccine available for humans, and mosquito control is the primary method used to prevent disease in people. There is a vaccine available for use in horses that is often used in at-risk species of captive birds.

Eastern and Western Equine Encephalomyelitis Virus

Eastern equine encephalitis (EEE) and Western equine encephalitis (WEE) are both caused by togaviruses. Clinical disease of EEE is most common in birds that are not native to North America, such as imported pheasants and cranes [33]. Clinical disease of WEE has been reported in pheasants, emus, chukars, English sparrows, chickens, and turkeys [33]. Many species of birds act as reservoirs for EEE and WEE. Chickens rarely develop disease from either of these viruses, and they do not typically develop high enough viremia to play a significant role in the transmission of the virus via mosquitos. Therefore, chickens are often used as sentinels for these diseases. The virus is transmitted through a mosquito bite; similar to West Nile virus, there is no direct transmission from birds to humans.

People are an accidental host to the EEE or WEE viruses and mortality can reach 75% if infected with EEE virus and 7% if infected with WEE virus [33].

Hypersensitivity Pneumonitis

Hypersensitivity pneumonitis is not an infectious disease but rather an allergic inflammation of the lungs in humans in response to certain antigens, such as feather dander, droppings, or moldy hay. The disease is sometimes called farmer's lung, bird breeder's lung, pigeon breeder's lung, or poultry worker's lung. It can present in acute, sub-acute, or chronic forms and can lead to death [34]. Poultry workers have been shown to have a higher prevalence of toxic pneumonitis, airway inflammation, and chronic bronchitis compared to controls [35]. Appropriate ventilation, cleaning of facilities, and respiratory protection, such as a mask, can reduce the likelihood of developing this problem.

References

1 Grunkemeyer, V.L. (2011). Zoonoses, public health, and the backyard poultry flock. *Vet. Clin. Exot. Anim.* 14: 477–490.

2 https://www.aphis.usda.gov/aphis/ourfocus/animalhealth/animal-disease-information/avian/avian-health (accessed 8 January 2018).

3 https://www.cdc.gov/salmonella/index.html (accessed 8 January 2018).

4 Mete, A., Giannitte, F., Barr, B. et al. (2013). Causes of mortality in backyard chickens in Northern California: 2007-2011. *Avian Dis.* 57 (2): 311–315.

5 https://www.aphis.usda.gov/aphis/ourfocus/animalhealth/nvap/NVAP-Reference-Guide/Poultry/National-Poultry-Improvement-Plan (accessed 8 January 2018).

6 https://www.cdc.gov/healthypets/resources/backyard-flock.pdf (accessed 8 January 2018).

7 Mermin, J., Hutwagner, L., Vugia, D. et al. (2004). Reptiles, amphibians and human Salmonella infection: a population-based, case-controlled study. *Clin. Infect. Dis.* 38 (Suppl 3): S253–S261.

8 https://www.cdc.gov/salmonella/general/index.html (accessed 8 January 2018).

9 https://www.epa.state.oh.us/portals/35/sludge/503_08_04_99.pdf (accessed 4 November 2019).

10 Shivaprasad, H.L. (2003). Pullorum disease and fowl typhoid. In: *Diseases of Poultry*, 11e (ed. Y.M. Saif), 568–582. Ames, Iowa, USA: Blackwell Publishing.

11 https://www.cdc.gov/salmonella/live-poultry-06-17/index.html (accessed 8 January 2018).

12 https://www.cdc.gov/salmonella/backyard-flocks-06-18/index.html (accessed 8 January 2018).

13 https://www.cdc.gov/campylobacter/ (accessed 8 January 2018).

14 https://www.cdc.gov/healthypets/pets/farm-animals/backyard-poultry.html (accessed 8 January 2018).

15 Keller, J.I., Shriver, G., Waldenstrom, J. et al. (2011). Prevalence of campylobacter in wildbirds of the mid-Atlantic region, USA. *J. Wildl. Dis.* 47 (3): 750–754.

16 Rutledge, M.E., Siletski, R.M., Weimin, G.U. et al. (2013). Characterization of campylobacter from resident Canada geese in an urban environment. *J. Wild. Dis.* 49 (1): 1–9.

17 https://www.cdc.gov/foodborneburden/ (accessed 8 January 2018).

18 Trung, N.V., Matamoros, S., Carrique-Mas, J.J. et al. (2017). Zoonotic transmission of mcr-1 Colistin resistance gene from small-scale poultry farms, Vietnam. *Emerg. Infect. Dis.* 23 (3): 529–532.

19 Barnes, H.J. and Nolan, L.K. (2008). Other bacterial infections. In: *Diseases of Poultry*, 12e (ed. Y.M. Saif), 891–970. Ames, Iowa, USA: Wiley Blackwell.

20 https://www.merckvetmanual.com/poultry/listeriosis/overview-of-listeriosis-in-poultry (accessed 8 January 2018).

21 McDougald, L.R. (2008). Cryptosporidiosis. Protozoal Infections. In: *Diseases of Poultry*, 12e (ed. Y.M. Saif), 1067–1120. Ames, Iowa, USA: Wiley Blackwell.

22 Sreter, T., Kovacs, G., DaSilva, A.J. et al. (2000). Morphologic, host specificity, and molecular characteristics of a Hungarian *Cryptosporidium meleagridis* isolate. *Appl. Env. Micro.*: 735–738.

23 Wang, R., Jian, F., Sun, Y. et al. (2010). Large-scale survey of cryptosporidium species in chickens and Pekin ducks (*Anas platyrhychos*) in Henan, China: prevalence and molecular characterization. *Avian Pathol.* 39 (6): 447–451.

24 Baroudi, D., Khelef, D., Goucem, R. et al. (2013). Common occurrence of zoonotic pathogen *Cryptosporidium meleagridis* in backyard chickens and turkeys in Algeria. *Vet. Parasit.* 196 (3–4): 334–340.

25 http://nasphv.org/documentsCompendiaPsittacosis.html (accessed 8 January 2018).

26 Dharma, K., Mahendran, M., Singh, S., and Sawant, P.M. (2011). Tuberculosis in Birds: Insights into the *Mycobacterium avium* Infections. *Vet. Med. Int.* 2011: 14. Art. No. 712369, http://dx.doi.org/10.4061/2011/712369.

27 http://www.who.int/csr/don/26-october-2017-ah7n9-china/en (accessed 8 January 2018).

28 https://www.aphis.usda.gov/aphis/ourfocus/animalhealth/animal-disease-information/avian/avian-influenza/ai (accessed 8 January 2018).

29 Fitzpatrick, A., Mor, S.K., Thurn, M. et al. (2017). Outbreak of highly pathogenic avian influenza in Minnesota in 2015. *J. Vet. Diagn. Invest.* 29 (2): 169–175.

30 https://www.merckvetmanual.com/poultry/newcastle-disease-and-other-paramyxovirus-infections/newcastle-disease-in-poultry (accessed 8 January 2018).

31 https://www.aphis.usda.gov/aphis/newsroom/news/sa_by_date/sa-2018/vrn (accessed 8 January 2018).

32 https://www.merckvetmanual.com/poultry/west-nile-virus-infection-in-poultry/overview-of-west-nile-virus-infection-in-poultry (accessed 8 January 2018).

33 https://www.merckvetmanual.com/poultry/viral-encephalitides/overview-of-viral-encephalitides-in-poultry (accessed 8 January 2018).

34 Hirschmann, J.V., Pipavath, S.N.J., and Godwin, J.D. (2009). Hypersensitivity pneumonitis: a historical, clinical, and radiologic review. *Radiographics* 29: 1921–1938.

35 Rylander, R. and Carvalheiro, M.F. (2006). Airways inflammation among workers in poultry houses. *Int. Arch. Occup. Environ. Health* 79 (6): 487–490.

11

Parasitic Diseases

Richard Gerhold

College of Veterinary Medicine, University of Tennessee, Knoxville, TN, USA

Introduction

Clinical parasitic disease in backyard poultry in general is less of an issue compared to commercially raised poultry due to the lower density of birds. When parasite-associated morbidity and mortality occur in backyard poultry, it is often due to poor husbandry and nutrition, overcrowding, or mixing of avian species or mixing of multiple age groups. This chapter contains common clinically significant parasites of backyard poultry, particularly birds in the order Galliformes, and thus is not an exhaustive list of avian parasites. Confirmatory testing for numerous parasites may require the submission of samples to a trained parasitologist. It is important to contact the respective laboratories prior to collection and shipment of samples to ensure proper protocols are followed to maximize parasite identification (Table 11.1).

Parasitic Causes of Diarrhea

Coccidiosis

Name of Disease: Coccidiosis

Clinical History: Although coccidiosis outbreaks have been reported from backyard poultry, the disease is most often observed in commercially raised birds. This is for two reasons: (i) parasite replication is self-limiting given the fixed number of asexual cycles and (ii) after infection, the host develops protective immunity. The disease most often occurs in immunologically naive animals or in animals that are stressed or crowded which both can result in overwhelming infections.

Causative Agent: Coccidiosis is the general term given to the disease caused by the lesions and clinical signs elicited by *Eimeria* spp., which are obligate intracellular protozoal parasites that infect and replicate within the host's intestinal epithelial cells.

Clinical Signs and Lesions: Mild to moderately affected birds have suppressed weight gain and diarrhea. Severely affected birds are depressed, have marked diarrhea (possibly with blood), ruffled feathers, and the birds often huddle together for warmth. Significant mortality can occur in untreated flocks. The lesions and clinical signs produced by the parasites are a function of the number of ingested oocysts, the immune status and age of the host, the site of infection, concurrent infections, and other factors [1].

Clinical coccidiosis in chickens is usually due to one of three species. Lesion with *Eimeria acervulina* causes raised white nodules in the duodenum, and *Eimeria maxima*

Table 11.1 List of laboratories that are known to perform parasitology tests on poultry samples.

Institution	Investigator	Laboratory address	Laboratory email	Laboratory phone number	Laboratory website
University of Tennessee	Rick Gerhold	University of Tennessee, CVM, 2407 River Dr., A233 Knoxville, TN 37996-4543	rgerhold@utk.edu	865-974-5645	http://www.vet.utk.edu/diagnostic/parasitology
Virginia Tech University	David Lindsay	VA-MD CVM, 1410 Prices Fork Rd. VA Tech Blacksburg, VA 24061	lindsayd@vt.edu	504-231-6302	http://www.vetmed.vt.edu/org/dbsp/faculty/lindsay.asp
Mississippi State University	Sue Ann Hubbard Kelli Jones	Poultry Research and Diagnostic Lab. MSU/CVM, 3137 Hwy. 468 W., Pearl MS 39208	hubbard@mvrdl.msstate.edu kjones@mvrdl.msstate.edu	601-932-6771	
Arkansas	Tom Yazwinski	Department of Animal Science, AFLS B110D, University of Arkansas, Fayetteville, AR 72701	yazwinsk@uark.edu	479-575-4398	
University of Georgia	Lorraine Fuller	Poultry Science Dept., 152 Poultry Science Bld. University of Georgia, Athens GA 30602-2772	alfuller@uga.edu	706-542-1367	
USDA, ARS	Eric Hoberg	US National Parasites Collection; Animal Parasitic Diseases, BARC-1180, 10300 Baltimore Ave., room 1180, Beltsville, MD 20705-2350	Eric.hoberg@ars.usda.gov	301-504-8588	

In general, most state animal health/veterinary diagnostic laboratories can run fecal examinations on poultry.

causes hemorrhage and mucosal reddening in the jejunum. *Eimeria tenella* causes hemorrhagic cecal cores, and often bloody feces are noted (Figure 11.1). Clinical disease in domestic turkeys is due to various different *Eimeria* species, especially *Eimeria adenoides* (which form dry firm cecal cores), and *Eimeria meleagrimitis* (forming petechiae and pseudomembranes in the ileum and jejunum).

Coccidia in game birds is often more prolific than in chickens and turkeys and can reach levels as high as 600 000–2 000 000 oocysts produced per oocyst ingestion [2, 3]. Oocyst production generally extends longer in game birds compared to chickens and turkeys, leading to increased environmental contamination [3]. Coccidiosis in ring-necked pheasants and chukars presents with gross lesions consisting of caseous cecal cores and hemorrhagic typhlitis.

In contrast, bobwhite quail usually lack cecal cores but instead have attenuated intestinal mucosa with marked enteritis and abundant edema.

Transmission Route: Oocysts are shed in the host's feces and, once outside the host, undergo sporulation. Following ingestion by another host animal, sporulated oocysts rupture, releasing sporozoites that infect the host's epithelial cells. Sporulation occurs more rapidly in ambient temperatures greater than 25 °C. Minimum sporulation time can be as little as 24 hours in warm, moist conditions.

Diagnostic Tests: Oocysts can be easily found on fecal floats or intestinal scrapes from affected regions of the intestines. Oocyst size and prepatent periods can vary depending on the *Eimeria* spp. infecting the birds [1] (Figure 11.2).

Differential Diagnosis: *Clostridium* infection, histomonosis, salmonellosis, cryptosporidiosis, dehydration, and pesticide intoxication.

Prevention and Control: Prevention of coccidiosis can be performed by removing bird feces and limiting mixing of young and older birds. Subclinical infections of coccidia can predispose birds to other parasitic and bacterial infections including *Clostridium* spp.; proper coccidial control is important for overall health.

The development of effective chemotherapy against coccidia was a major milestone in the evolution of the poultry industry; and without the use of these anticoccidial compounds, the broiler industry as we know it would not exist. Anticoccidial compounds generally fall into one of two categories. The first are polyether ionophores, which disrupt the proper intracellular and extracellular concentrations of the various cations and lead to cellular dysfunction in the parasite. The second group includes compounds that

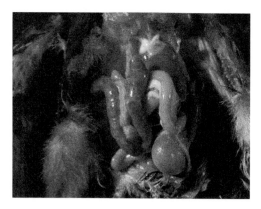

Figure 11.1 Necrohemorrhagic cecal cores in a two week old Americauna chick with severe coccidiosis from *Eimeria tenella*. *Source:* Photograph courtesy of Dr. Shelly Newman, University of Tennessee, Department of Biological and Diagnostic Services.

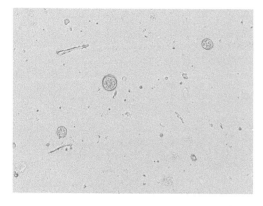

Figure 11.2 Sugar flotation generated *Eimeria* spp. oocysts from a chicken. Freshly defecated oocysts are unsporulated.

cause an enzymatic reaction. Ionophores generally have a lower rate of resistance development compared to the enzyme reaction drugs just listed and often allow some low-level cycling of the coccidia in the host, leading to host immunity [4]. Anticoccidial drugs belonging to the polyether ionophores include lasalocid, salinomycin, maduramicin, monensin, narasin, lonomycin, and semduramicin. Other drugs include amprolium, clopidol, diclazuril, decoquinate, robenidine, roxarsone, sulfadimethoxine/ormetoprin, salinomycin, semduramicin, and zoalene. The efficacy of these drugs is variable and may require some investigations to determine the most effective compound. Due to continual use of amprolium, resistance has been reported in numerous species including bobwhite quail [5]. Maxiban (narasin/nicarbazin) has been found to be toxic in turkeys and should not be used in this species. Live vaccines, consisting of infective oocysts of the important *Eimeria* species, are available for use in the poultry industry, providing an alternative to the use of anticoccidial drugs. The development of vaccines for coccidia is possible due to the fact that replication is self-limiting and infected birds develop protective cell-mediated immunity [6]. Protective immunity develops rapidly after exposure but depends on reinfection to reinforce the developing protection. There is no confirmed cross-protection between different species of *Eimeria* resulting in the requirement for multiple species of coccidia in vaccines. Given that *Eimeria* are species specific, separate and specific vaccine formulations are needed for each species of bird. Commercial vaccines are currently available for chickens and turkeys. Northern bobwhites and chukars administered low dose of *Eimeria lettyae* were protected against a high dose challenge, suggesting that vaccine development may be an option in game birds [7, 8].

Zoonotic Potential: None. *Eimeria* are species specific.

Histomonosis

Name of Disease: Histomonosis, histomoniasis, or blackhead

Clinical History: Blackhead is considered the most important parasitic disease for turkeys and is an important cause of mortality for numerous game birds. Recently mortality has been documented in backyard chickens [9].

Causative Agent: *Histomonas meleagridis* is a protozoal enteric pleomorphic flagellate. It loses the flagellum once it adheres to the intestinal wall and therefore has flagellated and amoeboid stages.

Clinical Signs and Lesions: Clinical signs include diarrhea, often having a sulfur yellow appearance, along with nonspecific findings of weight loss and ruffled feathers. Gross lesions generally include characteristic target shaped foci of necrosis of variable size in the liver (Figure 11.3).

The ceca are markedly thickened and the lumen is distended by a large amount of caseous necrotic and hemorrhagic material consistent with cecal cores (Figure 11.4).

Transmission Route: Ringneck pheasants are the natural host for *Histomonas*; however chickens can be patent host for the parasites including the *Heterakis* nematode that serves as a paratenic hosts for *Histomonas*. Earthworms and beetles can serve as paratenic hosts, harboring both the *Heterakis* nematode and histomonads. In high densities,

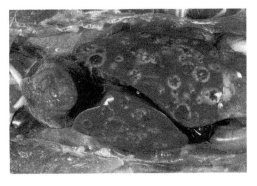

Figure 11.3 Gross histomonosis lesions in a wild turkey liver.

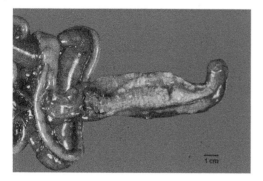

Figure 11.4 Histomonosis in a turkey with cecal lumen distended by a large amount of caseous necrotic and hemorrhagic material consistent with cecal cores.

transmission of histomonads can occur directly from bird to bird via cloacal drinking [10].

Diagnostic Tests: On fresh carcasses, the histomonads can often be identified using saline wet mounts of swabs or scrapes taken from necrotic cores. It is important to have a heat source, such as the microscope light to warm the histomonads. Histomonads have a single flagellum and their motion is characterized by slow agitating circular rotations. This is unlike trichomonads that have a fast undulating motion. If histopathology is performed, within the areas of necrosis and inflammation there are numerous round to oval, 10- to 20-µm-diameter protozoal organisms. Often the protozoa are surrounded by clear vacuoles, giving a halo appearance. Histomonads similar to trichomonads autolyze soon after death; thus, histopath is often unrewarding on birds that have been dead for more than 24 hours. In addition, affected cecal contents can be inoculated into Dwyer's media and shipped to diagnostic laboratories for identification. It is important to inoculate samples into prewarmed (≥30 °C) media and to keep media warm during shipment to ensure survival of histomonads [11]. The addition of tropical fish shipping warmer packets to the shipping container produces an ample heat source (Beckstead and Gerhold, unpublished data).

Differential Diagnosis: Coccidiosis, *Clostridium* infection, salmonellosis, cryptosporidiosis, dehydration, and pesticide intoxication

Prevention and Control: Turkeys, quail, grouse, or chukars cannot be raised in the same areas as chickens or pheasants. Additionally, the practice of raising game birds in houses previously used to house poultry tends to lead to blackhead outbreaks due to the environmental persistence of the *Heterakis* egg containing the histomonads. Various antihelmentics including benzamidazole products aimed at limiting *Heterakis* development have been useful in preventing outbreaks of blackhead [12].

Zoonotic Potential: None reported.

Cryptosporidiosis

Name of Disease: Cryptosporidiosis

Clinical History: Cryptosporidiosis may be seen infrequently in pen-raised quail and other birds.

Causative Agent: *Cryptosporidium baileyi* are coccidia organisms that invade host epithelial cells of the intestines and respiratory system.

Clinical Signs and Lesions: The most common clinical signs include diarrhea and dehydration. In addition to diarrhea, the parasites can infect the respiratory tract and cause respiratory disease. In respiratory infections of the parasite can lead to coughing, sneezing, and dyspnea.

Transmission Route: The oocysts are shed in the feces of infected birds and ingested from contaminated environments.

Diagnostic Tests: The oocysts are small with a diameter of approximately 5 µm. The oocysts have a pink hue when polarized, but they can be difficult to observe due to their small size. Fecal samples from suspected cases should be sent to trained parasitologists for identification.

Differential Diagnosis: Coccidiosis, *Clostridium* infection, salmonellosis, histomoniasis, dehydration, and pesticide intoxication

Prevention and Control: There are no known effective treatments for cryptosporidium. Removing feces and allowing the affected area to be exposed to direct sunlight are the most effective means of controlling outbreaks.

Zoonotic Potential: *Cryptosporidium baileyi* is specific to birds. Turkeys and chickens can be infected with *Cryptosporidium meleagridis*, which some sources say may be synonymous with *Cryptosporidium parvum*, which is zoonotic [1] (see chapter on zoonosis).

Oral Cavity and Respiratory Diseases

Trichomonosis

Name of Disease: Trichomonosis, trichomoniasis, crop canker, and frounce

Clinical History: Trichomonosis primarily affects pigeons, doves, birds of prey, domestic fowl, and birds in captive collections. The disease is frequently reported in doves and pigeons and is variably reported in other avian species.

Causative Agent: The flagellated protozoal parasite *Trichomonas gallinae*

Clinical Signs and Lesions: Trichomonosis is characterized by a rapid and progressive course. The intragular region (throats) of affected birds may appear to be bulging due to the canker and fluid often accumulates in the mouth most likely due to the inability to swallow. Affected birds may be observed attempting to aggressively ingest food; however, the mass precludes swallowing of food particles. The inability to ingest food leads to rapid weight loss and subsequent weakness and listlessness. Additionally, affected birds may be observed open-mouth breathing and gasping for air if the cankers obstruct respiration. Birds can die after 8–14 days of being infected in acute cases. Lesions initially appear as small white to yellow areas of necrosis within the oral cavity, crop, or esophagus. The cankers expand rapidly, often coalescing, to form large masses in the oral cavity and esophagus and often lead to complete obstruction of the oral cavity and esophagus. The virulence of *T. gallinae* is variable and the parasite can be found in clinically normal as well as diseased birds, so the presence of the parasite is not indicative of disease.

Transmission Route: Trichomonads are transferred from one avian host to another by direct contact or ingestion of contaminated food and water. Contaminated water is the most likely source of infection for chickens and turkeys. Predation of infected birds is a method of exposure for birds of prey.

Diagnostic Tests: Confirmatory testing can be performed by acquiring swabs of the oral fluid, mucus, or canker and performing wet mount examinations by light microscopy. The trichomonads have a characteristic undulating swimming motion (see Video 11.1 on website). A commercial media culture packet (InPouch™ TF) has been developed by BioMed Diagnostics (White City, Oregon, USA) for the culture of bovine trichomonads, but the packets work well for culture of *T. gallinae*. Polymerase chain reaction (PCR) testing is available for samples in which live trichomonads are not available for culture.

Differential Diagnosis: Gross lesions of avian trichomonosis are characteristic but not pathognomonic. Other diseases including avian pox, candidiasis, aspergillosis, oral *Capillaria* spp. infection, salmonellosis, and vitamin A deficiency can have similar gross findings.

Prevention and Control: Routine cleaning of birdfeeders and birdbaths with a 10% bleach solution in water and disposal of wet, moldy feed is recommended to help control outbreaks. Successful treatments in early infections include metronidazole and carnidazole [13]. Treatment of birds with fulminate trichomonosis is generally unrewarding. The intestinal trichomonad *Tetratrichomonas gallinarum* has also been found in numerous galliforms, but the pathogenicity of this parasite is incompletely known.

Crop Capillariasis

Name of Disease: Crop capillariasis, thread worm infection

Clinical History: Crop capillariasis is one of the more frequent causes of respiratory distress in quail. The parasite is found infrequently in other game birds.

Causative Agent: *Capillaria contorta* is a thread-like nematode parasite found in the oral cavity, crop, and esophagus of affected birds.

Clinical Signs and Lesions: The affected birds may be observed open-mouth breathing and gasping for air. The lesions are similar to trichomonosis and often the disease is misdiagnosed as trichomonosis if conformational wet mounts of the protozoa (trichomonads) are not performed. On necropsy, numerous thread worms can be seen especially with use of dissecting scope or magnifying lens.

Transmission Route: Birds are generally infected by ingesting embryonated eggs or the earthworm vector.

Diagnostic Tests: The eggs can be observed on fecal floats. The eggs are 55–60 μm long and 26–28 μm wide; contain two polar opercula; and are similar in appearance to *Trichuris* (whipworm) eggs except the polar plugs are offset in *Capillaria* (Figure 11.5).

The thread-like parasites are slender long worms that may be difficult to visualize grossly

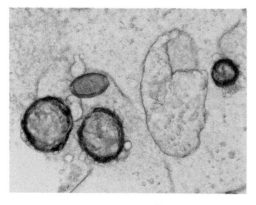

Figure 11.5 *Capillaria* eggs from sugar floatation of chicken feces (20×).

and may require magnifying glass or dissecting scope.

Differential Diagnosis: Avian pox, candidiasis, aspergillosis, trichomonosis, and vitamin A deficiency can have similar gross lesions.

Prevention and Control: The eggs are extremely environmentally resistant; treatment alone will not stop an outbreak. Other capillarids are found in the gastrointestinal tract and can cause weight loss and enteritis. Various antihelmentics including benzamidazole products have been successful; however, there are no approved products available, so prescription-based off-label use is indicated [14]. Prevention of infection is performed by removing feces and limiting access to earthworm vectors.

Syngamiasis

Name of Disease: Gapeworm infection, gapes, tracheal worm, *and* syngamiasis. Pheasants are most frequently affected and it is variably found in other poultry.

Causative Agent: *Syngamus trachea* is a bright red nematode.

Clinical Signs and Lesions: Pheasants are most frequently affected and clinical signs include gaping and gasping, listlessness, and lethargy.

Transmission Route: Eggs are passed up the trachea, swallowed, and then defecated. Eggs can be concentrated by earthworms and various other invertebrates that serve as paratenic hosts.

Diagnostic Tests: The eggs are approximately 80–100 μm in length with shallow polar plugs, similar to the morphology of *Capillaria* and *Trichuris*. These nematodes are easily seen on necropsy given their bright red color and the fact that the males and females are attached and form a characteristic "Y" shape (Figure 11.6).

Differential Diagnosis: Avian pox, candidiasis, aspergillosis, trichomonosis, crop capillariasis, and vitamin A deficiency can have similar gross lesions and clinical signs.

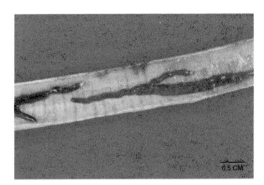

Figure 11.6 *Syngamus trachea* from trachea of wild turkey.

Prevention and Control: Treatments for gapeworm include benzimidazole antihelmentics including thiabendazole and fenbendazole [15]. In the US, thiabendazole is registered for control of gapeworms in pheasants [14].

Zoonotic Potential: None reported.

Dispharynxosis

Name of Disease: Dispharynxosis or proventricular worm

Clinical History: The disease is observed infrequently in ruffed grouse and other galliforms. Severity of disease is related to the number of worms infecting the bird.

Causative Agent: *Dispharynx nasuta* is a nematode.

Clinical Signs and Lesions: Infected birds are often listless, thin, but have an aggressive appetite. The nematode head penetrates the lamina propria of the proventriculus leading to swelling, ulceration, inflammatory infiltrates, caseous necrosis, squamous metaplasia, hemorrhage, and destruction of proventricular glands.

Transmission Route: Eggs are passed in feces and ingested by the required isopod intermediate hosts (pill bugs and sow bugs). The life cycle is completed when the birds ingest the isopod hosts.

Diagnostic Tests: The nematodes are relatively short (8 mm) and are generally found easily in the proventriculus on necropsy. The eggs are ellipsoidal and approximately 35 μm long and 21 μm wide and are embryonated in freshly defecated feces.

Differential Diagnosis: Avian pox, candidiasis, aspergillosis, trichomonosis, and crop capillariasis.

Prevention and Control: Prevention is mainly achieved by limiting feces of wild birds, to accumulate near captive birds and limiting isopod intermediate hosts. Successful treatment has occurred through use of ivermectin and benzimidazoles [16].

Note: Cryptosporidiosis can cause respiratory disease but see listing under causes of diarrhea.

Eyes and Associated Structures

Oxyspiruriasis

Name of Disease: Oxyspiruriasis, eye worm

Clinical History: *Oxyspirura* infection has been reported infrequently in back yard poultry. Nematodes in the genus *Oxyspirura* have been found in numerous galliforms and other avian families.

Causative Agent: *Oxyspirura* are approximately 15 mm long but can range from 8 to 22 mm and have a rounded anterior and pointed posterior.

Clinical Signs and Lesions: Infected birds can have swollen conjunctiva and birds are often seen scratching their eyes. If left untreated, the globe may be destroyed due to chronic inflammation.

Transmission Route: Birds are infected by ingesting infected cockroaches.

Diagnostic Tests: Diagnostics are performed by observing the nematodes in the eye or identification of nematode eggs in feces. Eggs are approximately 55–60 μm long and 45 μm wide and are embryonated in freshly defecated feces.

Differential Diagnosis: Trauma, foreign body

Prevention and Control: Prevention can occur by minimizing ingestion of arthropods. Ivermectin has shown efficacy in treatment of eyeworms in galliforms [17].

Central Nervous System

Toxoplasmosis

Clinical History: Toxoplasmosis is in theory infectious for all granivorous, insectivorous, and carnivorous birds. Infections are reported infrequently, which is perhaps due to lack of surveillance.

Causative Agent: *Toxoplasma gondii* is a coccidia in which felines are the definitive host.

Clinical Signs and Lesions: Clinical signs include incoordination, listlessness, seizures, and convulsions. Gross lesions are variable and can range from no lesions to pneumonia, encephalitis, and splenomegaly.

Transmission Route: Infection occurs by ingestion of oocysts in the environment or by ingestion of tissue cysts in muscle or other organs of intermediate hosts, such as mice.

Diagnostic Tests: Diagnosis of infected birds can be performed using sera in the modified agglutination test (MAT). Post-mortem diagnostics include histopath examination and PCR on affected tissues.

Differential Diagnosis: *Baylisascaris* infection, avian vacuolar myelinopathy, heavy metal and pesticide toxicosis, West Nile or equine encephalitis viruses, trauma, duck plague, *Leukocytozoon* infection, avian malaria, and botulism.

Prevention and Control: Limiting cat access to areas near the poultry is the most effective prevention. Sulfadiazine and pyrimethamine as well as diclazuril have been effective at treating toxoplasmosis in various avian species [18, 19].

Zoonotic Potential: Humans can be infected by ingestion of oocysts shed by domestic or wild cats or ingestion of tissue cysts in undercooked food.

Balisascariasis

Name of Disease: Baylisascariasis, raccoon roundworm infection, visceral larval migrans, neural larval migrans.

Clinical History: *Baylisascaris* is infectious for all birds. Infections are reported infrequently; however, outbreaks have been reported in captive collections.

Causative Agent: *Baylisascaris procyonis* is a nematode parasite of raccoons. The geographical distribution of *B. procyonis* has been increasing and the parasite has been detected in numerous locations in the US. Animals are infected by ingesting larvated eggs from the environment.

Clinical Signs and Lesions: Visceral and neural larval migrans of the larvae can result in numerous central nervous system (CNS) clinical signs similar to *Toxoplasma*. Postmortem diagnostics include histopath examination and PCR on affected tissues.

Transmission Route: Raccoons and domestic dogs can serve as definitive hosts for the parasite. Aberrant hosts are infected by ingesting larvated nematode eggs from the environment.

Diagnostic Tests: Post-mortem diagnostics include histopath examination and PCR on affected tissues.

Differential Diagnosis: Toxoplasmosis, avian vacuolar myelinopathy, heavy metal and pesticide toxicosis, West Nile or equine encephalitis viruses, trauma, duck plague, *Leukocytozoon* infection, avian malaria, and botulism.

Prevention and Control: Limiting raccoon access to yard and making the areas unattractive to raccoons, including removing excess pet, livestock, and poultry feed as the most effective prevention. Lids need to be secured on feed containers to ensure that raccoons or other wild animals cannot gain access to the feed [20].

Zoonotic Potential: Humans can be infected by ingestion of larvated eggs, which can lead to abherent migration.

Miscellaneous Parasites

Twenty-two nematode (roundworm) species belonging to various genera are found in galliforms. Ascarid eggs can be seen on fecal flotation (Figure 11.7). *Ascardia dissimilis* and other ascarids are frequently reported in birds in southeastern US. In heavy infections ascarids can interfere with intestinal passage of food (Figure 11.8).

Ascarids are relatively large and range from 3 to 10 cm in length. *Heterakis* spp. are cecal nematodes and in contrast to the larger size when compared to ascarids, *Heterakis* are short worms ranging from 0.5–2.0 cm in length. *Heterakis* can cause cecal inflammation in high numbers, but more importantly it is the vector of *H. meleagridis*, the cause of blackhead.

The trematodes *Athesmia* heterolecithodes and *Echinoparyphium recurvatum* have been reported to cause morbidity and mortality in galliforms. *Athesmia* heterolecithodes is found in the bile ducts of the liver and can obstruct bile flow resulting in enlargement and fibrosis of bile ducts. *E. recurvatum* is found in the small intestines and it has been reported to cause severe enteritis, emaciation, anemia, and mortality in chickens and domestic turkeys. The fluke is relatively small at approximately 2.5 × 0.5 mm. Since all the trematodes require a snail intermediate host, it would be more likely to find trematodes in birds in wet coastal areas compared to birds from dry, arid areas. Limiting access to marshes and standing water is the most effective control.

In severe cases of high parasite intensity, cestode infections can interfere with intestinal passage of food, otherwise there is limited disease associated with cestodes. Sometimes proglittids can be seen in fecal floats (Figure 11.9).

Haemoproteus meleagridis, *Leukocytozoon smithi*, and *Plasmodium hermani*, *Plasmodium kempi*, *Plasmodium* sp. are all vector borne protozoa that infect erythrocytes and muscle (*H. meleagridis)*, leukocytes, liver, and spleen (*L. smithi*), and erythrocytes (*P. hermani*, *P. kempi*, *Plasmodium* sp.) (Table 11.2) Proper vector control including eliminating stagnant water is needed to control these diseases.

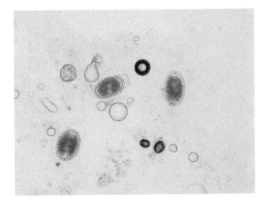

Figure 11.7 Mourning dove intestines impacted with ascarids.

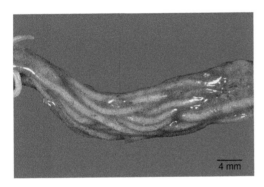

Figure 11.8 Ascarid eggs on fecal float from chicken (10×).

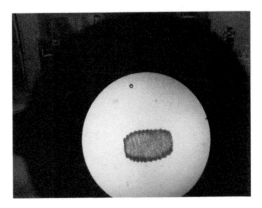

Figure 11.9 Tapeworm proglottid that just happened to be seen on a fecal float from a chicken with cestodiasis. *Source:* Photograph courtesy of Cheryl B. Greenacre.

Table 11.2 Important erythrocytic and leukocytic avian protozoa with corresponding vectors, organ involvement, and lesions.

Protozoa	Vector	Parasite development in avian host	Lesions
Haemoproteus meleagridis	*Culicoides* spp. (midges)	Asexual development (Merogony) within tissue and capillary endothelial cells; gametocytes found in RBC's	Myositis. Grossly with areas of pallor and hemorrhage.
Leukocytozoon smithi	*Simulium* and *Prosimulium* spp (Blackflies).	Merogony in liver and erythrocytes, gametocytes in leukocytes	Splenomegaly, hepatomegaly, tissue pallor, anemia. Liver can have central necrosis. Spleen and lung infiltrated with pigment-filled macrophages. Can have encephalitis and optic neuritis
Plasmodium hermani	*Culex nigripalpus* mosquitoes	Two stages of merogony in liver, spleen, brain, kidney, and lung followed by one stage of exoerythrocytic meronts in capillary endothelial cells. Then erythrocytic stages seen in erythrocytes.	Anemia, parasitemia, splenomegaly, hepatomegaly. Spleen and liver infiltrated with pigment-filled macrophages. +/− dilated capillary venules with edema.[a]
Plasmodium kempi	*Culex* spp. mosquitoes		
Plasmodium sp.	*Culex* spp. mosquitoes		

[a] Same vectors carry avian poxvirus so birds may be found with both diseases.

References

1 McDougald, L.R. and Fitz-Coy, S.H. (2013). Coccidiosis. In: *Diseases of Poultry*, 13e (eds. D.E. Swayne, J.R. Glisson, L.R. McDougald, et al.), 1147–1201. Ames Iowa: Wiley-Blackwell.

2 Ruff, M.D. (1985). Life cycle and biology of *Eimeria lettyae* sp. n. (protozoa: Eimeriidae) from the northern bobwhite, *Colinus virginianus* (L.). *J. Wildl. Dis.* 21: 361–370.

3 Gerhold, R.W., Guven, E., and McDougald, L.R. (2011). Oocyst production in *Eimeria lettyae* following low dose inoculations. *J. Parasitol.* 97: 525–526.

4 McDougald, L.R. (1993). Chemotherapy of coccidiosis. In: *Coccidiosis of Man and Domestic Animals* (ed. P.L. Long), 307–320. Boca Raton: CRC press.

5 Gerhold, R.W., Fuller, A.L., Lollis, L.A. et al. (2011). The efficacy of anticoccidial products against *Eimeria* spp. in northern bobwhites. *Avian Dis.* 55: 59–64.

6 Shirley, M.W., Smith, A.L., and Tomley, F.M. (2005). The biology of avian *Eimeria* with an emphasis on their control by vaccination. *Adv. Parasitol.* 60: 285–330.

7 Gerhold, R.W., Fuller, A.L., Beckstead, R.B., and McDougald, L.R. (2010). Immunization of northern bobwhites with a low dose of *Eimeria lettyae* provides protection against a high dose challenge. *Avian Dis.* 54: 1220–1223.

8 Fuller, A.L., Gerhold, R.W., and McDougald, L.R. (2011). Immunization of Chukar partridges against coccidia (*Eimeria kofoidi* and *Eimeria legionensis*) with low doses of live oocysts. *Avian Dis.* 55: 346–349.

9 Lollis, L.A., Gerhold, R.W., McDougald, L.R., and Beckstead, R.B. (2011). Molecular characterization of *Histomonas meleagridis* and other parabaslids in the United States using the 5.8S, ITS-1, and ITS-2 rRNA regions to identify genetic variation. *J. Parasitol.* 97: 610–615.

10 Hu, J. and McDougald, L.R. (2003). Direct lateral transmission of *Histomonas meleagridis* in turkeys. *Avian Dis.* 47: 489–492.

11 Gerhold, R.W., Lollis, L.A., Beckstead, R.B., and McDougald, L.R. (2010). Establishment of culture conditions for survival of *Histomonas meleagridis* in transit. *Avian Dis.* 54: 948–950.

12 McDougald, L.R. (2005). Blackhead disease (histomoniasis) in poultry: a critical review. *Avian Dis.* 49: 462–476.

13 Munoz, E., Castella, J., and Gutierrez, J. (1998). In vivo and in vitro sensitivity of *Trichomonas gallinae* to some nitroimidazole drugs. *Vet. Parasitol.* 78: 239–246.

14 McDougald, L.R. (2013). Internal parasites. In: *Diseases of Poultry*, 13e (eds. D.E. Swayne, J.R. Glisson, L.R. McDougald, et al.), 1117–1146. Ames Iowa: Wiley-Blackwell.

15 Everett, E.W. and Hwang, J.C. (1967). Anthelmintic activity of thiabendazle against the gapeworm (*Syngamus trachea*) in turkeys. *Avian Dis.* 11: 44–48.

16 Carreno, R. (2008). *Dispharynx, Echinuria,* and *streptocara*. In: *Parasitic Diseases of Wild Birds* (eds. C.T. Atkinson, N.J. Thompson and D.B. Hunter), 326–342. Ames, Iowa: Wiley-Blackwell.

17 Thomas-Baker, B. (1986). Ivermectin as a treatment for ocular nematodiasis in birds. In: *Proceedings of the Annual Meeting of the American Association of Zoo Veterinarians*, Chicago, Illinois, 99–100.

18 Lindsay, D.S., Glasser, R.B., Harrigan, D.N. et al. (1995). Central nervous toxoplasmosis in roller canaries. *Avian Dis.* 39: 204–207.

19 Work, T.M., Massey, B.A., Lindsay, D., and Dubey, J.P. (2000). Fatal toxoplasmosis in free-ranging endangered 'alala from Hawaii. *J. Wildl. Dis.* 36: 205–212.

20 Kazacos, K.R. (2001). *Baylisascaris procyonis* and related species. In: *Parasitic Diseases of Wild Mammals*, 2e (eds. W.M. Samuel, M.J. Pybus and A.A. Kocan), 301–341. Ames Iowa: University Press.

Further Reading

Permin, A. and Hansen, J.J. Epidemiology, diagnosis and control of poultry parasites. Food and Agriculture Organization of the United Nations http://www.fao.org/3/x0583e/x0583e.pdf (accessed 1 November 2019).

Jacob J. Internal parasites of poultry. Poultry Extension website. https://poultry.extension. org/articles/poultry-health/internal-parasites-of-poultry (accessed 26 Auegst 2020).

Macklin, K.S. and Hauck, R. Helminthiasis in Poultry (nematode and cestode). Merck Veterinary Manual. https://www.merckvetmanual.com/poultry/helminthiasis/helminthiasis-in-poultry (accessed 26 Auegst 2020).

12

Respiratory Diseases

Richard M. Fulton

Michigan State University Veterinary Diagnostic Laboratory, E. Lansing, MI, USA

Respiratory Diseases Common to Backyard Poultry

There are many respiratory diseases of poultry, but not all of them are covered in this chapter because the chance of them occurring in backyard poultry is highly unlikely. This chapter is divided into two parts: respiratory diseases that are common in backyard poultry (along with their occurrence) and those respiratory diseases that are not common in backyard poultry but could occur. This chapter does not include all of the respiratory diseases of poultry, so for further information the reader is referred to a more definitive text such as *Diseases of Poultry*, 14th Edition (D.E. Swayne editor, 2020). An additional, easily accessible reference source is the online version of the *Merck Veterinary Manual* at www. http://merckvetmanual.com.

Nonspecific Respiratory Disease (Extremely Common)

This condition is probably the most common respiratory disease of small flocks.

Clinical History

In the spring or fall of the year, when the weather is changing, the author receives many calls from small flock poultry owners concerned about their chickens rattling when they breathe. Snicking, which is like a reverse sneeze; sneezing; and, rarely, coughing are also observed in some flocks. The flock continues to be active, and feed and water intake remains normal.

Causative Agent

There is no known specific cause for this condition. Typically, none of these birds ever make it to necropsy or have diagnostic work performed. Likely causes for this condition include changes in the birds' local environment, such as dust or high levels of ammonia, but more than likely there is a change in the resident bacterial flora of the respiratory tract. This observation is based upon response to treatment (see "Prevention and Control").

Clinical Signs and Lesions

Typical clinical signs are described as all or some of the following: tracheal rales, snicks, sneezes, and coughing. The differentiating feature of this syndrome compared to infectious respiratory

Backyard Poultry Medicine and Surgery: A Guide for Veterinary Practitioners, Second Edition.
Edited by Cheryl B. Greenacre and Teresa Y. Morishita.
© 2021 John Wiley & Sons, Inc. Published 2021 by John Wiley & Sons, Inc.
Companion website: www.wiley.com/go/greenacre/medicine

disease is that the affected birds continue to be alert and active and continue to eat and drink.

Transmission Route

No transmission routes are known.

Diagnostic Tests

There is no known diagnostic test. A practitioner could proactively perform tracheal swabs of a normal flock and analyze the sample for the resident microflora including resident mycoplasmas. When or if the flock develops this syndrome, the tracheal swabs could be repeated and test results between the normal and affected flock compared.

Differential Diagnosis

Mycoplasmosis.

Prevention and Control

Maintain optimum environmental conditions. It is difficult to maintain proper humidity levels in manually ventilated or naturally ventilated poultry houses when there are huge temperature swings. During the spring and fall, temperature swings can be as large as 40 °F from morning to evening. This large temperature swing allows increases in poultry house humidity and thus ammonia levels because ventilation is typically set for the cool temperatures and not adjusted (opened up) or adjusted rapidly enough to match the outside temperature. The only way to control poultry house and litter moisture is through ventilation. Cooler air is brought into the house where it is warmed and picks up moisture. The warm moist air must be removed from the poultry house to remove the moisture. Build-up of moisture in the litter allows release of ammonia from poultry manure. Therefore, proper ventilation during these periods is extremely critical.

If untreated, the respiratory signs usually subside in 7–10 days. If the flock is treated with antibiotics, typically a member of the tetracycline family, the respiratory signs usually subside 3 days after treatment is initiated.

Mycoplasmosis (Very Common)

There are many mycoplasmas that infect poultry [1]. Not all mycoplasmas cause disease and many are considered commensal organisms. Furthermore, not all mycoplasmas cause respiratory disease. Many mycoplasmas that cause overt diseases in other species, such as turkeys and peafowl, can be silent infections in chickens. In addition to spread from animal to animal, mycoplasmas are typically passed from the hen to the chick or poult through the egg. This phenomenon is known as transovarial transmission. The lack of overt clinical signs in chickens combined with transovarial transmission and the ease of spread from bird-to-bird perpetuates these infections in backyard poultry flocks.

Mycoplasmosis Resulting from *Mycoplasma gallisepticum* (Very Common)

Clinical History

Clinical history varies with the type of poultry infected and whether the infection is complicated by other organisms. Uncomplicated infections with *Mycoplasma gallisepticum* (MG) in meat- and egg-type chickens are typically silent with no obvious clinical disease. Secondary infections with *Escherichia coli* typically cause elevated flock mortality. In broiler chickens, this condition is typically known as chronic respiratory disease (CRD) [2]. In turkeys and peafowl (peacocks and peahens), infection with MG alone typically presents as distended infraorbital sinuses and owners complain of birds with puffy or swollen faces. With secondary *E. coli* infections, there is an elevated death loss within the flock. Clinical history of mycoplasmosis often includes the recent addition of new poultry or adding birds back to the flock after they have been to a fair or exhibition.

Clinical Signs and Lesions

In uncomplicated infections in broiler- and egg-type chickens, there is a cough at most. There may be tracheal rales and/or snicks and sneezes. The lesion of uncomplicated MG presents as small to moderate amounts of yellow frothy material (proteinaceous exudate) within the air sacs; in other words, a mild airsacculitis. With secondary *E. coli* infections, overt illness results, and birds may cough, have decreased activity, have their contour feathers extended so they have a "puffed up" appearance, and appear sleepy and reluctant to move. There may be elevated flock mortality. Gross lesions of CRD present as sheets of white to yellow material (fibrin) over the surfaces of the pericardial sac, liver, and air sacs (fibrinous polyserositis).

In turkeys and peafowl, where the disease is called infectious sinusitis, the birds' infraorbital sinuses are often greatly distended. Pushing on the swollen sinuses may cause thick mucus to flow into the bird's mouth through the choanal cleft. If the sinuses are lanced or opened at necropsy, thick stringy mucus exudes from the interior. With secondary bacterial infection, the character of the sinus exudate may change to more caseous.

In small flocks infected with both MG and *Mycoplasma synoviae* (MS), the presenting complaint is often a higher than normal mortality rate and birds that have excess mucus exuding from the nares. MS is a joint pathogen in meat-type birds and often asymptomatic in egg-laying chickens.

Transmission Route

Transovarial or aerosol are the transmission routes. Mycoplasmas are easily carried on people's clothing and shoes. There have been cases reported of aerosol spread as far as one-half mile from an infected premise.

Diagnostic Tests

Culture and identification, polymerase chain reaction (PCR), and/or serology are used. The National Poultry Improvement Plan (NPIP) program uses either the serum plate agglutination test or the enzyme linked immunofluorescent antibody assay (ELISA) as basic screening tests for MG, and then positives can be followed up with the hemagglutination inhibition (HI) if needed. Culture is the gold standard for this organism. Most commercial poultry are MG free.

Differential Diagnosis

Pathogenic *E. coli*, Fowl cholera, infectious bronchitis, *Mycoplasma synoviae* (MS), turkey viral rhinotracheitis, or swollen head syndrome of chickens.

Prevention and Control

Only buy replacement birds from flocks that are known to be MG free. Establish a quarantine procedure for the flock, where birds that are purchased to add to the flock are kept in a separate area to ensure that they are free of disease. Quarantine procedures work to prevent not only mycoplasmas but many other diseases as well. Many small flock owners inadvertently cause their flocks to become infected with MG when they put new birds in their flock immediately after buying birds at sales and swap meets or someone gives them some "free" birds. Commercial vaccines are available; however, some of them (F-strain) can cause clinical disease in turkeys. Purchase only mycoplasma free poultry. Tylosin and tetracyclines have been effective at diminishing the effects of infection, although no antibiotic totally eliminates the organism. Clinical signs often reoccur after discontinuing antibiotic treatment.

Contact your local NPIP representative to discuss testing your flock for MG to prevent spread of this disease or read more about the NPIP Program Standards at www.poultryimprovement.org.

Mycoplasmosis Resulting from *Mycoplasma synoviae* (MS) (Uncommon)

Clinical History

Chickens develop a snick, sneeze, and/or tracheal rales soon after being added to an existing flock of chickens. MS is uncommon in backyard poultry of the Midwest. In general, almost all commercial egg-laying chickens are infected with MS after being placed in the egg-laying house. MS does not typically cause overt illness or production problems. The opposite is true in meat-type chickens and turkeys. When found in meat birds, multiple steps are taken to eliminate it from flocks because lameness, synovitis, and other production issues ensue.

Clinical Signs and Lesions

Clinical signs consist of a snick, sneeze, and/or tracheal rale. If an animal is sacrificed at this time, there may be a mild airsacculitis with a frothy exudate within the air sacs. In meat birds, swelling of the hock joints may be present [3].

Transmission Route

This disease is transmitted by the aerosol and transovarial routes.

Diagnostic Tests

Culture and identification, PCR, and/or serology is used.

Differential Diagnosis

Mycoplasma gallisepticum (MG), infectious bronchitis, or Newcastle disease.

Prevention and Control

Practice good biosecurity and only purchase mycoplasma-free poultry. Tylosin and tetracyclines have been effective at diminishing the effects of infection, although no antibiotic totally eliminates the organism.

Infectious Coryza (Common in the Southern United States and California)

Do not confuse this disease, infectious coryza, with the term "coryza" used through the years by poultry people to describe an upper respiratory infection. Infectious coryza is a defined disease phenomenon [4, 5].

Clinical History

Acute death in a flock of chickens, pheasants, or guinea fowl or the development of sick poultry with oculonasal discharge, facial edema, and/or swollen infraorbital sinuses (Figure 12.1). Although Infectious Coryza is common in the southern US and California, there have been some recent outbreaks in commercial egg flocks in Pennsylvania and Ohio.

Causative Agent

Avibacterium (Hemophilus) paragallinarum.

Clinical Signs and Lesions

Acute death or the development of respiratory signs including sick poultry with oculonasal discharge, facial edema, and/or swollen infraorbital sinuses. Infraorbital sinuses may

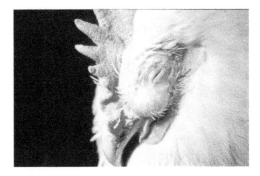

Figure 12.1 Chicken with swollen infraorbital sinuses due to *Avibacterium (Hemophilus) paragallinarum. Source:* Photograph courtesy of University of Tennessee pathology department website http://vetgrosspath.utk.edu.

contain mucus or a hard, yellow caseous material. Flocks that are infected are reported to have a distinct odor.

Transmission Route

This disease is transmitted by aerosol, ingestion, and/or people's clothing. The source of the bacteria is typically thought to be chronically infected sick or asymptomatic carriers.

Diagnostic Tests

Culture and identification are the tests used. To culture this organism, it is important to use the correct media or inform the laboratory that *A. paragallinarum* is suspected because it requires factor V for growth.

Differential Diagnosis

Fowl cholera (*Pasteurella multocida*), secondary bacterial infections following infections by mycoplasmas, ornithobacteria infection, or swollen head syndrome (extremely rare in the United States)

Prevention and Control

Depopulation to remove disease carriers is necessary. Cleaning and disinfection should be followed by a period, typically 3 weeks, where no poultry are allowed on the premise. This may also work to control mycoplasmosis. It is important to restock with *A. paragallinarum*–free stock. Treatment with sulfonamides, tetracycline, or erythromycin may be of some immediate help. Care should be exercised when treating egg-laying chickens since many antibiotics used in poultry cannot be used in chickens that lay eggs. (See Chapter 16 on removing the caseous material from the infraorbital sinus.) Vaccination may also be used as a preventative, although serotype-specific (A, B, or C) vaccines should match the serotype of the infecting bacteria; otherwise, vaccine failure may be expected.

Fowl Cholera (Very Common)

Clinical History

Fowl cholera, in its septicemic form, may be seen in small flocks as mortality events in chickens and turkeys. The septicemic form is more common in turkeys than in chickens. In chickens, where it causes accumulation of a hard inflammatory exudate, leading to subcutaneous masses, swollen eyes, ears, or wattles, it is a chronic disease [6, 7].

Causative Agent

Pasteurella multocida.

Clinical Signs and Lesions

Clinical signs consist of death without premonitory signs or subcutaneous masses, swollen eyes, ears, or wattles. Lesions of septicemia take the form of fibrin in multiple body cavities. Egg contents in the coelomic cavity of egg-laying birds that have been found dead has been described. Subcutaneous masses and swollen structures, on cross section, contain large amounts of yellow, easily crumbled material. In turkeys, a fibrinous bronchopneumonia is commonly found on necropsy.

Transmission Route

Pasteurella multocida is often introduced in a flock through bites from either cats or rats. Cats and rats carry *P. multocida* in their mouths as a commensal organism. Once in the flock, it can be spread through cannibalism and shed through bodily discharges.

Diagnostic Tests

Culture and sensitivity tests are used.

Differential Diagnosis

Septicemias caused by *E. coli* or *A. paragallinarum*.

Prevention and Control

Exclude cats and rats from poultry flocks. Commercial vaccines are available. It is important to determine the serotype of the infecting *P. multocida* because some vaccines are serotype specific. Serotypes 1, 3, 4, and 3×4 are the most common. Tetracyclines and sulfa drugs should be used during disease breaks. Antibiotic treatment is futile in the chronic form of the disease.

Infectious Laryngotracheitis (Not Uncommon)

Clinical History

Death loss, which can be dramatic, is often the first indication of infectious laryngotracheitis (ILT). The mortality rate may double each day the disease persists in a flock. Disease and mortality typically occur 7–10 days after returning from a poultry exhibit (county fairs, swap meets, breed shows, etc.) or after adding new birds to a flock. This disease is a disease of chickens but can also cause illness in flocks of peafowl and pheasants. Turkeys have only been infected experimentally. This disease is common in fairs and exhibitions where vaccinated and nonvaccinated birds are co-mingled.

Causative Agent

Infectious laryngotracheitis, also referred to as LT or ILT, is caused by *Gallid herpesvirus* 1. Clinical disease can occur because of wild-type viruses or from modified live virus vaccines. Vaccine viruses can cause disease as it passes from bird to bird in a vaccinated flock or from previously vaccinated birds when vaccine virus is shed and spread to nonvaccinated birds.

Clinical Signs and Lesions

Often the first clinical sign noticed by flock owners is mortality in their flock. The mortality rate in infected flocks can be explosive. Clinical signs can consist of death without any premonitory signs, coughing, head shaking, and dyspnea, and blood on the mouth, feathers, and chicken coop walls. Dyspnea typically consists of "pump handle" breathing. For example, when affected chickens inhale, they raise their head high. When they exhale, they lower their head. Thus, the movement mimics an old-fashioned well pump handle. Lesions consist of blood alone, fibrin alone, or a mixture of blood and fibrin within the larynx and proximal third of the trachea. Some cases of ILT may have conjunctivitis in addition to the tracheal lesions. In mild cases of ILT, a transmissible conjunctivitis may be the only presenting complaint [8].

Transmission Route

Aerosol exposure is the most common route of infection. ILT virus is transmitted by infected birds, from previously infected birds that have recovered, or by birds previously vaccinated with modified live vaccines. ILT is also known to be transmitted via fomites including clothing, shoes, and equipment.

Diagnostic Tests

Tests include histopathology, virus isolation, and PCR.

Differential Diagnosis

Viscerotrophic velogenic Newcastle disease, highly pathogenic avian influenza, septicemic pasteurellosis, acute infectious coryza, or infectious bronchitis.

Prevention and Control

Do NOT use modified live ILT vaccines because vaccination can result in latently infected carrier birds [9]. If vaccines are warranted, only genetically modified pox or turkey herpes virus (Marek) vaccines should be used. These vaccines contain only the protective portion of the ILT virus and not the whole virus. Genetically modified ILT vaccine is best used in chickens that are taken to poultry exhibits. Modified live ILT vaccines should not be used in backyard poultry. Biosecurity is also important in preventing ILT.

Respiratory Diseases Not Common to Backyard Poultry

Infectious Bronchitis (Rarely Seen)

Clinical History

Chickens show respiratory signs such as sneezing, snicking, tracheal rales, and/or cough [10]. Typically, affected chickens appear sick with reluctance to move and have a puffed-up appearance. If they are laying eggs, the eggs may have a hard shell with a wrinkled appearance (soft shells, shell-less eggs, and wrinkled eggs may be seen when birds are first coming into or going out of egg production). When infected very early in life, hens may become "false" layers. Their body develops normally but there is segmental aplasia of the oviduct, which leads to the inability of formed yolks to make it to completion and oviposition [11].

Causative Agent

Coronavirus.

Clinical Signs and Lesions

Sick chickens are reluctant to move, have a puffed-up appearance, and may appear sleepy. Lesions of uncomplicated infectious bronchitis may be hyperemia of the caudal third of the trachea resulting in rales (a wet sound to each breath) (Figure 12.2); (also see video online of the same two Plymouth Rock hens exhibiting rales). There may or may not be an increased amount of mucus within the trachea. Infectious bronchitis is often complicated by a secondary infection with *E. coli*. In these cases, lesions consist of bacterial septicemia with fibrin deposits over the pericardial sac, liver capsule, and within the body cavity [12]. A characteristic feature of this disease is the presence of wrinkled or abnormal shell surface of the egg in conjunction with respiratory rales.

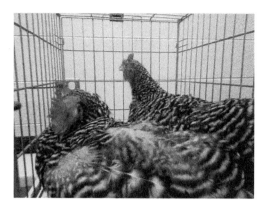

Figure 12.2 Two adult barred Plymouth rock hens with definitive diagnoses of infectious bronchitis virus (IBV) based on necropsy and ELISA testing of serum. Adult chickens were added to the flock about 10 days earlier. Note the fluffed appearance in both and the outstretched neck indicative of dyspnea in the hen on the right. Both exhibited "rales" a wet cough. See video with book to hear and see what "rales" with IBV looks like. *Source:* Photograph and video courtesy of C. Greenacre, University of Tennessee.

Transmission Route

Aerosol and/or oral routes.

Diagnostic Tests

High titers in nonvaccinated birds, virus isolation, and PCR are used.

Differential Diagnosis

Mycoplasmosis, mild strains of Newcastle disease, low pathogenic avian influenza, or infectious coryza.

Prevention and Control

Once identified as a flock problem, future flocks should be vaccinated with a serotype that protects against the field strain. Tetracycline or sulfa drugs could be used in cases of suspected secondary bacterial infections.

Pox (Diphtheritic, Wet Form) (Uncommon)

Clinical History

Increased mortality in a flock of chickens. This disease appears to spread slowly through the flock. Birds may exhibit dyspnea prior to death.

Causative Agent

Pox virus, most likely fowl pox. There are many different strains of pox viruses and they are typically named for the species that they infect naturally [13]. In poultry, fowl pox can infect both chickens and turkeys, while turkey pox only infects turkeys. Pox occurs as either dry pox (skin only) or wet pox (diphtheritic, affects mucous membranes). In chickens, wet pox can occur with fowl pox virus alone but may be complicated as a result of a dual infection with ILT virus and fowl pox virus.

Clinical Signs and Lesions

Dyspnea and increased flock mortality are the typical presenting clinical signs in wet pox. Wet pox causes lesions on the wet tissues (mucous membranes). It is called dry pox when it causes lesions on the dry skin, typically the nonfeathered areas of the body. The lesions of wet pox as they relate to respiratory disease present as a polypoid mass at the opening of the larynx and proximal trachea. Birds die when this mass occludes the trachea, thus suffocating the chicken (Figures 12.3 and 12.4) [14].

Transmission Route

Pox virus requires a break in the epithelium to infect an animal. This may occur because of dust or a different respiratory pathogen that disrupts the epithelium. Thus, during ILT infection, a break in the epithelium occurs and pox virus infects the epithelium at the break.

Diagnostic Tests

Histopathology, virus isolation, and PCR are used.

Differential Diagnosis

Infectious laryngotracheitis.

Prevention and Control

Vaccination and control of biting insects are important because pox virus can be spread from bird to bird by biting insects. The disease spread is usually slow enough that one can vaccinate in the face of an outbreak to prevent the spread of pox within the flock.

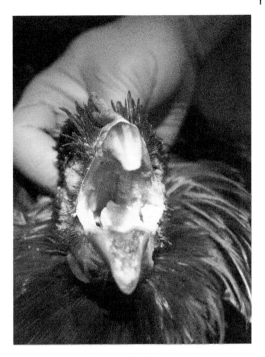

Figure 12.3 A 1-year-old Welsummer hen with fibrinonecrotic material involving the oropharynx and tongue consistent with the wet form of fowl pox. Eosinophilic intracytoplasmic inclusion bodies were demonstrated in the tissue of the tongue. *Source:* Photograph courtesy of Cheryl B. Greenacre, University of Tennessee.

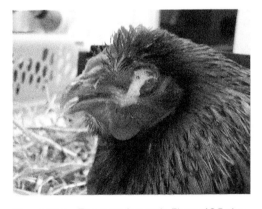

Figure 12.4 The same hen as in Figure 12.3 also had bubbly ocular discharge and severe dyspnea, probably due to concurrent bacterial infection (see video on website). *Source:* Photograph courtesy of Cheryl B. Greenacre, University of Tennessee.

Gape Worm (Uncommon in Poultry, Common in Game Birds)

Clinical History

Increased flock mortality in young poultry. Game birds, such as pheasants, quail, and partridges, are most often infected. Any backyard poultry may be at risk for this infection; however, it has only been reported in chicken, turkeys, guinea fowl, pea fowl, and geese. Affected live birds may breathe with their mouths open (gape). They may shake their heads or drag their open mouth on the ground as they walk.

Causative Agent
Syngamus trachea (see Chapter 11 on parasitology).

Clinical Signs and Lesions
Increased flock mortality in young birds is seen, as well as open mouth breathing, head shaking, and/or walking with their open mouth on the ground. Lesions consist of a reddish nematode parasite attached to the tracheal mucosa. Sites of attachment may consist of raised white nodules. The parasite may have a "Y" formation because the female parasite envelopes the male parasite as he is attached to the tracheal mucosa. In dead birds, the parasites may occlude the trachea (see Chapter 11 on parasitology).

Transmission Route
The infection is spread directly from bird to bird via ingestion of embryonated ova or larva or indirectly through the ingestion of an earthworm or insects containing the larva.

Diagnostic Tests
Gross lesions are diagnostic.

Differential Diagnosis
Any respiratory pathogen causing open mouth breathing such as wet pox and ILT.

Prevention and Control
Control of earthworms and other insect vectors is important in preventing the disease and its carry over between flocks. Safe-Guard® AquaSol for poultry (fenbendazole) has recently been approved for use in chickens.

Although treatment is off label, thiabendazole, mebendazole, cambendazole, and levamisole have shown effectiveness.

Aspergillosis (Uncommon)

Clinical History
In young birds this disease is called brooder pneumonia because the disease occurs during the time that birds are being brooded and the source of infection may be the brooding environment, which is usually dark, warm and moist. Typically, there is an increased flock mortality within the first 2 weeks of life [15]. In adult birds, the disease usually presents as one or a few birds with chronic illness and weight loss followed by death. Geese and turkeys are most commonly affected. Ducks are also susceptible to infection.

Causative Agent
Aspergillus fumigatus most commonly causes this disease, although other fungal species may cause the same lesions.

Clinical Signs and Lesions
In young birds, clinical signs may be open-mouth breathing and/or an increased mortality rate. Lesions in young birds consist of yellow, seed-like granules of granulomatous inflammation within the lung parenchyma. In older birds, clinical signs consist of chronic illness with weight loss followed by death. Lesions in these birds typically consist of a fungal airsacculitis. The air sacs, most commonly the cranial thoracic air sacs next to the lungs, are filled with large amounts of yellow, easily crumbled material. The surface may or may not have a gray fuzzy covering, which consists of fruiting bodies. In birds with acute death without premonitory signs, a plug of fibrin and fungal mycelia may be found blocking the tracheal bifurcation (syrinx) [16].

Transmission Route
Aerosol. In brooder pneumonia, birds can be infected while they are in the hatchery when

an infected egg explodes, spraying its contents and fungal spores throughout the incubator or setter/hatcher, or they can be infected during the brooding phase. As stated above, the brooder is an ideal place for fungi to grow. The source of fungal spores in the brooder is hard wood shavings: It is thought that the mycelia and spores are picked up on the trees when they are being processed in the forest.

Diagnostic Tests

Gross lesions provide a presumptive diagnosis, which can be confirmed by histopathology. A tease prep, using lactophenol blue, may be performed on the fuzzy growth on the air sacs.

Differential Diagnosis

Fowl cholera and *E. coli* septicemia.

Prevention and Control

Frequent candling of eggs in incubators and setters is important to detect embryos that may have died because of fungal infection. In older turkeys, dust control is important in preventing this condition. Providing environmental conditions that are not warm and damp is important in preventing this condition in ducks and geese.

References

1 Ferguson-Noel, N., Armour, N.K., Noormohammadi, A.H., et al. (2020). Mycoplasmosis. In: *Diseases of Poultry*, 14e (eds. D.E. Swayne, M. Boulianne, C.M. Logue, et al.), 907–965. Ames, Iowa: Wiley.

2 El-Gazzar, M. Mycoplasma gallisepticum Infection in Poultry, (Chronic Respiratory Disease, Infectious Sinusitis), (2020). https://www.merckvetmanual.com/poultry/mycoplasmosis/mycoplasma-gallisepticum-infection-in-poultry?query=mycoplasma%20poultry (accessed 29 October 2020).

3 El-Gazzar, M. Mycoplasma synoviae Infection in Poultry, (Infectious Synovitis), (2020). https://www.merckvetmanual.com/poultry/mycoplasmosis/mycoplasma-synoviae-infection-in-poultry?query=mycoplasma%20poultry (accessed 29 October 2020).

4 Blackall, P.J. and Soriano-Vargus, E. (2020). Infectious Coryza and related bacterial infections. In: *Diseases of Poultry*, 14e (eds. D.E. Swayne, M. Boulianne, C.M. Logue, et al.), 890–906. Ames, Iowa: Wiley.

5 Blackall, P.J. (2014). Overview of Infectious Coryza in Chickens. https://www.merckvetmanual.com/poultry/infectious-coryza/overview-of-infectious-coryza-in-chickens?query=coryza%20poultry . (accessed 29 October 2020)

6 Boulianne, M., Blackall, P.J., Hofacre, C.L., et al. (2020). Pasteurellosis and other respiratory bacterial infections. In: *Diseases of Poultry*, 14e (eds. D.E. Swayne, M. Boulianne, C.M. Logue, et al.), 831–889. Ames, Iowa: Wiley.

7 Sander, J.E. (2019) Fowl Cholera. https://www.merckvetmanual.com/poultry/fowl-cholera/fowl-cholera?query=fowl%20cholera (accessed 29 October 2020).

8 Garcia, M. (2020) Infectious Laryngotracheitis in Poultry. https://www.merckvetmanual.com/poultry/infectious-laryngotracheitis/infectious-laryngotracheitis-in-poultry?query=laryngotracheitis (accessed 29 October 2020).

9 Garcia, M. and Spatz, S. (2020). Infectious Laryngotracheitis. In: *Diseases of Poultry*, 14e (eds. D.E. Swayne, M. Boulianne, C.M. Logue, et al.), 189–209. Ames, Iowa: Wiley.

10 Jackwood, M.W., de Wit, S. (2020). Infectious Bronchitis. In: *Diseases of Poultry*, 14e (eds. D.E. Swayne, M. Boulianne, C.M. Logue, et al.), 167–188. Ames, Iowa: Wiley.

11 Espinosa, R.A. (2019). False Layer (in Poultry). https://www.merckvetmanual.com/poultry/disorders-of-the-reproductive-system/false-layer-in-poultry?query=false%20layer (accessed 29 October 2020)

12 Jackwood, M.W. (2019). Infectious Bronchitis in Poultry. https://www.merckvetmanual.com/poultry/infectious-bronchitis/infectious-bronchitis-in-poultry?query=infectious%20bronchitis%20virus (accessed 29 October 2020).

13 Tripathy, D.N. and Reed, W.M. (2020). Pox. In: *Diseases of Poultry*, 14e (eds. D.E. Swayne, M. Boulianne, C.M. Logue, et al.), 364–381. Ames, Iowa: Wiley.

14 Tripathy, D.N. (2019). Fowl pox in chickens and turkeys. https://www.merckvetmanual.com/poultry/fowlpox/fowlpox-in-chickens-and-turkeys?query=fowlpox (accessed 29 October 2020)

15 Arne, P. and Lee, M.D. (2020). Fungal Infections. In: *Diseases of Poultry*, 14e (eds. D.E. Swayne, M. Boulianne, C.M. Logue, et al.), 1109–1133. Ames, Iowa: Wiley.

16 Kromm, M., Lighty, M. (2020). Aspergillosis in Poultry, (Brooder Pneumonia, Mycotic Pneumonia, Pneumomycosis). https://www.merckvetmanual.com/poultry/aspergillosis/aspergillosis-in-poultry?query=aspergillosis (accessed 29 October 2020).

13

Avian Influenza and Viscerotropic Velogenic (Exotic) Newcastle Disease

Richard M. Fulton

Michigan State University Veterinary Diagnostic Laboratory, E. Lansing, MI, USA

Introduction

The following two diseases, avian influenza (AI) and viscerotropic velogenic Newcastle disease (vvND, exotic Newcastle disease [END], or virulent Newcastle Disease [VND]), rarely occur in backyard flocks, but nonetheless, the primary veterinarian should be familiar enough with the presentation and consequences of these diseases to be able to identify them when encountered and know what to do next [1, 2]. Easily accessible information in both of these diseases can be found at www.merckvetmanual.com [3, 4].

Avian Influenza

AI is also known as bird flu, fowl plague, fowl pest, and grippe.

Clinical History

The likelihood of AI occurring in backyard flocks is relatively low. The most likely premises are those that have waterfowl, that have access to wild migratory waterfowl, or flocks near bodies of water where migratory waterfowl and shore birds congregate. Clinical history for flocks with AI depends on the pathogenicity of the infecting AI virus. There may be complaints of mild respiratory signs in the affected flock such as a snick, like a reverse sneeze, cough, tracheal rales, or rattling when breathing and other general signs of illness. With more pathogenic strains of AI virus, known as highly pathogenic AI or HPAI, the owner may find a large amount of their flock dead with no previous clinical signs noticed.

Causative Agent

AI is caused by type A influenza viruses that occur in the avian species. Humans are infected with types A, B, and C influenza viruses, with types A and B being most common. Influenza viruses belong to the family Orthomyxoviridae. Influenza virus genomes are composed of eight segments of RNA. Segmentation of the genome allows swapping of gene segments between viruses and thus dramatic shifts in antigenic make-up of the virus (referred to as antigenic shift) can occur over short periods of time. AI viruses are enveloped; therefore, they are relatively easy to inactivate via such methods as soap and water, heat, sunlight, and most if not all disinfectants. On their envelopes are

Backyard Poultry Medicine and Surgery: A Guide for Veterinary Practitioners, Second Edition.
Edited by Cheryl B. Greenacre and Teresa Y. Morishita.
© 2021 John Wiley & Sons, Inc. Published 2021 by John Wiley & Sons, Inc.
Companion website: www.wiley.com/go/greenacre/medicine

two glycoproteins that project from their surface and allow further classification of these viruses. One glycoprotein is a hemagglutinin and the other is a neuraminidase. The hemagglutinin is responsible for allowing the virus to attach to a host cell. The neuraminidase is responsible for allowing newly formed viruses, assembled in the host cell, to escape from the cell. So far, 16 different hemagglutinins and 9 different neuraminidases have been identified on type A influenza viruses [3]. These proteins help identify the H (hemagglutinin) type and the N (neuraminidase) type of AI viruses. Each influenza virus has a single H type and a single N type, and they can occur in any combination. There can be an H1N1, an H1N2, an H1N3, an H2N1, an H3N1, an H4N1, and so on, so theoretically there can be 198 different AI viruses. The AI virus that most people are aware of is the Asian strain of H5N1, which has killed many poultry worldwide, made people sick and caused some people to die. It is endemic in Egypt, Vietnam, and Indonesia and cycles occasionally in other countries of Asia and Eurasia. To date, the Asian strain of H5N1 has not been identified in North America. An H5N1 strain has been found multiple times during surveillance of North American migratory waterfowl, but those viruses have not been classified as highly pathogenic or related to the Asian strain. In 2015, H5N2, with the N2 derived from a Eurasian virus, caused a poultry pandemic in the United States. Prior to infecting poultry in the Midwest, it was seen in small flocks in Washington, Oregon, Idaho, Kansas, and Montana [5].

Strains of AI differ in their ability to cause illness and death in domestic poultry. Historically, strains have been classified by their ability to kill a specific number of experimentally infected embryos or 6-week-old chicks. Those producing few signs and lesions and little or no dead animals were classified as low pathogenic AI viruses, referred to as LPAI. Those producing dramatic lesions and many dead animals were classified as highly pathogenic AI viruses, referred to as HPAI. Historically, only H5 and H7 viruses have caused catastrophic death loss in domestic poultry worldwide and have been classified as highly pathogenic AI viruses. Not all H5 and H7 AI viruses are highly pathogenic, BUT all H5 and H7 AI viruses have the potential to become highly pathogenic over time, as they pass from bird to bird. Recently, these viruses have been evaluated molecularly. It was discovered that a specific area on the H protein may be used as a predictor of high pathogenicity. Classic methods are still the most reliable, in the author's opinion, because in 2004 an H5N2 AI virus from a field case in a commercial egg-laying chicken flock was molecularly predicted to be a highly pathogenic type but proved to be avirulent in experimental chickens and caused few clinical signs in the commercial flock.

AI viruses can spread from waterfowl to domestic poultry, from pigs (where it is referred to as swine influenza) to domestic poultry, and more recently, as in the human pandemic H3N2, from humans to turkeys. H1N1 and H3N2 are typically found in swine populations, where they cause a respiratory disease of limited consequences. H1N1 and H3N2 cause little or no disease in chickens but cause commercial turkey breeder hens to stop laying eggs.

Clinical Signs and Lesions

AI viruses can infect any poultry at any age. They are thought to cycle in wild migratory waterfowl where they cause little or no disease. The problem occurs when they infect domestic poultry or a highly pathogenic strain develops. Clinical signs vary with the pathogenicity of the infecting AI virus. Signs of low pathogenic AI virus infection may consist of mild respiratory signs such as a snick, cough, tracheal rales, or rattling when breathing, occasionally diarrhea, with or without other general signs of illness such as inactivity, reluctance to move and a "puffed up" appearance caused by extension of the body feathers. Highly pathogenic viruses often cause rapid onset of illness with death occurring within <24 hours post infection. Clinical signs associated with highly pathogenic AI may also include central nervous system (CNS) signs such as tremors, torticollis, and opisthotonos and cessation of egg production but are often not noted because of the rapid onset of the disease followed by death.

Lesions of LPAI could be that of septicemia if AI is complicated by bacterial infection. LPAI may produce reddening of the tracheal mucosa with red, wet, heavy lungs. Lesions of HPAI reflect fulminant disease as seen in other catastrophic diseases such as viscerotrophic velogenic (exotic) Newcastle disease (vvND) and duck viral enteritis. It is impossible to differentiate HPAI from vvND by gross examination alone. Additional testing is required. HPAI causes edema, hemorrhage, and necrosis in skin and many visceral organs. Swelling of the face, neck, and feet may be present as well as swelling, hemorrhage, and cyanosis of the comb and wattle. Hemorrhages on the serosa and mucosal surface of the intestine are common. Hemorrhage in the proventriculus, ventriculus, and cecal tonsil may be present as well. The lungs are typically edematous and hemorrhagic.

Transmission Route

The virus is most typically transmitted by aerosol route from respiratory tract secretions but the virus may also be transmitted by fecal/oral route and, as with other avian pathogens, through fomites.

Diagnostic Tests

Diagnosis of AI must be confirmed via testing typically performed at diagnostic laboratories. Agar gel immunodiffusion (AGID) is typically used as a screening test because poultry are typically not vaccinated for AI. Currently, rapid virus identification tests are used in contrast to classic methods such as virus isolation. Certain antigen capture enzyme-linked immunosorbent assay (ELISA) test kits, like home pregnancy tests, have been proven effective in detecting AI virus from respiratory and cloacal swabs during acute infection.

National Animal Health Laboratory Network (NAHLN) laboratories are equipped with real time polymerase chain reaction (rtPCR) for AI virus matrix and for H5 and H7 identification. Further classification should be performed by more classic methods at the National Veterinary Services Laboratory in Ames, Iowa.

Differential Diagnosis

vvND, septicemic *Pasteurella multocida*, power failure in confined poultry, toxicant exposure and predation for HPAI, and other respiratory diseases for LPAI.

Prevention and Control

Vaccination for AI is not routinely practiced in the United States and is controlled by government agencies. Breeder turkeys are routinely vaccinated with H1N1 and H3N2 to prevent the dramatic egg production drop experienced during infection.

Newcastle Disease

ND is also known as ranikhet, avian pneumoencephalitis, and pseudo-fowl pest. vvND is also known as END, or VND.

Clinical History

The likelihood of ND occurring in backyard flocks is relatively low in most of the United States. California, however, has had occasional outbreaks of vvND in fighting chickens in the 1970s, 2002, 2003, and 2018/9. The majority of the 2003 and 2018/9 outbreak occurred in small household flocks in large cities. Worldwide, this disease is probably the most common disease of small household and village flocks. Throughout the world, vvND is known to spread from village to village, town to town, island to island totally decimating those poultry populations. Unlike the rest of the world, vvND is not endemic in the United

States and thus is commonly referred to as exotic ND. Clinical history for flocks with ND, like AI, depend on the pathogenicity of the infecting ND virus. Presenting complaints are respiratory disease with mild respiratory signs such as a snick, cough, tracheal rales, or rattling when breathing and other general signs of illness in milder forms. Complaints of CNS manifestations, such as torticollis, paresis, and paralysis, may be seen in addition to respiratory signs in more pathogenic strains in contrast to lack thereof in AI. Like AI, the owner may find a large amount of their flock dead with no previous clinical signs in infections of highly pathogenic strains of ND virus.

Causative Agent

ND, so named because one of the first outbreaks was identified in Newcastle-upon-Tyne in England, is caused by avian paramyxovirus serotype 1 (APMV-1). Like AI virus, APMV-1 is an enveloped RNA virus; however, its genome is not segmented. Like AI, APMV-1 viruses vary in the effects caused by their infection. They also are classified by their ability to kill experimentally infected embryos or 6-week-old chickens. The types of ND are referred to as lentogenic, mesogenic, or velogenic ND viruses. Lentogenic ND viruses are typically subclinical or cause mild respiratory signs. They are the most common strains of ND in the United States. Mesogenic ND viruses typically cause respiratory signs and occasional nervous system signs but with low mortality. These strains are occasionally found in the United States. Velogenic ND viruses cause high mortality often without previously noted clinical signs. Velogenic ND viruses are further classified as viscerotropic or neurotropic. vvND causes hemorrhagic gastrointestinal lesions, and neurotropic velogenic ND viruses cause high mortality typically after respiratory and nervous signs. vvND has occasionally been found in the United States and is thought to have arrived in smuggled birds including pet birds. Neurotropic velogenic ND appears to

cycle in flocks of cormorants found in some areas of the upper Great Lakes.

Clinical Signs and Lesions

As with AI, clinical signs depend on the pathogenicity of the infecting ND virus. Birds infected with lentogenic strains show mild or no respiratory signs, no CNS signs and no mortality. Reddening of the tracheal mucosa may be present in birds dying from other causes. Lesions of bacterial septicemia, such as fibrinous polyserositis and vasculitis, may be present in secondary bacterial infections. Birds infected with the mesogenic strains have moderate respiratory signs such as coughing, rattling when breathing, CNS signs, and general signs of illness such as inactivity, reluctance to move, and a "puffed up" appearance, and there may be some mortality in the flock. Lesions with mesogenic strains consist of reddening of the trachea, and lungs may be red and moist. There typically are no gross CNS lesions. Lesions of secondary bacterial infection may be present. Birds infected with velogenic strains are often found dead without previous clinical signs. Lesions of velogenic ND typically consist of hemorrhages of the gastrointestinal tract including esophagus, proventriculus, small and large intestine, and cecal tonsils. There may be facial edema and hemorrhage of the conjunctiva.

Transmission Route

The virus is typically transmitted by aerosol route from respiratory tract secretions, but the virus may also be transmitted by fecal/oral route and, as with other avian pathogens, through fomites.

Diagnostic Tests

Diagnosis of ND must be confirmed via testing, typically performed at diagnostic laboratories. NAHLN laboratories are equipped with rtPCR for ND virus matrix detection and fusion gene detection to predict velogenic character. Further classification should be performed by more classical methods at the National Veterinary Services Laboratory in Ames, Iowa. [6]

Differential Diagnosis

AI, septicemic *Pasteurella multocida*, power failure in confined poultry, toxicant exposure and predation for vvND, Marek disease, botulism, and toxicant exposure for paresis and paralysis. Other respiratory diseases should be considered in the differential for infections by milder strains of ND.

Prevention and Control

Vaccination for ND is not necessary in backyard flocks unless there is a known exposure in the area. There are many inexpensive and effective modified live vaccines available for ND. ND vaccines typically include infectious bronchitis vaccine virus as well. Vaccines should be applied at least twice to develop effective immunity. Poultry vaccines are typically applied through mass vaccination procedures including spraying of the vaccine or adding it in the drinking water. In backyard situations, eye drop method or water vaccination would be the easiest, most practical method of application. The B1 strain of ND virus is usually given for the first vaccine because it is a milder strain and causes little vaccine reaction. The second (booster) vaccine usually consists of La Sota ND virus, which produces better immunity but may cause more vaccine reaction.

References

1 Swayne, D.E., Suarez, D.L., and Sims, L.D. (2020). Influenza. In: Diseases of Poultry, 14e (eds. D.E. Swayne, M. Boulieanne, C.M. Logue, et al.), 210–256. Ames, Iowa: Wiley.

2 Miller, P.J. and Koch, G. (2020). Newcastle disease, other avian paramyxoviruses, and metapneumovirus infections. In: Diseases of Poultry, 14e (eds. D.E. Swayne, M. Boulieanne, C.M. Logue, et al.), 111–129. Ames, Iowa: Wiley.

3 Swayne, D.E. (2020). Avian Influenza. https://www.merckvetmanual.com/poultry/avian-influenza/avian-influenza (accessed November 2020).

4 Miller, P.J. (2014). Newcastle Disease in Poultry (Avian pneumoencephalitis, Exotic or velogenic Newcastle Disease). https://www.merckvetmanual.com/poultry/newcastle-disease-and-other-paramyxovirus-infections/newcastle-disease-in-poultry (accessed 4 January 2020).

5 Fitzpatrick, A., Mor, S.K., Thurn, M. et al. (2017). Outbreak of highly pathogenic avian influenza in Minnesota in 2015: lessons learned. *J. Vet. Diagn. Invest.* 29: 169–175.

6 Cattoli, G., Susta, L., Terregino, C., and Brown, C. (2011). Newcastle disease: a review of field recognition and current methods of laboratory detection. *J. Vet. Diagn. Invest.* 23: 637–656.

14

Musculoskeletal Diseases

Cheryl B. Greenacre

Department of Small Animal Clinical Sciences, College of Veterinary Medicine, University of Tennessee, Knoxville, Knoxville, Tennessee, USA

Introduction

The most common musculoskeletal disease of poultry is leg lameness due to a variety of causes including abnormalities in the foot, leg, hip, spine, central, or peripheral nervous system; reproductive system; or simply generalized illness (Figure 14.1). Less commonly, musculoskeletal abnormalities can involve the wing, neck, or beak of the bird. Diseases can include infectious (bacterial, viral) and noninfectious causes (trauma, congenital deformities, nutritional, neoplasia). A thorough history and physical examination are necessary, including a neurological examination, to arrive at a diagnosis. Nerve blocks are helpful to localize a lesion or, in cases of multiple lesions, can help differentiate which lesion is causing pain. One of the most helpful tools is radiography (see Chapter 9 on radiology) [1].

Diseases of the Foot

Pododermatitis (Bumblefoot)

Pododermatitis, or bumblefoot, is an inflammatory lesion primarily involving the plantar surface of the foot and ranges from mild inflammation with no bacterial involvement to severe with osteomyelitis with aerobic or anaerobic bacteria. The bacteria most often isolated are *Staphylococcus* sp., *Escherichia coli*, or *Anctinomyces* sp. Pododermatitis has many inciting causes including excess weight bearing from obesity, unequal weight bearing due to lameness causing lesions on the contralateral "good" foot, abnormal abrasions of the plantar surface from inappropriate substrate (too sharp or rough, wire, etc.), decreased blood supply to the foot (sometimes from lack of exercise), other trauma, or standing for prolonged periods of time, especially in ducks that are not provided adequate swimming opportunities (Figures 14.2 and 14.3). (See the chapter on husbandry regarding recommended litter for substrate.) Chronic inflammation can lead to infection as break down in the skin barrier occurs. Pus is thick and firm in birds because they possess heterophils (rather than neutrophils) that lack the enzyme myeloperoxidase to liquefy pus.

Obtain a thorough history including environment and substrate (Figure 14.3a,b). Perform a thorough physical examination by visually observing and palpating the plantar surface of the foot (Figure 14.4a–c). A thorough examination includes observing the bird stand and walk, palpating and examining the feet and hocks while the bird is standing and

Backyard Poultry Medicine and Surgery: A Guide for Veterinary Practitioners, Second Edition.
Edited by Cheryl B. Greenacre and Teresa Y. Morishita.

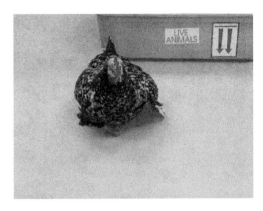

Figure 14.1 A two-year-old speckled Sussex hen presented for sudden onset of reluctance to ambulate. Initially it was suspected a leg abnormality was present but a thorough physical examination revealed an enlarged doughy coelomic cavity consistent with egg-related peritonitis. Within one week of oral antibiotics (trimethoprim-sulfamethoxazole), she was ambulating normally and continues to do well for over a year.

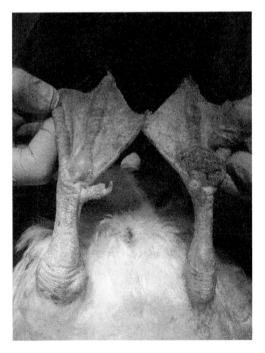

Figure 14.2 A seven-month-old Pekin duck presented with a swollen right hock with evidence of pododermatitis in the left foot from excessive weight bearing in the left foot to compensate for lameness in the right hock. At necropsy, the right hock was found to be septic.

also examining while holding the bird (either on its back or normal position but with legs dangling), making it easier to compare the hocks and plantar surfaces of the feet (Figure 14.5 and Video 14.1 of bird walking abnormally). Determine if any other factors are present that may be contributing or causing the pododermatitis. Perform radiographs to determine if osteomyelitis is present.

Pododermatitis is divided into varying grades depending on the literature source used but generally includes mild, moderate, and severe grades with the severe grades including osteomyelitis (Figures 14.6–14.11).

For mild cases of pododermatitis changing to a softer substrate, exercise to increase blood supply to the foot, soaking the affected foot in warm water, and the use of keratin softeners (used to soften corns on the feet of humans) to soften the callous may be all that is needed. The foot can also be soaked in a dilute chlorhexidine or iodine solution, but realize that chlorhexidine does not kill *Pseudomonas* spp. organisms. If there is a break in the skin, then soaking in a solution called Tricide (containing an antibiotic potentiator) with an antibiotic can speed healing.

If the tissues of the foot are infected with bacteria, then surgery may be indicated to remove pus or a large callous, but it must be performed under anesthesia with pain relievers administered (Figures 14.12a–d and 14.13). Be prepared for possible hemorrhage from the surgery site. If surgery is done and the lesion is opened, then an aerobic and anaerobic culture should be performed. Alternatively, a culture and sensitivity can be performed on an aspirate, but since the pus is thick, this technique may yield no growth.

Treatment can include parenteral antibiotics, wound management, and bandaging (Figure 14.14a–j).

Trauma to the Foot

Trauma to the dorsal surface of the foot is also possible, and typical wound management as

(a)

(b)

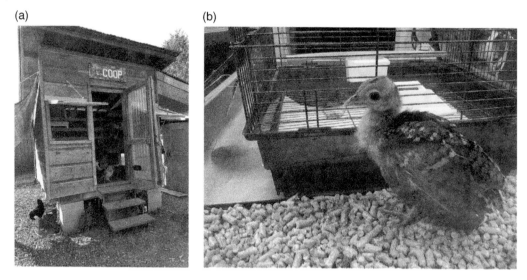

Figure 14.3 Examples of acceptable substrate to prevent foot and leg injury: (a) packed dirt and (b) pine pellet litter.

(a)

(b)

(c)

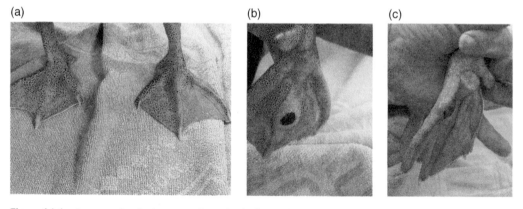

Figure 14.4 An example of why a complete physical examination is important. (a) With the bird standing, it is obvious there is a swelling of the #3 digit of the right foot. When the plantar surfaces of both feet are examined, it is discovered that not only does the (b) plantar surface of the right foot have an ulcerative lesion, but the (c) left #4 digit also has a swollen ulcerative area.

described here for pododermatitis or as described in the dermatology chapter can be used (Figure 14.15a–d).

Frostbite can occur in birds left outside in cold weather. It usually affects the tips of the comb or the toes. Slowly warm the body part and give supportive care. Keep the area clean and dry and apply ointment or cream until the tissue declares itself as definitely necrotic (usually approximately 10 days); then perform surgery if needed to remove necrotic areas. Sometimes antibiotics are needed (Figure 14.16a,b). Prevention includes avoiding exposure to cold weather, applying "booties" to feet or "hats" to combs, or sometimes petroleum jelly applied to the comb to provide moisture and a barrier. If you live in a cold area, consider purchasing breeds of chickens that are cold tolerant with small, flat combs, such as the Russian Orloff (see chapter on breeds for more information).

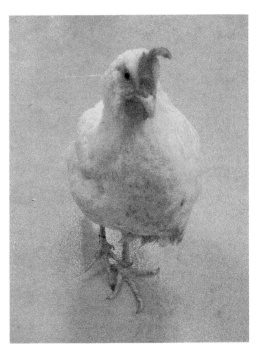

Figure 14.5 An eight-month-old white leghorn chicken with suspected *Mycoplasma synoviae* infection in the left intertarsal joint and the right hock. Note the swollen metatarsal area on the left foot compared to the right foot. This bird's right hock was very swollen (not visible in picture) and at necropsy was worse than the disease occurring in the left foot, hence the bird actually preferred to put its weight on the left leg rather than the right (see Video 14.2 on website).

Vitamin B2 (Riboflavin) Deficiency (Curled Toe Paralysis)

Vitamin B2 (riboflavin) deficiency causes "curled toe paralysis" in chicks where they sit on their hocks with their toe curled medially. Other signs include weakness, emaciation despite a good appetite, sitting on hocks, reluctance to walk or walking on hocks, and diarrhea. Chicks can develop clinical signs by 12 days of age on a deficient diet. Adults are less likely to show clinical signs (Figure 14.17a,b). Histopathologically, a demyelinating peripheral neuritis is seen with edema of the ischiatic and brachial nerves. Early treatment with riboflavin or vitamin B complex can reverse signs, but chronic cases may be left with permanent damage despite treatment. [2, 3]

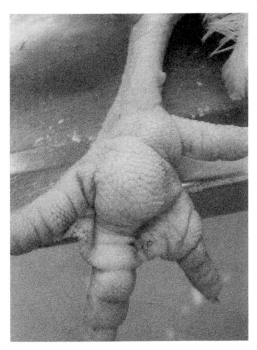

Figure 14.6 Normal foot of a white leghorn chicken. Note the clean, intact, textured surface.

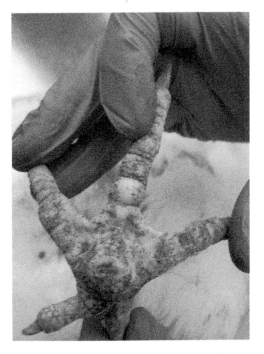

Figure 14.7 White leghorn chicken with mild pododermatitis. Note the 3 × 2 mm hard callous on the plantar surface of a thickened metatarsal pad.

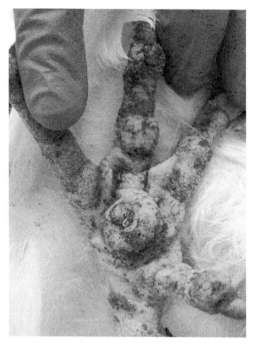

Figure 14.8 White leghorn chicken with moderate pododermatitis. Note the 5 x 5 mm hard callous with associated 10 × 10 mm swelling on the plantar surface of the metatarsal pad.

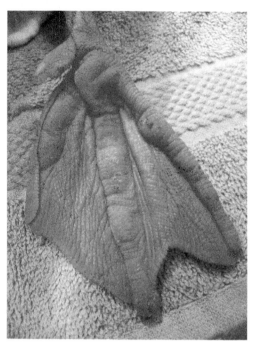

Figure 14.10 Pekin duck with mild pododermatitis. Note the 1 × 1 mm erosion on the digital pad of the #4 toe.

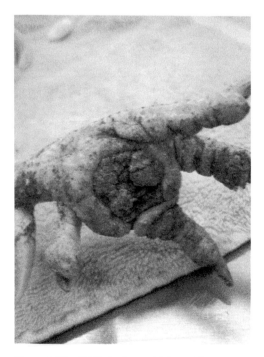

Figure 14.9 White leghorn chicken with severe pododermatitis. Note the 20 × 20 mm hard callous with associated 30 × 30 mm swelling on the plantar surface of the metatarsal pad.

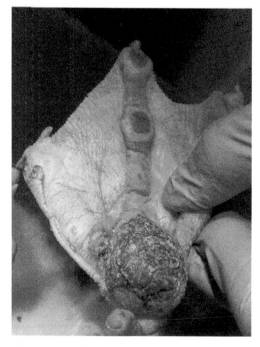

Figure 14.11 Pekin duck with severe pododermatitis. Note the 2 × 3 mm erosions on the plantar surface (digital pads) of the #3 toe and the 10 × 10 mm hard callous on the metatarsal pad.

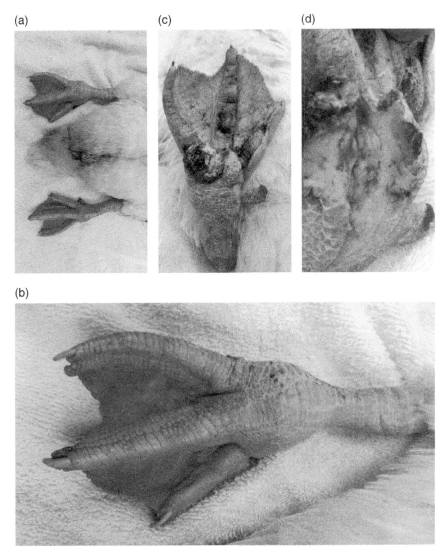

Figure 14.12 Adult Pekin duck presenting with severe pododermatitis of right intertarsal area. (a) Anterior surface of both feet showing swelling of right intertarsal area. (b) Close-up photograph of anterior surface of right foot. (c) Plantar surface of right foot showing swelling of intertarsal joint, and ulcerative and scabbed pododermatitis on plantar surface. (d) The owner elected euthanasia. At necropsy, the pododermatitis area is cut to show the thick fibrous tissue and deep infection. Diagnosis was septic intertarsal joint with chronic severe ulcerative pododermatitis.

Diseases of the Hock

Septic Joint

Causes of a septic joint are multiple, but the most common causes include *Staphylococcus aureus, Escherichia coli, Pasteurella multocida, Salmonella gallinarium, Mycoplasma synoviae,* and reoviruses [4]. The history may include an initial trauma, diarrhea, or respiratory disease that allowed the bacteria access to the joint either directly or through hematogenous spread. The bird usually presents with lameness either in one or multiple joints and an enlarged, warm joint (Figures 14.18 and 14.19). Aerobic and anaerobic culture, and maybe even

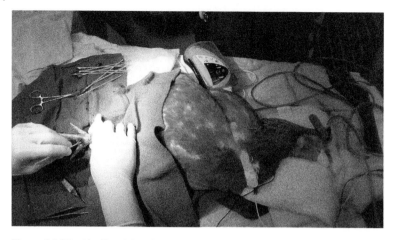

Figure 14.13 Ideally while a bird is under anesthesia adequate monitoring of heart rate, respiratory rate and depth of anesthesia should be constantly occurring. During surgery on this hen's foot, she was intubated, and the heart rate was monitored with a pulse oximeter placed on her comb, a Doppler probe on the radial artery of the wing (held in place with two tongue depressors taped together and used like a clothes-pin to hold the probe in place), an ECG (placed on left and right wing web near shoulder and left inguinal skin), and if needed a stethoscope was used. The respiratory rate was directly visualized as well as using an end-tidal CO_2 monitor (blue) placed between the endotracheal tube and the anesthetic tubing. Note the surgical area is aseptic, with sterile gloves, towels, and instruments used on an aseptically prepared foot and distal leg. The cotton tipped applicators were also sterile until placed at the edge of sterile field.

Mycoplasma culture or serology, aids in the diagnosis and choice of antibiotic. Radiographs help determine prognosis, the degree of osteomyelitis, and the duration of antibiotic therapy needed. The antibiotic chosen depends on the culture mainly but also with thought of treating a chicken; even if it is a pet, the species is covered by laws regarding antibiotic use in a food animal (see Regulatory Considerations for Medication Use in Poultry Chapter).

Prognosis is fair to poor, and often long-term therapy results in a joint with arthrodesis and limited range of motion but sufficient for the bird to walk around without putting undue stress and weight on the unaffected limb.

Perosis (Slipped Tendon)

Perosis, also known as "slipped tendon," refers to luxation of the gastrocnemius tendon causing the affected leg to be in a valgus position with an enlarged hock (Figure 14.20 a–d). Perosis is caused by a deficiency of choline, manganese, or biotin. Supplementing with

choline, manganese, and biotin, and suturing or tacking of the tendon sheath to keep the tendon in place have met with variable success [5]. Results of surgery are better if done when young, early in the clinical signs, and the leg is bandaged in flexion after surgery so that the bird can immediately use the leg and place it under their body. Careful not to bandage the leg in extension as this may create another deformity. Because it occurs at such a young age and the bird is growing fast, frequent rechecks, and bandage changes are necessary to provide the best bandage as the patient grows. Prognosis is usually poor.

Mycoplasmosis

There are three main species of *Mycoplasma* that can infect poultry. *Mycoplasma gallisepticum* (MG) causes respiratory disease in chickens, but an infectious sinusitis in turkeys. *Mycoplasma meleagridis* (MM) causes an airsacculitis and skeletal deformities in turkeys, and *Mycoplasma synoviae* (MS) causes

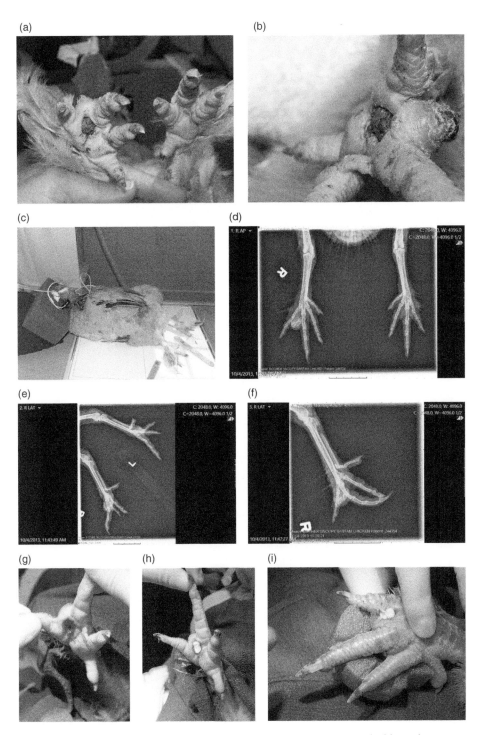

Figure 14.14 (a, b) An adult Welsummer hen with pododermatitis presented with an abscess ruptured through both the anterior and the plantar surface of the right foot between the third and fourth digit. (c) Endotracheally intubated under isoflurane anesthesia for a radiograph checking for osteomyelitis. (d) Ventrodorsal radiograph of both feet showing partially mineralized soft tissue mass between 3rd and 4th digits of right foot but no evidence of osteomyelitis. (e) Lateral radiograph of both feet showing partially mineralized soft tissue mass between 3rd and 4th digits of right foot, but no evidence of osteomyelitis. (f) Close-up view of radiograph of right foot. (g) Right foot after surgery to remove the abscess and debride the associated necrotic tissue. There was an expected amount of hemorrhage. (h) Right foot after amikacin-impregnated Gelfoam was placed in the lesion. (i) A polyethylene foam pad was cut to accommodate all four toes and leave a hole over the lesion area so that it could heal with air exposure and no mechanical pressure.

(j)

(k)

(l)

(m)

(n)

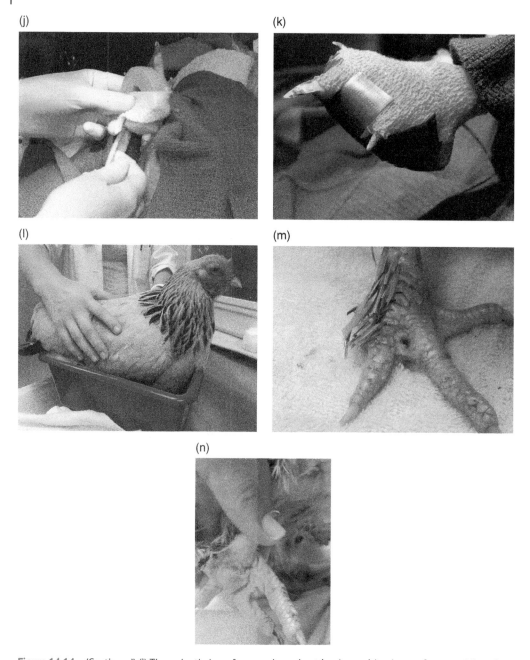

Figure 14.14 (Continued) (j) The polyethylene foam pad was kept in place with a layer of cast padding, then wrap. (k) Final bandage with a layer of duct tape on the plantar surface. (l) Hen during soaking of foot in warm chlorhexidine solution. This was done daily by the owner. (m) Anterior surface of right foot two weeks post-surgery and healing well. (n) Plantar surface of right foot two weeks post-surgery and healing well.

airsacculitis, mild upper respiratory infection, and synovitis/lameness in chickens and turkeys. MG is seen in backyard flocks and is of concern because it can easily spread to nearby commercial flocks and cause economic devastation for that commercial flock. Most commercial flocks are MG free. To participate in the National Poultry Improvement Plan (NPIP) a flock needs to be MG free. Transmission is through fomites.

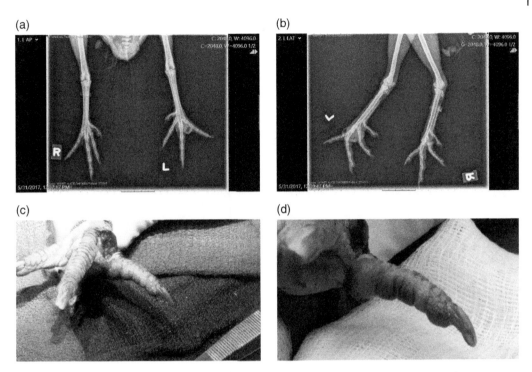

Figure 14.15 Same bird as Figure 14.13. (a) Ventrodorsal radiograph of both feet of chicken in Figure 14.13 showing mass with gas opacity between 3rd and 4th digit on the left foot. (b) Lateral radiograph showing mass between 3rd and 4th digit with gas opacity on the left foot. (c) Close up left foot during surgery after abscess removal. (d) Note in this view the left #4 toe has a blue discoloration with a definite line of demarcation indicating loss or decreased blood supply to this area from interrupted blood flow. This toe and foot healed very well and amputation of the toe was not necessary.

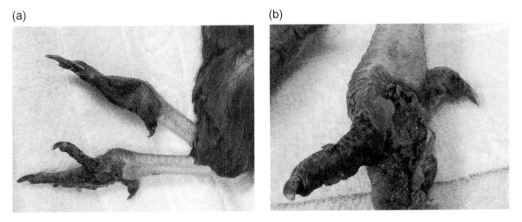

Figure 14.16 Two weeks previously this hen had stood in a puddle overnight that froze hard and caused necrosis due to frostbite of both feet. She was humanely euthanized. Usually frost bite affects the tips of combs or toes, not entire feet.

(a)

(b)

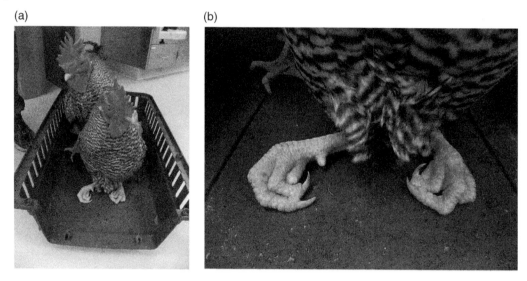

Figure 14.17 (a) Clutch of adult Plymouth Barred Rock Roosters presenting with varying degrees of curled toe paralysis that had been present since they were chicks. They also had varying degrees of ingrown comb/leader. Curled toe paralysis can be due to many possibilities but is usually thought to be associated with a deficiency in vitamin B2 (riboflavin).

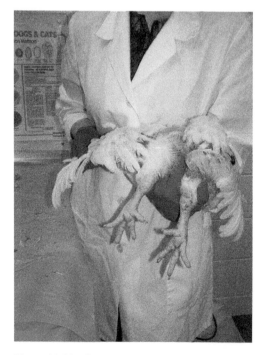

Figure 14.18 Demonstrating a method of holding a chicken to examine the hocks. This chicken has normal hocks.

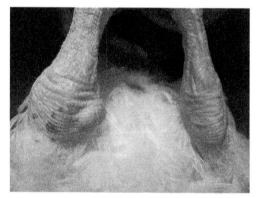

Figure 14.19 Enlarged and warm right hock in a duck due to a septic joint. Note that holding the bird in this position allows easy size comparison between the two hock joints.

Clinical signs relating to lameness caused by MM in turkeys usually occur in 1- to 6-week-old poults and include bowing, shortening, and twisting of the tarsometatarsal bone and associated hock swelling [6]. Morbidity is about 5–10%, with more males being affected. The main route of transmission is vertical

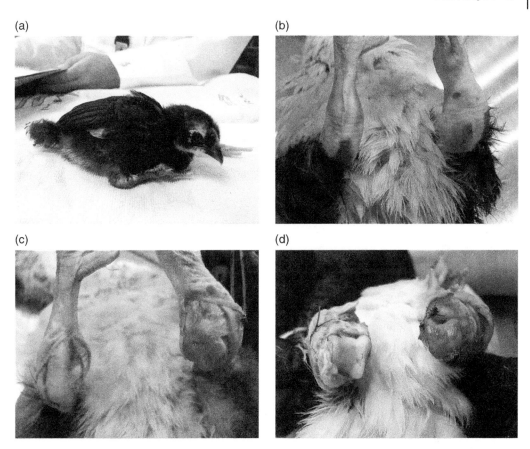

Figure 14.20 (a) Several-week-old sex-linked black star chick with perosis (slipped gastrocnemius tendon) of right leg showing typical stance. This age or sooner is the best age to perform corrective surgery. (b) Necropsy of a several-week-old duckling with perosis (slipped gastrocnemius tendon) of the left hock. Note the enlarged left hock with evidence of weight bearing on hock since was not weight bearing on the foot. (c) Note the lateral deviation of the tendon so that it does not sit within the groove of the distal tibotarsus and (d) also note the hyperemia and flattening of the condyle (the sutures seen were placed after death for practice of the surgical technique).

through the egg, but horizontal transmission can also occur either directly or indirectly. There are no vaccines for MM [6].

Clinical signs relating to lameness caused by MS in chickens or turkeys include an exudative synovitis, tenosynovitis, or bursitis of hock joints and foot pads [7] (Figure 14.21). Sometimes the sternal bursa or other joints are affected as well [7]. Morbidity is variable but is typically between 5% and 15% [7]. The main route of transmission is horizontal through the respiratory tract. A differential diagnosis is a septic joint due to other bacteria,

which tend to grow easily on aerobic and anerobic culture (see Septic Joints in this chapter). You can ask the laboratory to attempt growth of *Mycoplasma* spp. on special media, but it grows slowly and in chronic infections the organism may no longer be present [7]. Radiographs may help in that a septic joint due to other bacteria quickly progresses to include osteomyelitis visible on radiographs, whereas MS tends not to do this.

The best prevention is to depopulate and repopulate with clean stock. Treatment can be attempted with antibiotics (tetracycline,

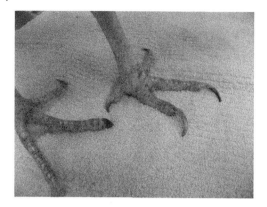

Figure 14.21 An eight month old white leghorn chicken with suspected *Mycoplasma synoviae* infection in the left intertarsal joint. Note the swollen metatarsal area on the left foot compared to the right foot.

spectinomycin, lincomycin, erythromycin, or tylosin), but birds remain carriers for life (see chapter on regulatory considerations for medication use in poultry).

Diseases of the Leg

Marek's Disease

Marek's disease (MD or MDV) is very common and affects only chickens. The causative agent is an alpha herpesvirus, but there three serotypes, four pathotypes, and many different strains of varying pathogenicity [8]. The prototype virus, the one that is associated with virulence or pathogenicity, is technically serotype 1, also known as *Gallid herpesvirus* 2 [8]. Serotype 1 is further subdivided into four pathotypes depending on virulence (mild, virulent, very virulent, and very virulent plus) [8]. MD causes a variety of clinical signs that have been divided into distinct pathological syndromes including what most people think of when they hear the words Marek's disease, which is fowl paralysis, but MD can also present as MD lymphoma, persistent neurological disease, skin leukosis, and ocular leukosis. Clinical signs of MD are generally seen in birds that are 10–20 weeks of age but can be seen as

young as 4 weeks of age. Be sure to obtain the exact age of the bird in weeks, as this will help later in helping to differentiate between MD and a very similar disease caused by avian leukosis virus (ALV).

MD is highly contagious and is transmitted horizontally either directly or indirectly by contact with virus via the airborne route. It can easily spread via fomites. Common sources are feathers, feather dander, secretions, and droppings (litter). Once a bird is infected, it sheds the virus indefinitely. The cell-free MD virus remains infectious for 4–8 months at room temperature and for at least 10 years at 4 °C (39 °F), which in a natural environment is practically indefinitely. Cleaning a plastic or metal cage of all debris and then disinfecting with a common disinfectant, such as a 1:10 dilution of household bleach, for 10 minutes, inactivate the organism [8].

Fowl Paralysis (Range Paralysis)

Clinical signs of unilateral paresis or paralysis are seen 3–4 weeks post infection, usually between the ages of 6–12 weeks but can be seen as young as 3–4 weeks of age and much older than 12 weeks. The typical stance is one leg stretched forward and the other pointing back (Figure 14.22a and Video 14.3). The classic, gross lesion that occurs with fowl paralysis is a unilateral enlargement of the sciatic plexus (the ischiadic nerve). A similar, but distinct syndrome is called transient paralysis that presents with a flaccid neck in young chickens. Sometimes birds that survive fowl paralysis go on to develop torticollis, crop stasis and dilation, or nervous tics associated with persistent neurological disease [8] (Figure 14.22b).

MD Lymphoma and other forms of MD

Outward clinical signs of MD lymphoma are usually subtle even with extensive neoplastic involvement and include weight loss, pale comb, anorexia, and diarrhea. The whitish to grayish focal nodular tumors or diffuse infiltration of mononuclear cells can involve a variety of tissues just like ALV and include ovary, lung,

(a)

(b)

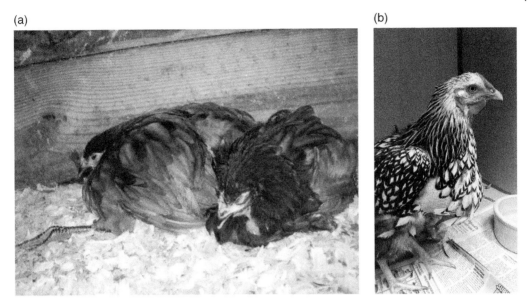

Figure 14.22 (a) Two lethargic 10-week-old blue Orpington chicks showing the typical stance of Marek's disease with one leg positioned forward and the other leg positioned backwards. The diagnosis was confirmed on necropsy with the typical lesion of unilateral sciatic (ishiadic) nerve enlargement. *Source:* Photograph courtesy of El Morse (see website for Video 14.3). (b) Young adult chicken with seer crop enlargement and stasis presumed to be associated with Marek's disease. A crop made of wrap around the neck helped minimally.

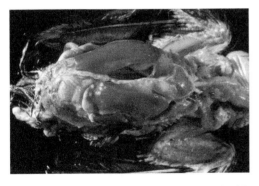

Figure 14.23 An 8-week-old chicken (pullet) with Marek's disease with diffuse hepatomegaly and multifocal nodular tumors in the liver. *Source:* Photograph courtesy of Dr. Linden Craig.

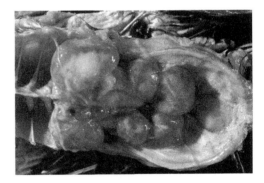

Figure 14.24 Same 8-week-old pullet as in Figure 11.28 that also had diffuse renalmegaly and multifocal nodular tumors in the kidney due to Marek's disease. *Source:* Photograph courtesy of Dr. Linden Craig.

heart, mesentery, kidney, liver, spleen, adrenal gland, pancreas, proventriculus, intestine, iris, skeletal muscle, and skin (Figures 14.23 and 14.24). When mononuclear infiltrates are found in the iris, this turns the affected iris a pale tan to gray instead of the usual yellow; this is called ocular lymphoma or "gray eye"

(Figure 14.25). Skin lymphoma presents as multiple, small (2×2mm) nodules associated with a feather follicle giving the skin a bumpy appearance. Organ distribution of MD lymphoma lesions is influenced by the genetic strain of the chicken and the strain of the virus.

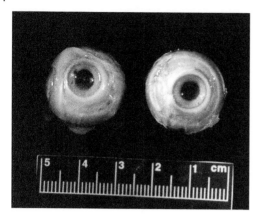

Figure 14.25 One-year-old male chicken (rooster) exhibiting the ocular form of Marek's disease with a light-colored tan/gray iris due to mononuclear cellular infiltrates as shown here in the eye on the left. The eye on the right is a normal yellowish color. *Source:* Photograph courtesy of Dr. Deb Miller.

Testing and Prevention of MD

Testing for MD can be done on 0.5 mL of serum using an inexpensive enzyme-linked immunosorbent assay (ELISA) test, or polymerase chain reaction (PCR) or virus isolation can be done on fresh tissue. This author is most familiar with sending samples to the Poultry Diagnostic and Research Center at the University of Georgia in Athens, Georgia (http://www.vet.uga.edu/avian). Other laboratories are available. Testing is helpful when trying to differentiate between MD lymphoma and ALV.

There is no treatment for MD. Prevention is by administering a polyvalent vaccine in the egg or at one day of age. There are several types of vaccine commonly used against MD either individually or in combination and include a low pathogenic serotype 1, a naturally avirulent Turkey Herpesvirus (HVT), and serotype 2 virus [8]. If purchasing chicks from a hatchery, always pay the slightly higher cost for a prevaccinated chick. Backyard poultry owners can purchase commercially available MD vaccine but they are in 1000–2000 dose vials that must be refrigerated or frozen prior to reconstitution and then used within one hour after reconsti-

tution and the remainder discarded appropriately. Understand that no vaccine is 100% protective and even "vaccinated" chicks can get the disease. The MD vaccines offer >90% protection, which is considered very effective. Much research has gone into MD-resistant strains of chickens, but even a "resistant" strain of chick should be vaccinated since even they can succumb to a virulent strain of MD [8]. Prior to the use of MD vaccines, mortality due to MD was as high as 60% [8].

ALV (Including Lymphoid Leukosis)

ALV is also known as leukosis/sarcoma group of diseases and causes a variety of tumors in chickens due to retroviruses [9]. Lymphoid leukosis (LL) is the most common form of this group of diseases, but many other neoplasia of chickens can also be caused by retroviruses including avian erythroblastosis, fibroma, fibrosarcoma, myoma, myxosarcoma, chondroma, osteoma, osteogenic sarcoma, squamous cell carcinoma, granulosa cell sarcoma, hemangioma, mesothelioma, meningioma, and glioma, to name a few [9]. This retrovirus is transmitted both horizontally and vertically. LL typically develops in chickens between 14 and 40 weeks of age but can occur later. Clinical signs of LL rarely develop before 14 weeks of age, which helps differentiate it from MD lymphoma, which usually occurs in younger chickens.

After clinical signs develop, chickens usually die within weeks. The clinical signs are nonspecific and include inappetence, weakness, diarrhea, dehydration, and emaciation. A predominant physical examination finding is a firm coelomic enlargement. Diagnosis is based on serology using ELISA or virus isolation on fresh tissue [9]. At gross necropsy, gray to white tumors are observed in the liver and other organs (Figures 14.26 and 14.27a,b). The clinical signs and gross pathological lesions are sometimes difficult to differentiate from those of MD, but LL does not occur before 14 weeks of age, whereas MD usually occurs at

10–12 weeks of age. There is no treatment and currently no vaccine. The best prevention is to test and cull positive breeder birds.

Reproductive Disease

Commonly, hens with reproductive disease have coelomic distention either due to fluid or soft tissue/organ enlargement, and they will present with lameness due to pain, weakness, illness, or simply due to the enlarged coelomic cavity that prevents normal ambulation

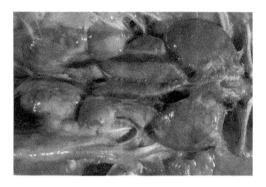

Figure 14.26 Kidney of a greater than one-year-old hen with suspected avian leukosis virus (ALV) due to age of the bird and gross and microscopic evidence of multiple organ tumors consistent with AVL. Note the similarity to the kidneys shown in Figure 14.24 of the eight-week-old chick with Marek's disease lymphoma. Source: Photograph courtesy of Dr. Danielle Reel.

(Figure 14.1 and Video 14.1). Reproductive disease in hens can include egg related coelomitis, retained egg, ectopic egg(s), right cystic oviduct, or neoplasia (Figure 14.28a–e) (see chapter on soft tissue surgery for further information). Perform a thorough physical examination and palpate the coelomic cavity. It should be soft in an egg-laying female, but not enlarged or fluctuant, nor enlarged and firm. If necessary perform radiographs to confirm enlarged coelomic cavity or to determine its cause. If necessary perform coelomocentesis to determine possible causes of "ascites" or excess coelomic fluid.

Valgus Deformities

There are many causes of valgus deformities in young chickens including slippery substrate, nutritional deficiencies (such as manganese deficiency), lack of exercise, and a diet too high in protein causing bones to grow faster than soft tissue. The lateral deviation can be at the intertarsal joint, tibiotarsus, at the hip, or a combination of the above (Figures 14.29 and 14.30a,b). Dyschondroplasia specifically refers to an abnormal persisting accumulation of cartilage at the growth plate common in meat type chickens, ducks, and turkeys and usually involves the tibiotarsus [10] Broiler-type breeds commonly have a valgus deformity at the intertarsal joint and/or

(a)

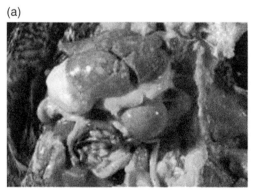

(b)

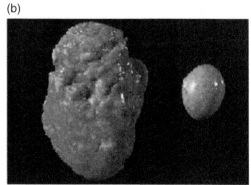

Figure 14.27 (a) A nine-month-old chicken hen with avian leukosis virus (ALV) evident by pale liver and pale spleen. (b) Close-up images.

(a) (b)

(c) (d) (e)

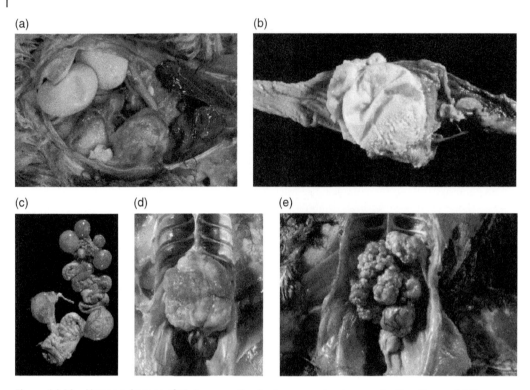

Figure 14.28 Necropsy images of birds presenting for lameness due to reproductive disease. (a) One-year-old chicken hen with egg related coelomitis and ectopic eggs due to a large egg causing egg impaction. *Source:* Photograph courtesy of Dr. Kim Newkirk. (b) An adult chicken hen with a retained egg (egg bound). *Source:* Photograph courtesy of Dr. M. Sula. (c) One-year-old chicken hen with right cystic oviduct. Note the cystic structure coming off the (bird's) right side of the cloaca as well as a normal and fully formed oviduct (with egg) and ovary on the left side. This chicken also presented with a cloacal prolapse. *Source:* Photograph courtesy of Dr. Linden Craig. (d) A six-month-old chicken hen with ovarian lymphoma from avian leukosis virus. *Source:* Photograph courtesy of Dr. Kim Newkirk. (e) A seven year-old turkey hen with ovarian carcinoma. *Source:* Photograph courtesy of Dr. Linden Craig.

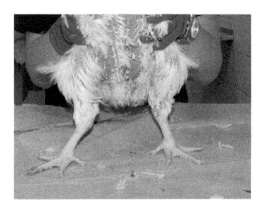

Figure 14.29 An eight-week-old chicken with an abnormal stance due to a valgus deformity of the right tibiotarsus.

the tibiotarsus of unknown cause but it is probably due to rapid growth. [10]. Often treatment includes slowing down the growth of the bird with a lower protein diet, which can be done by adding corn scratch to the diet at no more than 25% of the diet, or switching to an age-appropriate diet with slightly lower protein. Splay leg or spraddle leg is a lateral deviation at the hip that is usually associated with high humidity during incubation [10]. If caught early, lateral deviations of the leg can be bandaged (hobbled) to encourage the leg to be in a normal, usable position. Frequent, almost daily, bandage changes are necessary to keep up with the growth of the bird,

(a)

(b)

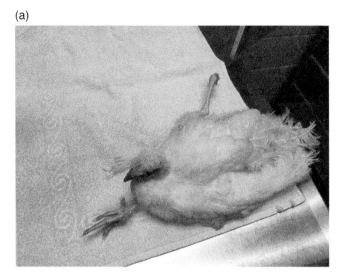

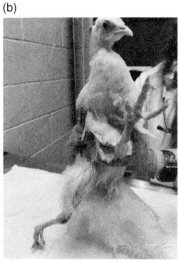

Figure 14.30 Juvenile white peahen with a severe valgus deformity of the right leg due to tibiotarsal rotation. (a) dorsal view, (b) ventral view. A dome osteotomy procedure was initially offered with a guarded prognosis until it was discovered on a complete physical examination that this bird also had a luxation of the left hip due to the long-term abnormal stance. The owner elected euthanasia since prognosis was grave for return to function (standing).

deterioration of the bandage, and reassessing the changing position of the leg. It is imperative that the bandage result in the leg being under the bird in a usable position or the bandaging itself can cause deviation of the hip over a period of just days in these young, quickly growing birds. Alternatively, an osteotomy, preferable a dome osteotomy which allows rotation in three dimensions, can be performed using external fixator pins, to correct a valgus or varus deviation in the bone.

Trauma to the Leg

Trauma is a very common presenting complaint in backyard poultry either from predator attack (dog, raccoon, etc.), being kicked by a horse, being accidently stepped on by the owner, or getting caught in some part of their enclosure and struggling (Figure 14.31a,b). Ducks can present for toe or foot trauma after being bitten by a snapping turtle (Figure 14.32a,b). Wounds can involve soft tissue only or soft tissue and bone. Wound

management is covered in the dermatological diseases chapter of this book. Fracture repair is covered next.

Fracture Repair

Radiographs should be taken before and after fracture repair and during the healing process to determine the type of repair needed, assess stability of the fracture after repair, assess the integrity of any bandage or hardware placed, and check for evidence of osteomyelitis (Figures 14.33–14.36). Frequent follow-up visits also allow for readjustments in the treatment plan.

Avian bones differ from mammalian bones in that they have a thin, brittle cortex, may be pneumatic (humerus and femur), and heal by mostly endosteal, and some periosteal, new bone growth. Generally, avian fractures heal faster than mammalian fractures at two o three weeks versus four to six weeks in mammals. The goal is to align the fracture as best as possible so that weight bearing can occur almost immediately so as not to cause excess stress and load on the unaffected limb. Pododermatitis

(a) (b)

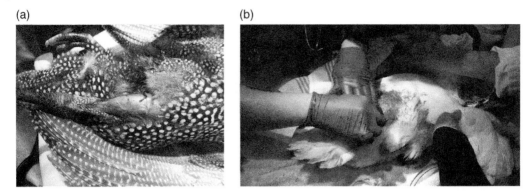

Figure 14.31 (a) Adult Guinea fowl attacked by a dog presented with a de-gloving injury over the left leg extending into the inguinal area. Wounds in a high motion area such as the inguinal area require long term, sometimes months of, wound care management. (b) Adult Pekin duck attacked by dogs showing typical wounds on rear dorsum. She was in shock and was receiving oxygen via a face mask while the wounds were being quickly assessed.

(a) (b)

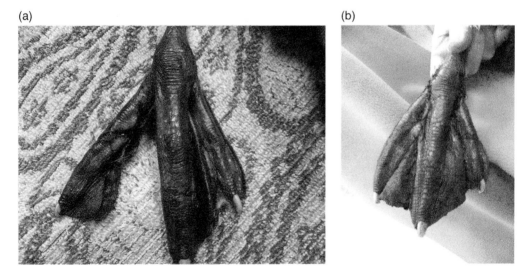

Figure 14.32 (a) An adult wild Canada goose presented with trauma to the webbing of one foot due to suspected snapping turtle bite. (b) After surgery to close the skin wounds. Care was taken to separately suture the two (anterior and plantar) layers of skin that make up the webbing of the foot.

needs to be prevented in the nonaffected leg or foot while the affected leg heals (Figure 14.2). This is best done by having the affected limb be usable as soon as possible, providing soft substrate, and watching for early signs of pododermatitis and taking steps to treat it early.

Ideally fractures need to have both rotational and bending forces controlled with the bone in as near to normal apposition as possible.

External fixation pins with or without an intramedullary (IM) pin tie-in usually provides the best fixation for most fractures in birds and can also be partially destabilized part way through the healing process to strengthen the bone and promote maximal healing. Since birds have thin brittle cortices, positive profile pins should be used for external fixation, not negative profile pins, in order to provide

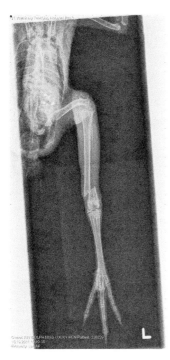

Figure 14.33 Ventrodorsal radiograph of the left leg of a less than one-year-old hen with an oblique distal tibiotarsal fracture that is close to but not involving the hock joint (tibiotarsal tarsometatarsal joint or intertarsal joint).

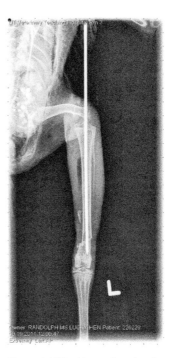

Figure 14.35 Ventrodorsal radiograph of the left leg of the chicken in Figure 14.33 immediately after open reduction. Only an intramedullary pin (IM) and external coaptation were used to repair this fracture and it healed well, although external fixation using an IM pin tie-in is considered ideal for fracture healing. The redundant part of the pin has not yet been trimmed.

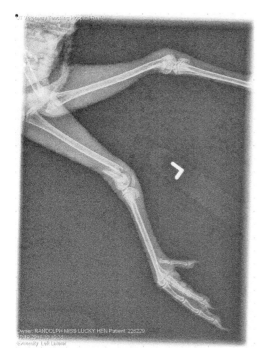

Figure 14.34 Lateral radiograph of left leg of hen in Figure 14.33.

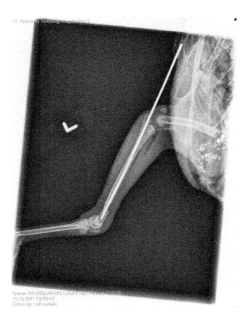

Figure 14.36 Lateral radiograph of the left leg of the chicken in Figure 14.33.

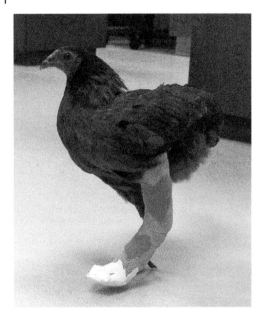

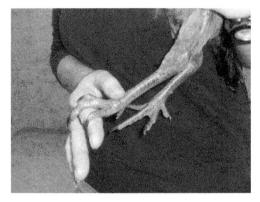

Figure 14.38 Same chicken as Figure 14.6 showing physical therapy in the form of gently extending the toes since this bird had some contracture. *Source:* Photo courtesy of Dr. Katherine Baine.

Figure 14.37 Same chicken from Figure 14.6 showing external coaptation used in conjunction with the IM pin. Note the flexed usable position of the bandaged leg. *Source:* Photo courtesy of Dr. Katherine Baine.

greater purchase of the bone, increase stability and lessen the chance for pin loosening.

An IM pin alone counteracts bending forces but not rotational forces; therefore ideally external fixation pins are also applied and tied-in to the IM pin. A splint, cast, or Robert-Jones bandage can be applied in conjunction with the IM pin tie-in, and suboptimally external coaptation can be used in conjunction with an IM pin without external fixation (Figure 14.37). Since the IM pin may pass through or near a joint, a smooth pin without threads is used to cause the least amount of trauma.

The connecting bar used to connect the external fixator pins can be made of lightweight materials such as polymethylmethacrylate (PMM), acrylic, plumber's putty, epoxy, or casting material. The freshly mixed soft PMM is usually syringed into a drinking straw or Penrose tube that has been impaled on the external fixator pins and held in place until the PMM hardens.

The integrity of the splint is directly proportional to its ability to counteract rotational forces. Place the bandage in flexion in as close to a normal position as possible so the bird can have immediate use of the limb, less abnormal forces placed on nearby joints, and rest with the leg under the body rather than out to the side (Figure 14.37). External coaptation (splint or Robert-Jones bandage) is sometimes used alone, but it is not ideal since there is a risk of bending and rotational forces causing less than ideal healing or even a false joint or malunion healing.

Other methods used in mammals to complement fracture repair can also be used in avian fracture repair such as physical therapy (Figures 14.38 and 14.39, and see website for Video 14.4 of chicken trained to go over a step).

Gastrocnemius Tendon Rupture

Gastrocnemius tendon rupture is not common in backyard poultry but can occur in meat type breeds of chickens typically older than 12 weeks. One or both hocks can be affected, and the bird presents sitting on the affected hock or hocks with the toes pointing ventrally [10]. The loose end of the tendon can be

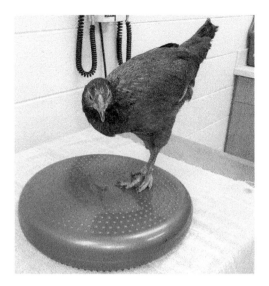

Figure 14.39 Same chicken as Figure 14.6 showing physical therapy in the form of training the chicken to step up to help extend the toes back to normal. See Video 14.4 on this book's accompanying website. *Source:* Photograph and video courtesy of Dr. Katherine Baine.

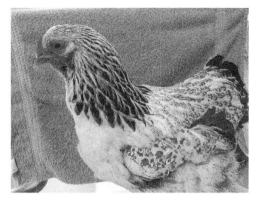

Figure 14.40 An adult hen with a figure-of-8 bandage placed on the left antebrachium to stabilize a radius and ulna fracture. Ideally for fracture healing, an IM pin, or an IM pin with an external fixator tie-in would have been placed, but due to cost and the bird not needing to fly, a bandage only was chosen by the owner. The fracture healed.

easily palpated bunched up on the posterior surface of the leg cranial to the hock. Also confirmatory is the lack of a gastrocnemius tendon attachment palpated at the hock. There will be a dark discoloration of hemorrhage under the skin in the affected area, or if it has been long enough, over three days, then a green discoloration since birds bruise green due to a lack of biliverdin reductase. Chronic lesions will also have some degree of fibrous tissue. The cause is unknown but may be related to infection with a reovirus causing a tenosynovitis. There is no treatment currently described for this disease.

Diseases of the Hip

Hip luxations occur uncommonly in birds due to the force needed for it to occur but are easy to palpate since the head of the femur will extend dorsal to the level of the hip. Treatment consists of performing a femoral head osteotomy

or pinning techniques have been described in avian textbooks.

Diseases of the Wing

If a wing droop is present, then a thorough physical examination should bear out the cause, such as fracture, brachial plexus avulsion, or soft tissue injury. Since backyard poultry do not need to fly, then fractures of the wing bones (humerus, radius, ulna) do not necessarily need to be in perfect alignment; many owners choose the less expensive method of external coaptation. A figure-of-8 bandage is used for fractures distal to the elbow, and a body wrap is included with the figure-of-8-bandage if the humerus is fractured (Figure 14.40). Primary repair with IM pins and external fixation devices and wound care are the same for poultry as other birds, keeping in mind the limitations set by the FDA regarding medication uses in poultry. Multiple avian textbooks describe these procedures. A partial or complete brachial plexus avulsion can occur during trauma if the wing is pulled away from the body and results in unilateral pectoral muscle atrophy (Figure 14.41).

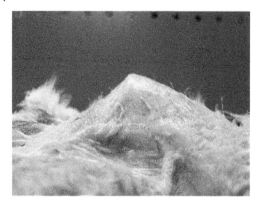

Figure 14.41 View of a bird at necropsy looking from the head caudally showing the pectoral muscle atrophy to the left of the bird's keel. This was due to brachial plexus avulsion.

For "angel wing," a condition brought on by a high energy diet in juvenile ducks, please refer to the anserform chapter.

Diseases of the CNS or PNS

Vitamin E Deficiency (Encephalomalacia)

Vitamin E deficiency can cause encephalomalacia as well as other diseases such as exudative diathysis, and nutritional myopathy in chicks. Encephalomalacia in chicks is characterized by ataxia or paresis but with rapid contraction and relaxation of the legs with forced movements, abnormal head and neck positions, and death [2]. Histopathological lesions include demyelination, neuronal degeneration, and marked hyperemia of meningeal, cerebral, and cerebellar vessels associated with ischemic necrosis [2]. Early treatment with can quickly reverse signs, otherwise the prognosis is poor.

Vitamin B1 (Thiamine) Deficiency (Star Gazing)

Vitamin B1 (thiamine) deficiency causes "star gazing" in chicks associated with anorexia, weight loss, ruffled feathers, ataxia, ascending paralysis, and opisthotonos. The term "star gazing" describes the typical position of the head drawn back while sitting on the hocks with the legs flexed due to paralysis of the anterior muscles of the neck [2]. Chicks can develop clinical signs as early as two weeks of age on a deficient diet, whereas adults take a lot longer. Histopathologically, a myelin degeneration of multiple nerves is observed, as well as hypertrophy of the adrenal glands and edema of the skin. Early treatment with thiamine or vitamin B complex can quickly reverse signs, but chronic cases may be left with permanent damage despite treatment [2, 3].

Botulism (Limberneck)

Botulism in backyard poultry usually involves ducks and other waterfowl but can also occur in other birds, including chickens, pheasants, and turkeys. It occurs from ingesting the type C exotoxin produced by the *Clostridium botulinum* bacteria often found in decaying meat and vegetation or in the associated maggots [11]. Clinical signs consist of an ascending flaccid paralysis of skeletal muscle that eventually leads to death by respiratory paralysis or drowning from the inability to keep the head above water. Morbidity and mortality are dose related: the higher the dose, the more acute and severe are the signs [12]. A high dose can result in clinical signs within hours, whereas a low dose may be associated with paralysis signs in one to two days. If not severe, spontaneous recovery can occur with supportive care. Confirming a diagnosis of botulism is difficult since there are no gross or histopathological signs, but the suspected ingested substance, crop contents, and gastrointestinal contents can be analyzed for toxins [12]. Treatment with antitoxin may be considered in valuable, individual birds since it was shown to be effective in birds but it only neutralized the free and extracellular bound toxin [12]. Preventing exposure to decaying meat and vegetation, removing cadavers promptly, and providing fresh food and water are the best preventative measures since both the bacteria and toxin are stable in the environment.

Avian Encephalomyelitis (Epidemic Tremor)

Avian encephalomyelitis (AE) is a disease with worldwide distribution that may be seen occasionally in unvaccinated flocks of chickens, but natural infections have also been documented in pheasants, quail, and turkeys [13–16]. AE is caused by an hepatovirus in the Picornaviridae family and usually affects chickens at one to three weeks of age. Clinical signs include initial depression and then progressive ataxia with tremors of the head and neck, hence the lay name of "epidemic tremors." Young birds will often lay on their sides with both legs stretched caudally. Birds exposed to the virus after 4 weeks of age are usually asymptomatic [13, 14, 16]. The morbidity in 1- to 2-week-old chicks is about 40–60% with a mortality rate of usually 25% but can be as high as 50%. Birds that recover are immune but have permanent ataxia, and some, weeks later go on to develop lens opacity (cataracts) and may become blind [13, 15, 17].

Transmission is usually vertical from the hen to the egg, hence the importance of vaccinating breeder hens at about 14 weeks of age before they start to lay. Infected laying birds may experience a 5–10% decrease in egg production. Horizontal transmission can also occur via the fecal-oral route to propagate in the intestines of young, 1- to 3-week-old chicks. Infected chicks can shed the virus for 5–21 days post infection [16].

Gross pathology signs are minimal except for white nodules observed in the muscularis of the ventriculus due to massive lymphocytic infiltration [13, 15].

Histopathologically, the changes that are strongly suggestive of AE are found in the brain/spinal cord and viscera and include a nonpurulent encephalomyelitis with a severe perivascular infiltrate, a ganglionitis of the dorsal root ganglion, and microgliosis [13, 15]. Aggregates of lymphocytes are also observed in the proventriculus, ventriculus, pancreas, and myocardium [13, 15, 16]. The peripheral nervous system is not involved as it is with MD, an important differential diagnosis. Other differential diagnoses include encephalomalacia due to vitamin E deficiency, toxins such as lead, Newcastle disease, and eastern equine encephalitis. Because the virus is nonenveloped, it is extremely resistant in the environment, lasting months in the soil and easily spread by fomites. Antibody tests (ELISA, ID, VN) can be used to determine exposure. An ELISA can be run on 0.5–1.0 mL of serum at laboratories (http://gapoultrylab.org or http://www.usu.edu/uvdl/htm/services/avian-testing), or virus isolation can be performed on fresh brain tissue.

Beak Deformities

Recently a paper was published demonstrating the use of a syringe casing and needles with a screw to slowly distract the mandible after osteotomy in a juvenile mute swan with mandibular deviation [18]. This procedure also worked well with a pullet with mandibular deviation using a small insulin syringe [19]. The sooner the procedure is performed, the better the prognosis (Figure 14.42).

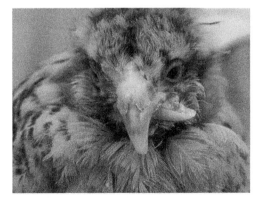

Figure 14.42 Several-week-old chick with deviation of the mandibular beak. Although a new distraction procedure is described for this condition that works well, this bird was deemed too severe and chronic for correction.

References

1 Ritchie, B.W., Harrison, G.J., and Harrison, L.R. (eds.) (1994). *Avian Medicine: Principles and Application*. Lake Worth: Wingers Publishing.

2 Andreasen, C.B. (2008). Staphylococcosis. In: *Diseases of Poultry* (ed. Y.M. Saif) (assoc. eds. A.M. Fadly, J.R. Glisson, L.R. McDougald et al.), 12e, 892–900. Ames, Iowa: Wiley Blackwell.

3 Schat, K.A. and Nair, V. (2008). Marek's disease. In: *Diseases of Poultry* (ed. Y.M. Saif) (assoc. eds. A.M. Fadly, J.R. Glisson, L.R. McDougald et al.), 12e, 1149–1196. Ames, Iowa: Wiley Blackwell.

4 Fadley, A.M., Nair, V., and Leukosis/Sarcoma Group (2008). *Diseases of Poultry* (ed. Y.M. Saif) (assoc. eds. A.M. Fadly, J.R. Glisson, L.R. McDougald et al.), 12e, 515–568. Ames, Iowa: Wiley Publishing.

5 Crespio, R. and Shivaprasad, H.L. (2008). Developmental, metabolic, and other noninfectious disorders. In: *Diseases of Poultry* (ed. Y.M. Saif) (assoc. eds. A.M. Fadly, J.R. Glisson, L.R. McDougald et al.), 12e, 1149–1196. Ames, Iowa: Wiley Publishing.

6 Olsen, G.H. (1994). Anseriformes. In: *Avian Medicine: Principles and Application* (eds. B.W. Ritchie, G.J. Harrison and L.R. Harrison), 1237–1275. Lake Worth: Wingers Publishing.

7 Chin, R.P., Yan Ghazikhanian, G., and Kempf, I. (2008). Mycoplasma meleagridis infection. In: *Diseases of Poultry* (ed. Y.M. Saif) (assoc. eds. A.M. Fadly, J.R. Glisson, L.R. McDougald et al.), 12e, 834–845. Ames, Iowa: Wiley Blackwell.

8 Kleven, S.H. and Ferguson-Noel, N. (2008). Mycoplasma synoviae infection. In: *Diseases of Poultry* (ed. Y.M. Saif) (assoc. eds. A.M. Fadly, J.R. Glisson, L.R. McDougald et al.), 12e, 845–856. Ames, Iowa: Wiley Blackwell.

9 Klasing, K.C. (2008). Nutritional diseases. In: *Diseases of Poultry* (ed. Y.M. Saif) (assoc. eds. A.M. Fadly, J.R. Glisson, L.R. McDougald et al.), 12e, 1121–1148. Ames, Iowa: Wiley Blackwell.

10 Bennett, R.A. (1994). Neurology. In: *Avian Medicine: Principles and Application* (eds. B.W. Ritchie, G.J. Harrison and L.R. Harrison), 723–747. Lake Worth: Wingers Publishing.

11 Gerlach, H. (1994). Bacteria. In: *Avian Medicine: Principles and Application* (eds. B.W. Ritchie, G.J. Harrison and L.R. Harrison), 949–983. Lake Worth: Wingers Publishing.

12 Dohms, J.E. (2008). Botulism. In: *Diseases of Poultry* (ed. Y.M. Saif) (assoc. eds. A.M. Fadly, J.R. Glisson, L.R. McDougald et al.), 12e, 879–885. Ames, Iowa: Wiley Blackwell.

13 Calnek, B.W. (2008). Other viral infections. In: *Diseases of Poultry* (ed. Y.M. Saif) (assoc. eds. A.M. Fadly, J.R. Glisson, L.R. McDougald et al.), 12e, 430–441. Ames, Iowa: Wiley Blackwell.

14 Gerlach, H. (1994). Viruses. In: *Avian Medicine: Principles and Application* (eds. B.W. Ritchie, G.J. Harrison and L.R. Harrison), 862–948. Lake Worth: Wingers Publishing.

15 http://www.merckmanuals.com/vet/poultry/avian_encephalomyelitis/overview_of_avian_encephalomyelitis.html (accessed 18 December 2013)

16 Ritchie, B.W. (ed.) (1995). Other avian viruses. In: *Avian viruses: Function and Control*, 413–438. Lake Worth: Wingers Publishing.

17 Bridges, C.H. and Flowers, A.I. (1958). Iridocyclitis and cataracts associated with an encephalomyelitis in chickens. *J. Amer. Vet. Med. Assoc.* 132: 79–84.

18 Carrasco, D.C., Dutton, T.A., Shimizu, N., and Forbes, N. (2016). Distraction osteogensis correction of mandibular ramus fracture malunion in a juvenile mute swan (Cygnus olor). *J. Avian. Med. Surg.* 30 (1): 30–38.

19 Brandao J. Personal communication. June 3, 2019.

15

Dermatological Diseases
Angela Lennox

Avian and Exotic Animal Clinic of Indianapolis, Indianapolis, IN, USA

Introduction

Dermatologic disease is sporadic in backyard poultry and most commonly involves ectoparasitism and trauma/wound management. Other infectious and noninfectious skin diseases can occur but are less frequently encountered in backyard flocks. Table 15.1 provides an overview of dermatologic diseases based on clinical presentation.

Husbandry

Skin quality is affected by a number of husbandry factors, including diet and sanitation. Research has focused on the effect of bedding type, size, and moisture on the development of footpad dermatitis in broiler chickens [1]. Not surprisingly, bedding moisture increased the incidence of foot lesions, particularly in younger birds. Another study compared three bedding types: wheat straw, chopped wheat straw, and wood shavings. Parameters measured were weight gain, food intake, and incidence of footpad necrosis. Weight gain and low footpad dermatitis scores were improved when birds were kept on wood shavings [1]. For backyard flocks, clean dry bedding, preferably not wheat straw, along with other appropriate husbandry measures is likely to decrease incidence of disease as well.

Most Common Dermatological Diseases of Backyard Poultry

Ectoparasitic Diseases

Many species of lice and mites infect birds [2, 3]. Lice are generally species specific, but mites often are not.

External parasites such as mites and lice are common in poultry. Prevention, checking your flock periodically for external parasites, and treating early helps prevent a larger flock outbreak. Other less common ectoparasites include bed bugs, chiggers, black flies, fleas, and ticks.

Lice

Lice species vary in color, size, and preferred area of the body they infect. The entire life cycle occurs on the host, and transmission is via close contact with affected birds. More than 40 species of lice have been identified in domestic fowl. The more common include the body louse (*Menacanthus stramineus*), shaft

Backyard Poultry Medicine and Surgery: A Guide for Veterinary Practitioners, Second Edition.
Edited by Cheryl B. Greenacre and Teresa Y. Morishita.
© 2021 John Wiley & Sons, Inc. Published 2021 by John Wiley & Sons, Inc.
Companion website: www.wiley.com/go/greenacre/medicine

Table 15.1 Diseases affecting the skin of poultry classified by clinical appearance

Lesion	Potential Etiology
Round lesions of unfeathered portions of the head and neck, and sometimes feet and vent; often scabbed	Poxvirus
Masses associated with feather follicles	Marek disease; Bacterial folliculitis
Lesions of the feet, especially the ventral aspects	Footpad dermatitis; trauma
Yellow thickening of skin	Xanthomatosis
Feather loss and lesions of the back of the head and back	Rooster or cage mate trauma
Focal skin irritation/inflammation	Ectoparasites; trauma
Skin wounds, often necrotic	Gangrenous dermatitis, trauma
Lesions and irritation of vent in older birds	Cage mate trauma,
Lesions and irritation of the vent in young birds	Infectious bursal disease
Pale discoloration of skin	Chicken anemia virus, other anemia
Lacerations and punctures; often of the head, neck, and extremities	Predator trauma
Visible ectoparasites	Usually lice, consider ticks, fly larvae
Swollen inflamed wattles, neck, and head, sometimes feet as well in visibly sick birds	Fowl cholera

Note that not all are commonly encountered in backyard poultry flocks.

louse (*Menopon gallinae*), head louse (*Culclotogaster heterographa*), and others [4]. More than one species can be on the bird at one time. The shaft louse lays its eggs on the shaft of the feather at the base (Figures 15.1a,b and 15.2). Lice may be clinically insignificant in older birds but can increase in number and cause debilitation in younger or sick birds. Lice infestation appears to be worse in the fall and winter.

Clinical signs include hyperemia and irritation of the skin of affected birds with small scabs and clots. A moth-eaten appearance to the feathers may be seen. Nits (louse eggs) are

(a)

(b)

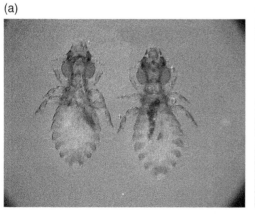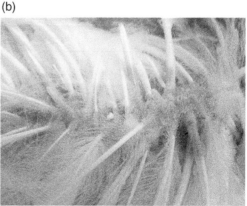

Figure 15.1 (a) Photograph of the common body louse of chickens, *Menacanthus stramineus*. *Source:* Photograph courtesy of Aly Chapman, University of Tennessee. (b) Photograph of yellowish body lice on a white chicken. *Source:* Photograph courtesy of Dr. Cheryl B. Greenacre.

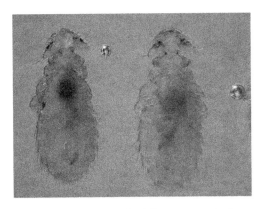

Figure 15.2 Photograph of the common shaft louse of chickens, *Menopen gallinae. Source:* Photograph courtesy of Aly Chapman, University of Tennessee.

laid in clumps at the base of feathers along the ventrum. The lice feed mainly on skin fragments and feather debris on the surface of the skin but can also feed on the blood inside of blood (pin, quill) feathers; otherwise they do not suck blood, since they are chewing lice. They spend their entire life cycle on the chicken. Lice are easily seen with the naked eye and are yellowish and flat bodied. Lice move fast in comparison to mites. Under the microscope, their big head with chewing mouth parts can be seen since they are chewing lice.

Treatment options are variable. Ivermectin is commonly used as a lice treatment in poultry, with reports of anecdotal success, although there are no studies to support this. Follow label directions for withdrawal times in food-producing poultry or contact FARAD (Food Animal Residue and Avoidance Database at http://farad.com). If selling the eggs commercially, the only allowed treatment is diatomaceous earth (DE).

Mites

Mites are much smaller than lice and feed on blood, feathers, and skin. Appearance is variable. They are capable of infecting any avian host. Some mites spend their entire life cycles on the bird, but some do not. For this reason, treatment of mites involves treating the envi-

ronment as well as the birds [4]. Some mites, including *Dermanyssus gallinae* feed at night and hide in cracks and joints of the enclosure during the day; therefore diagnosis can be difficult. Some mites can survive in the environment for up to 30 weeks without food, making premise treatment critical for effective eradication. More commonly encountered mite species include the chicken mite (*Dermanyssus gallinae*), the Northern fowl mite (*Ornithonyssus sylviarum*), and the scaly leg mite (*Knemidokoptes mutans*) (Figures 15.3–15.6). While not specifically zoonotic, temporary infestation of humans may occur.

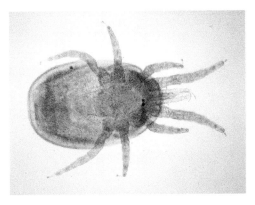

Figure 15.3 Photograph of *Dermanyssus gallinae,* the chicken mite, also known as the red chicken mite. *Source:* Photograph courtesy of Aly Chapman, University of Tennessee.

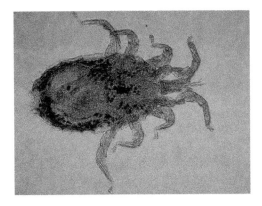

Figure 15.4 Photograph of *Ornithonyssus sylviarum,* the Northern fowl mite. *Source:* Photograph courtesy of Aly Chapman, University of Tennessee.

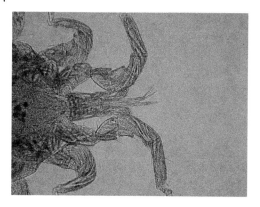

Figure 15.5 Close up photograph of the mouth parts of *Ornithonyssus sylviarum* showing the difference from the mouth parts of *Dermanyssus* spp. *Source:* Photograph courtesy of Aly Chapman, University of Tennessee.

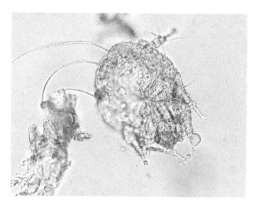

Figure 15.6 Photograph of *Knemidokoptes* spp., the scaly leg mite. *Source:* Photograph courtesy of Aly Chapman, University of Tennessee.

Ornithonyssus sylvarium (Northern Fowl Mite, Feather Mite) The Northern fowl mite is the most common external parasite in poultry, especially in cool weather climates. This mite spends its entire life cycle (egg to larva to nymphal stage to adult) on the chicken, which can take as little as a week in ideal conditions. Clinical signs of this mite infestation include soiled feathers around the vent, tail, and rear legs. Mites are commonly first discovered or seen on eggs. Heavy infestations can cause decreased egg production. Barely seen with the naked eye, the adults are a dark red to black with evidence of mites and eggs seen as a dark area at the base of feathers in the ventral regions (vent, ventral coelomic area, tail, ventral cervical area). Light-colored birds may have a darkening of the feathers from a build-up of mite feces. Diagnosis is based on typical clinical signs, seeing the mite grossly, or performing a tape prep of an affected area and examining for mites under the microscope. Mites can be transferred via fomites including crates, cages, clothing, and wild birds.

Dermanyssus gallinae (Chicken Mite, Red Mite, Roost Mite) This is the mite that feeds on poultry at night and then remains secluded during the day within the poultry house, making diagnosis difficult. This mite can live off the bird for 2–3 weeks. The life cycle can be completed in as little as 7–10 days with ideal conditions. Clinical signs include mild weight loss and decreased egg production. The mite is best seen using a magnifying glass and inspecting the birds and house at night.

A recent study showed mite populations were similar in hens that were raised caged or free range [5]. Another study compared mite populations between hens that were caged, free range, and free range with access to dust boxes containing sand and either DE, kaolin clay, or sulfur. All hens using dust boxes with any material showed a reduction in ectoparasites by 80–100% after 1 week compared to the other two groups. Ectoparasite populations recovered when dust boxes containing DE or kaolin clay were removed; however, sulfur provided a residual effect up to 9 months post removal [5]. Provision of dust boxes may be a simple and effective method of ectoparasite control for backyard flocks.

Studies into the efficacy of various acaricides in the treatment of ectoparasites in chickens have revealed some information. Tetrachlorvinphos with dichlorvos was the most effective at treating chickens naturally infected with Northern fowl mites, followed by Malathion dust and 10% garlic oil. Permethrin failed to reduce mite populations significantly [6].

Ivermectin is also commonly used to treat mite infestations in many species, including psittacine birds. Treatment in poultry anecdotally appears to be effective but only when combined with premises treatment for those mite species living extended periods off of the host.

Ticks

Although infestations are not common, the fowl tick, also known as the poultry tick (*Argas persicus*), can cause disease in chickens, ducks, and geese (Figure 15.7a,b). It is a yellowish brown (before blood meal) to slate-blue (after blood meal) soft bodied tick that tends to prefer warmer climates/seasons. Both nymphal stages and adults detach from the host after feeding and can be found in the nearby environment (Figure 15.8a,b). The soft tick *Argus persicus* has been shown to transmit the spirochete bacteria *Borrelia anserine,* which can severely affect poultry [7]. Clinical signs of weakness, decreased egg production, ascending paralysis, and death can be attributed to anemia, borreliosis, and also tick paralysis [8]. Some immunity to the paralysis-inducing toxins develops after previous exposure to the ticks, resulting in new or naïve birds being most affected. Treatment includes removing birds and treating the house using a high-pressure sprayer with carbaryl, coumaphos, malathion, permethrin, stirofos, or

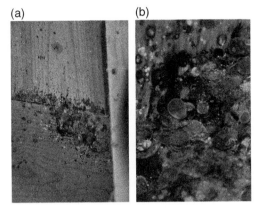

Figure 15.8 (a) Same soft bodied tick infestation as in Figure 15.7 showing the ticks in the environment crowding the crevices of the house. (b) Close-up image showing slate-blue colored soft bodied ticks in the environment. After feeding, the nymphal and adult stages leave the bird and hide in crevices in the chicken house. *Source:* Photographs courtesy of Dr. Abigail Duvall.

a mixture or stirofos and dichlorvos. Cracks and crevices of the house should then be filled in [9].

Other Ectoparasites

Other ectoparasites identified in poultry include bedbugs (*Cimex lectularius*), chiggers (larval mites of *Neoschongastia americana*), and sticktight fleas (*Echidnophaga gallinaceae*) (Figures 15.9–15.12). Recently, a henhouse was

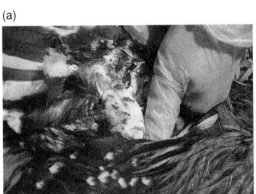
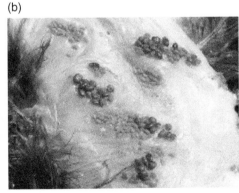

Figure 15.7 (a) Ventral surface of a chicken's wing showing severe soft tick infestation in a chicken. Although not confirmed, this infestation was thought to be due to *Argus persicus*, known as the fowl or poultry tick. (b) Close up image showing the yellowish brown bodies of ticks before a blood meal and the slate-blue color of ticks after they have had a blood meal. *Source:* Photograph courtesy of Dr. Abigail Duvall.

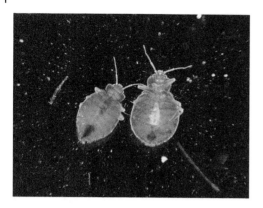

Figure 15.9 Photograph of bedbugs, *Cimex lectularius*, found to infect chickens and their environment. The dorsal aspect is shown on the left, the ventral aspect is shown on the right. *Source:* Photograph courtesy of Aly Chapman, University of Tennessee.

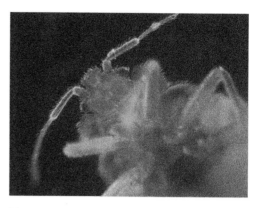

Figure 15.10 Close up photograph of the proboscis of a bedbug, *Cimex lectularius*. *Source:* Photograph courtesy of Aly Chapman, University of Tennessee.

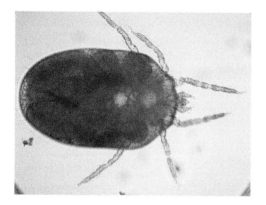

Figure 15.11 Photograph of the chiggers, the larval mite of *Neoschongastia americana*. *Source:* Photograph courtesy of Aly Chapman, University of Tennessee.

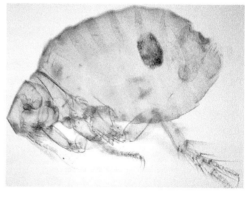

Figure 15.12 Photograph of the sticktight flea, *Echidnophaga gallinae*. *Source:* Photograph courtesy of Aly Chapman, University of Tennessee.

found to be infested with bed bugs and the hens were showing clinical signs of small, hard, white welts on the skin that became inflamed and pruritic. The bed bugs live in the cracks of the henhouse and come out to feed on the chickens at night. Diagnosis is based on grossly identifying the reddish-brown, oval to tear drop shaped, flattened bugs that are about ¼ to 5/8 in. in length.

Chiggers are most commonly encountered in turkeys in the southern states. Sticktight fleas cause skin irritation and possibly anemia.

Black flies (*Simuliidae*) can affect poultry (Figure 15.13) Large swarms of flies can produce anemia. Fowl ticks include a number of species that affect a wide range of poultry, birds and mammals. Some cause skin irritation and anemia [2].

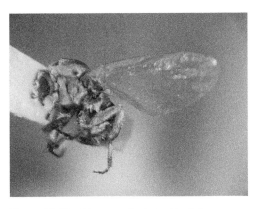

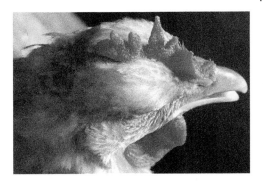

Figure 15.15 Chicken with feather loss over the dorsal cervical area due to conspecific aggression.

Figure 15.13 Photograph of the black fly, *Simuliidae* spp. *Source:* Photograph courtesy of Aly Chapman, University of Tennessee.

Trauma

Skin trauma results most commonly from other poultry and predators, including dogs, cats and wildlife such as raccoons, weasels, foxes, and larger birds of prey. Injuries range from mild to catastrophic. Hens frequently present with missing feathers and abrasions of the back and head created by the rooster during mating, or by attacks from dominant hens (Figures 15.14–15.17). In contrast, predator wounds are usually more severe and located around the face and neck or extremities. Fly strike is common in debilitated poultry with open wounds or fecal accumulation near the vent. Both severe injuries and the

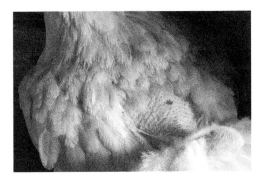

Figure 15.14 Chicken with feather loss over the dorsum due to conspecific aggression. Feather loss with or without skin lesions behind the head and over the dorsum are often caused by other poultry, including other roosters or dominant hens.

presence of maggots are frequently missed, as feathers often cover them. Injuries to digits occur, and can be caused by punctures or entrapment.

Initial therapy of the severely ill bird is aimed toward emergency stabilization and correction of shock. Fluid therapy is similar to that described in other avian patients. Vascular access is best accomplished in poultry via an intravenous catheter placed in the basilic (ulnar) vein or medial metatarsal vein; an alternative is an intraosseous catheter placed in the distal ulna or proximal tibiotarsus. Hypothermic patients are warmed externally and via infusion of warmed fluids. Antibiotic therapy is important. Selection should be based on results of culture and sensitivity when available and determined in part with legality and withdrawal times in mind (see Chapter 28). Unless not indicated based on culture and sensitivity, the author prefers the use of intravenous (or intramuscular) piperacillin (Zosyn) at 100 mg/kg IV q4–8h for severe bacterial infections with septicemia.

In general, pet poultry are good anesthetic and surgical candidates with impressive healing potential. The author has treated numerous cases of severe soft tissue and degloving injuries that have healed by second intention after weeks of supportive and wound care.

Sedation, anesthesia, and analgesia of avian species are well described, and the author has

(a)

(b)

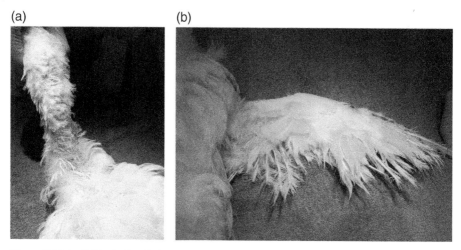

Figure 15.16 Pekin duck with feather loss over the (a) dorsal cervical area and (b) wing area (b) from conspecific aggression. This duck had a severe case of pododermatitis and could not compete well with the other ducks. *Source:* Photographs courtesy of Dr. Cheryl B. Greenacre.

(a)

(b)

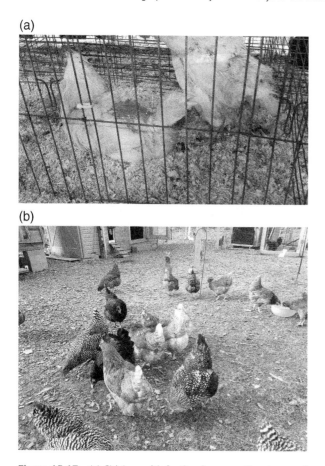

Figure 15.17 (a) Chicken with feather loss over the dorsum from the rooster repeatedly mounting this hen. (b) A potential enclosure set up with the rooster housed separately from the hens but still within visual and auditory contact. Note rooster in enclosure in background.

found that poultry do well with preanesthetic, induction, maintenance, and analgesic protocols described for psittacine birds. Many minor wounds can be addressed with sedation (the author recommends butorphanol 2–3 mg/kg and midazolam 0.5 mg/kg IM) with lidocaine 2 mg/kg as a local or regional block (Figures 15.18–15.20). Other surgical techniques are described in another chapter, and whenever possible strive for primary wound closure (Figure 15.21). As for any

therapeutic agent, legal ramifications including drug withdrawal times and appropriate drug use must be kept in mind.

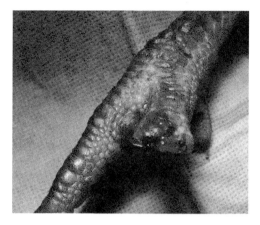

Figure 15.20   Toe shown in Figure 12.5 after amputation, which was easily accomplished with sedation and local analgesia without general anesthesia.

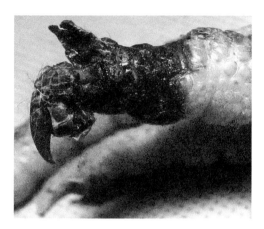

Figure 15.18   Toe lesions are common in poultry and may be caused by various traumatic episodes. This chicken's toe has a black necrotic area.

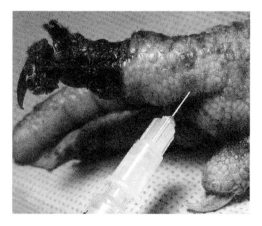

Figure 15.19   Toe shown in Figure 12.5 during instillation of a local analgesic.

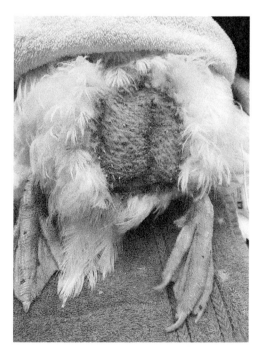

Figure 15.21   Primary closure of a surgical skin incision using an intradermal suture pattern provides excellent healing. A simple continuous or Ford-interlocking skin suture pattern also works well.

Wound Management

If the wound is due to predator attack, then antibiotics are needed to prevent sepsis. The bird may be in shock and supportive care including subcutaneous or intravenous fluids, warmth, quiet, and administration of pain relievers are usually necessary. Cleaning and debridement of the wound may need to wait a few hours until the patient has been stabilized. If the wound is older than 3 days, it will show some evidence of green bruising. Birds bruise green due to the lack of biliverdin reductase. If the wound punctures into the coelomic cavity, there may be subcutaneous emphysema present. Some wounds are extensive and may take a few days to fully declare viability of tissue and may take months to fully heal especially if an area of high movement such as the inguinal area. Various types of bandages and compounds have been used, but the most important aspect of wound management is daily reassessment of the wound. Pharmaceutical-grade honey works well for wound healing and can be used in egg-laying birds without worry of drug use in an egg-laying bird. In general, chickens heal skin wounds very well given enough time.

Tie-over bandages work well on large wounds because the constant tension brings the wound

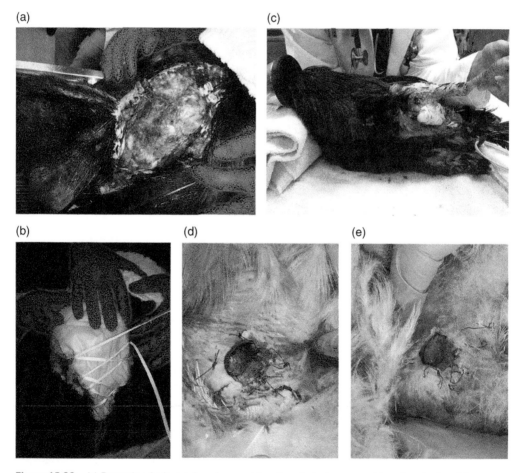

Figure 15.22 (a) Example of a large dorsal wound in a female turkey caused by a tom turkey. (b) Application of a tie-over bandage over the same wound. (c) A tie-over bandage works well in high-movement areas such as the inguinal area wound in this rooster. (d) A tie-over bandage also works well for deep, contaminated wounds that need to heal by second intention such as this conspecific aggression wound near the cloaca (cloaca to the right) that 3 days later (e) was kept clean by the bandage and showed signs of healing. Some of the suture loops needed to be replaced due to loss.

edges together. They are also easy for the owner/client to replace daily after cleaning, gently debriding, and applying a fresh layer of ointment/cream to the wound. Tie-over bandages are held in place with umbilical tape that is laced through many loops made of suture placed all around the edges of the wound. The suture loops are placed approximately 1 cm outside the wound edge in normal skin (Figure 15.22a–e).

Less Common Dermatological Diseases of Backyard Poultry

Infectious Diseases

A number of infectious diseases specifically target the integument; in others, skin is secondarily affected. Most diseases listed here are included for completeness, but are seldom encountered in backyard poultry flocks. The incidence of many can be reduced with ideal husbandry, including proper nutrition, sanitation, and by avoiding overcrowding and exposure to predators.

With the exception of trauma and ectoparasitism, biopsy and histopathology greatly aid diagnosis. Diagnostic tests available for viral diseases of poultry include serology, polymerase chain reaction (PCR), and viral isolation. Culture and sensitivity help identification of bacterial pathogens.

Some vaccines are available in small quantities for viral diseases of backyard fowl. Many large poultry suppliers sell birds already vaccinated for diseases, in particular for Marek disease. (Vaccination of backyard poultry is discussed in Chapter 30.)

Marek Disease

Marek disease is an oncogenic cell-associated herpesvirus-induced neoplastic disease that causes T-cell lymphoma in various tissues in chickens [10]. Unlike many other infectious diseases that are primarily problems in production facilities, it is commonly encountered in backyard poultry flocks. The most common form of Marek disease produces organ neoplasia and enlargement. A dermatological form of the disease produces reddened enlargement of feather follicles, which consist of aggregates of lymphocytes (Figure 15.23a,b). Transmission occurs through shedding of secretions and feather fol-

(a)

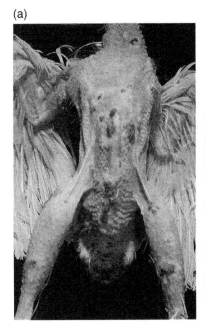

(b)

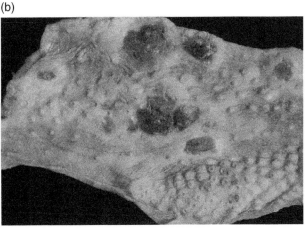

Figure 15.23   (a) A 1.5-year-old chicken hen with the cutaneous form of lymphoma. (b) Close up breast skin of this chicken. The hen also had hepatic lesions. *Source:* Photograph is courtesy of Dr. Kim Newkirk.

licle dander, and recent work has shown that viral particles can be found in skin epithelial cells as well [11]. Infected nonsymptomatic carrier birds may shed the virus for life. Diagnosis of this cutaneous form is via biopsy and histopathology of affected feather follicles. Due to the prevalence of Marek disease in flocks, serology is likely less useful. Prevention is through acquisition of vaccinated birds from reputable breeders. There is no known treatment for Marek disease. Birds with confirmed disease should be isolated and the premises thoroughly cleaned and disinfected, although the organism can live years in the environment.

Fowl Pox (Pox, Avian Pox)

Viral pox diseases affect nearly every species of bird. In poultry, chickens and turkeys can be affected [12]. Pox is caused by a large DNA poxvirus referred to specifically as fowl poxvirus and turkey poxvirus in these species. The virus produces typical round "pox-like" lesions of the integument, most commonly the unfeathered portions of the head or neck (Figure 15.24a–d). Decreased weight gain and egg production often result. Lesions may also occur on the feet or vent. Respiratory pox infections can produce dyspnea and ocular or nasal discharge. Pox scabs are desquamated in the environment and are infectious to other birds for many months. Transmission also occurs via cannibalism and spread by vectors such as mosquitoes. Onset is gradual and often not noticed until cutaneous lesions are detected. Diagnosis is confirmed via histopathology. Acquisition of birds from reputable breeders can prevent exposure to

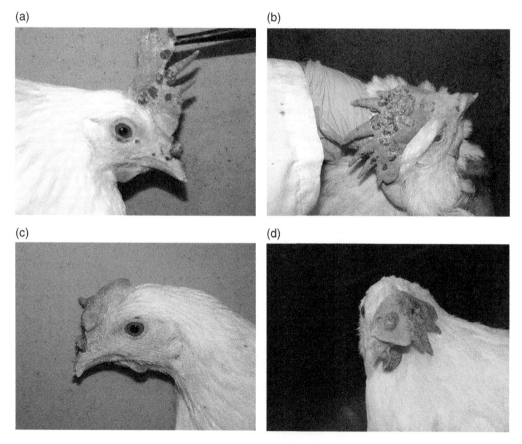

(a)

(b)

(c)

(d)

Figure 15.24 Dry fowl pox lesions commonly occur on the beak, nostrils, eyelid, comb, face, and/or neck. *Source:* Photographs courtesy of Dr. Robert Porter.

this disease. Pox vaccine is available. Treatment is supportive. Affected birds should be isolated from the rest of the flock.

Chicken Anemia Virus (Chicken Infectious Anemia, Blue Wing Disease, Anemia Dermatitis Syndrome)

While ubiquitous in production birds, chicken anemia virus (CAV) is uncommon in backyard flocks. This circovirus produces severe anemia in young chicks, which results in anorexia, lethargy, and pale tissues including the skin [13]. Hematocrit values typically range from 6% to 27%. Gangrenous dermatitis and a blue discoloration can be noted as well [14]. Adult infected birds do not develop disease but infect the young via egg transmission. Transmission also occurs via the orofecal and possibly respiratory route. Diagnosis is histopathology, serology, and PCR. Treatment is supportive and includes fluid therapy, blood transfusion in severely affected birds, and treatment of secondary gangrenous dermatitis. Purchasing birds from a reliable source can help prevent exposure to this disease. Vaccines are available for breeder flocks.

Infectious Bursal Disease (Gumboro Disease)

This viral disease is included in diseases of the integument, as clinical signs include vent picking and trauma, along with trembling, ataxia, and diarrhea [15]. Infectious bursal disease (IBD) is a highly contagious viral disease caused by a birnavirus that primarily affects lymphoid tissue including the bursa of Fabricius. It is a disease of young chickens, most commonly 3–6 weeks old. The virus persists in the environment for months, is resistant to many disinfectants, and therefore is difficult to eradicate. Transmission is via exposure to virus in feces, feed, and water and associated with fomites.

IBD is not commonly diagnosed in backyard flocks, and acquisition of birds from reliable sources can prevent exposure. Diagnosis is via histopathology and serology. Treatment is usually unrewarding, but improved husbandry may mitigate severity of the disease. Vaccines are available for breeder flocks.

Gangrenous Dermatitis (Necrotic Dermatitis)

This term refers to several disease presentations characterized by sudden onset of cutaneous skin wounds and cellulitis often over the wings, thighs, breast, and head. It is usually accompanied by septicemia and toxemia. Lesions are associated with a number of bacteria, including *Clostridia* sp., *Staphylococcus* sp., and *Escherichia coli*. Other factors include concurrent viral disease (in particular, CAV and IBD in young birds), nutritional insufficiency, poor sanitation, cannibalism, or mechanical trauma. Large outbreaks in flocks are thought to be due to immune deficiency and may be associated with warm, humid conditions [14]. Recent outbreaks reported in the literature in broiler facilities have been linked to clostridial infection and production of bacterial endotoxins. These birds often demonstrated antibody titers to other infectious diseases as well [16].

While outbreaks are unlikely in backyard flocks, individual birds are susceptible to the same syndrome when wounds are infected with bacteria.

A complete blood count can identify birds that are septicemic (leukocytosis, left shift, presence of heterophil toxicity). Many birds have anemia secondary to infection and inflammation, which can be severe. Histopathology can identify necrosis, and culture of lesions may help identify specific bacterial agents. Therapy includes antimicrobials, ideally identified on culture and sensitivity, fluid support, blood transfusion in severely anemic birds, and eventual surgical debridement of wounds. Ideal husbandry and prevention of overcrowding can aid prevention. Vaccination of breeder birds against other viral diseases has been helpful as well.

Fowl Cholera

This disease is caused by *Pasturella multocida* and can produce inflammation and swelling of the face, wattles, neck, and footpads. Birds are generally sick and depressed due to septicemia. Caseous dermatitis and cellulitis are identified histopathologically. The most likely source is chronically infected but asymptomatic birds and rodents. Antibiotic therapy based on culture and sensitivity is ideal; however, sulfa drugs and penicillins are frequently listed as drugs of choice [17].

Noninfectious Diseases

Breast Blister

These fluid-filled lesions of the sternal bursa are sometimes noted in the ventral aspect of the keel bone of large, heavy bodied birds. They are thought to be related to repeated trauma and may become secondarily infected [18]. Surgical excision is indicated for large and/or infected cysts. As large, heavy bodies meat breeds are more prone to breast blister and other debilitating degenerative diseases, the keeping of these breeds as pets should be discouraged.

Xanthomatosis

This disease features abnormal subcutaneous accumulation of intracellular cholesterol [19]. Lesions are usually firm and yellow, but in early stages may be soft with straw-colored fluid (Figure 15.25). In the past, xanthomatosis in production birds was thought to be associated

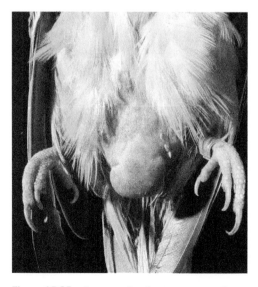

Figure 15.25 An example of cutaneous xanthoma in a parrot. The hallmark of this tumor is the presence of cholesterol clefts on histology and a typical bright yellow color grossly. The tumor would look similar no matter the avian species. *Source:* Photograph courtesy of Dr. Kim Newkirk.

with contamination of feed fat with hydrocarbons. However, xanthomatosis is associated with repeated trauma in other bird species and may be seen in poultry as well. Diagnosis is via biopsy and histopathology. Treatment includes investigating and removing sources of trauma. Lesions are usually self-limiting, but surgical removal may be indicated in birds with larger debilitating lesions. In psittacines, xanthomas are highly vascular and must be removed with care; the same cautions are likely valid for poultry as well. Prevention measures include ideal husbandry and prevention of trauma.

Cutaneous Melanoma

Although rare, melanoma can be seen in poultry as a pigmented dermal mass that can metastasize throughout the body (Figure 15.26). Diagnosis is confirmed via biopsy. Excisional biopsy can be done but this tumor commonly metastasizes and prognosis is guarded. A melanoma vaccine has been attempted in other avian species with variable success. Realize that some breeds of chickens, particularly the Silkie breed normally has melanosis, or black pigmented skin, periosteum, and peritoneum, and should not be confused with melanoma (Figure 15.27)

Feather Cysts

Dysplastic feather and follicles are occasionally encountered in turkeys. Cysts are firm and yellow (Tsang Long, personal communication).

Frost Bite

Necrosis of distal extremities such as the comb, toes, or even feet after below freezing weather can be the result of frostbite. Once the tissue declares as nonviable, it can be amputated, if possible or necessary (Figure 15.28a,b).

Ingrown Comb (Ingrown Leader)

An ingrown comb or leader is a congenital deformity resulting in an abnormal comb that has varying degrees of involuted or proliferative comb tissue at the caudal end (Figure 15.29a,b). The cause is unknown but may be due to abnormal incubation temperature or humidity

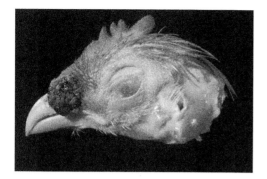

Figure 15.26 A 3-year-old chicken hen at necropsy with cutaneous melanoma on the beak and metastasis to the lung and bone. *Source:* Photograph courtesy of Dr. Linden Craig.

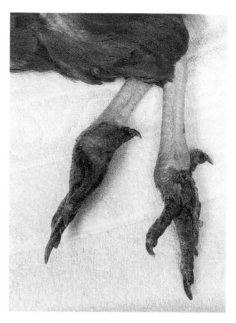

Figure 15.28 Severe necrosis of both feet of a chicken secondary to frostbite that occurred approximately 1 week earlier. The chicken had stood in water that froze overnight.

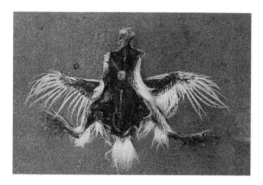

Figure 15.27 A 6-week-old white Silkie hen demonstrating the normal melanosis, or pigmented skin, of this breed. The skin, periosteum, and peritoneal lining are all pigmented. *Source:* Photograph courtesy of Dr. Linden Craig.

or due to dietary deficiencies since it is seen in entire clutches. The affected comb can be kept clean by the owner to prevent infection in the ingrown areas, or surgery can be performed to remove the abnormal, highly vascular tissue.

(a)

(b)

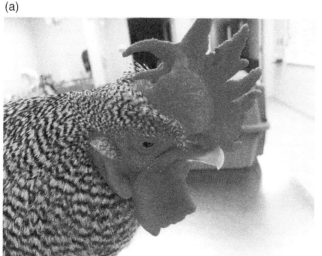
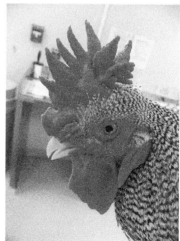

Figure 15.29 Examples of ingrown comb or leader in Plymouth barred rock roosters from the same clutch showing the variations of (a) ingrown comb with some having proliferative tissue as well (b).

References

1 Cengiz, O., Hess, J.B., and Bilgili, S.F. (2001). Effect of bedding type and transient wetness on footpad dermatitis in broiler chickens. *J. Appl. Poult. Res.* 20 (4): 554–560.

2 Foreyt, W.J. (2013). Parasites of birds. In: Veterinary Parasitology Reference Manual, 6e, 153–166. Ames: Wiley-Blackwell.

3 Hinkle, N.C. and Corrigan, R.M. (2013). External parasites and poultry pests. In: Diseases of Poultry, 13e (eds. D.E. Swayne, J.R. Glisson, L.R. McDougald, et al.), 1099–1116. Ames Iowa: Wiley-Blackwell.

4 Charlton, B.R. (ed.) (2000). Parasites and pests. In: Avian Disease Manual, 5e, 146–150. Kennett Square, PN: American Association of Avian Pathologists.

5 Martin, C.D. and Mullens, B.A. (2012). Housing and dustbathing effects on northern fowl mites (*Ornithonyssus sylviarum*) and chicken body lice (*Menacanthus stramineus*) on hens. *Medical and Vet. Entomol.* 26 (3): 323–333.

6 Yazwinski, T.A., Tucker, C.A., Robins, J. et al. (2005). Effectiveness of various acaricides in the treatment of naturally occurring *Ornithonyssus sylviarum* (northern fowl mite) infestations of chickens. *J. Appl. Poult. Res.* 14 (2): 265–268.

7 Lisbôa, R.S., Teixeira, R.C., Rangel, C.P., Santos, H.A. et al. (2009) Avian Spirochetosis in chickens following experimental transmission of *Borrelia Anserina* by Argas (Persicargas) Miniatus. *Avian Diseases*. U.S. National Library of Medicine.

8 Rosenstein, M. (1976). Paralysis in chickens caused by larvae of the poultry tick. *Argas Persicus*. Avian Diseases 20.2: 407–09 (JSTOR. American Association of Avian Pathologists, Inc. 2017).

9 Philips, J.R. Fowl Ticks. (2013). https://www.merckvetmanual.com/poultry/ectoparasites/fowl-ticks (accessed 3 November 2019).

10 Charlton, B.R. (ed.) (2000). Avian Viral Tumors: I. Marek's disease. In: Avian

Disease Manual, 5e, 22–23. Kennett Square, PN: American Association of Avian Pathologists.

11 Heidari, M., Fitzgerald, S.D., Zhang, H.M. et al. (2007). Marek's disease virus-induced skin leukosis in scaleless chickens: tumor development in the absence of feather follicles. *Avian Dis.* 51: 713–718.

12 Charlton, B.R. (ed.) (2000). Fowl pox. In: Avian Disease Manual, 5e, 43–46. Kennett Square, PN: American Association of Avian Pathologists.

13 Charlton, B.R. (ed.) (2000). Chicken infectious anemia. In: Avian Disease Manual, 5e, 30–31. Kennett Square, PN: American Association of Avian Pathologists.

14 Charlton, B.R. (ed.) (2000). Gangrenous dermatitis. In: Avian Disease Manual, 5e, 92–93. Kennett Square, PN: American Association of Avian Pathologists.

15 Eterradossi, N. and Saif, Y.M. (2013). Infectious Bursal disease. In: Diseases of Poultry, 13e (eds. D.E. Swayne, J.R. Glisson, L.R. McDougald, et al.), 219–246. Ames Iowa: Wiley-Blackwell.

16 Li, G., Lillehoj, H.S., Lee, K.W.A. et al. (2010). An outbreak of gangrenous dermatitis in commercial broiler chickens. *Avian. Pathol.* 29 (4): 247–253.

17 Cholera, A. (2011). The merck veterinary manual. www.merckvetmanual.com (accessed 26 August 2012).

18 Nowaczewski, S., Rosinski, A., Markiewicz, M., and Kontecka, H. (2011). Performance, foot-pad dermatitis and haemoglobin saturation in broiler chickens kept on different types of litter. *Archiv. fur. Geflugelkunde.* 75 (2): 132–139.

19 Charlton, B.R. (ed.) (2000). Integument disorders. In: Avian Disease Manual, 5e, 200. Kennett Square, PN: American Association of Avian Pathologists.

16

Reproductive Diseases
Eric Gingerich[1] and Daniel Shaw[2]

[1] *Diamond V, Cedar Rapids, IA, USA*
[2] *Veterinary Medical Diagnostic Laboratory, University of Missouri, Columbia, MO, USA*

Reproductive disease is very common in back-yard chickens since they are usually egg layers and they typically live longer than the average commercial chicken. Some very common, and then less common, causes of reproductive disease in backyard laying hens is outlined here.

Common Causes of Reproductive Disease

Uterine Prolapse/Vent Prolapse of Egg Layers

Clinical History: Layers of any age are susceptible and will be seen with blood-stained vent areas or blood-stained eggs. Mortality may be seen.

Cause of Condition: This condition is caused by cannibalistic behavior of pen mates. Some strains of breeds of layers are more cannibalistic than others. High light intensity, non–beak-trimmed hens, nutrient deficits, or stressful conditions such as crowding or inadequate nesting space can promote this problem.

Clinical Signs and Lesions: Lesions of a blood-tinged vent area, uterus prolapsed, and possibly tissues missing (consumption by pen mates) will be seen (Figure 16.1). Blood-tinged eggs can also be seen.

Transmission Route: This condition is not infectious.

Diagnostic Tests: Diagnosed by observations of lesions.

Differential Diagnosis: Wounding or trauma to the oviduct by other means than pecking needs to be ruled out.

Prevention and Control: Proper beak trimming helps. An adequate nutritional plane can reduce cannibalistic tendency. It also helps to reduce the light intensity, especially during the egg laying process. In commercial settings provide one nest box for every four birds. In the backyard setting this disease is not as common since the birds are not as crowded.

Oviduct Impaction

Clinical History: Birds that have oviduct impaction have been in production and then will cease production and become progressively lethargic, depressed, and lose weight. Depending on the amount of exudate in the oviduct, a duck-walking gait may be seen. This condition occurs most often in older layer birds.

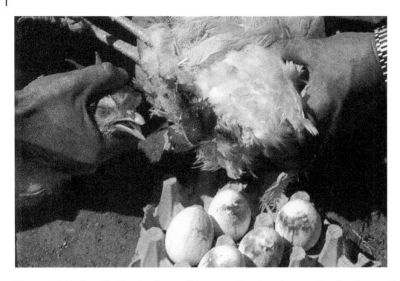

Figure 16.1 Cannibalism/peckout of the vent showing the contributing factor of a sharp beak. Note the blood on the eggs and on the beak of the bird doing the pecking.

Cause of Condition: It is thought that the older birds' reproductive tracts weaken with age and allow a greater amount of bacteria into the oviduct by retrograde peristalsis. Also with age, the amount of time the oviduct is everted during oviposition in increased allowing more time for exposure to bacteria. Generally, *Escherichia coli* is thought to be the causative agent involved, although other bacteria such as *Staphylococcus aureus, Klebsiella pneumoniae,* and *Salmonella* spp. have been implicated.

Clinical Signs and Lesions: Depression, lethargy, and loss in body weight are clinical signs. Upon necropsy, one will find an extended oviduct filled with caseous material [1] (Figure 16.2). Exposure of the oviduct lumen to bacteria from retrograde peristalsis of exposed oviduct during oviposition is thought to be the mechanism of disease. Palpation or radiography of the abdomen can detect the caseous mass in the oviduct.

Transmission Route: This condition is not infectious.

Diagnostic Tests: Necropsy lesions.

Differential Diagnosis: There are many different causes for cessation of egg laying and all of these should be considered as differential diagnoses. There will be a normal amount of this condition in all flocks and it will be seen increasingly with the age of the flock.

Prevention and Control: For prevention, maintaining clean nesting conditions will indeed aid in reducing the degree of oviduct exposure to bacteria during oviposition. Therapy using antibiotics orally has not been met with success. Surgery to remove the caseous mass has been done successfully.

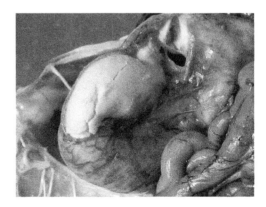

Figure 16.2 Necropsy of a chicken with oviduct impaction. Note the caseous debris in the oviduct.

Egg Bound, Egg Binding

Clinical History: The typical history with this condition is that the bird has stopped laying, she is having difficulty walking, and an egg may be seen in the cloaca.

Cause of condition: The underlying causes and contributing factors can include an excessively large egg (double yolk, large eggs in older hens), low blood calcium (hypocalcemia), calcium tetany, trauma to the uterus, vagina, or vent due to pecking, obesity, or stimulation into production before the bird's pelvis has matured.

Clinical Signs and Lesions: The lesion is a shelled egg lodged in the uterus or vagina but the hen is not able to lay it [1] (Figure 16.3).

Transmission Route: This condition is not infectious.

Diagnostic Tests: Palpation or radiography can be used to diagnose this condition.

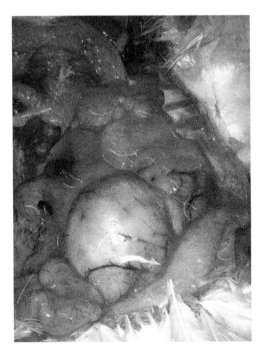

Figure 16.3 Necropsy of chicken with egg impaction and regression of the ovary.

Differential Diagnosis: This condition must be differentiated from other causes of cessation of egg laying.

Prevention and Control: Prevention lies with avoiding the causes and contributing factors such as avoiding double yolks by using a standard lighting schedule, controlling obesity, and excessively large eggs by routine body weight monitoring and controlling nutrient intake accordingly, feeding adequate calcium levels, and preventing cannibalism and wounding of the vent.

A veterinarian should undertake treatment of this condition. It may involve (1) lubricating the canal and attempting to ease the egg out or (2) imploding the egg by extracting the contents (ovocentesis) or (3) surgery to perform a salpingohysterectomy. Parenteral calcium in the form of calcium gluconate intramuscularly initially, and then calcium glubionate or calcium carbonate orally should also be given.

Retained Cystic Right Oviduct

Clinical History: Normally, no outward signs of disease will be seen with this condition. The prevalence of this condition is fairly rare in commercial chickens but is seen more often in backyard chickens.

Cause of Condition: Two Muellerian ducts are present early in the developing bird embryo [1]. The left duct develops into the oviduct and the right duct regresses. Occasionally in chickens, the remnant of the right duct becomes dilated with an accumulation of watery fluid.

Clinical Signs and Lesions: No outward signs of a problem typify this condition until a necropsy is performed and the retained, cystic right oviduct is found. Upon necropsy, a large, fluid-filled sac will be seen (Figure 16.4). This condition is seen at a higher incidence in some strains of layers than others.

Transmission Route: This condition is not infectious.

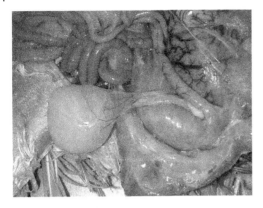

Figure 16.4 Persistent cystic right oviduct.

Diagnostic Tests: The condition is identified during postmortem examination. A radiograph and ultrasound would show a fluid-filled structure suggesting this disease.

Differential Diagnosis: This condition is differentiated from ascites by the presence of the membranous wall of the remnant right oviduct containing the fluid rather than the fluid being free in the body cavity. Sometimes during coelmic centesis it is difficult to ascertain if the fluid being aspirated is loose in the coelmic cavity or is from inside the cystic duct.

Prevention and Control: This is an error in embryonic development and not preventable.

Egg Yolk Peritonitis (Egg-Related Coelomitis)

Clinical History: The yolk-laden ova on the ovary are delicate structures surrounded by a thin membrane called the vitelline membrane. Rough handling of pullets or hens in production, sudden excitement inducing vigorous activity, etc. may cause trauma to the body wall that ruptures one or more of the yolks on the ovary. The vitelline membrane may also become weak secondary to bacterial septicemia or systemic viral infections and rupture.

Causative Agent: Free yolk is very irritating to the body cavity linings and induces a severe inflammatory response that results in peritonitis usually without microbial infection.

Clinical Signs and Lesions: An affected hen may be depressed and off feed. When examined at surgery or at necropsy the coelomic area contains thick friable yellow exudate that is adhered to the serosal linings (Figure 16.5).

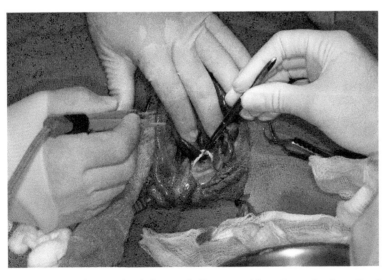

Figure 16.5 Yellow exudate being surgically removed from the coelomic cavity of a one year old bantam silkie hen with egg yolk peritonitis. One soft shelled egg and the collapsed remains of 6 other eggs were also removed. The hen continues to do well over a year after surgery. *Source:* Photograph courtesy of Dr. Cheryl Greenacre.

If the hen had been off feed for very long, the ovary may show evidence of involution.

Transmission Route: This is not initially an infectious disease. A secondary bacterial infection, usually with *E. coli*, may occur.

Diagnostic Tests: The condition is usually diagnosed at necropsy. Radiographs may show multiple radiopaque densities in the intestinal peritoneal cavity area. Ultrasound may help to further identify these masses. Coelomocentesis may provide fluid that can be evaluated for bacteria, yolk material, and inflammatory cells.

Differential Diagnosis: Airsacculitis caused by primary agents such as *Mycoplasma* sp., respiratory borne bacterial infections, respiratory viral infections (infectious bronchitis [IB] virus (IBV), paramyxovirus 1, etc.), coccidiosis, and carcinomatosis (Figure 16.6).

Prevention and Control: Hens that are producing eggs should be handled carefully. Precautions should be used when amongst the birds to prevent or minimize startling of the flock. Individual hens can be administered antibiotics and/or surgery can be performed to remove some of the irritating egg material with or without performing a salpingohysterectomy, but the prognosis is fair to poor depending on the severity.

Internal Layer

Clinical History: Soft-shelled or fully formed eggs may be found in the body cavity of some hens at necropsy (Figure 16.7). This may be an incidental finding when examining dead hens from the laying flock.

Cause of Condition: An increase in the number of hens with internally laid eggs may be seen with abrupt changes in day length (example: artificial lights to control day length are off for a number of days then on again when the problem is found) or infectious bronchitis infection.

Clinical Signs and Lesions: Usually there are only one or two eggs in the body cavity and the affected hens display no signs. Some hens, however, may accumulate several eggs and adopt a penguin-like posture. The presence of the egg and the amount of development indicate how far it traveled down the oviduct before reverse peristalsis caused it to be expelled into the body cavity. There is minimal reaction to the presence of the egg if the shell membranes or shell are intact. Rupture of the membrane and release of the content into the body cavity can induce an inflammatory response. The internally located egg may be shrunken and have a caseous consistency due to absorption of water from it while it is present

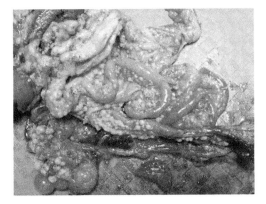

Figure 16.6 Carcinomatosis in an adult hen either of ovarian or pancreatic origin. Note the multiple masses that should not be confused with egg related peritonitis. *Source:* Photograph courtesy of University of Tennessee pathology department website http://vetgrosspath.utk.edu.

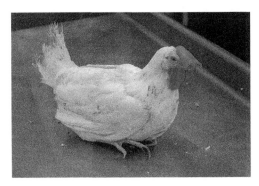

Figure 16.7 Hen weak from hypocalcemia.

in the body cavity. If there is an inflammatory response, the egg may be surrounded by thick caseous deposits of inflammatory exudate. Sectioning of the mass will reveal the egg structure in the center.

Transmission Route: The condition is not infectious.

Diagnostic Tests: The condition is identified during postmortem examination. Radiographic and ultrasonographic evaluation can suggest the egg material is loose in the coelomic cavity, but sometimes this is difficult to determine definitively.

Differential Diagnosis: The condition may have to be differentiated from salpingitis or severe airsacculitis.

Prevention and Control: In most cases, this is an error in the function of the oviduct and cannot be prevented. Otherwise, give consistent day lengths to the flock. Also, avoid the occurrence of infectious bronchitis (see the chapter on respiratory disease).

Zoonotic Potential: None.

False Layer Syndrome

Clinical History: The condition is also called ovulating, non-laying syndrome. Layer flocks fail to reach their normal peaks in egg production with no clinical signs.

Cause of Condition: Damage to the oviduct tissue during the early development stages (first 3 weeks of life) from a nephropathogenic IBV and the inability of the oviduct to function. The ovary continues to function normally. Layer flocks affected by this condition are usually found in areas where broiler flocks are infected by certain nephropathogenic strains of IBV. Also, the condition has been found in multiage pullet growing facilities where nephropathogenic strain of IBV has established itself.

Clinical Signs and Lesions: Birds appear to have expected comb development and pelvic spread. The left oviduct may swell with an accumulation of fluid. Some birds may develop a "duck walk" due to the very large size of the fluid-filled left oviduct. A portion of the oviduct may be atretic.

Transmission Route: Infectious bronchitis virus is transmitted by droplets from the respiratory tracts of infected chickens. The virus in these droplets may be spread by fomites or dust and become airborne again and breathed in by other chickens.

Diagnostic Tests: Finding birds with a functioning ovary but nonfunctional left oviduct. The causative strains of IBV may be detected in preparations of the respiratory tract or cecal tonsil material from 2- to 4-week-old pullets.

Differential Diagnoses: Any condition or disease that can reduce peak production.

Prevention and Control: The main effort in control has been to improve early immunity to IBV infection by vaccination at young age with a mild, broad spectrum vaccine such as the Ma5 vaccine or Georgia 08 vaccine. In addition, the first normally applied IB vaccine should be given by 18 days of age. Biosecurity in regard to preventing exposure to fomites that have been exposed to other flocks that are carrying the causative agent is important.

Zoonotic Potential: None.

Less Common Causes of Reproductive Disease

Paratyphoid Oophoritis

Clinical History: Infection with *Salmonella* sp. may involve the ovary and attached yolks. Inflammation of the ovary, when gravid, frequently leads to debilitation and death of the hen.

Causative Agent: *Salmonella* spp.

Clinical Signs and Lesions: The infection may cause debilitation and death of the hen. In the gross examination, the follicles of the ovary are covered by tan-white caseous exudate. The yolk material loses its normal translucence and the follicles shrink. The inflammation may spread to involve the entire coelomic area.

Transmission Route: Infection with *Salmonella* sp. may occur vertically through the egg of latently infected hens. It may also occur horizontally through contact with or ingestion of contaminated materials such as fomites, feed, rodents, etc. [2]

Diagnostic Tests: Bacterial culture should be used to identify the causative agent. *Salmonella* group D isolates should be reported to your state veterinarian.

Differential Diagnosis: Other bacterial infections caused by organisms such as *E. coli* and *Pasteurella multocida* can cause a similar changes.

Prevention and Control: Antibiotic therapy will help control the spread of the infection in a flock. Replacement hens should be obtained from breeding flocks that have been tested and found negative for the presence of the group D *Salmonella* sp. Flocks monitored under the National Poultry Improvement Plan (NPIP) are free of this group of *Salmonella* sp.

Zoonotic Potential: Many of the *Salmonella* sp. have the potential of causing egg contamination that may lead to human infection.

Decreased Egg Production/ Cessation of Laying

Clinical History: With this condition, a noticeable drop in number of eggs collected from one day to the next. This happens quite often in backyard flocks due to a variety of reasons.

Cause(s) of condition: Numerous causes of reduced egg production are possible including infectious (infectious bronchitis, *Mycoplasma gallisepticum* [MG], egg drop syndrome [EDS], Newcastle disease, and avian influenza), nutritional (water deprivation, inadequate calcium, phosphorus, sodium, protein, or vitamin intake), and environmental (declining day length, excessive heat, excessive cold).

Clinical Signs, Lesions, and Diagnostic Tests: Variable depending on the cause.

Prevention and Control: To prevent and control the possible infectious disease causes see each specific disease section, but in general it helps to provide adequate nutrient intakes at all times and phases of life to support normal egg laying and ensure adequate water is available to the birds at all times. Provide a warming device for water in the cold months.

Feather Loss

Clinical History: This condition consists of laying hens that lose varying degrees of feather cover over the laying period until they cease egg production and molt. The amount of feather loss involves the interaction of several factors.

Cause(s): There are several factors that may influence the degree of feather loss in hens. Malnutrition is a leading cause and can include inadequate amino acid intake throughout lay especially the sulfur-containing amino acids methionine and cysteine, inadequate sodium intake that can influence feather pecking activity and cannibalism, or inadequate vitamin or trace mineral intake that leads to poor feather growth and quality. In commercial chickens, the beak trimming quality can influence the degree of feather loss. Longer beaks yield more feather pecking. Stresses such as crowding (inadequate floor, perch, nest, feeder, or waterer space), group size, and external parasite load can also increase feather pecking activity of the flock and pen mates. Other stresses include egg production and egg size level, for example, high egg production or larger than normal egg size reduces the amount of amino acids for feather growth and maintenance.

Clinical Signs and Lesions: Normal feather loss progression over the period of lay starts with neck feather loss and progresses to loss of feathers over the crop, over the breast, then the back. Normal percentage of the body covered with feathers from point-of-lay through one lay cycle is outlined in Table 16.1. Higher percentage feather losses can be seen due to the causative factors listed above.

Transmission Route: This condition is not infectious.

Diagnostic Tests: Physical examination findings.

Differential Diagnosis: Varied.

Prevention and Control: To avoid excessive feather losses, (1) beak trim birds to avoid feather pecking/pulling, (2) feed a complete ration that fulfills the birds' needs for protein, energy, vitamins, and minerals, (3) avoid overcrowding and inadequate floor, perch, nest, feeder, or waterer space, and (4) control external parasites.

Table 16.1 Normal percentage of the body covered with feathers from point-of-lay through one lay cycle is outlined

Part of Lay Cycle/Weeks of Age	Percentage of Body COVERED With Feathers
Start of lay/18 weeks of age	100
30 weeks of age	95%
40	90
50	85
60	80
70	75
80	70

Lighting

Clinical History: This is a relatively common problem among backyard flock owners, especially newcomers.

Cause(s) of Condition: Birds reproductive systems are sensitive to lighting differences in day length and intensity. Increasing day length stimulates reproductive development and production, whereas decreasing day length destimulates the reproductive system. In nature, the springtime increasing day length stimulated bird populations to reproduce when conditions were becoming more favorable for hatchling survival and the declining day lengths of fall and winter prevented birds from reproducing when conditions were not favorable. Lighting effects can come from either natural day length or artificial sources of light. Stimulation with light promotes the growth of the ovaries and oviduct and induces birds to lay. Destimulation with decreased photoperiod or light intensity cause birds to cease egg production and begin molting.

Diagnostic Tests: An array of serologic tests can be done to determine if one of the infectious agents is the cause of the egg production lost.

Differential Diagnosis: Some infectious disease conditions can mimic loss of egg production such as infectious bronchitis, *M. gallisepticum*, etc. in a subtle way with very few clinical signs.

Prevention and Control: Obtain information on the sunrise and sunset times in your area to aid in setting time clocks. Use lighting program information from the various poultry breeder organization you got them from.

Molting

Clinical History: Members of the flock will be seen out of production, lose feathers, regenerate their feathering, and regain egg production.

Cause(s) of Condition: Molting is a natural process whereby the laying hen rests her reproductive tract to renew and renovate the oviduct for another cycle of laying. This occurs in nature when day lengths decline in the fall and the ovary is destimulated.

Clinical Signs and Lesions: The molting layer will lose most all its feathers during a molt in the following order: neck, breast, body, wings, and tail. The primary wing feathers are lost first followed by the secondary wing feathers. Some hens will completely cease egg production while others may continue to lay. As the replacement of feathers takes a lot of nutrients, egg production will not be at a normal rate.

Diagnostic Tests: A diagnosis of molting can be made if evaluations of management factors involving feed, lighting, air quality, water, and diseases that will result in loss of egg production are ruled out.

Differential Diagnosis: Lack of adequate nutrition, declining day length, poor air quality, excessive cold, excessive heat, lack of water, and a variety of disease agents (Newcastle, avian influenza, infectious bronchitis, etc.) that result in loss of egg production.

Prevention and Control: Commercial egg producers and some backyard flock owners perform planned molts to synchronize egg production and improve egg quality and numbers. A planned molt consists of reducing the day length (reduced to 8 hours) and reducing nutrient intake (feeding 50 g of growing type ration per bird per day, for example) to bring birds out of production then rest them. Once they have rested for about 3 weeks after ceasing egg production, the day length is increased to 14 hours and lay ration is full fed. Weekly day length increases of 30 minutes are then given until a total of 16 hours is reached.

Calcium Depletion, Calcium Tetany, Hypocalcemia, Caged Layer Fatigue

Clinical History: Cage layer fatigue is a term used to describe leg weakness and acute deaths in chickens in cages caused by inadequate calcium levels in the blood stream. Calcium is required for muscle function, bone formation, and egg shell formation. This condition may be seen even in floor birds under certain conditions. It is seen most often in young hens early in production.

Cause(s) of Condition: Calcium depletion is rarely caused by feed formulation errors. It is more commonly associated with feed manufacturing errors such as ingredient separation during manufacture, delivery, or feeding. Insufficient calcium particle size to stay in the gut during the night may occur. Inadequate feed intake may not support the level of egg production. This is a problem that may occur if the hens are fed a complete ration and allowed to forage. The ingestion of forage of inadequate nutrient composition will dilute the value of the desired ration and potentially lead to nutritional inadequacies. Vitamin D is required for absorption of calcium from the intestine.

Clinical Signs and Lesions: Affected hens are weak and unable to stand (Figure 16.8). Very few postmortem lesions may be evident. Hens that die may have a completely shelled egg in the shell gland. Dead hens may have soft bones. The ribs are most likely to display the softness since they are thin structures and more susceptible to effects of loss of calcium. On a flock basis, there may be a decline in egg

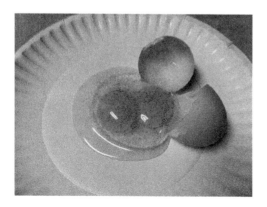

Figure 16.8 Example of a double-yolked egg.

numbers and egg shell quality may decrease. Bone deformities such as a curved keel bone and bent ribs develop in a hen with soft bones over time.

Diagnostic Tests: Knowledge of the flock history, clinical signs, and postmortem findings are usually sufficient to diagnose the problem. Response to treatment helps confirm the diagnosis.

Differential Diagnosis: Botulism.

Prevention and Control: Calcium depletion is rarely caused by feed formulation errors. It is more commonly associated with feed manufacturing errors such as ingredient separation during manufacture, delivery, or feeding. Insufficient calcium particle size to stay in the gut during the night may occur. Large particle limestone or oyster cannot usually be used in pelleted feed or crumbles. Inadequate feed intake may not support the level of egg production. This is problem that may occur if the hens are fed a complete ration and allowed to forage. The ingestion of forage of inadequate nutrient composition will dilute the value of the desired ration and potentially lead to nutritional inadequacies. It is important to feed a ration appropriate for the stage of production. Vitamin D is required for absorption of calcium from the intestine. A deficiency of vitamin D is uncommon in hens that are allowed access to sunlight. It should be noted, however, that vitamins may deteriorate over time. Feeds should be stored in cool dry conditions and used as soon as possible to insure freshness.

Broodiness

Clinical History: Broodiness denotes the behavior of the hen when she desires to sit on a nest.

Causative Agent: This usually occurs after a group of eggs (clutch) has been laid.

Clinical Signs and Lesions: At this time, the hen will seek dimly lit secluded areas where her or other eggs are located. The bird will become secretive and quiet.

Differential Diagnosis: This behavior is rarely seen in breeds of chickens selected for high rates of egg production. Few of the species of game birds kept in captivity display broodiness. The instinct may, however, be very strong in some breeds of chickens and turkeys. This may be a desired quality if breeding your own chickens.

Prevention and Control: Prevent access to dimly lit areas and hiding places. Remove all eggs form nests and floor as soon after laying as possible. Normal egg pick up should be twice in the morning and once in the afternoon.

Shell-Less Eggs

Clinical History: This condition is characterized by finding fully formed eggs in the nest area with no shell, on the shell membrane.

Cause(s) of Condition: Certain diseases that affect the oviduct function such as infectious bronchitis, MG, or EDS due to adenovirus 127 will result in numerous shell-less eggs. Nutrient deficits such as calcium, phosphorus, or vitamin D3 or excessive intakes of phosphorus or vitamin D3 may lead to an increase in the finding of shell-less eggs. A normal increase in shell-less eggs will be seen in older layer flocks.

Clinical Signs and Lesions: Clinically, one will find an increased number of shell-less eggs.

Diagnostic Tests: Various tests to rule out the possible etiologies.

Differential Diagnosis: Other possible diseases that need to be ruled out are infectious bronchitis, MG infection, and EDS.

Prevention and Control: Prevention starts with preventing those diseases that may cause shell-less eggs: IB, MG, and EDS.

Providing adequate levels of nutrients, especially calcium and phosphorus, is also important.

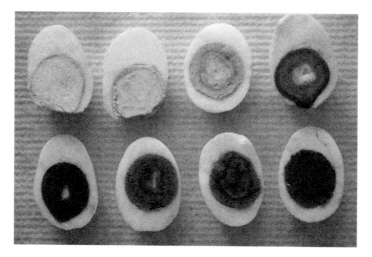

Figure 16.9   Discolored yolks from copper contamination of the soil.

Double Yolking, Double Yolks

Clinical History: Normally seen in young flocks just starting into production. There can be a very high incidence in a flock with perhaps up to 20% of eggs.

Cause(s) of Condition: Double yolking is caused by excessive stimulation with light caused by either an excessive increase in day length or an excessive increase in light intensity. Excessive intake of the amino acid methionine can also induce this condition.

Clinical Signs and Lesions: Unusually large eggs will be seen. When broken out, two yolks will be found (Figure 16.9).

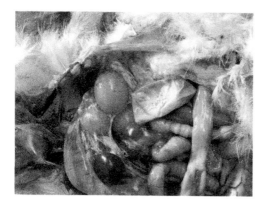

Figure 16.10   Shell membrane from partially absorbed egg in body cavity.

Transmission Route: This condition is not contagious.

Differential Diagnosis: Excessive egg size with a single yolk.

Prevention and Control: Use a controlled lighting program of both day length and intensity to prevent double-yolking. Removing the inciting cause(s), excess day length, excess light intensity, or excess methionine, may help reduce this problem.

Discolored Yolks/Blood Spots/Meat Spots

Clinical History: In this condition, discolored yolks, bloodspots, meat spots, and other abnormalities of the internal contents of the egg occur without any indication of a problem with the flock.

Cause(s) of Condition: Certain materials eaten by the bird may cause discolored yolks. For example, high copper levels in the soil caused discolored yolks that after a rain allowed the hens to drink high levels of copper from the water puddles (Figure 16.10). Gossypol, a natural component of cottonseed meal, can result in extreme discoloration of egg yolks as well as production loss.

Blood spots are the result of a stress on the hen such as a thunderstorm or sudden excitement such as a dog attack. Inadequate vitamin K can also be a contributing factor. Blood spots are much more common in brown egg layers than white egg layers. Some genetics companies have placed much more emphasis on eliminating blood spots from their lines of layers than others.

Meat spots are the result of a piece of tissue from the ovary or oviduct becoming incorporated into an egg during ovulation. The incidence is much higher in brown egg layers than white. Some genetics companies have put much more effort into reducing meat spots in their lines of birds than others.

Clinical Signs and Lesions: Normally, there are no outward signs of anything wrong with the flock.

Transmission Route: Usually, the agent causing a yolk discoloration problem is ingested. Blood and meat spots are not transmittable.

Diagnostic Tests: For yolk discoloration, chemical assays can be run on the yolk to determine the cause. For blood and meat spots, visual observation is diagnostic.

Prevention and Control: For yolk discoloration, do not allow birds to have access to water puddles after a rain. Control the intake of feedstuffs to avoid possible causative agents. For blood spots provide a nutritionally sound diet complete with adequate vitamin fortification. Avoid stressors that excite the flock. Use strains of layers with a low incidence of blood spots. Break out eggs in a bowl before use. For meat spots use strains of layers with a low incidence of meat spots. Break out eggs in a bowl before use. (See the chapter on egg diagnostics.)

Zoonotic Potential: Depending on the chemical causing the yolk discoloration, illness may be seen in the consumer of the eggs. There is no zoonotic potential with blood or meat spots.

Abnormally Shaped Eggs

Clinical History: Various shaped eggs will be seen during the lay cycle of most all flocks.

Causative Agent: In many cases, it is not known what causes these abnormal shapes. In some cases the cause may be due to a change in lighting schedule that disrupts the ovulation pattern resulting in double ovulation with two eggs developing at one time. Two eggs side-by-side in the uterus results in a slab-sided shaped egg. Infectious bronchitis or EDS virus infection will cause a variety of misshapen eggs.

Clinical Signs and Lesions: Misshapen or "wrinkled" egg shells seen. Other clinical signs are usually not seen unless infectious bronchitis or EDS is involved in which case respiratory signs and lesions along with egg production loss will be seen cause it.

Transmission Route: If caused by infectious bronchitis, fomites may transfer the virus from one flock to another.

Diagnostic Tests: Have a veterinary diagnostic lab perform tests for infectious bronchitis and EDS.

Prevention and Control: Prevention of misshapen eggs may be accomplished by using a consistent lighting schedule and preventing infectious bronchitis.

Zoonotic Potential: Normally not an infectious or toxic condition. IB and EDS are not zoonotic agents.

Shell Color Loss

Clinical History: Shell color loss is only noticeable in brown egg layer flocks. As flocks age, brown shell color loss will occur. Also, the different strains of layers will have differing rates of lighter color eggs than others.

Cause(s) of condition: The protoporphyrin-IX pigment that is secreted from the epithelial cells lining the uterus during the

90 minutes just prior to oviposition is responsible for the brown eggshell color. Strain of bird, age of bird, and stress levels can affect the shade of brown of the eggshell. Nicarbazin, a coccidiostat, if fed to brown egg layers will result in a temporary total loss of shell color while the material is present in the diet. The diseases EDS and infectious bronchitis result in total shell color loss as well. The pigment loss will recover with IB but may take up to 6 weeks.

Clinical Signs and Lesions: If IB is the cause then see respiratory signs and egg production loss, whereas with EDS and nicarbazin poisoning usually only see egg production loss.

Diagnostic Tests: Virus isolation and serology are used to determine if IB or EDS is the cause of the loss of color. An assay of the feed can be performed to test for nicarbazin poisoning.

Prevention and Control: Preventing shell color loss involves (1) keeping stress level of the flock to a minimum, (2) control diseases such as EDS and IB through vaccination and biosecurity efforts, and (3) avoiding nicarbazin contamination of feed.

Zoonotic Potential: None of the causes have zoonotic potential.

Poor Egg Shell Quality

Clinical History: Eggshell characteristics are affected by a variety of nutritional, infectious, and physical influences.

Cause(s) of Condition: Factors that interfere with calcium utilization, such as inadequate mineral supplementation, inappropriate phosphorus levels in feed, inadequate vitamin A or D levels in feed, may lead to defects in the egg shell such as thinness. Roughness or shells with a "sandpaper" consistency may appear in flocks early or in the middle stages of production. This condition may be associated with inadequate vitamin supplementation, especially vitamins A and D.

Body checks are cracks that occur in the eggshell while it is still developing in the shell maker gland. The cracks are covered by secretion of additional shell material in the shell maker gland and appear as ridged areas over the original breakage sites. The shell is weak in these areas and more subject to breaking. This damage may occur after excessive vigorous activity in the flock.

Soft ends of the eggshell are occasionally seen early in production. The cause of this condition is not known. It may be associated with strain of chicken or nutritional factors.

Clinical Signs and Lesions: The problems can occur at any age and may not be associated with clinical signs in the hen unless associated with a systemic disease condition.

Diagnostic Tests: Diagnosis is based on location and characteristics of the shell changes. Serological evaluation for certain viral diseases such as infectious bronchitis and paramyxovirus 1 infection may help determine if a challenge from one these agents may have occurred.

Prevention and Control: Include animal movement, vaccines, and disinfectant use.

Worms in Egg

Clinical History: The avian roundworm, *Ascaridia galli*, or tapeworm segments may occasionally be found by a consumer in an egg.

Causative Agent: Intestinal parasitism of the hen.

Clinical Signs and Lesions: The hens are not usually sick.

Transmission Route: It is believed that the worm has migrated from the cloaca up the oviduct and becomes incorporated into the egg.

Diagnostic Tests: The worms can be detected by candling the eggs.

Prevention and Control: Hygromycin B and an aqueous suspension of fenbendazole are currently the only deworming compounds approved for use in chickens producing eggs for human consumption. They are not effective against tapeworms. No medications are available for treating tapeworms in chickens. If there is a concern the eggs should be candled and any that contain the parasite discarded.

Zoonotic Potential: Roundworms and tapeworms of chickens do not parasitize humans.

Egg Drop Syndrome

Clinical History: This disease has recently been detected in the United States.

Causative Agent: An adenovirus, EDS-76 or adenovirus 76 is the cause of this disorder.

Clinical Signs and Lesions: Clinically, a dramatic drop in egg production without clinical signs of illness characterizes this disease. Egg quality also declines dramatically with a loss of pigmentation and shell quality. A large number of shell-less eggs are seen. Pullets may be infected but will not show any clinical signs.

Transmission Route: This virus may be transmitted vertically from infected parent stock to their progeny. The virus then can become active when the bird reaches sexual maturity. The virus can also be transmitted horizontally by fomites contaminated with the virus to different locations. The virus may be shed in the feces and enter through the oral route.

Diagnostic Tests: For diagnosis, virus isolation, or the recently developed PCR assay, from the uterus should be attempted. Hemagglutination inhibition (HI) tests can also be used diagnostically.

Differential Diagnosis: One must use the diagnostic laboratory to differentiate between diseases such as avian influenza, Newcastle disease, IB, and MG.

Prevention and Control: In countries where EDS is prevalent, an effective inactivated vaccine is available for use.

Zoonotic Potential: There is no known human disease from the EDS virus.

References

1 Crespo, R. and Shivaprasad, H.L. (2008). Developmental, metabolic, and other noninfectious disorders. In: Diseases of Poultry (ed. Y.M. Saif) (assoc. eds. A.M. Fadly, J.R. Glisson, L.R. McDougald et al.), 12e, 1149–1196. Ames, Iowa: Blackwell Publishing.

2 Shivaprasad, H.L. and Barrow, P.A. (2008). Pullorum disease and fowl typhoid. In: Diseases of Poultry (ed. Y.M. Saif) (assoc. eds. A.M. Fadly, J.R. Glisson, L.R. McDougald et al.), 12e, 620–636. Ames, Iowa: Blackwell Publishing.

17

Gastrointestinal and Hepatic Diseases

Teresa Y. Morishita[1] and Robert E. Porter, Jr[2]

[1] College of Veterinary Medicine, Western University of Health Sciences, Pomona, CA, USA
[2] Department of Veterinary Population Medicine, Veterinary Diagnostic Laboratory, College of Veterinary Medicine, University of Minnesota, St. Paul, MN, USA

Gastrointestinal diseases are common in floor-raised backyard chickens. One way to clinically assess the gastrointestinal health of poultry is to observe their feces. Chickens have two different physical forms of feces. The feces of clinically healthy chickens are brown in color and are well formed in consistency [1]. There is often a white portion on the surface of the feces. This white portion, often referred to as the white cap, is not any excreta from the digestive system but rather is nitrogenous waste excreted as solid uric acid (Figure 17.1). The other excreta from clinically healthy chickens are the excreta from the ceca. These cecal droppings are loose and tenacious in physical form and are dark (Figure 17.1). While an occasional cecal dropping is normal, an increased observation of cecal droppings has been associated with stress [1]. The loose cecal droppings should be distinguished from diarrhea. Diarrhea is defined as an increased amount, increased frequency, and/or change in consistency of feces [1]. Depending on the cause of the diarrhea and the pathogenicity of the infectious agent involved, the color can vary from yellowish brown to bloody [1]. Hence, periodic monitoring of feces on the floor can help to detect early gastrointestinal disease and to determine the normal conditions in the flock.

Approaching the Sick Poultry Patient

A physical examination is most important to access the general physical state of the patient and to determine the chronicity of the disease state. Emaciation can be evaluated by palpation of the breast muscles to determine if a prominent keel bone is present [2]. Assessment of feather quality also provides clues as to the nutrition provided to the flock [2]. Numerous feather lines, called stress bars, appear as clear areas that are visible transversely across the feather vane and appear if the bird was provided inadequate nutrition on a long-term basis [2]. The presence of a pasty vent, fecal material adhered to the vent feathers, could indicate past and/or current diarrhea [2].

To evaluate the gastrointestinal health of poultry, the following samples should be collected and associated diagnostic tests should be performed:

1) Collect uncoagulated blood for hematology for general health assessment [2, 3]
2) Collect serum for clinical biochemistry evaluation and serological monitoring of diseases [2, 3]

Backyard Poultry Medicine and Surgery: A Guide for Veterinary Practitioners, Second Edition.
Edited by Cheryl B. Greenacre and Teresa Y. Morishita.
© 2021 John Wiley & Sons, Inc. Published 2021 by John Wiley & Sons, Inc.
Companion website: www.wiley.com/go/greenacre/medicine

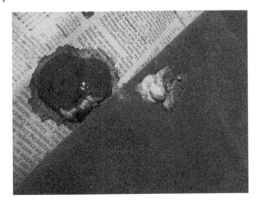

Figure 17.1 Normal chicken feces generally consists of semisolid green to brown excreta admixed with a cap of white urates. Note the looser normal cecal dropping on the left.

3) Collect feces for evaluation of intestinal parasites and repeat collection at 3 to 4-week intervals [2]
4) If diarrhea is observed, the feces should also be cultured for bacteria such as *Salmonella* and should be collected at successive periods as shedding can be intermittent [2]. Feces can also be collected for detection of enteric viruses that can be performed at a state diagnostic laboratory, but for most backyard flocks this may be cost prohibitive for the owner unless there is mass mortality and
5) If a bird dies, it is important to perform a necropsy, especially if more than one bird has died [2]

While there are conditions, such as intestinal parasitism, that primarily affect the gastrointestinal tract, conditions of other systems, such as respiratory disease, might present with gastrointestinal signs (e.g., diarrhea). This chapter is organized to assist the veterinary practitioner to first look for clinical signs, followed by descriptions of diseases that can be considered by biopsy or necropsy. While the primary purpose of backyard poultry medicine is to keep the individual bird alive, diagnostic tests on euthanized or sick birds may be indicated if the health of large numbers of birds is at stake.

Lesions of the Oropharynx

Examination of the oral cavity should be performed during a physical examination [2]. The oral cavity can be observed by grasping the lower beak and drawing it ventrally while stabilizing the head. The mucosa should be pink and smooth. Diseases that can occur in backyard poultry include whitish yellow plaques in the mouth of birds [2]. The top five differential diagnoses for poultry include fowl pox, candidiasis, trichomoniasis, vitamin A deficiency, and aspergillosis [4]. One can gently scrape the mucosa to identify the causative agent via cytology, or biopsy of the lesions can identify fowl pox. If malnutrition is suspected, samples of the feed should be collected and submitted for vitamin analysis. Balanced commercial diets are readily available for backyard poultry.

Fowl Pox

Fowl pox is a relatively slow-spreading viral disease of chickens and turkeys that is characterized by eruptions and scab-like lesions on the skin, combs, wattles, and inside the mouth, as well as diphtheritic or plaque-like lesions in the mouth, esophagus, and the upper part of the trachea. The causative agent is a poxvirus belonging to the *Poxviridae* family, subfamily Chordopoxvirinae, genus *Avipoxvirus*, species *Fowl pox virus,* a large double-stranded DNA virus with a biconcave core. There are a number of strains within the group that differ in their specificity for and pathogenicity to various species of birds [5]. The disease spreads slowly in a flock with an incubation period of 4–10 days. Infection occurs to the injured or lacerated skin through mechanical transmission of the virus. Mosquitoes have been shown to spread the disease in chicken flocks. Flies can deposit the virus in the eye or in open wounds or lacerations. The mucosa of the upper respiratory tract and oropharynx are highly susceptible to the virus, and infection can occur in the absence of skin trauma or injury [6].

Clinical Signs

Fowl pox has two forms: the cutaneous (dry) and membranous (wet) forms. In the cutaneous form, formation of nodules on the comb, wattle, eyelids, and other unfeathered areas of the body occurs. These nodules increase in size and can coalesce to form large brown to yellow scabs. These lesions eventually form scabs that dry up and drop off. The membranous form, referred to as wet pox, is characterized by raised fibrinous plaques or nodules on the mucous membranes of the oropharynx, esophagus, or upper part of the trachea (Figure 17.2). These lesions may coalesce to form an adherent membrane that covers the ulcerated areas. Lesions in the oropharynx often make it difficult for birds to eat or drink. High mortality resulting from suffocation can occur if the lesions occlude the upper trachea, particularly the glottis (tracheal plugs) [7].

Diagnosis

A presumptive diagnosis is based on the presence of scabs on the skin, comb, wattles, or other unfeathered areas of the body, or yellowish plaques on the mucous membranes of the oropharynx or esophagus. A definitive diagnosis can be made by histopathological examination of the scabs, or by virus isolation on the chorioallantoic membrane of embryonated eggs (dropped CAM method) [6, 7].

Treatment

There is no specific treatment that is effective against the poxvirus. Good management, including mosquito control, reduces stress in infected flocks. Vaccination is presently the only method of controlling fowl pox. There are two types of live virus vaccines used to immunize birds. Fowl pox vaccine of chick embryo origin is used to vaccinate birds of four weeks of age and older. Fowl pox vaccine of tissue culture origin is milder and can be used to vaccinate chicks as young as one day of age. The pigeon pox vaccine is mild and can be used in chickens of any age. Pox vaccines should be administered by the wing-web method in chickens. A thigh stick is usually used in turkeys because they tend to tuck their heads under their wings when resting and the face can come into contact with the vaccine strain and cause a vaccine reaction on the head. Cannibalism should also be controlled in a flock to reduce transmission of poxvirus [6, 7].

Candida albicans Infection (Candidiasis)

Candida albicans is a mycotic infection affecting a wide variety of birds and occurs primarily in the upper digestive tract, especially the oropharynx and crop. This yeast infection is fairly common and is usually the result of long-term (one to two weeks) administration of oral antibiotics. Candidiasis has also been referred to as crop mycosis, crop mold, and thrush. *C. albicans* is yeast that forms pseudohyphae in tissues. This yeast is ubiquitous and overgrowth is usually controlled by normal bacterial microflora in the digestive tract. This condition is often associated with other diseases, usually those of the digestive or respiratory tract. In addition, long-term oral antibiotics, especially

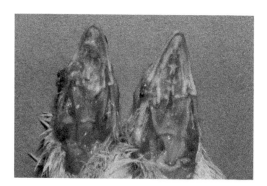

Figure 17.2 Raised friable plaques on the mucous membranes of oropharynx, and choana of a chicken with wet pox.

when administered in drinking water, can alter microflora of the upper digestive tract and promote yeast growth [8]. *Candida* is not transmitted from bird to bird and can often affect more than one bird if the flock has been treated with long-term oral antibiotics.

Clinical Signs

There are no specific signs but birds may appear unthrifty. Lesions commonly occur in the crop, which has a fine, white pseudomembrane lining on its mucosal membrane, giving it a "Turkish towel" appearance (Figure 17.3). The oral cavity and/or esophagus can also be affected. The pseudomembrane is often friable and can be peeled off the mucosa. Other diseases may resemble candidiasis. The five top differentials for white patches/plaques in the oropharynx of birds are candidiasis, trichomoniasis, the wet form of fowl (avian) pox, aspergillosis, and vitamin A deficiency. A differential diagnosis for a roughened crop lining besides candidiasis is capillariasis.

Diagnosis/Prevention/Treatment

Diagnosis for candidiasis is usually made using gross and histopathological lesions (Figure 17.4), although fungal culture can also be considered. Candidiasis can be prevented by focusing on primary husbandry or infectious

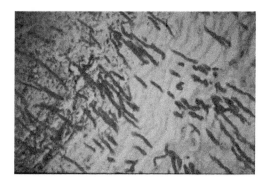

Figure 17.4 Candidiasis of chicken crop. In histologic section there is epithelial hyperplasia and the crop epithelium is infiltrated with linear pseudohyphae consistent with *C. albicans* (periodic acid–Schiff stain).

disease problems and avoiding unnecessary use of antibiotics, especially in young birds; copper sulfate or nystatin might be an effective treatment [8].

Lesions of the Crop

Abnormalities in the crop that can be detected during a physical examination include crop enlargement. Gallinaceous birds that have recently eaten have a full crop, which feels doughy on palpation. This is normal and should disappear within a couple of hours. However, if the crop does not decrease in size, it could indicate crop stasis. A crop wash can be collected for cytological evaluation and culture, if needed. Radiographs can also be performed to determine whether the crop is enlarged by a space-occupying mass (e.g. neoplasm or foreign body). A bird with an enlarged crop should be treated gently because excessive handling and manipulation can cause aspiration pneumonia if there is excessive crop fluid. The crop can be enlarged as a result of excess fluid, from an impaction resulting from indigestible materials or tumor, or from ingestion of a foreign body. A fecal examination or crop wash cytology preparation may reveal the presence of crop worms.

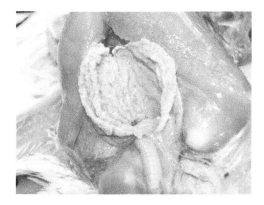

Figure 17.3 Turkey poult with moderate to severe crop infection caused by *Candida albicans*. Note the white pseudomembrane lining the open crop.

Pendulous Crop

The crop can become enlarged and filled with fluid. Crop washes do not recover any fungal elements, only foul-smelling liquid. The exact cause of pendulous crops is not known and there may be a genetic component as it has often been observed in related birds. Surgical reduction can be attempted but its effectiveness has not been documented.

Crop Impaction

Poultry have been known to ingest items out of curiosity or as a response to stress. Ingestion of poorly digestible items (e.g. grass, newspaper, sawdust shavings/wood chips, and feathers) has been known to cause crop impaction [9]. Impaction can also occur when poultry are exposed to new environmental substrates, especially floor substrates. Surgical removal of the impaction is necessary to alleviate the problem; however, the condition may not be recognized by the owner until the bird is near death.

Candidiasis

As described in the Oropharynx section, candidiasis is one of the most common crop diseases occurring for poultry.

Crop Worms (Capillariasis)

Although there are several nematode species that can be found in the crop, *Capillaria annulata* and *Capillaria contorta* are the most prevalent and are diagnosed most often in gamebirds (pheasants, partridges, and quail), but can also occur in turkeys. These nematodes are long and slender, are often referred to as threadworms, and are less than 60 mm long. These nematodes generally have a 30-day life cycle from ovum to adult. Adults embedded in the crop mucosa produce ova that are shed in the feces. The ovum must mature in the intermediate host (earthworm for *C. annulata*) or while free in the environment (*C. contorta*) [10].

Diagnosis

When embedded in the crop mucosa in large numbers, the affected birds can be depressed, weak, and emaciated. There can often be a history of sudden death without previous signs. Affected birds might gasp and appear as if they are having trouble breathing. With light infections, one may observe crop stasis or increased white fluid in the crop. In mild infections, the crop mucosa can be covered with a thin, white film; while in heavy infections, the entire crop wall can be thickened, fluid-filled, with a rough, irregular mucosa covered by a thick white, fibrinonecrotic exudate. The infection can extend beyond the crop into adjacent regions of the esophagus.

Treatment

Fenbendazole and levamisole are approved for treating *Ascaridia* and *Heterakis*, and are effective against *Capillaria*, but are not labelled for *Capillaria*. As infections are most severe in floor-raised birds, rotating, or moving pens to decrease the build-up of ova in the soil is recommended. Moreover, the soil should be dry and well drained to decrease the number of earthworms [11].

Lesions of the Intestines

Intestinal disease is usually manifested as diarrhea or weight loss. Adherence of excessive feces to the vent feathers (pasty vent) indicates repeated bouts of diarrhea (Figure 17.5). In addition to the physical examination, the quality of the feces provides potential clues as to the causative agent. When diarrhea is present, it is important to consider the age of the affected bird and other clinical signs. In poultry, there are many diseases, while not primarily intestinal diseases, that can affect the gastrointestinal system to cause diarrhea. To work-up diarrhea cases, a fecal examination

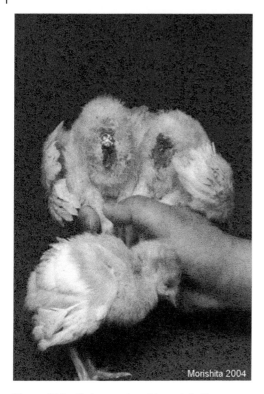

Figure 17.5 Turkey poults with vent feathers stained with feces.

and fecal bacterial culture are the primary diagnostic tools. Feces can be examined by zinc sulfate or sugar flotation to identify parasitic ova/oocysts. Fecal culture can determine whether *Salmonella* is present, especially in young birds, but culture may have to be performed over several sampling periods because *Salmonella* is shed intermittently. In addition, physical visualization of the feces can help with differential diagnoses. Blood analysis can identify potential blood loss if feces are not readily available. Serum should be collected to determine the presence of respiratory pathogens that can cause diarrhea.

Salmonella Pullorum

Salmonella pullorum infection is an infectious, egg-transmitted disease affecting chicks and turkey poults. This disease is often associated with white diarrhea and high mortality in young birds, whereas adults are nonsymptomatic carriers of infection. This disease has been known as bacillary white diarrhea or pullorum disease. *S. pullorum* is a gram-negative, rod-shaped bacterium that is usually poultry specific and is closely related to *Salmonella gallinarum*, the causative agent of fowl typhoid. These two bacteria share surface antigens and the pullorum test can be used to identify reactors to both pullorum disease and fowl typhoid [12].

Young chicks and turkey poults are particularly affected and infection is often fatal. Older birds are more resistant and may not show clinical signs or may serve as inapparent carriers but can transmit this infection through the egg to the hatchling [13]. Infected hatchlings can also transmit the infection horizontally to other birds in the hatcher. This disease is monitored through the National Poultry Improvement Plan (NPIP) in the United States. Many states provide training for flock owners or veterinarians to become certified blood testers for pullorum-typhoid.

Because this disease is primarily egg-transmitted, the concern for backyard flocks is that infected hens lay infected eggs, which hatch to produce infected chicks. Infected chicks that do not die can produce infected eggs at sexual maturity to repeat the cycle. Hence, this disease is of concern for flock owners who hatch their own breeding stock.

Peak mortality occurs about two to three weeks after hatching and can begin prior to 10 days of age.

Clinical Signs

In severe cases, dead chicks can be found in the hatcher. Pasty white vents (cloaca) are noted in affected birds, which appear chilled and are reluctant to eat. Adult birds that are necropsied occasionally have misshapen ovaries, pericarditis, and peritonitis, but some have no lesions. Young birds may have no gross lesions if the infection is peracute. White to gray nodules in the heart, liver, cecum, and gizzard may be seen. Moreover, cecal plugs, firm, caseous, yellow cores found in the lumen of the cecum, are

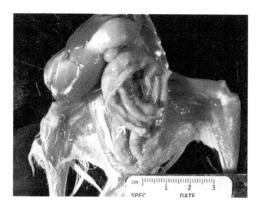

Figure 17.6 Salmonellosis is often associated with formation of caseous cecal cores, particularly in young birds. Note that the open cecum contains an inflammatory core.

characteristic of this disease (Figure 17.6). Septic arthritis, including swollen hock and wing joints, has been noted in some birds; urates accumulate in the ureter as a result of dehydration. Birds may also have septicemia with hepatosplenomegaly (hepatitis).

Diagnosis

Bacterial culture of sick birds (definitive) and blood testing (whole blood plate test) in adult breeder birds are needed to identify reactors. The same killed Salmonella antigen is used to detect antibodies to both *S. pullorum* and *S. gallinarum* (fowl typhoid) in the whole blood plate test. A tube agglutination test is preferred for turkeys [12]. A differential diagnosis should include fowl typhoid; colibacillosis; chilling or overheating associated with white diarrhea; omphalitis (navel infection) caused by *Escherichia coli*, *Pseudomonas*, or *Staphylococcus*. To prevent this disease, birds should be purchased only from NPIP-approved hatcheries. This disease may be common in backyard flocks.

Treatment

This disease is reportable, so backyard flocks are euthanized, rather than treated, under the supervision of the state regulatory agency [12].

Salmonella Gallinarum

Fowl typhoid, which is caused by a gram-negative, non-motile rod-shaped bacteria *S. gallinarum*, is an infectious disease that primarily affects chickens and turkey. It has many features similar to pullorum disease as both of these bacteria share surface antigens and hence cross-agglutinate on the pullorum test [12]. This disease usually affects young adults or mature chickens and is occasionally reported in chicks and poults. Ducks, geese, peacocks, pheasants, and turkeys are more resistant than chickens. Fowl typhoid usually affects chickens that are older than 12 weeks with reported losses of up to 50% [8, 14].

Similar to pullorum disease, fowl typhoid is egg transmitted; however, it is most frequently transmitted horizontally between adults. As with other *Salmonella* infections, it can also be spread between houses by rats, wild birds, and humans, which serve as fomites. Adults have a higher mortality when compared with pullorum disease, which mostly causes mortality in young birds.

Clinical Signs

If chicks and poults are infected, clinical signs include dead or dying birds in the hatcher with whitish, pasty vents; anorexia; and labored breathing. Growing and mature birds usually have an acute disease, with dead birds found on the nest or floor. Affected birds can also show a drop in feed consumption, depression with pale combs, high fever with associated open-mouth breathing, and greenish diarrhea. Lesions in chicks and poults are similar to pullorum disease. Adult birds may have bile-stained (bronze) livers, occasionally with necrotic foci, enlarged dark spleens, hepatosplenomegaly, and enteritis.

Diagnosis

Bacterial culture is definitive, and it is best to use a whole blood plate agglutination test to check for reactors to both pullorum disease and fowl typhoid [14]. To prevent this disease, purchase chicks and poults from NPIP-approved hatcheries. NPIP serologic monitoring of breeder flocks eliminates breeder sources of infection.

Treatment

As this is a reportable disease in the United States, reactor birds are reported to the state regulatory agency and culture-positive birds are euthanized, rather than treated.

Paratyphoid *Salmonella* Infection

Paratyphoid *Salmonella* infection is characterized by lesions of septicemia and caused by one of over 2000 paratyphoid *Salmonella* species, *Salmonellae,* which have a wide host range. Over 250 Salmonella species have been isolated from chickens. This is a disease that usually occurs in poultry, and many may carry the bacterium but not demonstrate any clinical signs. The infection can be devastating in chicks, poults, and gamebirds of less than three weeks of age. Infected birds are intermittent fecal shedders [15]. Moreover, eggshells may become contaminated by these carrier birds; hatchery contamination can occur from infected hatchlings; and rats and mice can perpetuate this disease on the farm. One particular strain, *Salmonella enteritidis (SE)*, can be vertically transmitted from hen to egg and has been associated with foodborne illness in humans when contaminated raw eggs are pooled and improperly cooked [16]. Transmission of SE in feces can be enhanced when infected hens are stressed by molting, which at one time was induced by feed deprivation [15].

Clinical Signs

While most birds do not display any clinical signs, affected birds are listless and huddle together. They have diarrhea and pasting of feces on the vent [17, 18]. Diagnosis is made by culturing the agent from the intestines and organs such as the liver. It may be difficult to prevent this disease because a wide variety of animals can serve as carriers.

Infectious Bursal Disease

Infectious bursal disease, often referred to as IBD or Gumboro disease, is a highly contagious viral disease of three- to six-week-old chickens characterized by high mortality, anorexia, diarrhea, and depression. The virus has a preference for lymphoid tissue, primarily the bursa of Fabricius, and may cause prolonged immunosuppression of chickens. The causative agent is a virus belonging to the genus Birnavirus, which replicates in B lymphocytes, is very stable, and persists for long periods in poultry houses, even when they have been thoroughly cleaned and disinfected. This disease spreads rapidly within a flock by direct contact, inhalation, or contaminated feed and water. The darkling beetle can also spread the virus [19].

Clinical Signs

Clinical signs can be seen in 48–72 hours after infection. Initially, affected chicks appear depressed, have ruffled feathers, and a whitish or watery diarrhea may be present. As the disease progresses, anorexia, dehydration, trembling, and death can occur. Vent picking can be observed. In affected flocks, morbidity may reach 100% and mortality may vary from 0% to 30%. The subclinical form of IBD has no clinical signs, but immunosuppression occurs to make the birds more susceptible to other diseases, such as *E. coli*, coccidiosis, necrotic dermatitis, and necrotic enteritis. These birds may have poor responses to vaccination. Necropsy reveals dehydration, hemorrhages in the thigh and pectoral muscles, and a bursa of Fabricius that is swollen and hemorrhagic or edematous [20]. The bursa atrophies to approximately one-third of the original weight by day 8 postinfection. Kidneys can be swollen with urate retention in ureters.

Diagnosis

In acute IBD, a presumptive diagnosis can be made based on the lesions observed in the bursa of Fabricius and clinical signs that are typical of IBD. A positive diagnosis of IBD can be made by histological examination of the bursa or by virus isolation. The bursa and spleen are the tissues of choice for isolation of IBD virus. There is no specific treatment that changes the onset of immunosuppression after infection. When secondary infections are present, specific treatment for the secondary disease is suggested. As the IBD virus is very stable in the poultry house environment, good sanitation procedures are essential in helping to reduce exposure in subsequent flocks [19]. The best method to control IBD in chickens is by vaccination at 1 day of age and revaccinated at 7–14 days. IBD vaccination is rarely practiced in small chicken flocks.

Coccidiosis

Coccidiosis, which is caused by the protozoan parasite *Eimeria* spp., affects the intestinal tract of poultry. These parasites are species specific, so coccidia that infect chickens do not infect turkeys and vice versa. Most outbreaks involve infection with two or more species of Eimeria.

Infections are more common in floor-raised birds but can occur in caged birds. The life cycle is initiated by ingestion of sporulated oocysts (eggs) and usually takes four to six days to complete. A single, mature oocyst (egg) contains four sporocysts, and each sporocyst contains two sporozoites (eight sporozoites in each oocyst), which can sporulate in less than 48 hours (under warm and moist conditions). These infected oocysts are then consumed by the bird [21].

Clinical Signs
Affected birds display pale combs and wattles from blood loss in the intestines, ruffled feathers, depression, blood in droppings, and shivering. The mortality rate may increase, particularly in young birds. Decreased egg production can occur in adult birds. Each species affects a different part of the intestines, so lesions vary depending on the *Eimeria* involved.

Eimeria tenella causes marked cecal hemorrhage and cecal cores in chickens.

Diagnosis
Diagnosis is made by observing gross lesions and fecal floatation, or by confirming the presence of intestinal sexual or asexual forms of coccidia by histopathology. Alternatively, segments of infected intestine can be opened and the mucosa can be gently scraped with a glass coverslip. A coverslip is then placed on the glass microscope slide and the oocysts can be observed using a ×40 objective lens [22].

Treatment/Prevention
To control coccidiosis in the flock, anticoccidial drugs that kill (coccidiocidal), or decrease the growth rate (coccidiostat) of coccidia should be used on a semi-annual rotational basis to avoid resistance build-up in the parasite. In addition, live, attenuated coccidial vaccines containing up to six species of *Eimeria* have been used on farms with severe infections. Effective control includes killing oocysts in the environment or preventing contact with viable oocysts (using deep litter and salting the floor with 60–80 lb of rock salt per 100 ft^2 before placing litter). Litter should not be recycled between flocks, or at least the top 3 in. of used litter should be removed and replaced [23] (see Chapter 11).

Hemorrhagic Enteritis (HE)

Hemorrhagic enteritis is an acute disease of young turkeys of four weeks of age or older and is characterized by depression, massive hemorrhage into the intestinal tract, and sudden death. Mortality is variable but can be high. In the subclinical form, HE is characterized by immunosuppression and secondary bacterial infection, especially from *E. coli*. HE is generally considered to be the most immunosuppressive viral infection of turkeys that is caused by a type II adenovirus, a double-stranded RNA virus with an icosahedral morphology [24]. Transmission of the virus occurs by ingestion of contaminated feces. Contaminated litter may infect subsequent flocks in the same house, as the disease recurs in houses in which it has occurred previously. Equipment and boots may carry infected fecal material from farm to farm. There is no evidence of egg transmission.

Clinical Signs

Clinical signs are usually observed in affected turkeys of 6–12 weeks of age but may occur as early as 4 weeks. In the classical form of the disease, HE is characterized by rapid onset with depression, bloody droppings, and death. All signs usually occur within 24 hours. Dark-red to brownish blood is found on the skin and feathers around the vents of dead or dying birds. In the subclinical form of the disease, there are no clinical signs of HE, but viral-induced immunosuppression can promote secondary *E. coli* infection. At necropsy, the intestines are distended, dark in color, and full of red or brownish blood. Spleens of infected birds are characteristically enlarged, fragile, and mottled. In subclinical cases, mild enteritis may be present in addition to lesions of colibacillosis [25].

Diagnosis

A presumptive diagnosis can be made based on clinical signs and lesions. Confirmation of the diagnosis can be accomplished by submitting spleens for histopathology [26]. Serology may also help support the diagnosis.

Treatment/Prevention

There is no satisfactory treatment of affected birds. Supportive care and good management help to minimize losses. Convalescent antiserum given within 24 hours of the onset of signs may prevent heavy losses. Secondary *E. coli* infections may be treated with antibiotics. A good biosecurity program should include an all-in/all-out procedure and thorough cleaning and disinfection of the premises [25]. Vaccination with a live, avirulent HE vaccine has been effective in reducing the clinical signs

that result from HE. A variety of HE vaccines are commercially available.

Roundworms (Ascariasis)

Ascaridia galli, a nematode residing in the upper small intestine of chickens and turkeys, causes the common roundworm infection. Young birds, less than three months of age, are most susceptible to intestinal damage and lightweight egg breeds (e.g. Leghorns) are more susceptible to infection than heavy meat-type breeds (e.g. Plymouth Rocks). In caged birds, infection can occur from exposure to contaminated flies. The life cycle is direct and takes 30 days to complete [27]. The eggs contaminate the environment and can remain infective for 160 weeks on the ground.

Clinical Signs

Parasitized birds can show depression, weight loss, diarrhea, and decreased growth. Lowered egg production can occur in cases of heavy infection [27]. Worms in the small intestine can occasionally cause death by blockage/impaction [28]. Gross lesions can include a reddened intestinal mucosa (enteritis). Thin birds show atrophy of the breast muscle and decreased body fat [2]. Ascarids can migrate to the oviduct and become incorporated in the egg prior to shell formation [28, 29]. Necropsy reveals worms that are large, yellow-white, and 5–11 cm long. Fecal flotation needs to be performed using zinc sulfate or sodium nitrate solutions.

Diagnosis

Confinement and cage rearing have reduced problems with most intestinal parasites. Using deep litter (4–6 in. of wood shavings) reduces exposure to parasite eggs, and proper clean up between flocks reduces future infections [23]. It is important to evaluate new birds for such parasites before introducing them to the flock.

Treatment

Piperazine is the treatment of choice (see Chapter 11).

Cestode (Tapeworm) Infections

Tapeworms are usually of no clinical significance in poultry, although these parasites may have a minor effect on growth rates [30]. Seven species affect chickens and all require an intermediate host to complete the life cycle. *Choanotaenia infundibulum* and *Raillietina cesticillus* are the most commonly found tapeworms in caged pullets or layers because of consumption of an intermediate host (housefly or beetle). Gross lesions of heavy tapeworm burden are usually striking, but the infection likely has little clinical effect. There is no effective chemical treatment. Butynorate (Tinostat) is no longer available. Prevention should focus on control of intermediate host: Flies, beetles, and ants. Heavy tapeworm infections indicate that there is a need for fly or darkling beetle control on the premises [31].

Capillariaisis (*Capillaria obsignata*)

Capillaria obsignata, is a 0.5–1.8 cm long threadlike nematode that primarily affects the small intestine of chickens, with a direct life cycle of about 18 days. Eggs are infective for up to 102 weeks in the environment. Usually, young adults display signs, and the effects of the infection can diminish as the bird ages. Infected birds are often in poor condition and may have diarrhea, weight loss, pale combs and wattles, and decreased egg production [32, 33]. "Platinum egg yolks," white egg yolk caused by a decreased absorption of vitamin A and carotenoids in the intestine, can occur. Unless there is a severe infection, mortality is minimal.

Adult worms partially burrow into the small intestines and cecum to cause hemorrhagic enteritis, and the intestinal wall may become thickened in severe cases. Affected layers can have decreased egg production and pale egg yolks.

Diagnosis
For heavy infections, diagnosis can be made by scraping the intestinal mucosa and placing it

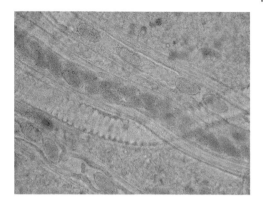

Figure 17.7 Mucosal scraping of the intestinal mucosa reveals *Capillaria* worms containing distinctive bioperculate ova.

onto a glass slide for microscopic evaluation (Figure 17.7). For light to moderate infections, wash intestinal scrapings through a fine mesh screen (100 mesh) to observe the worms. Regular and proper sanitation should prevent infections.

Treatment
Birds that are in lay should be supplemented with vitamin A to maintain egg yolk color. Fenbendazole can be effective as treatment [34] (see Chapter 11).

Necrotic Enteritis

Necrotic enteritis is a common enteritis of chickens that causes depression and sudden death. The disease is observed less often in turkeys and older chickens. Broiler chickens are most often affected. This disease often occurs concurrently or following an outbreak of coccidiosis or occasionally ascariasis [35]. The etiologic agent is *Clostridium perfringens*, type A and C, which produce alpha and beta toxins that cause necrosis of the intestinal mucosa. This gram-positive bacillus requires anaerobic conditions for culture [18, 36].

Clostridium is ubiquitous and infection is probably initiated by changes in intestinal pH, damage from coccidiosis, and gut stasis that promote conditions for growth of *C. perfringens*.

Necrotic enteritis has been associated with feed containing wheat, which possibly causes alterations of the intestinal pH [37]. This disease usually occurs when birds are around three weeks of age.

Although *Clostridium* may be found in the soil, its spores can reach high concentrations in litter that is not replaced periodically and infection can recur in contaminated houses [18].

Clinical Signs
In affected birds, sudden death can occur, or birds can appear weak and hold their heads down. The small intestines are swollen and are filled with a tan to yellow, thick pseudomembrane ("Turkish towel") (Figure 17.8a,b). Moreover, water in the crop and marked dehydration may occur in affected birds [38].

Diagnosis/Prevention
Diagnosis can be made based on history (recent coccidiosis outbreak), gross lesions, and optional bacterial culture. To prevent future outbreaks litter should be changed periodically; a coccidial prevention program should be established; and wheat midlings should be avoided in the ration. Moreover, the birds should be assessed for infectious bursal disease that could immunocompromise the flock.

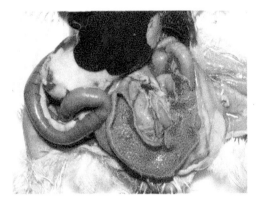

Figure 17.8 Necrotic enteritis in a three-week-old broiler chicken. The dilated small intestine is lined by a tan pseudomembrane of fibrinoecrotic exudate.

Treatment
The use of ionophore anticoccidials, such as monensin, has helped reduce the occurrence of necrotic enteritis. During outbreaks of necrotic enteritis, birds may be treated with a gram-positive spectrum antibiotic [39].

Avian Mycobacteriosis

Avian mycobacteriosis, also known as avian tuberculosis, avian TB, TB, or mycobacteriosis, is a chronic bacterial infection that forms visceral granulomas (nodules) in a variety of mature/adult birds, resulting in progressive wasting and death. The causative agent is *Mycobacterium avium*, subspecies *avium*, a nonmotile, non–spore-forming bacterial rod that stains acid-fast. It is highly resistant to pH, water, cold, and many disinfectants [40]. The granulomas (tubercles) of *M. avium* often develop in the intestinal tract. Tubercles rupture to release bacteria into intestinal lumen and subsequently into the feces. Infected feces contaminate feed, water, and litter [18]. *M. avium* is also zoonotic for humans [41]. Transmission takes place via ingestion of contaminated feed, water, and litter. Affected birds show progressive wasting with occasional diarrhea. However, birds can die suddenly without premonitory signs. On necropsy, birds appear lightweight to emaciated, with marked atrophy of breast muscle and no internal body fat (Figure 17.9a). White to gray nodules in the intestine, spleen, liver, and bone marrow may be present (Figure 17.9b) [42].

Diagnosis
A diagnosis can be made based on history, gross lesions, and histopathology. Histologic sections show characteristic granulomatous inflammation with acid-fast bacterial rods in the center of the lesion. To prevent outbreaks, all-in/all-out breeder programs to eliminate infected birds are recommended. Thoroughly dry-clean and disinfect houses and equipment between flocks. Keep young and old birds separated and cull affected birds [8].

(a)

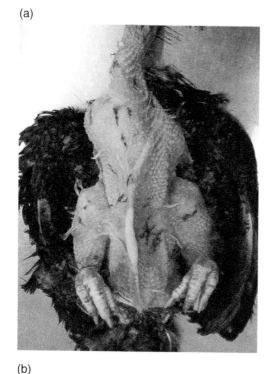

(b)

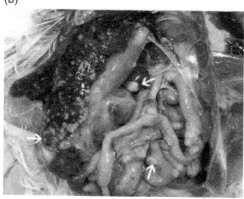

Figure 17.9 Aged laying hens with mycobacteriosis are often emaciated (a) with granulomas (arrows) (b) on liver, spleen, and intestine.

Avian Chlamydiosis

Avian chlamydiosis, also referred to as psittacosis or ornithosis, is an acute to chronic infectious disease that can cause systemic, pulmonary, and enteric lesions. This agent is a public health concern as a zoonosis and is reportable in some states [43]. The causative agent, *Chlamydia psittaci*, (formerly known as *Chlamydophila psittaci*), order Chlamydiales, is an obligate intracellular gram-negative bacterium that occurs in a wide variety of birds. Until recently, the microorganism had been referred to as Chlamydia.

Most outbreaks occur in young birds. This disease is extremely rare in poultry and is only occasionally diagnosed in turkeys. Infected birds can act as carriers by intermittently shedding the agent in oculonasal secretions and feces. Young birds can contract infection by ingesting nasal secretions or fecal material.

Clinical Signs

Clinical signs are often quite mild with low-grade respiratory signs or diarrhea. Turkeys may show signs of depression, weakness, anorexia, weight loss, nasal discharge, or marked yellowish green diarrhea. Necropsied birds may show fibrinous pneumonia, airsacculitis, hepatitis, pericarditis, peritonitis, and splenitis [44].

Diagnosis

Chlamydiosis can be diagnosed by culture in embryonated chicken eggs, antigen capture assay on tracheal swab, or by performing a complete necropsy and histopathology examination. Macchiavello stain has been used to identify intracytoplasmic elementary (infectious) *Chlamydia* bodies in impression smears of the lungs, spleen, and liver [45]. Other diseases to consider include *Mycoplasma gallisepticum*, *Pasteurella multocida*, avian influenza (AI), and aspergillosis. There is no vaccine for chlamydiosis, so thorough cleaning and disinfection, as well as all-in/all-out management to prevent infection in young birds is recommended. *Chlamydia* is prevalent in pigeons, so caution should be used if free-living or captive pigeons are present on the same farm (see Chapter 10).

Ulcerative Enteritis

Although this is a common bacterial enteric disease of domestic bobwhite quail and other upland game birds, such as pheasants, chickens, and turkeys can also be affected. The lesions are characterized by multifocal discoid ulcers in the small intestine and multifocal hepatic necrosis [46]. The causative agent is *Clostridium colinum*, a gram-positive, spore-forming bacterial rod, and is spread in the feces of infected birds [47]. *C. colinum* is hardy and can persist in the soil or litter for several months. *C. colinum* spreads rapidly from bird to bird and via flies that have been in contact with contaminated feces. The disease is rare in birds that are raised in cages.

Clinical Signs

Affected quail are usually 6–10 weeks of age and have white, watery diarrhea with subsequent sudden death. Birds that do not die suddenly are depressed with closed eyes and ruffled feathers. Infected birds are thirsty and huddle around the drinkers. The course of disease lasts about two weeks and can result in nearly 100% mortality in bobwhite quail [11]. Lesions are prominent in most affected birds and include fluid-filled distended crops and deep punctate to discoid ulcers that are tan to gray in color in the small intestine (Figure 17.10). These ulcers often penetrate the entire wall of the intestine to result in peritonitis and adherence of intestinal loops. The liver may or may not contain pale foci of necrosis on the capsule and on cut surfaces. Birds that live for more than 10 days can become emaciated.

Diagnosis is usually made using history and gross lesions. The organism has specific growth requirements and bacterial isolation is generally not needed for a diagnosis. Affected birds can be treated with bacitracin, the antibiotic of choice, in the water at 0.25–0.50 g per gal of water for 7–10 days. Penicillin and tetracyclines can also be effective [48]. Ulcerative enteritis rarely occurs in birds that are raised on wire. If free-range is desired and if this disease occurs on the farm, rotation of pens on a regular basis can reduce exposure to *Clostridium* spores.

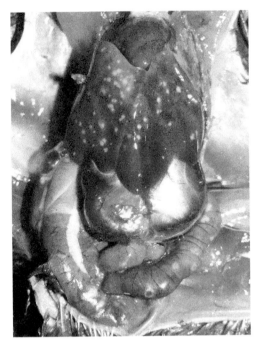

Figure 17.10 Four-week-old Bobwhite quail with ulcerative enteritis. Note the pale, necrotic foci in the small intestine and liver.

Newcastle Disease (ND)

Newcastle disease is an acute, rapid-spreading, contagious disease of birds of all ages characterized by lesions in the respiratory tract, visceral organs, and brain. It causes minor to severe mortality in susceptible flocks, depending on the pathogenicity of the virus. The causative agent belongs to the family Paramyxoviridae, subfamily Paramyxovirinae, genus *Avulavirus*, species *Newcastle disease virus*, and is a negative sense single-stranded RNA (ssRNA) virus. The agent is a paramyxovirus, an enveloped ssRNA virus with helical capsid symmetry (100–150 nm diameter). There are nine serogroups of avian paramyxovirus and ND virus is PMV-1 [49]. ND viruses are classified according to their pathogenicity for chickens. Pathogenicity is determined by inoculating virus directly into the brain of one-day-old chicks, intravenously into the six-week-old chickens, or by characterizing amino acid sequences in the fusion protein. The velogenic strains produce severe disease and high mortality in susceptible birds. The mesogenic strains cause respiratory disease or marked drop in egg production in field infections but with lower mortality. The lentogenic strains (e.g. B-1 and LaSota) only produce a mild respiratory disease. They are commonly used for vaccine production. The lentogenic strains can cause a moderate respiratory disease in broilers and pullets, particularly if complicated by secondary *E. coli* infection. Additionally, chicken embryos that are inoculated via the allantoic sac with Newcastle disease virus have different mean death times depending on whether the virus is velogenic (death in less than 60 hours), mesogenic (60–90 hours), or lentogenic (greater than 90 hours to kill embryo) [49, 50].

The virus is present in the discharges from the respiratory and intestinal tracts. Therefore, the infectious ND virus can be transmitted by aerosol droplets, contaminated feed and water, off-farm movement of poultry, and infected wild birds. The greatest potential for spread of Newcastle disease is via humans and contaminated equipment.

Clinical Signs

Clinical signs vary with the age of the birds, strain of ND virus, the immune status of the birds, and the environmental conditions. In young birds that have little or no maternal antibodies, or have not been vaccinated, the signs can be severe. Birds under stressful conditions are also more susceptible to severe clinical signs. The velogenic form spreads rapidly through a susceptible flock. Birds may be found dead without any signs. Initially, depressed birds are observed with increased respiration. There is progressive weakness and prostration. The birds develop a watery greenish diarrhea. A marked cough, gasping respiration, and nasal and eye discharge are often present. Comb and wattles may turn dark and bluish, and birds may develop swollen heads. Birds that survive the initial acute phase show involvement of the nervous system. Egg production drops sharply and deformed eggs may

be present. Mortality is usually over 90% in a susceptible flock [50]. For the mesogenic form, the clinical signs are similar to the velogenic form but less severe. Mortality may vary from 5% to 50%, depending on the age of birds and environmental conditions. Nervous signs may occur but are not common. The lentogenic form is characterized by mild respiratory signs and a sudden drop in egg production. The egg production returns to normal within a few weeks and birds completely recover from the disease. In young susceptible birds, severe respiratory disease can occur. Lesions found on necropsy vary depending on the strain of the infecting virus. With the velogenic strain, there are varying degrees of congestion and hemorrhages in visceral organs, including the proventriculus, ceca, and small intestines [51]. Chickens and turkeys that are infected while in lay usually have egg yolk in the abdominal cavity (egg yolk peritonitis). With the mesogenic form, hemorrhages may occur in the proventriculus and less commonly in the small intestines. There is clear fluid present in the nasal passages, larynx, and trachea. In the lentogenic form, no clinical signs or a mild tracheitis may be seen in early cases [52]. A presumptive diagnosis can be made based on the clinical signs, lesions, and serological tests. A positive diagnosis of the causative virus can only be made by isolation and identification of the virus by embryonated egg inoculation. Specimens for attempting isolation of the virus should be selected from birds that show early clinical signs of the disease. Swabs should be taken from the trachea, cloaca, and brain [50].

Treatment

There is no effective treatment against the ND virus. Broad-spectrum antibiotics may help to prevent secondary bacterial infections. Good management practices to reduce any additional stress on the birds aids in recovery. Prevention of Newcastle disease involves a sound biosecurity program and an effective vaccination program. Keep unauthorized personnel out of the poultry area and maintain a good clean out and sanitation procedure. Frequency and timing of Newcastle vaccination depend on the type of bird and the incidence of Newcastle disease in the area [53]. Chickens can be vaccinated with the Type B vaccine strain at 1 day, 14 days, and 6 weeks of age. Laying chickens can be vaccinated with the LaSota strain at 13–16 weeks and then every 60 days during production. The Newcastle vaccine is usually administered in combination with the infectious bronchitis vaccine. Turkeys can be vaccinated with B, Type, B, Strain at three weeks and then revaccinated with the LaSota strain at eight weeks (see Chapter 13 for more information).

Avian Influenza

Avian influenza is an infectious respiratory disease of poultry, especially turkeys, and is characterized by respiratory symptoms, depression, and lowered feed and water consumption. In laying birds, there is a severe drop in egg production and hatchability. Avian influenza is a type A orthomyxovirus, an 80–120 nm diameter, icosahedral enveloped ssRNA virus, that can infect a wide variety of birds, including most game birds. The virus can be inactivated in three hours at 56 °C and 30 minutes at 60 °C. In warm weather, the virus can survive for 35 days in water, soil, manure, and on contaminated equipment. In cold climates, the virus can survive for up to three months [54]. The virus is found most often in wild waterfowl and shore birds, which serve as natural reservoirs by carrying and transmitting the virus, usually without showing clinical signs, so exposure to backyard flocks with such free-living birds should be reduced [55]. The AI virus is rapidly destroyed by most commercial disinfectants. The virus exists in high pathogenic (HPAI, ability to cause severe disease) and low pathogenic (LPAI, mild disease) forms that are categorized by both live bird inoculation and determination of amino acid sequences at the hinge region of the hemagglutinin molecule. Avian influenza viruses are also characterized by the glycoproteins attached to the surface of the viral envelope. One glycoprotein is hemagglutinin (H), of which 16 types can be encoded by the viral genome. A second glycoprotein is neuraminidase (N). The genome of the AI virus can encode for one of nine different N types. AI virus is primarily described by the H and N types on the virus surface. The AI virus has the ability to change form through antigenic drift (point mutation in the H or N) or antigenic shift (two or more viruses with differing H and N types sharing genomic segments to create a new virus with a novel combination of H and N expressed on the virus envelope). HPAI usually take the form of H5 and H7 [56, 57]. The virus is transmitted by direct contact between infected and susceptible birds and indirect contact, including aerosol droplets or exposure to virus-contaminated boots, clothing, or equipment.

Clinical Signs

Poultry that have been infected with LPAI can show decreased egg production, respiratory signs (coughing, sneezing), or no clinical signs at all. Secondary infections with *E. coli* can increase the flock mortality. HPAI can cause rapid death without clinical signs, or signs can involve the respiratory (cough, sneeze), nervous (paralysis, ataxia), and digestive systems (diarrhea), and decreased egg production. Edema of the head and neck is commonly observed. Poultry that have been infected with LPAI may have no gross lesions or can have fibrinous exudates in the trachea, sinuses, air sacs, and conjunctiva. The oviduct can be inactive or shrunken. With HPAI infection, lesions are severe. The comb or wattle may be shrunken, ulcerated, or cyanotic (purple). Edema of the face and feet along with hemorrhages on the shanks are commonly observed. Hemorrhages or fibrinous exudates can cover the pericardial sac, mesentery, air sacs, abdominal fat, trachea, intestine, and oviduct. In addition, hemorrhage and necrosis can be observed in the cecal tonsils and proventricular glands [58].

Diagnosis

Diagnosis of LPAI is based on serology (agar gel immunodiffusion test) and virus isolation to differentiate the infection from other diseases such as colibacillosis, Newcastle disease, and infectious bronchitis. HPAI is diagnosed by observing the extreme clinical signs and must be differentiated from exotic ND. Nine- to ten-day embryonated chicken eggs are inoculated via the allantoic sac to cultivate the virus [59]. Polymerase chain reaction analysis can also be performed on cloacal or oral swabs of ill or dead birds [57].

Treatment

There is no practical treatment for AI virus infections except to prevent secondary bacterial infection. Antibiotic treatment has been used to reduce the effects of concurrent bacterial infections. As the disease is spread from infected bird to susceptible bird and by contaminated boots and equipment, strict biosecurity is important. In outbreaks that involve highly pathogenic subtypes, eradication programs are used to control the disease. In low pathogenic cases, use of a killed vaccine (autogenous) has been allowed. Random vaccination is not permitted by the United States Department of Agriculture (see Chapter 13 for more information).

Heterakis Gallinarum (Cecal Worm)

Heterakis gallinarum, a cecal worm that is found in chickens, turkeys, and pheasants, can harbor the protozoan *Histomonas meleagridis*, the causative agent of blackhead in turkeys, in its eggs. Hence, chickens can serve as a possible source of infection for turkeys if the turkeys are raised in proximity to chickens. *H. gallinarum* are thin, white, 0.5–1.5 cm long worms that can reach the infective stage at two weeks or less, depending on ambient temperature, and can remain infective for up to 230 weeks [60]. *H. gallinarum* eggs are occasionally ingested by earthworms, which can also serve as a source of infection when ingested by poultry. Affected birds usually have no clinical signs other than the presence

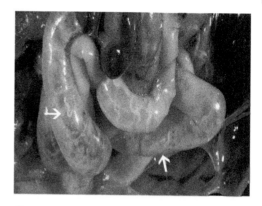

Figure 17.11 Open cecum of adult floor-raised hen distended with cecal worms (*Heterakis gallinarum* arrows).

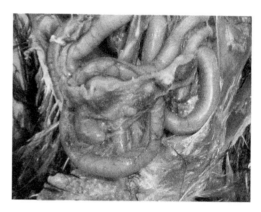

Figure 17.12 Adult chicken with cecal worms (*Heterakis*). The nematode can occasionally invade the cecal wall to form inflammatory nodules.

of worms in the ceca (Figure 17.11); however, in heavy infections *H. gallinarum* or related species can imbed in the cecal mucosa to form mural granulomas (Figure 17.12). Prevention is similar to that described for ascarids [8, 61] (see Chapter 11 for more information).

Cloacal Prolapse

The cloaca (vent) of the laying hen temporarily everts when an egg is laid. The cloaca can become permanently everted and inflamed if is traumatized by other hens (cannibalism, pecking, peckout, etc.) or if the egg being laid is particularly large relative to the cloacal lumen. Birds dying from peckout/prolapse show hemorrhage around the vent area and most of the intestinal tract can be absent as a result of removal by other birds. Factors affecting the severity and incidence of cloacal prolapse include strain of bird, the quality of beak trim, quality of ration, amount of floor, feeder, or drinker space, high light intensity, and large egg size. Young birds early in lay are more susceptible to cloacal prolapse because the cloacal lumen has not become fully expanded to accept relatively large eggs. Additionally, vent trauma and cloacal prolapse in floor-raised chickens can be decreased by offering perches and obstacles to provide protection for hens, and by maintaining adequate nest: hen ratios (one nest: four hens) to decrease fighting for nest space [8].

Diseases of the Liver

Liver disease may be detected using biochemical tests. Physical examination can reveal an enlarged liver [62]. A normal-size liver should not be palpable past the keel bone [2, 62]. Palpation of part of the liver extending past the keel bone can indicate hepatomegaly [2]. Radiographs may also indicate liver enlargement. Marek's disease is a common cause of liver disease in some backyard flocks.

Other liver lesions include the masses seen in avian mycobacteriosis and should be the primary differential for nodular lesions in the liver along with colibacillosis. Crater-like lesions are unique with histomoniasis being one of the most common diseases.

Some peracute bacterial diseases, which cause septicemia, may cause a slight liver enlargement. Acute bacterial diseases can cause multifocal white spots in the liver with colibacillosis being the most common. While not as common, white spots on the liver can indicate larvae migrations in the liver from severe roundworm infections.

Perihepatitis, manifested as a white film around the liver, can be caused by bacterial diseases with chlamydiosis, salmonellosis, and colibacillosis being top differentials. These tissues should be cultured and also placed in formalin for histopathology.

Marek's Disease (MD)

Marek's disease is a herpesvirus infection that causes lymphoma of T lymphocytes and is ubiquitous throughout the world. Tumors can occur in the nerves, ovaries, testes, viscera, eyes, muscles, and skin. Leg paralysis resulting from Marek's disease is often referred to as range paralysis. The disease is caused by a cell-associated herpesvirus (double-stranded DNA virus, hexagonal enveloped virus). There are three serotypes of the MD virus: serotype 1, the oncoviruses (tumor-causing); serotype 2, the non-oncogenic viruses; and serotype 3, the herpes virus turkey (HVT) [63]. The virus is intranuclear (cell-associated) and normally cannot live outside the host cell, as it is protected from the environment by the host epithelium. Infectious virus is only produced in the feather follicle epithelium and spreads by direct or indirect contact between birds. The infectious virus contaminates the premises through infected molted feathers and dander. Birds become infected when they inhale dust that contains the virus. Contaminated dust may remain infectious for several months. Many apparently normal birds are carriers and can transmit the infection. Some birds have been found to shed virus from skin for as long as 18 months. Darkling beetles may also act as a mechanical vector [64].

Clinical Signs

In acute outbreaks, birds become severely depressed, anorectic, and uncoordinated followed by unilateral or bilateral paralysis of legs and wings. Many birds become dehydrated, emaciated, and eventually die. The extremities affected include the legs, wings, and neck. In an infected flock, mortality gradually builds and generally persists for 4–10 weeks. Ocular Marek's disease is characterized by decreased pupil size and irregular diameter, and the iris becomes gray ("gray eye"). A number of factors influence the extent of losses in affected flocks, such as virus strain, dosage, route of exposure, and genetic resistance of the host. Immunosuppression can occur as a long-term effect. Gross lesions can usually be found in one or more peripheral nerves, particularly the sciatic and brachial nerves. Affected nerves are characterized by loss of cross-striations, gray or yellow discoloration, and may be swollen (Figure 17.13). Lymphoid tumors may be found in the gonads, heart, liver (Figures 17.14 and 17.15), lungs, kidneys, spleen, bursa, intestines, muscles, and skin. Skin lesions are not readily seen until feathers are removed, and the feather follicles may be enlarged and pale. The cloacal bursa is usually not involved.

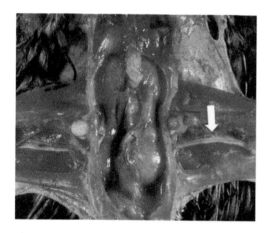

Figure 17.13 Eight-week old Barred Rock chicken with Marek's disease. Note the enlarged kidney (lymphoma). The right sciatic nerve is of normal thickness while the left sciatic nerve (arrow) is swollen, pale and has lost cross-striations.

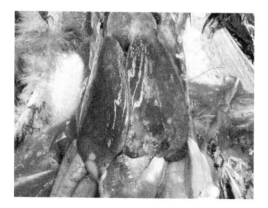

Figure 17.14 Hepatic lymphoma (hepatomegaly) can be seen in Marek's disease.

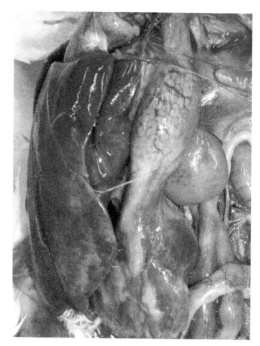

Figure 17.15 Nineteen-week-old pullet with hepatosplenomegaly caused by the lymphoid leukosis virus.

Diagnosis

A presumptive diagnosis is made based on the presence of tumors and the observed paralysis; however, gross necropsy and histopathology are important to arrive at a definitive diagnosis and to differentiate Marek's disease from other forms of paralysis or recumbency [65].

Treatment/Prevention

There is no specific treatment for chickens with Marek's disease and the emphasis is on prevention. Vaccination against MD is effective in controlling the disease. Marek's disease vaccine is usually administered on day 1. Three types of vaccines are commercially available: The HVT serotype 3, natural occurring avirulent isolates of serotype 2, and non-oncogenic strains of serotype 1 (Rispens) [66]. For backyard flocks, the HVT vaccine is commonly used.

Lymphoid Leukosis (LL)

Lymphoid leukosis is a viral disease of chickens that is characterized by the formation of tumors (lymphoma of B lymphocytes) in internal organs. Under natural situations, lesions are seen mainly in sexually mature birds because of the long incubation period (270 days) of the virus. The causative agent is an RNA virus (80–120 nm diameter) belonging to the avian type C oncoviruses [67].

The most common route of vertical transmission of the LL virus is from the infected oviduct to the progeny through the egg. Chicks infected through the egg are immunotolerant (serum antibody negative, viremia positive) and have a high incidence of tumors [68]. There is some horizontal transmission of the virus from bird to bird at a young age; these birds are only temporarily viremic and do develop antibody to the virus. Usually, only a small number of LL-infected birds develop lesions; the others remain as carriers and shedders [69]. LL is rarely seen in large-scale poultry production because of elimination of the oncovirus from primary breeder flocks.

Clinical Signs

Clinical signs usually do not appear before four months of age and are nonspecific. Affected birds may appear pale, emaciated, and dehydrated. The comb may become shriveled, and occasionally cyanotic. There is a drop in egg production and loss of appetite. The abdomen is often enlarged and feathers are sometimes spotted with urates and bile. LL virus can also cause erythroblastosis (anemia, hepatosplenomegaly), myeloblastosis (bone marrow, leukemia, and hepatomegaly), and myelocytomatosis (deformation of flat bones of the skull and mandible) [67]. LL virus can also induce proliferation and activation of osteoblasts in bone; a disease known as osteopetrosis, characterized by formation of new bone on the periosteum and endosteum of long bones. These bones are heavier and thicker than normal. Lymphoma that is characterized by tumors or organ enlargement occurs in the organs, especially the liver and spleen (hepatosplenomegaly) (Figure 17.15). Tumors can also develop in the kidneys, lungs, ovaries, testicles, bursa of Fabricius, heart, and bone marrow [70]. Tumors vary in size and are soft, smooth, glistening, and gray to white.

Diagnosis/Treatment/Prevention

A presumptive diagnosis can be made based on the presence of tumors and the age of the birds. Usually with LL, lesions are seen in birds of four months and older, whereas, in birds affected with Marek's disease, lesions may appear as early as four weeks of age. A positive diagnosis requires histological examination. There is no effective treatment and no vaccine is available. It is helpful to cull all birds that are obviously affected. The best prevention method is the laboratory detection of infected breeders. Breeding leukosis-free offspring from leukosis-free breeders can eventually lead to eradication of the disease. An ELISA is available to test egg albumin or serum for the presence of avian leukosis antigen.

Colibacillosis

Colibacillosis is an infectious disease caused by the gram-negative rod *E. coli* as the primary pathogen or as a secondary invader that causes septicemia, peritonitis, cellulitis, omphalitis, salpingitis, and airsacculitis. Colibacilosis, also referred to as *E. coli* infection, coligranuloma, or colisepticemia, is caused by *E. coli* that are serotypes 01, 02, or 078, but are also often untypeable. *E. coli* is ubiquitous and is present in the intestines of birds and mammals [71]. It is disseminated in feces, and infections often result from management failures. Birds may be infected by direct contact with dirty litter and hatchers or contaminated egg shells.

Clinical Signs

Affected birds usually display nonspecific signs and include ill-thrift, ruffled feathers, enlarged and swollen navels (Figure 17.16), decreased appetite, depression, diarrhea, and pasting of feathers around the vent. Depending

(a)

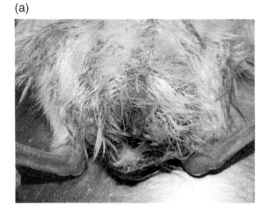

(b)

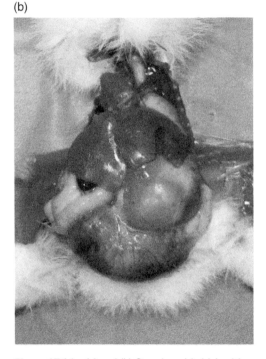

Figure 17.16 (a) and (b) One-day-old chick with omphalitis (a) and yolk sacculitis (b) from colibacillosis.

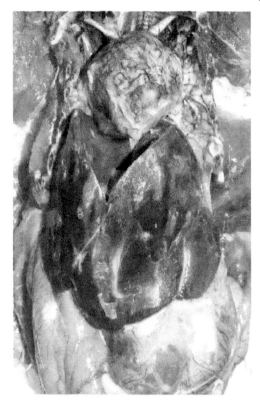

Figure 17.17 Nine-week-old turkey hen with fibrinous pericarditis, perihepatitis, and airsacculitits resulting from colibacillosis.

on the body system that is affected, there can be a variety of lesions, including airsacculitis, perihepatitis, and pericarditis, resulting from secondary invasion of *E. coli* into a primary subacute to chronic respiratory disease [72]. A white, friable material covers the air sacs, liver, and pericardial sac (Figure 17.17). The respiratory form of *E. coli* infection in juvenile birds is often preceded by *Mycoplasma*, Newcastle disease, or infectious bronchitis. Newly hatched birds have omphalitis (swollen, red, and crusted navels), which is caused by contamination of egg shells through a dirty setter, feces-covered eggs, or excessive moisture during storage of eggs. Cases of omphalitis resulting from colibacillosis should be differentiated from those caused by other bacteria [73–75]. Birds may also have septicemia with hepatosplenomegaly (hepatitis), hemorrhages, and necrosis in affected organs [76]. Hepatitis and cecal cores were observed in turkeys with colibacillosis [77]. Septic birds can develop hypopyon (exudate within the eye). Infected laying hens commonly develop salpingitis, in which the oviduct is filled with yellow, caseous exudate, with or without peritonitis [78–80] (Figure 17.18). Cellulitis ("scabby hip") with yellow exudate can accumulate underneath the skin of the hip, leg, and breast, particularly in broiler chickens [81].

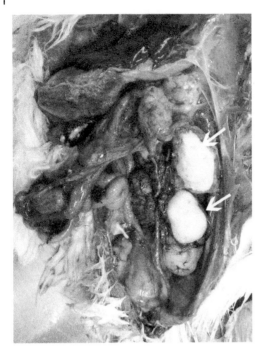

Figure 17.18 Colibacillosis is the most common cause of salpingitis in laying hens. Note enlarged and exudate-filled oviduct (arrows).

Diagnosis/Treatment

Histopathology, along with bacterial culture of affected organs, is required for diagnosis. Many *E. coli* strains are resistant to antibiotics, so a combination of treatments have been attempted for large flocks including: (i) Combining 200 g Neomycin and 200 g Terramycin per ton of feed for seven days, followed by two weeks of probiotic in the feed; (ii) adding either household bleach (6–10 oz per gal stock metered at 1 oz per gall drinking water) or iodine disinfectant (8–12 oz per gal stock) for 10 days to reduce bacterial load in the water; and (iii) fog the house with a fine mist of VirconS (1% solution) or chlorine dioxide (0.5% with no activator) twice a day for four to five days in order to reduce aerosolized bacteria. To prevent outbreaks, a vigorous sanitation program in the breeder house, hatchery, and at the grow-out facility is recommended. Reducing aerosolized dust, routinely removing dead birds, and avoiding overcrowding in the poultry house are strategies to reduce outbreaks.

Visceral Gout/Urolithiasis

Gout/urolithiasis is a condition commonly seen in older layer flocks and is often related to kidney failure. On occasion, gout can be a very significant part of flock mortality, sometimes as high as 0.5% per week, but it is often associated with sporadic low-grade mortality. Kidneys can be damaged by low phosphorus diets, water deprivation, high vitamin D3 in the ration, or excessive calcium before sexual maturity (15–16 weeks) [82]. A nephrotropic infectious bronchitis (e.g. Australian T or Italian strain) can cause similar lesions. Losses resulting from gout tend to be chronic with the number of affected birds dependent on the way in which the renal damage was induced in the flock. The strain of bird can also affect the severity and incidence of gout. Birds with gout usually show no clinical signs before death or are emaciated. The lesions of gout are associated with the accumulation of urates (uric acid is the primary nitrogenous excretory product of birds) on the surfaces of the internal organs (visceral gout) (Figure 17.19) as well as within joint spaces and along synovial membranes (articular gout). The urates are gritty and white as opposed to the inflammatory exudates that result from bacterial infections such as colibacillosis, which are yellow and friable [4]. Portions of kidney are atrophic or absent and contralateral portions are often swollen (compensatory hypertrophy) [83]. Birds can be treated, with varying success, by adding ammonium sulfate or ammonium chloride to the ration but these treatments do not cure gout and may cause wet droppings and deterioration of shell quality [84]. Gout can be prevented or minimized by providing proper calcium and phosphorus nutrition throughout the growing process (1% calcium and 0.50–0.45% available phosphorus), starting layer levels of calcium feeding at the proper time (one week prior to first egg), and avoiding water deprivation at the housing [85].

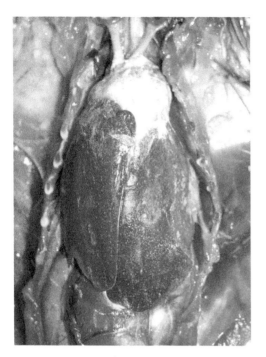

Figure 17.19 Visceral gout with c halk-like urate deposits on pericardial sac and liver capsule.

Histomoniasis

Histomoniasis is a protozoal disease that affects the cecum and liver of gallinaceous birds and has also been referred to as blackhead, infectious enterohepatitis, and *H. meleagridis* infection. The disease has been diagnosed in peafowl and turkeys, and occasionally in chickens [86]. The causative agent, *H. meleagridis*, is a flagellated ameboid protozoan that replicates in the ameboid state in the cecum and liver. The infection is often carried in eggs of the cecal worm *Heterakis gallinae* [87], which are shed in feces and consumed by earthworms. The cecal worm or earthworms were often considered a required intermediate host, but recent research indicates that turkeys can transmit the protozoan directly from bird to bird, in the absence of cecal worms and earthworms, through the phenomenon of cloacal drinking, by which contaminated fecal material in litter is carried into the colon by rhythmic contractions of the cloaca or vent [88].

Clinical Signs/Diagnosis

Lesions are usually present in ceca at eight days post-infection and liver lesions are present by 10 days. Birds that are affected can appear to die suddenly in good condition or exhibit progressive wasting. Fecal material can be yellow in color as well as containing flecks of blood. The birds are depressed, with closed eyes, huddling, and ruffled feathers. The ceca are often enlarged, pale, thick-walled, firm, and contain abundant gray to tan, friable material (cecal cores) [89]. Peritonitis can occur if inflammation penetrates the cecal wall. The liver is enlarged and contains multifocal to coalescing circular, and occasionally concentric, dark red rings with a yellow center that resemble an archery target (hence the term "target lesion") (Figure 17.20). Some birds in early stages of infection have cecal lesions without liver lesions [89]. The classical gross lesions are often diagnostic. Additionally, histomonads in liver and cecum can be observed in tissue impressions and histologic sections (Figure 17.21).

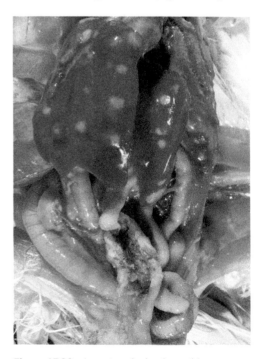

Figure 17.20 Immature laying hen with *Histomonas meleagridis* infection with round, target-like, necrotic foci in liver and enlarged ceca filled with fibrinous to caseous material.

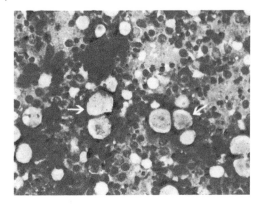

Figure 17.21 Wright-Giemsa-stained section of chicken liver reveals multiple round amoeba (arrows) consistent with *Histomonas meleagridis*.

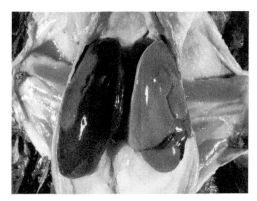

Figure 17.22 Obese hen with enlarged fatty liver that has ruptured, resulting in fatal pericapsular hemorrhage.

Treatment

There is no effective treatment that is commercially available. The emphasis is on prevention. Few preventive medications are commercially available. Good sanitation is the key to prevention. Keep chickens and turkeys separated [23].

Regularly deworm turkey flocks to decrease the population of cecal worms. Birds should be raised on litter or sandy, dry soil to minimize exposure to earthworms [23] (see Chapter 6 for more information).

Fatty Liver Syndrome

Fatty liver is caused by an imbalance of energy (positive energy gain) and protein intake. Fatty liver is observed most often in caged laying hens and occasionally in breeder turkey hens. Caged layers are particularly prone to fatty liver because of minimal exercise accompanied by high caloric intake [90, 91]. Obese backyard laying hens are also susceptible to developing fatty livers. The liver is enlarged, pale orange, soft, friable, and easily fractured (Figure 17.22). Rupture of the fatty liver with hemorrhage into the abdominal cavity or around the liver capsule is a common cause of death in laying hens [8]. Treatment with choline chloride, vitamin K, biotin, and vitamin E in the feed for two weeks has been used to control mortality with varying results and is certainly not necessary in small flocks, in which the problem is excessive calorie intake. Prevention is effected by means of an adequate diet with proper energy and protein levels [90]. Similar changes in small flocks are best prevented by monitoring body weights and feed intake, and by limiting access to high fat treats (e.g. egg noodles and cheese).

References

1 Morishita, T.Y. (1994). *Can you judge a Fecal sample by its color?* In: *Proceedings of the 43rd Western Poultry Disease Conference*, Sacramento, California (27–28 February, 1 March, 1994), 7.

2 Morishita, T.Y. (1999). Clinical assessment of chickens and waterfowl in backyard flocks. *Vet. Clin. North Am. Exot. Anim. Pract.* 2 (2): 383–404.

3 Ison, A.J., Spiegle, S.J. and Morishita, T.Y. (2004). Poultry blood collection. In: *Poultry Health Resources* (ed. T.Y. Morishita), Factsheet 2019-13. Pomona, CA: Western University.

4 Morishita, T.Y. (1990). *Establishing a differential diagnosis for backyard poultry flocks*. In: *Proceedings of the 1990 Annual Conference of the Association of Avian*

Veterinarians, Association of Avian Veterinarians, Phoenix, Arizona (10–15 September, 1990), 136–146.

5 Schnitzlein, W.M., Ghildyal, N., and Tripathy, D.N. (1988). Genomic and antigenic characterization of avipoxviruses. *Virus Res.* 10: 65–76.

6 Tripathy, D.K. and Reed, W.M. (2003). Pox. In: *Diseases of Poultry*, 11e (ed. Y.M. Saif), 253–269. Ames, IA: Iowa State University Press.

7 Dhillon, A.S. (1993). Fowl pox outbreaks in commercial layers. In: *Vineland Update No. 45*, 1–3. Vineland NJ: Vineland Laboratories.

8 Porter, R.E. (2012). *Diseases of backyard poultry*. In: *Proceedings Minnesota Veterinary Medical Association 114th Annual Meeting, Hilton Hotel, Minneapolis, MN*, pp. 1–26, 201.

9 Morishita, T.Y., Aye, P.P., and Harr, B.S. (1999). Crop impaction resulting from feather ball formation in caged layers. *Avian Dis.* 43: 160–163.

10 McDougald, L.R. (2020). Internal Parasites. In: *Diseases of Poultry*, 14e (eds. D.E. Swayne, M. Boulianne, L.R. McDougald, et al.), 1157–1191. Ames, IA: Wiley Blackwell.

11 Porter, R.E. (2008). *Common diseases of Gamebirds*. In: *Proceedings South Dakota Veterinary Medical Association Regional Continuing Education Meeting, Brookings, SD* (15 March 2008), 1–24.

12 United States Department of Agriculture, Animal and Plant Health Inspection Service (2018). 145.14 *Salmonella pullorum* testing. In: *National Poultry Improvement Plan and Auxilliary Provisions*, 14–16. US Government Printing Office.

13 Hinshaw, W.R., Upp, C.W., and Moore, J.M. (1926). Studies on transmission of bacillary white diarrhea in incubators. *J. Am. Vet. Med. Assoc.* 68: 631–641.

14 Gast, R.K. and Porter, R.E., Jr. (2020). Salmonella infections. In *Diseases of Poultry*, 14e (eds. D.E. Swayne, M. Boulianne, L.R. McDougald, et al.), 719–753. Ames, IA: Wiley Blackwell.

15 Porter, R.E. Jr. and Holt, P.S. (1993). Effect of induced molting on the severity of intestinal lesions caused by Salmonella enteritidis infection in white Leghorn chickens. *Avian Dis.* 37: 1009–1016.

16 Macri, N., Porter, R.E., and Holt, P.S. (1997). The effect of induced molting on the severity of acute intestinal infection caused by Salmonella enteritidis. *Avian Dis.* 41: 117–223.

17 Brown, D.D., Ross, J.G., and Smith, A.F.G. (1976). Experimental infection of poultry with Salmonella infantis. *Res. Vet. Sci.* 20: 237–243.

18 Porter, R.E. Jr. (1998). Bacterial enteritides of poultry. *Poult. Sci.* 77: 1159–1165.

19 Benton, W.J., Cover, M.S., and Rosenberger, J.K. (1967). Studies on the transmission of the infectious bursal agent (IBA) of chickens. *Avian Dis.* 11: 430–438.

20 Boulianne, M., Brash, M.L. Charlton, B.R. et al. (eds.) (2013). Infectious bursal disease. In: *Avian Disease Manual*, 7e, 55–57. Jacksonville, FL: American Association of Avian Pathologists.

21 Bowman, D.D. (2014). Protista. In: *Georgi's Parasitology for Veterinarians*, 10e (ed. D.D. Bowman), 87–121. St. Louis, MO: Elsevier Saunders.

22 Long, P.L. and Reid, M.W. (1982) *A guide for the diagnosis of coccidiosis in chickens*. Research Report 404, August 1982, The University of Georgia College of Agriculture Experiment Stations, pp. 1–17.

23 Morishita, T.Y. (1995). Poultry management 101: poultry management topics for avian veterinarian. In: *Section 7: Practice Management*, Main Conference Proceedings, Association of Avian Veterinarians Annual Conference, Philadelphia, Pennsylvania, 327–331.

24 Zhang, C. and Nagaraja, K.V. (1989). Differentiation of avian adenovirus type-II strains by restriction endonuclease fingerprinting. *Am. J. Vet. Res.* 9: 1466–1470.

25 Boulianne, M., Brash, M.L. Charlton, B.R. et al. (eds.) (2013). Hemorrhagic enteritis of turkeys. In: *Avian Disease Manual*, 7e, 12–14. Jacksonville, FL: American Association of Avian Pathologists.

26 Gross, W.H.B. and Domermuth, C.H. (1975). Spleen lesions of hemorrhagic enteritis of turkeys. *Avian Dis.* 3: 455–466.

27 Norton, R.A., Hopkins, B.A., Skeeles, J.K. et al. (1992). High mortality of domestic turkeys associated with *Ascaridia dissimilis*. *Avian Dis.* 36: 469–473.

28 Morishita, T.Y. and Schaul, J.C. (2006). Parasites of birds. In: *Flynn's Parasites of Laboratory Animals* (ed. D.G. Baker), 217–302. Ames, Iowa: Blackwell Publishing Professional.

29 Reid, W.M., Mabon, J.L., and Harshbarger, W.C. (1973). Detection of worm parasites in chicken eggs by candling. *Poult. Sci.* 52: 2316–2324.

30 Botero, H. and Reid, W.M. (1969). The effects of the tapeworm *Raillietina cesticillus* upon body weight gains of broilers, poults and on egg production. *Poult. Sci.* 48: 536–542.

31 Boulianne,M., Brash, M.L. Charlton, B.R. et al. (eds.) (2013). Nematodes, cestodes and trematodes. In: *Avian Disease Manual*, 7e, 158–162. Jacksonville, FL: American Association of Avian Pathologists.

32 Wakelin, D. (1965). Experimental studies on the biology of *Capillaria obsignata*, Madison, 1945, a nematode parasite of the domestic fowl. *J. Helminthol.* 39: 399–412.

33 McDougald, L.R. (2020). Internal parasites, 14e (eds. D.E. Swayne, M. Boulianne, L.R. McDougald, et al.), 1157–1191. Ames, IA: Wiley Blackwell.

34 Norton, R.A., Yazwinski, T.A., and Johnson, Z. (1991). Research note: use of fenbendazole for the treatment of turkeys with experimentally induced nematode infections. *Poult. Sci.* 70: 1835–1837.

35 Al-Sheikhly, F. and Al-Saieg, A. (1980). Role of coccidia in the occurrence of necrotic enteritis of chickens. *Avian Dis.* 24: 324–333.

36 Shane, S.M., Gyimah, J.E., Harrington, K.S., and Snider, T.G. III (1985). Etiology and pathogenesis of necrotic enteritis. *Vet. Res. Commun.* 9: 269–287.

37 Branton, S.L., Reece, F.N., and Hagler, W.M. Jr. (1987). Influence of a wheat diet on mortality of broiler chickens associated with necrotic enteritis. *Poult. Sci.* 66: 1326–1330.

38 Hemboldt, C.F. and Bryant, E.S. (1971). The pathology of necrotic enteritis in domestic fowl. *Avian Dis.* 15: 775–780.

39 Boulianne, M., Brash, M.L., Charlton, B.R. et al. (eds.) (2013). Necrotic enteritis. In: *Avian Disease Manual*, 7e, 117–118. Jacksonville, FL: American Association of Avian Pathologists.

40 Thoen, C.O., Karlson, A.G., and Himes, E.M. (1981). Mycobacterial infections in animals. *Rev. Infect. Dis.* 3: 972.

41 Falkinham, J.O. (1994). Epidemiology of Mycobacterium infections in the pre- and post-HIV era. *Res. Microbiol.* 145: 169–172.

42 Mutalib, A.A. and Riddell, C. (1988). Epizootiology and pathology of avian tuberculosis in chickens in Saskatchewan. *Can. Vet. J.* 29: 840–842.

43 Schlossberg, D., Delgado, J., Moore, M.M. et al. (1993). An epidemic of avian and human psittacosis. *Arch. Intern. Med.* 153: 2594–2596.

44 Page, L.A. (1958). Experimental ornithosis in turkeys. *Avian Dis.* 3: 51–66.

45 Edson, M., Stobierski, M.G., Smith, K.A. et al. (1995). Public veterinary medicine: compendium of chlamydiosis (psittacosis) control, 1995. *J. Am. Vet. Med. Assoc.* 12: 1874–1880.

46 Bickford, A.A. (1985). Comments on ulcerative enteritis. *Am. J. Vet. Res.* 36: 586.

47 Berkhoff, H.A. (1985). *Clostridium colinum* sp. nov., nom. rev., the causative agent of ulcerative enteritis (quail disease) in quail, chickens, and pheasants. *Am. J. Vet. Res.* 36: 583–585.

48 Kondo, F., Tottori, J., and Soki, K. (1988). Ulcerative enteritis in broiler chickens caused by *Clostridium colinum* and in vitro activity of 19 antimicrobial agents in tests on isolates. *Poult. Sci.* 67: 1424–1430.

49 Aldous, E.W. and Alexander, D.J. (2001). Detection and differentiation of Newcastle disease virus (paramyxovirus type 1). *Avian Pathol.* 30: 117–128.

50 Beard, C.W. and Easterday, B.C. (1967). The influence of the route of administration of Newcastle disease virus on host response. I. Serological and virus isolation studies. *J. Infect. Dis.* 117: 55–61.

51 Hamid, H., Campbell, R.S.F., and Parede, L. (1985). Studies of the pathology of velogenic Newcastle disease: virus infection in non-immune and immune birds. *Avian Pathol.* 20: 561–575.

52 Hamid, H., Campbell, R.S.F., and Lamichhane, C. (1990). The pathology of infection of chickens with the lentogenic V4 strain of Newcastle disease virus. *Avian Pathol.* 19: 687–696.

53 Alexander, D.J., Aldous, E.W., and Fuller, C.M. (2012). The long view: a selective review of 40 years of Newcastle disease research. *Avian Pathol.* 41 (4): 329–335.

54 Shaw, M.L. and Palese, P. (2013). Orthomyxoviridae. In: *Fields Virology*, 6e (eds. D.M. Knipe and P.M. Howley), 1487–2456. Philadelphia, PA: Lippincott Williams and Wilkins.

55 Ito, T., Okazaki, K., Kawaoka, Y. et al. (1995). Perpetuation of influenza a viruses in Alaskan waterfowl reservoirs. *Arch. Virol.* 140: 1163–1172.

56 Alexander, D.J. (2000). Review of avian influenza in different bird species. *Vet. Microbiol.* 74: 3–13.

57 Spackman, E., Senne, D.A., Meyers, T.J. et al. (2002). Development of a real-time reverse transcriptase PCR assay for type a influenza virus and the avian H5 and H7 hemagglutinin subtypes. *J. Clin. Microbiol.* 40: 3256–3260.

58 Swayne, D.E. and Suarez, D.L. (2000). Highly pathogenic avian influenza. *Rev. Sci. Tech.* 19: 463–482.

59 Woolcock, P.R., McFarland, M.D., Lai, S. et al. (2001). Enhanced recovery of influenza virus isolates by a combination of chicken embryo inoculation methods. *Avian Dis.* 45: 1030–1035.

60 Fedynich, A.M. (2008). *Heterakis* and *Ascaridia*. In: *Parasitic Diseases of Wild Birds* (eds. C.T. Atkinson, N.J. Tomas and D.B. Hinter), 388–412. Ames, IA: Wiley-Blackwell.

61 Griner, L.A., Migaki, G., Penner, L.R. et al. (1977). Heterakidosis and nodular granulomas caused by *Heterakis* isolonche in the ceca of gallinaceous birds. *Vet. Pathol.* 14: 582–590.

62 Spiegle, S.J, Ison, A.J. and Morishita, T.Y. (2004). Performing a physical exam on a Chicken. In: *Poultry Health Resources* (ed. T.Y.Morishita), Factsheet 2019–10. Pomona, CA: Western University.

63 Schat, K.A. (1985). Characteristics of the virus. In: *Marek's Disease* (ed. L.N. Payne), 77–112. Boston: Martinus Nijhoff.

64 Sharma, J.M. (1991). Current status of Marek's disease in the field. In: *Proceedings of Avian Tumor Virus Symposium*, 26–33. Seattle, WA: American Association of Avian Pathologists.

65 Boodhoo, N., Gurung, A., Sharif, S. et al. (2016). Marek's disease in chickens: a review with focus on immunology. *Vet Res.* 28; 47 (1):1–19.

66 Witter, R.L. (1985). Principles of vaccination. In: *Marek's Disease* (ed. L.N. Payne), 203–250. Boston: Martinus Nijhoff.

67 Purchase, H.G. (1987). The pathogenesis and pathology of neoplasms caused by avian leukosis viruses. In: *Avian Leukosis* (ed. G.F. de Boer), 171–196. Boston, MA: Martinus Nijhoff.

68 Doughtery, R.M. and DiStifano, H.S. (1967). Sites of avian leucosis virus multiplication in congenitally infected chickens. *Cancer Res.* 27: 322–332.

69 Gavora, J.S., Spencer, J.L., and Chambers, J.R. (1982). Performance of meat-type chickens test-positive and – negative for lymphoid leucosis virus infection. *Avian Pathol.* 11: 29–38.

70 Spencer, J.L., Gilka, F., Gavora, J.S. et al. (1984). Distribution of group specific antigen of lymphoid leucosis virus in tissues from laying hens. *Avian Dis.* 28: 358–373.

71 Gross, W.G. (1994). Diseases due to *Escherichia coli* in poultry. In: *Escherichia coli in Domestic Animals and Humans* (ed. C.L. Gayles), 237–259. Tucson, AZ: CAB International.

72 Morishita, T.Y. (1994). *Respiratory syndromes in backyard poultry*. In: *Association of Avian Veterinarians Annual Conference* (Reno, Nevada, 28–30 September 1994), 35–44. (Core Seminar Proceedings).

73 Morishita, T.Y. (2010). *Enterococcosis*. In: *The Merck Veterinary Manual*, 10e, 2419–2420. Whitehouse Station, NJ: Merck & Company, Inc.

74 Morishita, T.Y. (2010). Staphylococcosis. In: *The Merck Veterinary Manual*, 10e, 2466. Whitehouse Station, NJ: Merck & Company, Inc.

75 Morishita, T.Y. (2010). Streptococcosis. In: *The Merck Veterinary Manual*, 10e, 2468. Whitehouse Station, New Jersey: Merck & Company, Inc.

76 Nakamura, K., Maeda, M., Imada, Y. et al. (1985). Pathology of spontaneous colibacillosis in a broiler flock. *Vet. Pathol.* 22: 592–597.

77 Morishita, T.Y. and Bickford, A.A. (1992). Pyogranulomatous typhlitis and hepatitis in market turkeys. *Avian Dis.* 36: 170–175.

78 Davis, M.F., Ebako, G.M., and Morishita, T.Y. (2003). A Golden comet hen (Gallus gallus forma domestica) with an impacted oviduct and associated colibacillosis. *J. Avian Med. Surg.* 17: 91–95.

79 Morishita, T.Y. (1996). Common infectious diseases in backyard chickens and turkeys (from a private practice perspective). *J. Avian Med. Surg.* 10 (1): 2–11.

80 Morishita, T.Y. (1995). Common reproductive problems in the backyard chicken. In: *Section 11: Topics in Clinical Medicine, Main Conference Proceedings, Association of Avian Veterinarians Annual Conference, Philadelphia, Pennsylvania*, 465–467.

81 Johnson, L.C., Bilgili, S.F., Hoerr, F.J. et al. (2001). The influence of *Escherichia coli* strains from different sources and the age of broiler chickens on the development of cellulitis. *Avian Pathol.* 30: 475–479.

82 Siller, W.G. (1981). Renal pathology of the fowl-a review. *Avian Pathol.* 10: 187–262.

83 Chandra, M. (1985). Occurrence and pathology of nephritis in poultry. *Acta-Vet.* 35: 319–328.

84 Stevens, V.I. and Salmon, R.E. (1989). Effect of chronic acid load as excess dietary protein, ammonium chloride, sulfur amino acid or inorganic sulfate on the incidence of leg problems in turkeys. *Nutr. Rep. Int.* 48: 477–485.

85 Morishita, T.Y. (1997). *Doctoring the fowl patient*. In: *113th Annual Convention, Ohio Veterinary Medical Association, Annual Conference Proceedings*, Hyatt Regency, Columbus, Ohio (20–23 February, 1997), vol. 4, 319–321.

86 McDougald, L.R. (2000). New developments in research on black head disease in chickens. *World Poultry*, (Supplement) 8: 1–3.

87 Lee, D.L. (1969). The structure and development of *Histomonas meleagridis* in the female reproductive tract of its intermediate host, *Heterakis gallinarum* (Nematoda). *Parasitology* 59: 877–884.

88 Gibbs, B.J. (1962). The occurrence of the protozoan parasite *Histomonas meleagridis* in the adults and eggs of the cecal worm *Heterakis gallinae*. *J. Protozool.* 9: 288–293.

89 Clarkson, M.J. (1962). The progressive pathology of *Heterakis*-produced histomonasis in turkeys. *Res. Vet. Sci.* 3: 443–449.

90 Butler, E.J. (1976). Fatty liver disease in the domestic fowl. A review. *Avian Pathol.* 5: 1–14.

91 Klasing, K.C. and Korver, D.R. (2020). Nutritional diseases. In *Diseases of Poultry*, 14e (eds. D.E. Swayne, M. Boulianne, L.R. McDougald, et al.), 1257–1285. Ames, IA: Wiley Blackwell.

18

Cardiovascular Diseases

Hugues Beaufrère[1] and Marina Brash[2]

[1] Department of Clinical Studies, Ontario Veterinary College, University of Guelph, Guelph, ON, Canada
[2] Animal Health Laboratory, University of Guelph, Guelph, ON, Canada

Diagnosing Cardiovascular Diseases in Backyard Poultry

General Considerations

There are a number of differences between the avian and the mammalian heart, some of which have clinical implications in the pathophysiology and diagnosis of poultry cardiovascular diseases [1] (Table 18.1).

The avian cardiovascular system is highly efficient but commercial poultry have been intensely selected for increased growth and production, and the high energy and oxygen demand to even meet the basal metabolic requirements may be close to its physiological maximum [2–4]. Selection for fast growth and heavy birds has also introduced developmental abnormalities in cardiac tissue and mismatching between body mass and heart mass [5]. Consequently, heavy meat-type galliformes (turkeys and broilers) do not thermoregulate well and readily experience periods of dyspnea and tachycardia with mild stress and exercise and are far more susceptible to cardiovascular diseases than other species and breeds. In fact, a high number of these kinds of birds have subclinical cardiac disease [3]. Furthermore, already compromised animals may collapse easily during examination and restraint. They may also be poor anesthetic candidates and preoxygenation and preliminary therapy (abdominocentesis and/or diuretics) are recommended before diagnostic procedures can be considered. In broilers and turkeys, cardiovascular diseases may be the most common cause of mortality [6]. In backyard poultry flocks raised for meat, cardiovascular diseases such as ascites syndrome may still be encountered in small flocks of broilers and other chicken breeds because most are genetically related to commercial broilers of the White Plymouth Rock breed. However, cardiac disease tends to be relatively rare in backyard poultry flocks [7]. A recent two year small flock disease surveillance project conducted at the Animal Health Laboratory (AHL), University of Guelph, Guelph, Ontario, produced similar results with 2.45% of primary diagnoses involving the cardiovascular system [8, 9].

In addition to general signs of disease, specific clinical signs of cardiovascular diseases include dyspnea, exercise intolerance, cyanosis or hypoperfusion (bluish or pale comb, wattles, ricti, or periorbital skin, and increased

Backyard Poultry Medicine and Surgery: A Guide for Veterinary Practitioners, Second Edition.
Edited by Cheryl B. Greenacre and Teresa Y. Morishita.
© 2021 John Wiley & Sons, Inc. Published 2021 by John Wiley & Sons, Inc.
Companion website: www.wiley.com/go/greenacre/medicine

Table 18.1 Some avian cardiovascular anatomical and physiological peculiarities which differ from mammals.

Avian cardiovascular system peculiarities
Muscular unicuspid right AV valve
No chordae tendinae in the right AV valve
Tricuspid (poorly defined) left AV valve
Muscular ring around aortic valve
Negative cardiac mean electrical axis (except broilers, Pekin ducks)
Ring of Purkinje fibers around aorta and right AV valve
Depolarization of epicardium precedes endocardium
Higher heart rate, arterial blood pressure, cardiac output
Larger heart
Smaller cardiac muscle fibers
Absence of T-tubules in cardiac myocytes
Absence of M-bands connecting myosin filaments
Ascending aorta on the right
Two cranial vena cava
Brachiocephalic arteries larger than aorta
Cartilage/ossification at base of aorta
No cerebral arterial circle of Willis
Renal portal system

AV: atrioventricular.

comb capillary or ulnar vein refilling time), ascites, syncope, collapse, and sudden death. Cardiac auscultation may reveal muffled heart sounds, murmurs, or rhythm abnormalities but is usually not as rewarding in birds as it is in mammals because of their rapid heart rate. Normal heart rates are listed in Table 18.2. Arterial catheterization for direct blood pressure measurement is challenging in poultry because of their relatively atrophied wings. However, indirect blood pressure measurement using a Doppler unit, while inaccurate in small to medium sized birds, seems more reliable in larger birds but may be closer to the mean rather than to the systolic arterial blood pressure [16]. Observing trends in indirect blood pressure may be useful.

Laboratory Ancillary Diagnostics

Apart from assessing the general health of the backyard poultry patient, clinical pathology tests may reveal specific changes associated with cardiovascular diseases. Erythrocytosis, described as a packed cell volume (PCV) greater than 35% (note: the PCV is lower in poultry than in other birds), may be caused by chronic hypoxia resulting from persistent ventilatory-perfusion mismatching (e.g. congenital cardiac malformation, ascites syndrome, pulmonary pathology) and increased oxygen demands (e.g. ascites syndrome). Leukocytosis may be seen in bacterial myocarditis and valvular endocarditis. Cardiovascular microfilariae may be observed on the blood smear. Poultry are large enough for arterial blood samples and blood gas analyses may help pinpoint an oxygenation problem. Myocardial damage can lead to a rise in creatinine kinase (CK) (and cardiac CK isoenzyme) and cardiac troponin T (only 68% sequence homology with humans which may affect diagnostic tests accuracy). Electrolyte disorders (Ca, Mg, K, Na), hypoproteinemia, and hyperuricemia can also cause arrhythmia and cardiac diseases. Bile acids are frequently elevated with hepatic congestion secondary to congestive heart failure. Lipoprotein abnormalities may also be diagnosed in conjunction with some degenerative lesions but have to be interpreted in the context of the egg-laying cycle and the genetic selection lines [15]. Finally, ascitic and effusion fluid should always be analyzed and can provide useful information. Cardiac-induced ascitic (coelomic) fluid is a pure or modified transudate, thus having low protein and cellular content and a low specific gravity. Blood culture may be valuable to isolate causative agents of cardiac bacterial infections and can be performed with only 0.5–2 ml of blood.

Electrocardiography

Electrocardiography (ECG) is invaluable to investigate conduction disorders and arrhythmia. The avian ECG is typically obtained by

Table 18.2 Published reference intervals for selected electrocardiographic parameters in different backyard poultry species on lead II.

Species	Chicken [10] (white leghorn)	Chicken [11] (broilers)	Turkeys [12]	Chukar partridge [13]	Pekin duck [14]	Guineafowl [15]
n	72	300	50	10	50	8
Age	6 mo	4–5 wk	20 wk	Mature	12–18 mo	6–12 mo
Anesthesia	None	Isoflurane	None	None	None	None
Heart rate (bpm)	180–340	270–450	146–266	200–435	200–360	300–376
Mean electrical axis (°)	Negative −(91 to 120)	Mainly positive 0–180	Negative −(75 to 120)	Negative −(60 to 139)	Mainly positive −160 to +95 (mean: +147)	Negative −(12 to 108)
P duration	0.035–0.046		0.021–0.061	0.006–0.034	0.015–0.035	
R amplitude			−0.305 to 0.279			
PR interval	0.073–0.089		0.054–0.122		0.04–0.08	0.024–0.056
QRS duration	0.02–0.028	22.8–48.4	0.038–0.066	0.019–0.021	0.028–0.044	0.03–0.05
(Q)rS amplitude	Females: 0.10–0.33 Males: 0.795 (mean)	−0.96 to +0.78	0.276–3.736	0.26–0.94	0.35–1.03	−0.17 to 0.39
ST interval	0.119–0.149			0.106–0.138		0.018–0.042
T amplitude	Females: 0.03–0.19 Males: 0.255 (mean)		0.1–0.65	0–0.38	0.04–0.40	0.15–0.41
QT interval			0.142–0.198	0.106–0.138	0.08–0.12	0.106–0.134
T duration	0.119–0.145				0.03–0.07	

Note: To obtain a 95% interval, all published results in the form of mean ± SD were reported as mean ± 2SD and in the form of mean ± sem were reported as mean ± 2sem √n, when only the range was published, it was reported as is. Values are in seconds for wave and intervals duration, and mV for amplitudes. n = number of birds examined.
Source: [10–15].

placing two cranial electrodes on each propatagium and one (left) or two caudal electrodes on the knee web, just cranial to the legs, using needles or clips. Each lead evaluates the cardiac electrical activity on a different plane and a standard examination classically includes three bipolar leads (I, II, and III) and three augmented unipolar leads (aVR, aVL, aVF). Recordings need to be performed at a minimum speed of 100 mm/s to better assess the morphology of the QRS complexes. In contrast to mammals, the cardiac mean electrical axis is usually negative in birds, which gives negative QRS complexes on lead II (Figure 18.1). In broilers and Pekin ducks, however, the mean electrical axis is most commonly positive [11, 13]. The mean electrical axis is affected by changes in heart position and relative dilation of cardiac chambers and is one of the most commonly modified parameters identified on the ECG with common poultry cardiac diseases. A T_a wave

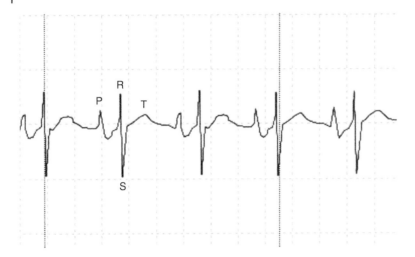

Figure 18.1 ECG from a normal chicken in lead II. Note the typical negative QRS complex.

(auricular T wave related to atrial repolarization) is normal in some species [18]. The Q wave is absent in chickens, small in turkeys, and prominent in Pekin ducks [1, 10, 12, 14]. In lead II, the QRS complex often shows a prominent S wave and a small R wave. This differs from mammals, in which the R wave is usually more prominent [19]. Normal variations of the QRS complex, however, have been documented in chickens, especially in broilers [11]. In addition, the P and T waves are often fused [19]. Measurements are normally performed on lead II and reference values have been determined for some poultry species [10–15, 20–22]. (Table 18.2). Interpretation of the ECG should be methodical and include an evaluation of the heart rate, cardiac rhythm, mean electrical axis, and measurements. The reader is referred to more exhaustive references for further information on avian ECG [18, 23]. Anesthesia and stress may induce alterations of the normal ECG such as atrioventricular (AV) blocks and sinus tachycardia or bradycardia. Broilers have a normally high prevalence of arrhythmias especially under anesthesia [24]. Common ECG abnormalities in chickens include mean QRS axis deviation, ventricular premature contractions, and AV blocks.

Diagnostic Imaging

Whole-body or thoracic radiographs (large galliforme and anseriforme species) are useful for a preliminary assessment of cardiovascular diseases. However, no reference intervals for cardiac radiographic measurements are available in commonly seen poultry species. Radiographic signs that may be observed in cardiovascular diseases include an enlarged cardiac silhouette (cardiomegaly or pericardial effusion), an enlarged hepatic silhouette (hepatic congestion), pulmonary edema, and a decrease in coelomic details and airsac space (ascites). Angiocardiography using radiography, fluoroscopy, or computed tomography (CT) scan may be of value to diagnose cardiomegaly or vascular abnormalities (e.g. aneurysms) and can be performed with an injection of 2–3 ml/kg of intravenous contrast (e.g. iohexol) over three seconds [25, 26]. Diagnostic imaging procedures should be started immediately or a few seconds after the injection to obtain high concentration of contrast in blood during radiographic exposure. Coelioscopy through the left or right thoracic approach, or interclavicular approach may be performed to identify pericardial diseases. However, endoscopic procedures are more challenging in chickens than in other birds as a result of the reduced airspace present, the heavy muscles, the degree of subcutaneous and abdominal fat, the size of the liver, and the potential presence of developing ovarian follicles on the left.

Echocardiography is the diagnostic imaging method of choice for assessing the cardiovascular function in birds and the procedure in chickens presents certain peculiarities. Cardiac chamber dimensions, myocardial contractility, and hemodynamic function can be evaluated in a non-invasive manner with a cardiac ultrasound examination, which does not require anesthesia in most cases. As in other birds, a 7.5 MHz or higher frequency probe with a microcurved or small straight transducer is appropriate in most cases. Sonographic windows are limited in birds because of the extensive airsac system surrounding cardiovascular structures, the fact that the heart lies in a ventral indentation of the keel bone, the high heart rate of birds, and the relatively small size of the imaged structures. While only the ventromedial transcoelomic sonographic approach can be performed in most raptors and parrots, an additional transcoelomic approach, the parasternal approach, can be used in galliformes either caudally to the ribs, because the ribs have limited caudal extension, or between the sternal ribs through the large window of the sternum present in poultry, but the optimal approach is not always consistent and depends on individuals, age, and breeds [25, 27, 28]. These two approaches allow a more complete echocardiographic examination in chickens than in most other avian species with the possibilities of performing unidimensional M-mode for assessing ventricular contractility (Figure 18.2), two-dimensional B-mode for evaluating chamber dimensions in longitudinal and transverse views, spectral Doppler for flow velocities, and color flow Doppler for the detection of valvular insufficiency. The most commonly used approach in chickens and turkeys is the parasternal

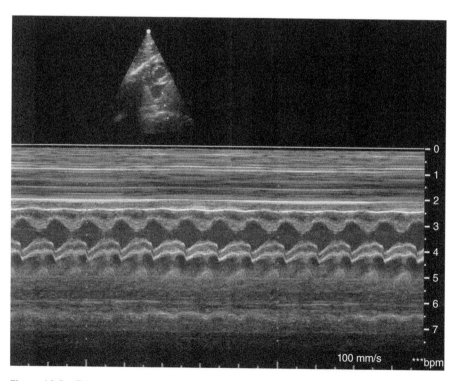

Figure 18.2 Echocardiogram in M-mode through a parasternal approach showing chicken left ventricle.

approach. The probe is positioned either in front of the stifle joint on either side of the thorax with the bird standing (intercostal approach) or behind the pelvic limb and the last rib, again with the bird standing, and the probe angled cranially [28–30] (Figure 18.3). For the ventromedial approach, the probe is placed on the midline behind the caudal border of the keel and angled cranially dorsal to the keel. The heart is imaged through the liver, which is used as an acoustic window [23, 25]. Echocardiographic

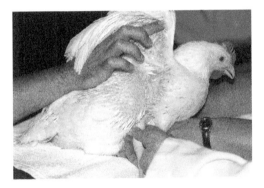

Figure 18.3 Performing an echocardiogram in a chicken showing the parasternal approach.

reference values have been produced through the parasternal approach and fast-growing chickens have smaller cardiac measurements than slow-growing chickens relative to their body weight [28, 31, 32] (Table 18.3). There are no echocardiographic studies or report or reference intervals for echocardiographic parameters in the various breeds commonly seen as backyard poultry [7]. It is also noteworthy that most reference values have been obtained from birds younger than two to three months and limited information is available for older birds. Nevertheless, the evaluation of the relative sizes of the cardiac chamber and their functional assessment is probably more clinically useful than taking echocardiographic morphometric measurements, which appear to show low reliability in birds [33]. No standardized echocardiographic examination with a clear description of the different views have been described in chickens but the classically obtained views include transverse views (short axis two-chamber views) at the level of the ventricles and a longitudinal view (long axis four-chamber view) through the parasternal approach, and a longitudinal

Table 18.3 Published reference intervals (in centimeters) for selected echocardiographic parameters in different backyard poultry species using a parasternal approach.

Species	Broiler chicken [30, 32]	Leghorn chicken [38, 30]	Turkey [29]
n	30	5	34
Age	6 wk	7 wk	4 wk
Anesthesia	None	None	None
LVDS	0.17–1.27	0.22–0.30	0.01–0.54
LVDD	0.81–1.25	0.63–0.71	0.44–1.05
FS-LV (%)		32.6–54	37–93
RVDS	0.06–0.50		
RVDD	0.00–0.97		
IVSD	0.25–0.69	0.17–0.35	0.14–0.38

LVDS: left ventricular diameter in systole; LVDD: left ventricular diameter in diastole; FS-LV: fractional shortening of left ventricle; RVDS: right ventricular diameter in systole; RVDD: right ventricular diameter in diastole; IVSD: interventricular septum width in diastole.

Note: To obtain a 95% interval, all published results in the form of mean $\pm$ SD were reported as mean $\pm$ 2SD and in the form of mean $\pm$ sem were reported as mean $\pm$ 2sem $\sqrt{n}$, when only the range was published, it was reported as is. n = number of birds examined.

Source: [28–30, 32].

horizontal (four-chamber) (Figure 18.4) and a vertical (two-chamber) (Figure 18.5) view through the ventromedian approach. The echocardiographic examination is more easily performed, and the views obtained are of better resolution, in birds with cardiac disease because the presence of coelomic fluid and hepatic congestion provides better acoustic windows. In anseriformes, the transcoelomic ventromedian

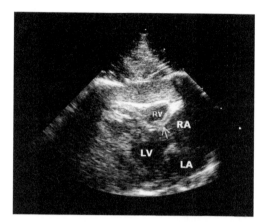

Figure 18.4 Echocardiogram of chicken showing the long axis view. LV, left ventricle; RV, right ventricle; LA, left atrium; RA, right atrium; arrow: right atrioventricular valve.

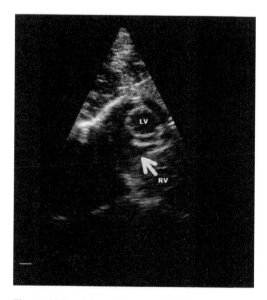

Figure 18.5 Echocardiogram of chicken showing the short axis view. LV, left ventricle; RV and arrow, right ventricle.

approach is typically used [34]. Transesophageal echocardiography uses a small transducer at the tip of a long flexible tube and consists of imaging the heart from inside the proventriculus and esophagus [35]. The examination must be performed under anesthesia and has overall a superior resolution than transcoelomic techniques but the equipment is expensive and not widely available. Chickens, turkeys, and ducks are easily imaged using this technique as they are large birds.

Therapeutics

The use of drugs in poultry is controversial as only a few first-generation medications are legally approved and withdrawal times are not determined for many therapeutic agents. Furthermore, legislation regarding antimicrobial use in poultry being raised for meat or eggs for human consumption may vary according to country so it is important to understand the regulations of the country where the poultry are being raised. In some countries, veterinarians prescribing extra-label drugs for poultry can access or are required to provide withdrawal interval recommendations based on information contained in the global Food Animal Residue Avoidance Database (gFARAD). In addition, there is increased recognition of the need to use antimicrobials designated critically or highly important to human medicine cautiously in poultry because of development and transfer of resistance among bacteria. Specific cardiac medications are probably less problematic and medical treatment may not be practical with the exception of valuable or companion poultry patients, that are not being raised for the production of meat or eggs. Draining of ascitic or pericardial fluid is recommended to alleviate signs of dyspnea or cardiac tamponade. Drug dosages for selected cardiovascular therapeutics in birds are shown in Table 18.4 [36]. Veterinarians should focus more on prevention, management, and breed selection to limit cardiovascular diseases that are only prevalent in fast-growing and heavy

Table 18.4 Selected cardiovascular drugs in poultry.

Drug	Dose	Comments
Furosemide	2.5 mg/kg IM 5 mg/kg PO 0.015% in food	Loop diuretic
Spironolactone	1 mg/kg PO	Diuretic, aldosterone receptor antagonist
Enalapril	1–5 mg/kg	Angiotensin conversion enzyme inhibitor
Digoxin	0.004–0.02 mg/kg PO q24h	Digitalic, inotrope
Pimobendan	0.25–0.5 mg/kg	Phosphodiesterase inhibitor, inotrope
Atenolol	25 ppm in food 10–30 mg/kg PO q24h (Turkey)	β-blocker
Propranolol	0.1–0.2 mg/kg	β-blocker
Diltiazem	15 mg/kg PO q12h	Calcium channel blocker
Lidocaine	2.6–6 mg/kg IV	Antiarrhytmic, short half-life
Atorvastatin	5–10 mg/kg PO q12h	Statin, lipid lowering agent

Note: Dosages are based on pharmacodynamic studies (but not pharmacokinetic) in chickens and turkeys [34]. Some dosages are empirical or based on other avian species. Therapeutic plasma levels monitoring is recommended for valuable or companion poultry birds.

birds. Educate owners regarding the importance of not breeding birds with genetic forms of cardiac disease.

Common Cardiovascular Diseases of Backyard Poultry

Dilated Cardiomyopathy in Turkeys

Clinical History
Also known as round heart disease or spontaneous cardiomyopathy of turkeys, it is most commonly encountered in 1–4-week-old turkeys and usually peaks at two weeks. The prevalence is typically 0.5–3% in commercial turkey flocks but can be higher [37]. Young fast-growing males are more susceptible. While rare, the disease has also been described in wild turkeys [38].

Causative Agent
The exact cause of the disease is unknown in turkeys. It has been demonstrated that some of these turkeys show an abnormal troponin T structure and dysregulation of some cardiac enzymatic pathways. Some toxic compounds such as furazolidone and antitrypsin

may also have been implicated in some cases [37, 39]. Genetic factors, previous myocarditis, hypoxia during incubation, and other environmental and dietary factors have also been proposed to play a role in the etiology [39–41].

Clinical Signs and Lesions
In many cases, affected birds die suddenly. They may also show abdominal distension resulting from ascites, respiratory signs, other signs of congestive heart failure, and non-specific signs such as listlessness, lethargy, ruffled feathers, and impaired growth. Gross lesions include cardiomegaly, which is caused by dilation of both ventricles, congested and edematous lungs, congested liver, hypertrophic left ventricle (in older animals), ascites, and hydropericardium [40]. Right ventricular dilation may be the only observable gross lesions in early cases. Histopathologic lesions include degeneration of myocardial myofibers with vacuolation, secondary endocardiosis, focal infiltration of lymphocytes, and secondary hepatic changes associated with heart failure [40, 42].

Transmission Route
Not applicable.

Diagnostic Tests
The combination of clinical signs, age, and fast-growing types of turkeys should raise a strong suspicion of dilated cardiomyopathy. Radiographs show an enlargement of the cardio or cardiohepatic silhouette and organomegaly or ascites as a result of passive congestion. On the ECG, the following changes, associated with dilation and hypertrophy of the ventricles, can be identified: Increased R wave amplitude, negative T wave, and rotation of the mean electrical axis [19, 43]. Reports of the use of cardiac ultrasound have been limited in turkeys. Dilation of the cardiac chambers (more than double in chamber measurements), reduced ventricular fractional shortening (to 14%), pericardial effusion, and ascites can be expected on echocardiography [29].

Differential Diagnosis
Other causes of congestive heart failure, congenital cardiac abnormalities, restrictive cardiomyopathy, valvular insufficiency.

Prevention and Control
Slowing the growth rate of susceptible lines by dietary manipulation and avoiding hypoxic condition in pre- and post-hatching periods may reduce the incidence of the disease [6, 40].

Zoonotic Potential
Not applicable.

Ascites(Coelomic Fluid)/Pulmonary Hypertension Syndrome in Broilers

Clinical History
This syndrome is one of the most common causes of mortality in commercial flocks of broilers, with an average prevalence of approximately 4.7%, which can go as high as 15–20% in certain roaster chicken flocks [6, 38, 40]. The condition can be exacerbated by rearing at high altitude and additional genetic and environmental factors (intensive rearing, fluctuating temperatures, too cold or too hot temperatures, activity, hypoxia during incubation, ventilation, electrolytes

supplementation) may promote its occurrence [3]. Affected chickens are usually younger and males seem to be more susceptible. The disease is expected to be less common in backyard flocks but may occur if meat-type poultry are raised (broilers and related breeds).

Causative Agent
This metabolic disease is associated with growth and production and has increased in frequency with selection for a higher and faster muscle mass production and different body conformation. The ascites is caused by right-heart congestive heart failure and valvular insufficiency. The physiopathogenesis is associated with an increased workload of the heart and oxygen demand coupled with an overall insufficient pulmonary capillary capacity and decreased respiratory efficiency in chickens compared to other birds. This quickly leads to pulmonary hypertension, which in turns leads to right ventricular hypertrophy and ultimately to dilation. With the dilatory changes affecting the right ventricle, the right atrioventricular valve, which extends from its wall, develops insufficiency, which in turns increases the preload and leads to systemic congestion and ascites by increased hydrostatic pressure. Some researchers also argue that left-heart dysfunction plays a major role in the pathogenesis and that chronic hypoxemia and pulmonary hypertension are secondary to chronic left heart failure. In addition, the elevated PCV triggered by the chronic hypoxia may increase blood viscosity and increase the resistance to the flow [3, 4, 6, 41, 43]. Hypoxia and increased metabolic rate are the two most important factors that influence the development of this condition [45].

Clinical Signs and Lesions
Birds present with impaired growth and lethargy. Specific signs may include coelomic distension caused by ascites, dyspnea, cyanosis, pale comb, and acute death (Figure 18.6). Some birds can die from pulmonary edema caused by pulmonary hypertension. Gross lesions may include dilated and hypertrophic right ventricle, ascites, pericardial effusion, pericardial thickening, organ congestion, dilation of pulmonary

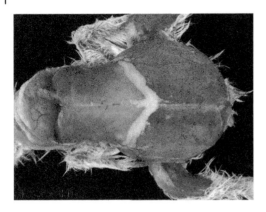

Figure 18.6 Gross necropsy of ascites syndrome in a broiler. *Source:* Photo courtesy of Dr. Oscar J. Fletcher, North Carolina State University.

veins, and a shrunken, fibrotic liver when chronic [6, 39–41]. Ascitic (coelomic) fluid is typically clear yellow but can also be cloudy with gelatinous or fibrin clots. In advanced cases, histologic lesions other than associated with systemic congestion include myocardial myofiber degeneration with swelling, focal necrosis, edema, and fibrosis [42].

Transmission Route
Not applicable.

Diagnostic Tests
A loss of abdominal detail and an enlarged cardiac and/or cardiohepatic silhouette are present on radiographs. Coelomic fluid analysis is consistent with a pure or modified transudate but can still show clots of fibrin and proteins because of associated chronic coelomitis. On ECG, the heart rate is usually decreased and there may be an increase in S-wave amplitude and ventricular fibrillation associated with right-heart dilation and a right deviation of the mean electrical axis (which becomes negative) [9, 19, 44, 46]. These chickens consistently show an increased PCV and serum troponin T level is elevated (normal is <0.50 ng/ml, n = 20, age one to two months) [44, 47, 48]. Echocardiographic findings include right and left atrioventricular valves regurgitation, reduction in fractional shortening of the left ventricle, dilation of cardiac chambers, and pericardial effusion [30, 32].

Differential Diagnosis
Other causes of ascites in chickens: Vascular damage (toxins, nutritional deficiencies), blockage of lymph drainage (ovarian adenocarcinoma), increased vascular pressure (portal hypertension resulting from advanced hepatic disease), hypoproteinemia, congenital abnormalities, sodium toxicosis, and other causes of right-sided and bilateral cardiac failure (valvular endocarditis, congenital cardiac abnormality, atherosclerosis, toxic, dilated cardiomyopathy, restrictive cardiopathy). Other causes of coelomitis can induce production of coelomic fluids as well.

Prevention and Control
Genetic factors increase bird susceptibility and selection against this syndrome may be useful [3, 49]. The prevalence of the disease can be lowered by decreasing growth rate [50], restricting food intake, modifying food type (pelletized diet seems to increase feed efficiency and then metabolic demand) [51], and minimizing sources of decreasing oxygen availability (fluctuating temperatures, too low or too high temperatures, altitude [above 1500 m is inappropriate for meat-type chickens], concomitant respiratory diseases such as fungal pneumonia) and minimize the use of electrolyte supplements [6, 39, 40]. As a result of the low individual value of broilers, treatment has rarely been reported but, experimentally, furosemide has been shown to reduce mortality and L-arginine supplementation appears to reduce the incidence of the disease [52, 53]. Treatment with β2-agonists may reduce the ventilatory-perfusion mismatch by inducing bronchodilation, hence reducing mortality [44]. The use of L-carnitine, antioxidants, and omega-3 fatty acids have been mentioned to reduce the incidence of ascites but scientific evidence is either lacking or inconclusive [3, 54]. However, it must be kept in mind that pharmacologic interventions may have limited results as the disease is associated with high metabolic demand in birds with poor cardiovascular and respiratory efficiency.

Zoonotic Potential
Not applicable.

Editor's Vignette (CBG)

An approximately six-month-old White Leghorn broiler chicken presented with a sudden onset of dyspnea, lethargy, and exercise intolerance. A physical examination identified a mildly thin bird, with severe coelomic distension due to coelomic fluid and a Grade III/VI heart murmur. Approximately 200 ml of coelomic fluid (about one fourth to one third of the fluid present) was removed by coelomocentesis. Dilated cardiomyopathy was diagnosed based on echocardiogram. Treatment with digoxin (this was before the advent of pimobendan), enalapril, and furosemide improved respirations and myocardial contractility, and decreased coelomic distension dramatically. Later, the bird required the addition of the potassium-sparing drug spironolactone. With periodic rechecks, including recheck echocardiograms, and minor adjustments in medications, this bird went on to live to eight years of age despite our initial grave prognosis. This outcome is not typical.

Aortic Rupture/Dissecting Aneurysm in Turkeys

Clinical History

The disease is mostly encountered in growing turkeys of 7–24 weeks of age and primarily affects males [40]. Mortality is approximately 1–2% in commercial turkey flocks but has been as high as 50% in the past.

Causative Agent

As with most poultry cardiovascular diseases, the exact cause of aortic dissecting aneurysm is uncertain. Systemic hypertension (common in meat-type turkeys, especially young males), atherosclerosis, absence of *vasa vasorum* in the abdominal aorta, genetic factors, connective tissues disorders, peas in the ration (peas' toxin β-aminopropionitrile causes aortic rupture experimentally by interference with collagen formation), and dietary deficiencies, notably in copper (also demonstrated in ratites) may contribute to the pathogenesis [6, 39, 40]. Hypertension is thought to be the most significant risk factor.

Clinical Signs and Lesions

Turkeys usually die acutely from severe internal hemorrhage. On necropsy, the head, skin, and muscles appear anemic, blood may be noticed in the mouth, and massive hemorrhage, coagulated blood is found in the intestinoperitoneal cavity, and the aorta is torn longitudinally between the external iliac and ischiatic arteries [40, 41]. Less commonly, the rupture may occur in the ascending and "thoracic aorta" with blood present around the heart (hemopericardium) (Figure 18.7). Histologically, there may be a separation of the tunica intima and media from the adventitia with the presence of folds, degenerative changes in the media, and inflammatory cells infiltration. Intimal thickening, a fibrous intimal plaque, and disintegration of elastic laminae may be observed at the rupture site [40].

Transmission Route

Not applicable.

Diagnostic Tests

An aneurysm, if large enough, should be expected to be identified on angiography but antemortem diagnosis has not been reported

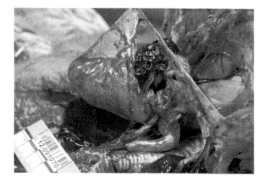

Figure 18.7 Gross necropsy of turkey with atrial rupture. The pericardial sac was distended with hemorrhage (hemopericardium). *Source:* Photo courtesy of Ms. Megan MacAlpine, University of Guelph.

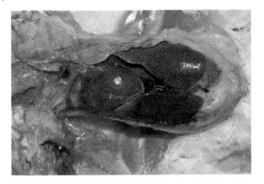

Figure 18.8 Hemopericardium and lacerated liver with coelomic hemorrhage in a chicken that sustained a keel bone fracture.

because of the low individual value of meat-type turkeys. Turkeys are large birds; therefore indirect blood measurement using a Doppler unit is expected to be more reliable than in smaller birds and may help pinpoint a hypertensive problem.

Differential Diagnosis
Sudden death syndrome of turkeys, acute presentation of spontaneous dilated cardiomyopathy, other causes of hemopericardium i.e. secondary to trauma (Figure 18.8).

Prevention and Control
Minimizing stress and excitement and slowing growth in susceptible birds may reduce the incidence of the disease. Treatments are uncommonly reported but reserpine, an antihypertensive drug, and propranolol may have favorable preventative effects in susceptible birds [55, 56].

Zoonotic Potential
Not applicable.

Sudden Death Syndrome of Broilers

Clinical History
Broiler chickens of one to eight weeks of age, mainly males (about 70% of cases), are affected. The prevalence depends on genetic, environmental, and dietary conditions and approximates to 0.5–4% [39, 40, 57].

Causative Agent
The cause is unknown but is thought to be associated with ventricular fibrillation and tachycardia as a result of electrolytic or other metabolic imbalances. Recent investigations have shown a possible link with changes in intracellular calcium as a result of genetic mutations [58].

Clinical Signs and Lesions
As the name implies, birds die acutely with no premonitory signs and exhibit a short violent wing-flapping seizure at time of death. The disease is also termed flip-over disease because dead birds are frequently found on their back. Birds are in good body condition at necropsy and no specific lesions are seen but edematous lungs, enlarged liver, and contracted heart ventricles are common findings. There is typically food in crop, gizzard, and atonic intestinal tract suggesting birds had been eating prior to death. Histopathologic lesions are not specific [40, 57].

Transmission Route
Not applicable.

Diagnostic Tests
As a result of the acuteness of the disease and the unknown etiology, the identification of birds at risk may not be possible. Birds dying of sudden death syndrome show ventricular fibrillation on electrocardiogram [19].

Differential Diagnosis
Sudden death from pulmonary hypertension syndrome, rupture of right atrium, heart defects, and other non-cardiac causes (e.g. fatty liver hemorrhagic syndrome).

Prevention and Control
Feed restriction and other nutritional modifications (mash, lower caloric density, implementation of lighting programs slowing growth) may lower the incidence. Stress, bright light, and overcrowding should be limited [40, 57].

Zoonotic Potential
Not applicable.

Sudden Death Syndrome of Turkeys

Clinical History
Heavy meat-type turkeys are mainly affected by this syndrome and almost exclusively males are susceptible. The disease is common in turkeys of 8–15 weeks of age. Mortality is usually around 0.8–1.8% but can reach 6–10% [40, 41].

Causative Agent
As in most poultry cardiovascular diseases, the etiology lies in the intense selection for meat production and the cardiovascular system of turkeys may not be able to meet the extra demand induced by exercise, stress, and other environmental factors, leading to hypotension, lactic acidosis, circulatory shock, and death. Systemic hypertension and hypertrophic cardiomyopathy also appear to play a role in this syndrome [39, 41].

Clinical Signs and Lesions
As in chicken broilers, there are no premonitory signs and birds usually die following a brief wing-flapping period. Gross lesions are consistent with generalized passive congestion and perirenal hemorrhage (other name of the disease) and birds are generally in good condition. The left ventricle and interventricular septum are often hypertrophied. Contrary to a ruptured aneurysm, free blood is usually not found in the intestinoperitoneal cavity but the perirenal hemorrhage may be related to small aortic tears nonetheless. Microscopic lesions are not specific [40].

Transmission Route
Not applicable.

Diagnostic Tests
Because birds die acutely, antemortem diagnosis is rarely made. Cardiac ultrasound may be able to detect cardiac changes associated with hypertrophic cardiomyopathy. Indirect arterial blood pressure measurement may reveal increased blood pressure in susceptible males.

Differential Diagnosis
Ruptured aortic aneurysm, ruptured atrium, acute presentation of dilated cardiomyopathy, non-cardiac causes of sudden death (e.g. obstructive pulmonary disease caused by aspergillosis).

Prevention and Control
Avoid stress and excitement of susceptible male birds.

Zoonotic Potential
Not applicable.

Less Common Cardiovascular Diseases

Round Heart Disease in Chickens

Clinical History
The condition is seen in mature chickens but the prevalence is extremely rare nowadays and the disease has not been seen for several decades [41].

Causative Agent
A nutritional deficiency is thought to contribute to the disease but the etiology is unknown.

Clinical Signs and Lesions
Birds typically die acutely and clinical signs are rarely seen [59]. Gross lesions are characterized by an enlarged heart with hypertrophy of the left ventricle and yellowish color, ascites, and excess gelatinous fluid in the pericardial cavity [40, 42, 59] (Figure 18.9). Histologic lesions include primarily myocardial myofiber degeneration with swelling and vacuolation [42].

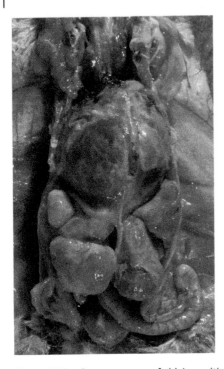

Figure 18.9 Gross necropsy of chicken with dilated cardiomyopathy with multifocal myocarditis. This seven-year-old chicken also had concomitant marked bilateral cystic thyroid hyperplasia and hepatic sarcoma. *Source:* Photo courtesy of Dr. Linden Craig, University of Tennessee.

Transmission Route
Not applicable.

Diagnostic Tests
Published information is rare on the antemortem diagnosis of this disease but is presumed to be difficult because birds usually die abruptly without premonitory signs.

Differential Diagnosis
Sudden death syndrome of broilers, ascites syndrome of broilers.

Prevention and Control
Appropriate nutrition.

Zoonotic Potential
Not applicable.

Infectious Cardiopathies

Clinical History
All backyard poultry species and breeds are thought to be susceptible to infectious cardiopathies and the prevalence is generally accepted to be low. Some pathogens are more species specific than others (e.g. viruses in chickens).

Causative Agent
A wide variety of pathogens have been reported to cause cardiac diseases (Table 18.5). Among bacteria, *Enterococcus*, *Staphylococcus*, *Pasteurella*, and *Erysipelothrix* are more commonly isolated from valvular endocarditis. *Escherichia coli* is frequently involved in pericarditis and myocarditis. Avian chlamidiosis is frequently associated with pericarditis and myocarditis in ducks and turkeys. Epicarditis is usually caused by *Salmonella* spp. or *E. coli* [18, 42, 60]. Chronic bacterial infection in other organ systems (e.g. salpingitis and bumblefoot) can lead to bacteremia and subsequent cardiac infection. Infectious agents colonizing cardiac tissues cause destruction of valves and other cardiac structures, leading to valvular insufficiency, impaired cardiac function and the likelihood of septic embolism. Marek's disease virus (gallid herpesvirus 2) and avian retroviruses can induce lymphoid tumors in the heart or vascular tumors [42]. Marek's disease virus may also promote atherosclerosis in chickens. A recent two-year small flock disease surveillance project conducted at the Animal Health Laboratory (AHL), University of Guelph, Guelph, Ontario, identified Marek's disease as the most commonly diagnosed primary viral disease in 10.6% of the chicken postmortem submissions. Marek's disease was the highest ranked etiological cause of mortality or morbidity which is an indicator of the high prevalence of Marek's disease in Ontario small poultry flocks.

One of the chickens had extensive ventricular epicardial hemorrhage at necropsy (Figure 18.10a) and this chicken and five more

Table 18.5   Infectious agents reported to cause cardiovascular lesions in poultry.

Pericarditis/epicarditis	Myocarditis
Listeria monocytogenes	*Escherichia coli*
Riemerella anatipestifer (turkeys, ducks, and other waterfowls)	*Salmonella* spp.
Chlamydophila psittaci (ducks, turkeys)	*Listeria monocytogenes*
Mycoplasma gallisepticum	*Pasteurella multocida*
Salmonella spp.	*Mycobacterium* spp.
Escherichia coli	*Aspergillus* spp.
Reovirus	West Nile virus
Pericardial effusion	Eastern equine encephalitis virus
Fowl adenovirus (serotype IV)	Avian leucosis virus
Reovirus	Parvovirus (geese and Muscovy ducks)
Endocarditis	Avian encephalomyelitis virus
Enterococcus spp.	Reovirus
Streptococcus spp.	Avian paramyxovirus 1 (Newcastle disease virus)
Staphylococcus spp.	Avian influenza
Pasteurella multocida	*Sarcocystis* spp.
Erysipelothrix rhusopathiae	*Leucocytozoon* spp.
Pseudomonas aeruginosa	*Toxoplasma gondii*
Escherichia coli	
Reovirus	
Intravascular/intracardiac parasites	Cardiac neoplasias
Splendidofilaria spp.	Marek's disease virus
Chandlerella spp.	Avian leukosis virus
Cardiofilaria spp.	Reticuloendotheliosis virus
Paronchocerca spp.	
Sarconema spp. (swans and geese)	
Schistosomes (geese)	

of the 26 chickens with Marek's disease had histologic evidence of cardiac neoplasia (Figure 18.10b) and a seventh chicken had the characteristic histologic atherosclerotic vascular lesions. Based on the results from this small flock disease surveillance project, the likelihood of identifying pale raised or flat tumor nodules in the heart at necropsy are low, requiring histologic evaluation of tissues for confirmation of heart involvement.

In addition, avian leucosis virus, avian influenza virus, and avian avulavirus-1 (previously known as avian paramyxovirus-1 or Newcastle disease virus) can cause myocarditis in chickens and other avian species [61, 62]. Fungal infections can reach the heart via emboli or by extension of adjacent airsacculitis lesions. Protozoan parasites mainly induce myocarditis as a result of the presence of cysts in myofibers. Nematodes (filarioid nematodes) and trematodes (schistosomes) localized in the vascular system are mainly found in wild galliformes and anseriformes but can be a concern to backyard poultry, and some species have

(a)

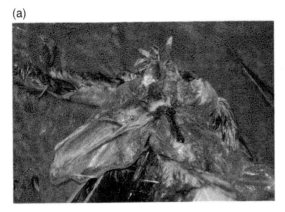

(b)

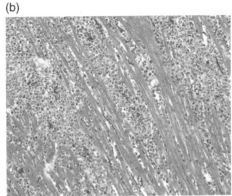

Figure 18.10   (a) This small flock hen was found dead. Most of the ventricular epicardium is ridged and coated with paintbrush hemorrhage. Both lungs are red/dark red and firm. There is a focal pale area on the liver and a large soft mass in the vaginal wall. The intestinal wall is also thickened. (b) Histologically, there is marked infiltration of the heart endocardium, myocardium and to a lesser extent, the epicardium by neoplastic T-lymphocytes as confirmed by immunohistochemistry. There was also locally extensive myocardial and epicardial hemorrhagic necrosis, which would explain the reddened epicardium noted at necropsy. Other tissues including brain, eye, sciatic nerve, gastrointestinal tract, respiratory tract, and reproductive tract were also affected. H&E stain, magnification ×200.

been recovered in chickens and domestic ducks and geese [63, 64].

Clinical Signs and Lesions

Clinical signs may not be specific but congestive heart failure or arrhythmia can be documented as a result of ensuing valvular insufficiency and myocardial involvement respectively. Birds are also frequently lethargic and may show dyspnea. Restrictive pericarditis can also lead to heart failure and ascites. Gross lesions of erysipelas, peracute-acute *Pasteurella multocida* or *Reimerella anatipestifer* infection or avian influenzamay include petechial or ecchymotic epicardial hemorrhages (Figure 18.11). Gross lesions of bacterial cardiopathies may also include pericardial exudate (Figure 18.12), granulomatous, or nodular inflammatory deposits on the valves and on the endocardium (Figure 18.13), and lesions elsewhere in the coelom, such as perihepatitis and coelomitis.

Transmission Route

Bacterial and viral infectious agents, for the most part, do not have an intrinsic cardiac tropism

and, for more specific information, the reader is invited to consult respective chapters on infectious diseases. Backyard flocks are naturally exposed to avian chlamydiosis through its wild bird reservoir (e.g. pigeons, gulls, egrets). The definitive host of *Sarcocystis falcatula* is the Virginia opossum, and cockroaches can serve as mechanical vectors. The definitive host of

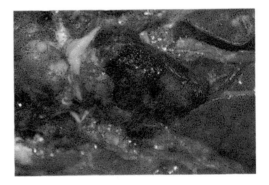

Figure 18.11   Petechial hemorrhages of the epicardial fat and ecchymotic hemorrhages of the epicardium of the heart of a duck with acute erysipelas. Other bacterial septicemias, including fowl cholera (*Pasteurella multocida*), *Reimerella anatipestifer*, and viremias including avian influenza can present similarly.

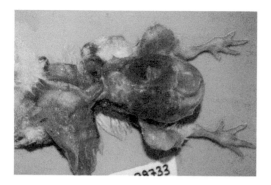

Figure 18.12 Fibrinous pericarditis, perihepatitis and serositis secondary to *Escherichia coli* infection in a young chicken. These systemic bacterial infections can be caused by single or multiple bacterial etiologies.

Toxoplasma gondii is the domestic cat. Some infectious pathogens are transmitted by arthropod vectors (*Leucocytozoon* by simuliidae, West Nile virus by *Culex*, and Eastern equine encephalitis by *Culisetta*, intra-cardiovascular parasites). Schistosomes penetrate hosts through the skin from a water environment.

Diagnostic Tests

CBC may reveal leukocytosis and biochemistry may reveal elevation in CK or troponin T in the case of myocardial involvement. Blood culture can be attempted to isolate a bacterial organism.

Blood smear examination may identify microfilaria and blood stages of *Leucocytozoon* (gametocyte). Electrocardiography findings are not specific and may show augmented P, T, S, and/or R wave, prolonged segment intervals, axis deviation, ventricular premature contraction, ventricular tachycardia, and arrhythmias [18, 19]. These changes are consistent with alterations of electrical conduction in the heart and myocardial ischemia. Valvular vegetation may be identified on a cardiac ultrasound examination and signs of congestive heart failure, valvular regurgitation, and myocardial dysfunction may also be evident. If the flock is experiencing elevated morbidity or mortality, necropsy and additional diagnostic testing including but not limited to, histology, bacteriology, and virology may also be required in order to identify an etiology.

Differential Diagnosis

Other infectious processes, other cardiac diseases and causes of congestive heart failure (ascites syndrome, turkey dilated cardiomyopathy). On necropsy, pericardial urate deposition (Figure 18.14) can resemble fibrinous pericarditis.

Prevention and Control

Antimicrobials targeting the causative agents are indicated but most of these medications

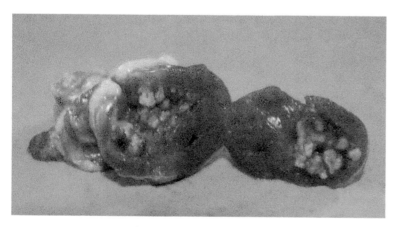

Figure 18.13 Valvular and mural endocarditis in a broiler, note the dilated right ventricle and thickened right ventricular wall. *Staphylococcus aureus* was recovered from the tissues. *Source:* Photo courtesy of Ms. Megan MacAlpine, University of Guelph.

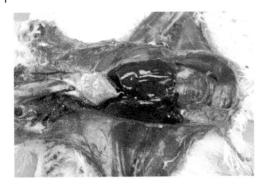

Figure 18.14 Pericardial urate deposition in a very dehydrated chicken. Note the purple leg muscles. The urate deposits are typically bright white and are soft or granular. The liver capsule may also be coated with a fine bright white stippling of urates and there may also be small white plaques in the lungs and surrounding soft tissues.

cannot be given to poultry from which eggs or meat are destined for human consumption because of an undetermined withdrawal period. For more information, please refer to the paragraph on Therapeutics. Vaccines are available for selected bacterial and viral agents however, are typically available only in large quantities as they are intended for commercial poultry operations.

Zoonotic Potential
Some bacterial pathogens causing cardiac lesions have zoonotic potentials (e.g. *E. coli*, avian chlamydiosis).

Nutritional and Toxic Cardiopathies

Clinical History
Younger poultry birds are more commonly affected by nutritional deficiencies and excess. Most non-nutritional cardiac toxicoses are of iatrogenic origin.

Causative Agent
Some noncurrent antimicrobials used to cause cardiac diseases: Furazolidone (nitrofuran) causes dilated cardiomyopathy, and ionophores (e.g. monensin, salinomycin), still commonly used, may cause myocardial necrosis.

Doxorubicin and ethanol also have cardiac toxicities in poultry. Toxicities may also be caused by minerals in excess, such as silver, cobalt, selenium, lead, sodium, and potassium. Vitamin E/selenium deficiency may cause myofiber degeneration and Vitamin D3 toxicity leads to cardiac mineralization. Plant toxicities may be encountered with *Cassia*, *Crotalaria*, rapeseed meal (erucic acid, glucosinolate), and avocado (persin). Environmental toxins, such as chlorinated biphenyls and dioxin, have been involved in some poultry cases [6, 42, 65].

Clinical Signs and Lesions
Signs are usually non-specific. Furazolidone toxicity causes similar signs to dilated cardiomyopathy in turkeys and has been used in experimental induction of this disease. Sodium toxicity may induce ascites and edema similar to the ascites syndrome in chickens. Potassium deficiency and toxicity may lead to cardiac arrhythmia. Chlorinated biphenyls, dioxin, and cresol may cause hydropericardium.

Transmission Route
Not applicable.

Diagnostic Tests
History and diet analysis are used for diagnosis. Myocardial lesions may lead to changes in the electrocardiogram and increase plasma muscle enzymes and troponin T. Dilated cardiac chambers, ascites, and hydropericardium may be detected on echocardiography.

Differential Diagnosis
Furazolidone toxicity cannot be distinguished from dilated cardiomyopathy in turkeys, sodium toxicosis causes similar signs and lesions to ascites syndrome in chickens.

Prevention and Control
Not applicable.

Zoonotic Potential
Not applicable.

Atherosclerosis

Clinical History

Atherosclerosis mainly affects older birds and seems to be more common in male than in female poultry birds. Chickens, quails, and turkeys are susceptible and have been used as experimental models. Turkeys seem to be the most susceptible galliforme species to spontaneous atherosclerosis. Some lines are hypertensive and lesions have even been found in wild turkeys [66, 67].

Causative Agent

Atherosclerosis is a chronic inflammatory fibroproliferative vascular disease characterized by the buildup of atheromatous materials containing numerous compounds including inflammatory cells (mainly macrophages), lipid, calcium, and collagen on the luminal surface of the arteries in response to multiple forms of endothelial injuries, which, in chickens, include Marek disease (which also affects lipid metabolism) [40, 41, 68]. Risk factors have not been completely characterized in poultry but age, gender, specific breeds [restricted ovulatory (RO) chicken, susceptible-to-experimental-atherosclerosis (SEA) quails], inbreeding (some experimental lines of chickens and quails), and dietary factors may have a role in the pathogenesis. Hypertension may also be a risk factor in turkeys [67]. Cholesterol feeding induces atherosclerosis in poultry [69, 70].

Clinical Signs and Lesions

Clinical signs are associated with arterial stenosis, myocardial infarction, aneurysm, and thromboemboli. However, they are uncommonly recognized in spontaneous disease and birds may die acutely or never show clinical manifestation. In some cases, atherosclerotic lesions may predispose turkeys to aneurysm and aortic rupture but the two conditions seem to be different clinical entities overall. Atherosclerotic lesions develop mainly in the coronary arteries, aorta, and brachiocephalic trunks in poultry. Advanced atherosclerotic lesions are composed of a necrotic and lipid core (atheroma) covered by a fibrous cap (fibroatheroma). Spontaneous lesions are rarely advanced in chickens [41, 69].

Transmission Route

Not applicable.

Diagnostic Tests

Dyslipidemia may be a risk factor for the development of atheromatous plaques, such as an increase in cholesterol and LDL. Chickens have a normally high cholesterol level. Some lines of chicken are deficient in HDL but this does not necessarily correlate with more severe lesions [71]. Atherosclerotic lesions are usually not detectable in birds using current imaging modalities except when calcified, but may promote cardiac dysfunction and congestive heart failure.

Differential Diagnosis

Aortic rupture/aneurysm in turkeys, vasculitis, fibromuscular dysplasia.

Prevention and Control

Limiting risk factors by increasing activities and decreasing fat in the diet. Omega 3 fatty acids may be useful dietary supplements [72].

Zoonotic Potential

Not applicable.

Acknowledgments

We thank Dr. Caryn Reynolds (DoveLewis Veterinary Emergency and Specialty Hospital, Portland, Oregon) for performing echocardiographies on broiler chickens and Dr. Joao Brandao (Oklahoma State University) for performing electrocardiograms on broiler chickens for the first edition of this chapter.

References

1 Smith, F.M., West, N.H., and Jones, D.R. (2000). The cardiovascular system. In: *Sturkie's Avian Physiology* (ed. G.C. Whittow), 141–232. London: Academic Press.

2 Decuypere, E., Bruggeman, V., Barbato, G., and Buyse, J. (2003). Growth and reproduction problems associated with selection for increased broiler meat production. In: *Poultry Genetics, Breeding and Biotechnology* (eds. W. Muir and S. Aggrey), 13–28. Wallington, UK: CABI Publishing.

3 Baghbanzadeh, A. and Decuypere, E. (2008). Ascites syndrome in broilers: physiological and nutritional perspectives. *Avian Pathol.* 37 (2): 117–126.

4 Olkowski, A.A. (2007). Pathophysiology of heart failure in broiler chickens: structural, biochemical, and molecular characteristics. *Poult. Sci.* 86 (5): 999–1005.

5 Al Masri, S., Kattanek, M., Richardson, K.C. et al. (2017). Comparative quantitative studies on the microvasculature of the heart of a highly selected meat-type and a wild-type Turkey line. Tang D, editor. *PLoS One* 12 (1): e0170858.

6 Julian, R. (2002). Cardiovascular disease. In: *Poultry Diseases*, 5e (eds. F. Jordan, M. Pattison, D. Alexander and T. Faragher), 484–495. London, UK: W.B. Saunders.

7 Krautwald-junghanns, M.-E., Moerke-Schindler, T., Vorbruggen, S., and Cramer, K. (2017). Radiography and ultrasonography in the backyard poultry and waterfowl patient. *J. Avian Med. Surg.* 31 (3): 189–197.

8 Brochu, N.M., Guerin, N.T., Varga, C. et. al. (2019). A two-year prospective study of small poultry flocks in Ontario, Canada, part 2: causes of morbidity and mortality. *J. Vet. Diagn. Invest.* 31 (3): 336–42.

9 Cadmus, K.J., Mete, A., Harris, M. et al. (2019). Causes of mortality in backyard poultry in eight states in the United State. *J. Vet. Diagn. Invest.* 31 (3): 318–26.

10 Sturkie, P. (1949). The electrocardiogram of the chicken. *Am. J. Vet. Res.* 10 (35): 168–175.

11 Olkowski, A.A., Classen, H.L., Riddell, C., and Bennett, C.D. (1997). A study of electrocardiographic patterns in a population of commercial broiler chickens. *Vet. Res. Commun.* 21 (1): 51–62.

12 McKenzie, B.E., Will, J.A., and Hardie, A. (1971). The electrocardiogram of the turkey. *Avian Dis.* 15 (4): 737–744.

13 Uzun, M., Yildiz, S., and Onder, F. (2004). Electrocardiography of rock partridges (*Alectoris graeca*) and chukar partridges (*Alectoris chukar*). *J. Zoo Wildl. Med.* 35 (4): 510–514.

14 Cinar, A., Bagci, C., Belge, F., and Uzun, M. (1996). The electrocardiogram of the Pekin duck. *Avian Dis.* 40 (4): 919–923.

15 Hassanpour, H., Zarei, H., and Hojjati, P. (2011). Analysis of electrocardiographic parameters in helmeted guinea fowl (*Numida meleagris*). *J. Avian Med. Surg.* 25 (1): 8–13.

16 Zehnder, A.M., Hawkins, M.G., Pascoe, P.J., and Kass, P.H. (2009). Evaluation of indirect blood pressure monitoring in awake and anesthetized red-tailed hawks (*Buteo jamaicensis*): effects of cuff size, cuff placement, and monitoring equipment. *Vet. Aneasth. Analg.* 36 (5): 464–479.

17 Alvarenga, R.R., Zangeronimo, M.G., Pereira, L.J. et al. (2011). Lipoprotein metabolism in poultry. *World's Poult. Sci. J.* 67: 431–440.

18 Lumeij, J. and Ritchie, B. (1994). Cardiology. In: *Avian Medicine: Principles and Applications* (eds. B.W. Ritchie, G.J. Harrison and L.R. Harrison), 695–722. Lake Worth, FL: Wingers Publishing.

19 Martinez, L., Jeffrey, J., and Odom, T. (1997). Electrocardiographic diagnosis of cardiomyopathies in Aves. *Poul. Av. Biol. Rev.* 8 (1): 9–20.

20 Hassanpour, H., Hojjati, P., and Zarei, H. (2011). Electrocardiogram analysis of the normal unanesthetized green peafowl (*Pavo muticus*). *Zoo Biol.* 30 (5): 542–549.

21 Goldberg, J. and Bolnick, D. (1980). Electrocardiograms from the chicken, emu, red-tailed hawk and Chilean tinamou. *Comp. Biochem. Physiol. Comp. Physiol.* 67 (1): 15–19.

22 Szabuniewicz, M. and McCrady, J.D. (2010). The electrocardiogram of the Japanese (*Coturnix coturnix japonica*) and bobwhite (*Colinus virginianus*) quail. *Zentralbl. Vet.* 21 (3): 198–207.

23 Fitzgerald, B. and Beaufrere, H. (2016). Cardiology. In: *Current Therapy in Avian Medicine and Surgery* (ed. B. Speer), 252–328. Saint Louis, MO: Elsevier.

24 Olkowski, A.A. and Classen, H.L. (1998). High incidence of cardiac arrhythmias in broiler chickens. *J. Vet. Med. Ser. A* 45 (1–10): 83–91.

25 Pees, M., Krautwald-Junghanns, M.E., and Straub, J. (2006). Evaluating and treating the cardiovascular system. In: *Clinical Avian Medicine* (eds. G.J. Harrison and T.L. Lightfoot), 379–394. Palm Beach, FL: Spix Publishing.

26 Beaufrère, H., Rodriguez, D., Pariaut, R. et al. (2011). Estimation of intrathoracic arterial diameter by means of computed tomographic angiography in Hispaniolan Amazon parrots. *Am. J. Vet. Res.* 72 (2): 210–218.

27 Krautwald-junghanns, M.-E. and Pees, M. (2011). Ultrasonographic imaging of normal structures: cardiovascular system. In: *Diagnostic Imaging of Exotic Pets* (eds. M.-E. Krautwald-junghanns, M. Pees, S. Reese and T.N. Tully), 42–46. Hannover, Germany: Schlutersche Verlagsgesellschaft mbH & Co.

28 Martinez-Lemus, L.A., Miller, M.W., Jeffrey, J.S., and Odom, T.W. (1998). Echocardiography evaluation of cardiac structure and function in broiler and Leghorn chickens. *Poult. Sci.* 77 (7): 1045–1050.

29 Einzig, S., Staley, N.A., Mettler, E. et al. (1980). Regional myocardial blood flow and cardiac function in a naturally occurring congestive cardiomyopathy of turkeys. *Cardiovasc. Res.* 14 (7): 396–407.

30 Olkowski, A.A., Abbott, J.A., and Classen, H.L. (2005). Pathogenesis of ascites in broilers raised at low altitude: aetiological considerations based on echocardiographic findings. *J. Vet. Med. A Physiol. Pathol. Clin. Med.* 52 (4): 166–171.

31 Martinez-Lemus, L.A., Miller, M.W., Jeffrey, J.S., and Odom, T.W. (2000). Echocardiographic study of pulmonary hypertension syndrome in broiler chickens. *Avian Dis.* 44 (1): 74–84.

32 Deng, G., Zhang, Y., Peng, X. et al. (2006). Echocardiographic characteristics of chickens with ascites syndrome. *Br. Poult. Sci.* 47 (6): 756–762.

33 Beaufrère, H., Pariaut, R., Rodriguez, D. et al. (2012). Comparison of transcoelomic, contrast transcoelomic, and transesophageal echocardiography in anesthetized red-tailed hawks (*Buteo jamaicensis*). *Am. J. Vet. Res.* 73 (10): 1560–1568.

34 Mitchell, E.B., Hawkins, M.G., Orvalho, J.S., and Thomas, W.P. (2008). Congenital mitral stenosis, subvalvular aortic stenosis, and congestive heart failure in a duck. *J. Vet. Cardiol.* 10 (1): 67–73.

35 Beaufrere, H., Pariaut, R., Nevarez, J.G. et al. (2010). Feasibility of transesophageal echocardiography in birds without cardiac disease. *J. Am. Vet. Med. Assoc.* 236 (5): 540–547.

36 Fitzgerald, B.C., Dias, S., and Martorell, J. (2018). Cardiovascular drugs in avian, small mammal, and reptile medicine. *Vet. Clin. North Am. Exot. Anim. Pract.* 21 (2): 399–442.

37 Crespo, R. and Shivaprasad, H. (2008). Developmental, metabolic, and other noninfectious disorders. In: *Diseases of Poultry*, 12e (eds. Y. Saif, A. Fadly, J. Glisson, et al.), 1149–1195. Ames, IA: Blackwell Publishing.

38 Frame, D.D., Kelly, E.J., and Van Wettere, A. (2015). Dilated cardiomyopathy in a Rio Grande wild turkey (*Meleagris gallopavo*

intermedia) in southern Utah, USA, 2013. *J. Wildl. Dis.* 51 (3): 790–792.

39 Charlton, B., Bermudez, A.J., Boulianne, M. et al. (2008). Cardiovascular diseases. In: *Avian Disease Manual*, 6e (eds. B. Charlton, A.J. Bermudez, M. Boulianne, et al.), 174–178. Madison, USA: American Association of Avian Pathologists, Inc.

40 Crespo, R. and Shivaprasad, H. (2013). Developmental, metabolic, and other noninfectious disorders. In: *Diseases of Poultry*, 13e (eds. D. Swayne, J. Glisson and L. McDougald), 1233–1270. Ames, IA: Wiley.

41 Julian, R.J. (2005). Production and growth related disorders and other metabolic diseases of poultry – a review. *Vet. J.* 169 (3): 350–369.

42 Fletcher, O. and Abdul-Aziz, T. (2008). Cardiovascular system. In: *Avian Histopathology*, 3e (eds. O. Fletcher and T. Abdul-Aziz), 98–129. Madison, USA: American Association of Avian Pathologists, Inc.

43 Czarnecki, C. and Good, A. (1980). Electrocardiographic technic for identifying developing cardiomyopathies in young turkey poults. *Poult. Sci.* 59: 1515–1520.

44 Currie, R.J. (1999). Ascites in poultry: recent investigations. *Avian Pathol.* 28 (4): 313–326.

45 Olkowski, A.A. and Classen, H.L. (1998). Progressive bradycardia, a possible factor in the pathogenesis of ascites in fast growing broiler chickens raised at low altitude. *Br. Poult. Sci.* 39 (1): 139–146.

46 Odom, T.W., Hargis, B.M., Lopez, C.C. et al. (1991). Use of electrocardiographic analysis for investigation of ascites syndrome in broiler chickens. *Avian Dis.* 35 (4): 738–744.

47 Maxwell, M.H., Robertson, G.W., and Moseley, D. (1995). Serum troponin T concentrations in two strains of commercial broiler chickens aged one to 56 days. *Res. Vet. Sci.* 58 (3): 244–247.

48 Maxwell, M.H., Robertson, G.W., and Moseley, D. (1995). Serum troponin T values in 7-day-old hypoxia-and hyperoxia-treated, and 10-day-old ascitic and debilitated,

commercial broiler chicks. *Avian Pathol.* 24 (2): 333–346.

49 Dey, S., Parveen, A., Tarrant, K.J. et al. (2018). Whole genome resequencing identifies the CPQ gene as a determinant of ascites syndrome in broilers. Xu P, editor. *PLoS One* 13 (1): e0189544.

50 Kamely, M., Karimi Torshizi, M.A., and Rahimi, S. (2015). Incidence of ascites syndrome and related hematological response in short-term feed-restricted broilers raised at low ambient temperature. *Poult. Sci.* 94 (9): 2247–2256.

51 Hasani, A., Bouyeh, M., Rahati, M. et al. (2018). Which is the best alternative for ascites syndrome prevention in broiler chickens? Effect of feed form and rearing temperature conditions. *J. Appl. Anim. Res.* 46 (1): 392–396.

52 Wideman, R.F., Ismail, M., Kirby, Y.K. et al. (1995). Supplemental L-arginine attenuates pulmonary hypertension syndrome (ascites) in broilers. *Poult. Sci.* 74 (2): 323–330.

53 Wideman, R.F., Ismail, M., Kirby, Y.K. et al. (1995). Furosemide reduces the incidence of pulmonary hypertension syndrome (ascites) in broilers exposed to cool environmental temperatures. *Poult. Sci.* 74 (2): 314–322.

54 Walton, J.P., Julian, R.J., and Squires, E.J. (2001). The effects of dietary flax oil and antioxidants on ascites and pulmonary hypertension in broilers using a low temperature model. *Br. Poult. Sci.* 42 (1): 123–129.

55 Boucek, R.J., Gunja-Smith, Z., Noble, N.L., and Simpson, C.F. (1983). Modulation by propranolol of the lysyl cross-links in aortic elastin and collagen of the aneurysm-prone turkey. *Biochem. Pharmacol.* 32 (2): 275–280.

56 Waibel, P.E., Burger, R.E., and Krista, L.M. (1962). Influence of reserpine and antibiotics on incidence of dissecting aneurysm in turkeys as induced by beta-aminopropionitrile. *Poult. Sci.* 41 (5): 1554–1559.

57 Siddiqui, M., Khan, K., and Khan, L. (2009). Sudden death syndrome – an overview. *Vet. World* 2 (11): 444–447.

58 Basaki, M., Asasi, K., Tabandeh, M.R., and Aminlari, M. (2016). Polymorphism identification and cardiac gene expression analysis of the calsequestrin 2 gene in broiler chickens with sudden death syndrome. *Br. Poult. Sci.* 57 (2): 151–160.

59 Riddell, C. (1997). Developmental, metabolic, and other noninfectious disorders. In: *Diseases of Poultry*, 10e (ed. B. Calnek), 913–950. Ames, IA: Iowa State University Press.

60 Chadfield, M.S., Christensen, J.P., Christensen, H., and Bisgaard, M. (2004). Characterization of streptococci and enterococci associated with septicaemia in broiler parents with a high prevalence of endocarditis. *Avian Pathol.* 33 (6): 610–617.

61 Schmidt, R.E., Hubbard, G.B., and Fletcher, K.C. (1986). Systematic survey of lesions from animals in a zoological collection. *J. Zoo Anim. Med.* 17: 8–41.

62 Gilka, F. and Spencer, J.L. (1990). Chronic myocarditis and circulatory syndrome in a White Leghorn strain induced by an avian leukosis virus: light and electron microscopic study. *Avian Dis.* 34 (1): 174–184.

63 Bartlett, C. (2008). Filarioid nematodes. In: *Parasitic Diseases of Wild Birds* (eds. C. Atkinson, N. Thomas and D. Hunter), 439–462. Ames, IA: Wiley Blackwell.

64 Huffman, J. and Fried, B. (2008). Schistosomes. In: *Parasitic Diseases of Wild Birds* (eds. C. Atkinson, N. Thomas and D. Hunter), 246–260. Ames, IA: Wiley Blackwell.

65 Fulton, R. (2008). Other toxins and poisons. In: *Diseases of Poultry*, 12e (eds. Y. Saif, A. Fadly, J. Glisson, et al.), 1231–1258. Ames, IA: Blackwell Publishing.

66 Krista, L. and McQuire, J. (1988). Atherosclerosis in coronary, aortic, and sciatic arteries from wild male turkeys (*Meleagris gallopava silvestris*). *Am. J. Vet. Res.* 49 (9): 1582–1588.

67 Pauletto, P., Scannapieco, G., Vescovo, G. et al. (1988). Catecholamine-induced cardiovascular disease in the spontaneously hypertensive and atherosclerotic turkey. *Method. Find. Exp. Clin. Pharmacol.* 10 (6): 357–362.

68 Beaufrere, H. (2013). Atherosclerosis: comparative pathogenesis, lipoprotein metabolism and avian and exotic companion mammal models. *J. Exot. Pet Med.* 22 (4): 320–335.

69 Moghadasian, M.H. (2002). Experimental atherosclerosis: a historical overview. *Life Sci.* 70 (8): 855–865.

70 Xiangdong, L., Yuanwu, L., Hua, Z. et al. (2011). Animal models for the atherosclerosis research: a review. *Protein Cell* 2 (3): 189–201.

71 Poernama, F., Subramanian, R., Cook, M.E., and Attie, A.D. (1992). High density lipoprotein deficiency syndrome in chickens is not associated with an increased susceptibility to atherosclerosis. *Arterioscler. Thromb.* 12 (5): 601–607.

72 Petzinger, C., Heatley, J.J., Cornejo, J. et al. (2010). Dietary modification of omega-3 fatty acids for birds with atherosclerosis. *J. Am. Vet. Med. Assoc.* 236 (5): 523–528.

Section 4

Specialized Care and Surgery

19

Emergency and Critical Care

Jennifer E. Graham and Elizabeth A. Rozanski

Department of Clinical Sciences, Cummings School of Veterinary Medicine at Tufts University, North Grafton, MA, USA

Introduction

Emergency presentations of chickens may include acute and chronic conditions. Important considerations for the veterinarian include origin/use of the bird (production, pet, display, etc.), duration and nature of illness (acute, chronic, insidious onset), extent of disease, potential for recovery, and financial commitment of the owner. Patient status at presentation helps determine the appropriate range and depth of stabilization required prior to any necessary diagnostic testing. It is vital that the veterinarian is aware of zoonotic diseases of poultry and state and federal laws regarding poultry species; for example, reportable diseases and appropriate drug use in food animals. See Chapters 1, 10, and 28 for detailed information on these topics. Separate equipment and housing should be used for birds with suspected contagious disease and all equipment and cages should be thoroughly disinfected after use to minimize risk of disease transmission. Temporary housing must be available with capability to provide oxygen therapy, nebulization, or heat support as needed. This chapter will review aspects of emergency care for chickens including triage and patient assessment, diagnostics, supportive care procedures, and common emergency presentations.

Triage and Patient Assessment

Cardiopulmonary Resuscitation

Basic life support is the most important component of CPCR (cardiopulmonary cerebral resuscitation) and should be started as soon as CPA (cardiopulmonary arrest) has been identified (Figure 19.1) [1]. Unresponsiveness, apnea or agonal breathing, and lack of cardiac sounds on auscultation are all signs of potential or impending CPA. Establishing the "ABCs" (airway, breathing, circulation) of cardiopulmonary resuscitation (CPR) is crucial, although there has been debate about using the "CAB" (compressions, airway, breathing) approach instead. Chest compressions should be initiated as soon as possible; however, the effectiveness of these compressions is lower in birds than mammals.

Chest/Cardiac Compressions

If cardiac arrest is identified, cardiac compressions should be initiated. Adopting a different technique than mammals for cardiac compression

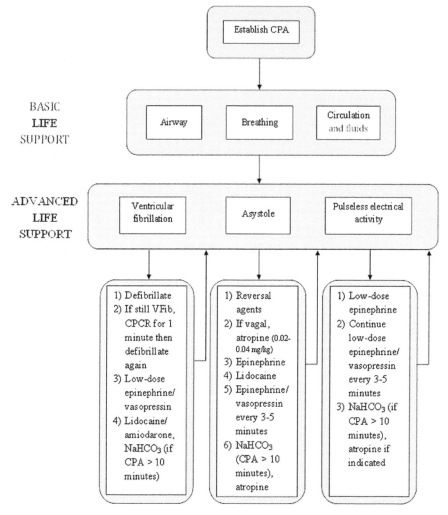

Figure 19.1 Steps for cardiopulmonary resuscitation in the critical avian patient. *Source:* Figure courtesy of Claudia Kabakchiev and Hugues Beaufrere.

may be more effective, such as making cardiac compressions on the lateral and dorsal aspect of the thorax rather than over the keel [2]. An attempt to approximate the normal heart rate, i.e. >120 compressions/minute, is recommended. Cardiac activity can be monitored with electrocardiography (ECG) and a Doppler probe can determine effectiveness of compressions.

Ventilation

Any obstructing material should be removed from the oral cavity and the bird should be intubated with an appropriately sized uncuffed endotracheal (ET) tube. If a suspected upper airway obstruction that cannot be relieved, an air sac cannula should be placed (see Airway Obstruction). Mechanical ventilation with 100% oxygen at 10–20 breaths/minute is recommended. If an ET tube or air sac cannula cannot be placed, ventilation can be encouraged by moving the wings up and down or lifting the sternum.

Advanced Life Support

Advanced life support is recommended when the ABCs have been established. It includes the use of emergency drugs, fluid therapy, and defibrillation if needed. To maintain appropriate circulation, intravenous or intraosseous access is needed (see Vascular Access) [3]. Fluid therapy can be initiated once intravascular or intraosseous access has been established (see Fluid Therapy Plan). If there is an anesthesia-related cardiac arrest, reversal agents for any administered sedatives should be given. Atropine should be administered if there is bradycardia or a vagal arrest; otherwise, epinephrine is one of the first drugs to be used in CPA cases [4]. If ECG is available for patient monitoring, then emergency drugs can be used based on the ECG findings. CPRC in birds usually results in an unfavorable outcome but should always be attempted if permitted by the owner, particularly in previously healthy animals that have just collapsed or during any routine anesthesia.

Physical Examination

Physical examination is like other avian species apart from restraint; see Chapter 8 for information on restraint and physical examination in poultry. Careful observation of the bird prior to handling is recommended. The observational exam is key in determining the length, depth, and fashion of the physical examination and further diagnostics that the patient will tolerate. Many abnormalities may be obscured by the camouflage of the feathers, but upon observation and exam, these signs can be obvious or pronounced. Note any increased respiratory effort (Figure 19.2) or tail bob, posture and awareness of the bird, and any musculoskeletal or neurologic abnormalities (Figure 19.3), such as a wing droop or head tilt. If a bird is showing signs of hemorrhage, head trauma, seizures, open fractures, extreme respiratory difficulty or weakness, emergency care should be given prior to performing a complete physical examination.

Weight determination, accurate to the gram, is a necessary part of the chicken physical examination. While many birds may willingly

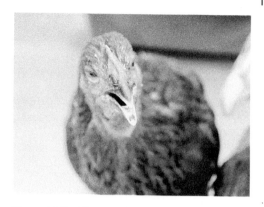

Figure 19.2 The open beak breathing in this hen is consistent with respiratory distress. *Source:* Photograph courtesy of Yuko Sato.

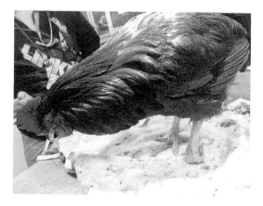

Figure 19.3 Proprioceptive deficits in a rooster.

step onto a scale, some birds may remain calmer when lightly wrapped in a towel or weighed in a carrier. All equipment for physical examination should be ready prior to restraint. This preparation will minimize handling and examination time and therefore patient stress. If the patient is debilitated, an examination is performed in a stepwise fashion with small breaks given to the bird between handling, examination, diagnostics, and treatments. Care should be taken to hold the bird upright if the bird is showing signs of respiratory distress or if any fluid or masses are palpated in the coelomic cavity (Figure 19.4). Dorsal recumbency decreases tidal volume by 40–50% and increases breathing frequency by 20–50% in conscious chickens [5]. Oxygen therapy prior to, during, or after physical

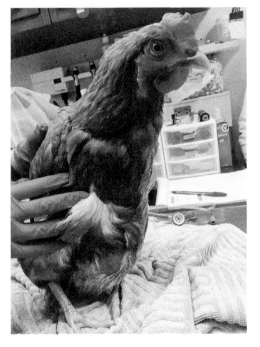

Figure 19.4 Severe coelomic distention caused by ascites in a hen with reproductive disease.

examination may be beneficial in the patient suffering debilitation, shock, or respiratory compromise. If oxygen therapy is needed, an oxygen cage delivering 50–80% humidified oxygen concentration or a facemask with 50 ml/kg/min flow rate can be used.

Replacement of luxations and closure of open wounds may need immediate attention to ensure a positive outcome but stabilizing the patient may require initiating fluid therapy and shock treatment prior to in-depth wound care. Initially, a light nonadherent wrap can be placed to minimize bleeding and further trauma to open wounds. When the patient is stable, complete wound care may require analgesia, sedation, or anesthesia (Figure 19.5). Examine the oral cavity, ears, and nares closely for any signs of blood, a sign of head trauma. Additional references are available concerning triage and patient assessment [6–10].

Vascular and Hematologic Effects of Blood Loss in Chickens

Chickens showing signs of hypovolemic blood loss shock need immediate fluid therapy (see Fluid Therapy). It is unclear if phases of shock as described in mammals apply to birds. Chickens have been reported to have a rate of

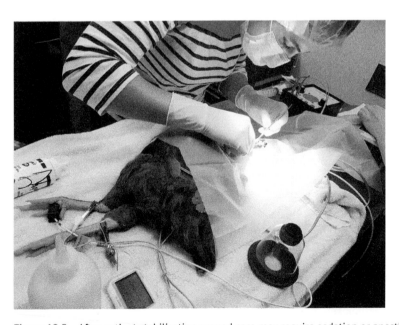

Figure 19.5 After patient stabilization, wound care may require sedation or anesthesia.

post-hemorrhagic fluid mobilization twice that of mammals and lack a phase of shock irreversible to transfusion [11]. Small reductions in blood volume in the chicken are associated with large reductions in blood pressure. Concomitant with the fall in pressure is a reduction in cardiac stroke volume with either an increased or static heart rate. Total peripheral resistance (TPR) either falls or is unchanged during hemorrhagic hypotension in chickens and resistance to flow through skeletal muscle is not affected. Hematologic changes noted during hemorrhage in chickens include progressive hyperkalemia, hyperglycemia, and hemodilution (indicated by linear falls in hematocrit, hemoglobin, and plasma protein concentration). Plasma sodium, plasma osmolality, arterial pH, and P_{O_2} are unchanged but there is a significant fall in arterial P_{CO_2} [11]. Generally, birds with decompensatory or terminal shock exhibit bradycardia with low cardiac output, severe hypotension, pale or cyanotic mucous membranes, absent capillary refill time, weak or absent pulses, hypothermia, oliguria to anuric renal failure, pulmonary edema, and a stupor to comatose state; CPA commonly occurs at this stage [8].

Monitoring Techniques

Blood pressure, ECG (see Chapter 18), pulse quality, capillary refill time, and body temperature are physical examination parameters that may be useful in assessing patient status [12–14].

Blood Pressure
Systolic blood pressure measurements obtained with a Doppler flow detector from the ulnar vessels can be performed in birds and systolic blood pressure has been found to correlate well with direct blood pressure measurements in ducks (*Anas platyrhynchos*) [12]. Although direct arterial blood pressure is not commonly performed in avian species due to the invasive nature of the procedure, normal systolic, mean, and diastolic arterial blood pressure in chickens is 99 ± 13, 84 ± 13, and 69 ± 15 mmHg, respectively [15]. Guidelines for fluid therapy for hypovolemia are based on blood pressure measurements as is used with mammals and psittacine birds. Birds should be treated for hypovolemic shock when indirect Doppler blood pressures are below 90 mmHg systolic [8].

Pulse Quality and Capillary Refill Time
Pulse quality and capillary refill time (CRT) help guide therapy in poultry patients. The deep radial artery, which runs alongside the ulnar vein, or the metatarsal artery as it crosses the dorsal surface of the tibiotarsal-tarsometatarsal joint, can be used to assess pulse quality. A weak or thready pulse can be a sign of shock while an absent pulse can indicate cardiac asystole, peripheral vasoconstriction due to cold, hypovolemia, or hypotension [6]. Oral mucous membrane assessment for CRT can be challenging due to the presence of pigmentation. Eyelid or vent eversion is an alternative mucous membrane for assessment of membrane color. Ulnar vein turgidity is useful for determining vascular perfusion; the vessel should refill immediately when depressed, which is not visually detectable [16]. If vessel refill is visualized, the bird is estimated to be approximately 5% dehydrated. If a 1-second refill time of the ulnar vein is seen, the patient is approximately 10% dehydrated or in shock. Comb refill time is approximately two seconds. See Chapter 8 for further details.

Body Temperature
Body temperature is less often used when assessing the critical avian patient but should be a consideration when determining the need for supplemental heat. The normal core body temperature of a chicken is about 105.0–109.4 °F (40.6–43.0 °C) [16]. Remote sensing constant readout thermometers can be used to measure body temperature in anesthetized patients when placed in the esophagus to the level of the heart. Remote sensing thermometers or conventional digital thermometer can

be carefully inserted into the cloaca in unanesthetized birds to measure body temperature. While cloacal temperature monitoring can be accurate, it is dependent on body temperature and cloacal activity over time [17].

Sample Collection

Samples for hematologic and biochemical analysis are preferably obtained prior to treatment for best diagnostic ability. However, the patient's needs must be prioritized. Poultry in shock must be stabilized prior to extensive diagnostic sampling. If blood can be safely obtained, it is ideal to collect baseline samples for hematology and chemistry analysis prior to treatment. A conservative minimum database includes determination of packed cell volume, total solids, and estimated white blood cell count. Venipuncture sites in poultry include the medial metatarsal vein, jugular vein (the right jugular vein is larger), and cutaneous ulnar or basilic vein. While total blood volume varies based on species, in general, 1% of total body weight can be safely collected from the healthy chicken [10, 18]. In the compromised patient, this should be reduced to 0.5% of total body weight. Once the bird is stable, venipuncture for heavy metal testing, infectious disease and additional sample collection, radiographs

or computed tomography (CT), respiratory washes, endoscopy with biopsies, and other tests can determine the cause and extent of disease. A fecal parasite examination should ideally be performed on all patients.

Diagnostic Imaging

Radiography

Radiographs can be a high return, low risk diagnostic procedure in stable poultry. Properly positioned radiographs allow for visualization of organ size and location, evaluation of the lungs/air sacs, detection of heavy metal foreign bodies, fractures, the presence of an egg within the reproductive tract, GI (gastrointestinal) abnormalities, and other pathology (Figure 19.6). Radiographs can be taken without anesthesia in the tractable poultry patient; see Chapter 9. Restraint boards and masking or paper tape can be utilized for positioning of poultry to minimize exposure of personnel to radiation. Two-view whole body radiographs are recommended with additional views taken of extremities if indicated. Additional oblique views of the head are also indicated in cases of skull trauma. A baseline view of the feet affected by podo- dermatitis can guide prognosis and treatment. When available, horizontal beam radiography is preferable to lateral radiographic positioning

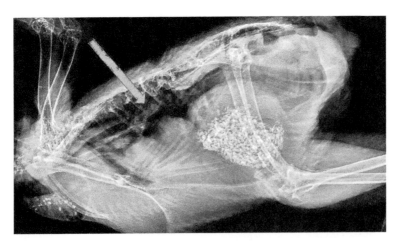

Figure 19.6 Lateral radiographic projection of a chicken in respiratory distress. Arrow points to increased soft tissue density and scalloping in the region of the caudal lung.

of birds with coelomic fluid. Contrast radiography or fluoroscopy may be helpful imaging modalities in some cases.

Ultrasonography

Air sacs and the boney keel can make imaging of avian species challenging. Imaging is best obtained with the probe placed midline caudal to the sternum and feathers can be wetted and parted prior to gel application. Ultrasound may be most helpful when coelomic fluid is present and can help facilitate coelomocentesis. The heart, liver, sections of the GI tract, and active reproductive tissue are normally visible. It is difficult to image the spleen, kidneys, and inactive reproductive tract. Ultrasound-guided aspirates can be performed to assess abnormal tissues when indicated (Figure 19.7). Although imaging the lungs via ultrasound is not often useful in avian patients, large granulomas or masses close to the body wall may be visualized in some instances.

Advanced Imaging

CT and MRI (Magnetic Resonance Imaging) can be useful in some avian patients. Evaluation of sinuses, skull, and respiratory tract can best be made with CT. MRI is most helpful to assess soft tissue structures including the brain. CT is advantageous in many patients due to the short time required for imaging versus MRI.

Endoscopy

Endoscopy is generally performed on an anesthetized patient. Rigid and small flexible endoscopes are used to directly evaluate the avian respiratory and gastrointestinal tracts. The choanal slit and internasal septum can be examined if the bird is showing signs of upper respiratory disease. The length of the trachea can be examined with special focus on the syrinx to detect foreign body obstruction or granulomas. If a bird is showing obvious signs of upper airway obstruction, an air sac cannula should be placed before anesthetic induction to provide an alternative source of oxygen and anesthetic gases while the trachea is examined. Endoscopy of the air sacs and lungs is indicated if lower respiratory disease is suspected. Endoscopy of the gastrointestinal tract can usually be performed to the level of the ventriculus by way of a small flexible endoscope or with a rigid endoscope by way of an ingluviotomy. Coelomic endoscopy in poultry is complicated by the presence of the large gastrointestinal and reproductive tracts. Direct visualization, biopsies, and swabs for culture or cytology can be obtained via endoscopy.

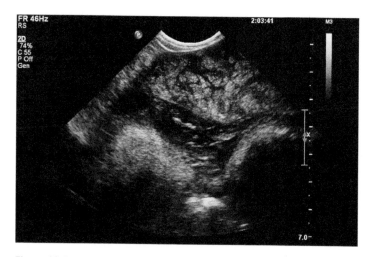

Figure 19.7 Ultrasound of the coelom of a chicken revealed a large mass with mixed echogenicity suspected to be an impacted oviduct. Fine needle aspirate was consistent with egg contents.

Fluid Therapy

Vascular Access

Fluids can be administered orally (PO), subcutaneously (SC), intravenously (IV), or intraosseously (IO). Administration of PO or SC fluids is reserved for the stable patient that is less than 5% dehydrated and standing. Oral fluid administration requires a bird that can maintain an upright body position and has a functional gastrointestinal tract to avoid regurgitation and aspiration of fluids. The inguinal site, where the inner thigh meets the body wall, or the lateral flank are preferred for administration of subcutaneous fluids. Other potential subcutaneous fluid administration sites include the axillary region, midback, and intrascapular area. Subcutaneous fluid administration requires avoidance of fluids entering the coelomic cavity and air sac system.

Intravascular administration of fluids (IV or IO) is essential in treatment of the critical avian patient. Sites for intravenous catheterization include the medial metatarsal vein (Figure 19.8), the ulnar vein and the jugular vein [10]. Ulnar vein catheterization is a pre-ferred site because fluids and drugs can be administered here without regard for the renal portal system. A figure-of-eight bandage can secure the ulnar catheter after it has been glued or sutured in place. The catheter site should be checked daily. Catheterization of the medial metatarsal vein is usually well tolerated by poultry. Intravenous catheters can be challenging to maintain in birds due to fragility of vessels, lack of dermal tissues for catheterization, and patient temperament.

Intraosseous catheterization has advantages when compared with intravenous catheterization of the avian patient based on ease of placement and maintenance. Intraosseous catheters usually consist of a small gauge needle, such as a spinal needle, placed in the distal ulna or proximal tibiotarsus. Pneumatic bones such as the femur and humerus should not be used for IO catheters [10]. Intraosseous catheters can be maintained for 3–5 days and require the same aseptic technique as IV catheters during placement and maintenance. Placement is similar to that of a normograde insertion of an intramedullary pin. IO catheter placement is particularly challenging in older laying hens with hyperostotic endocytosis of long bones.

Fluid Types and Indications

Fluids are classified as crystalloids or colloids. Crystalloids are further divided into hypotonic, isotonic, and hypertonic. Only 25% of crystalloids remain in the circulation after a short time; as such, they should be considered interstitial rehydrators. Lactated Ringer's solution (LRS), Normosol-R, and PlasmaLyte-A are balanced buffered solutions that closely approximate the extracellular fluid composition and can be used in most situations. The 0.9% saline is not buffered and unbalanced and is generally restricted for patients with metabolic alkalosis. LRS is hypo-osmolar to avian plasma and should not be used at high intravenous rate (e.g. resuscitation) but is appropriate for SC administration as it may be absorbed more readily than isotonic solutions. PlasmaLyte-A

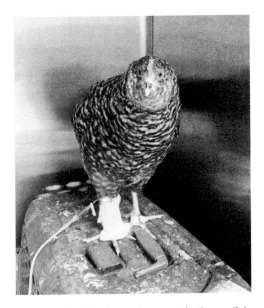

Figure 19.8 IV catheter placement in the medial metatarsal vein of a chicken.

7.4 is the closest fluid to avian plasma composition in terms of pH, osmolality, and electrolyte concentrations. Hypertonic saline is an intravascular expander equivalent to that of colloids at one fourth the volume and is used in resuscitation and in combination with crystalloids and colloids. Dextrose 5% is primarily used as a carrier for constant rate infusion of drugs or as a source of pure water. A variety of additives can be added to fluids or in separate IV lines with a dedicated syringe pump when intravenous or intraosseous catheters are in place. Most replacement fluids are deficient in potassium and should be supplemented after initial stabilization or hypokalemia may develop after a few days.

Colloids are intravascular expanders that increase the plasma colloidal pressure by pulling interstitial fluids into the intravascular space. Colloids are indicated for hypotension, hypovolemia, hypoproteinemia, significant hemorrhage, when colloidal pressure is low, and in fluid resuscitation. Coagulopathy, pneumonia, congestive heart failure, and renal failure are all contraindications for colloid administration.

Fluid Therapy Plan

The objectives of fluid replacement therapy are to replace fluid deficits to correct perfusion and hydration without inducing fluid overload, to anticipate fluid loss and provide maintenance needs, and to correct electrolytes and acid-base abnormalities. Additionally, the fluid therapy plan should be monitored and reassessed while underlying conditions are diagnosed and treated.

Fluid therapy is divided into three stages: resuscitation, rehydration, and maintenance. If the bird has signs of hypoperfusion, shock, or active hemorrhage, emergency fluid resuscitation is required.

Resuscitation

Fluids used in resuscitation include isotonic balanced crystalloids and/or a combination of hypertonic saline (7.5% NaCl), crystalloids, and colloids. A goal for fluid resuscitation is to use the least amount of fluid to reach the desired effect and to achieve fast intravascular volume expansion and reverse the hypotensive state. The authors regularly use 3 ml/kg of 7.5% NaCl mixed with 5 ml/kg of colloid given over 10 minutes followed by crystalloids bolused at 10 ml/kg [7]. Crystalloid boluses may be repeated every 10–15 minutes until improvement of clinical markers is seen or until blood pressure is greater than 90 mmHg. Atropine (0.2 mg/kg IV) and epinephrine (0.02 mg/kg IV) may also be used if non-responsive. At this stage, blood work, electrolytes, and blood gas analysis may help assess other causes of non-responsive shock (e.g. hypoglycemia, hypocalcemia).

Rehydration and Maintenance

For the rehydration phase of the fluid therapy plan, once perfusion has been restored and the degree of dehydration estimated, the rate of fluids should be calculated. The volume of fluids for deficit correction is determined by the formula:

$$\%\text{dehydration} \times \text{kg} \times 1000 \text{ ml}$$

Usually 50–100% of estimated loss may be replenished within the first 24 hours. To this, maintenance requirements (around 3 ml/kg/h) and anticipated losses should be added. In general, the more rapid the fluid loss, the more rapid the replacement should be, especially when pre-renal azotemia has been identified. Consequently, total fluid deficit may be replenished in 4–10 hours if acute dehydration is suspected. The choice of fluid type is usually guided by acid base and electrolyte abnormalities. Most avian patients are in metabolic acidosis with dehydration or various illness which makes PlasmaLyte the fluid of choice [19]. LRS may be used instead but is slightly hypotonic to avian plasma. For vomiting and loss of KCl and metabolic alkalosis, 0.9% NaCl is the fluid of choice. Monitoring the patient's response to fluid therapy is important as calculations are only rough estimates. Body weight gives a good estimate of the amount of rehydration. Since fluid deficits and requirements are difficult to estimate and clinical endpoints challenging to assess in birds, rehydration may continue for another 24–48 hours using a lower rate. If an IV or IO catheter is not well tolerated, the maintenance phase can be performed subcutaneously, and the catheters removed.

The fluid "surgical rate" under anesthesia is typically 10 ml/kg/h to treat the anesthetic-induced hypotension and anticipated fluid loss due to oxygen flow and evaporation through the surgical sites.

Blood Transfusion

Blood is considered a colloid with the added benefit of providing blood cells and coagulation factors. While chickens are intolerant to large acute blood loss (LD_{50} for acute blood loss in chickens is 40–50% of blood volume), they can withstand a large blood loss if removed slowly [11]. Fluid mobilization in the chicken does not require an increase in precapillary resistance and because the chicken does not exhibit intense precapillary constriction, unlike that noted in mammals, it is spared some of the deleterious effects of inadequate tissue perfusion [11]. If severe hemorrhage or anemia is present, birds may benefit from homologous blood transfusions (Figure 19.9).

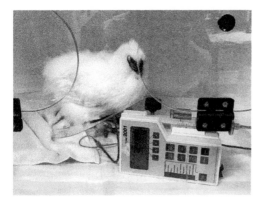

Figure 19.9 Administration of a blood transfusion to an anemic silkie chicken.

The transfusion (usually 10% of blood volume taken from a donor bird, as higher volume is generally not feasible unless several donors are available) is typically administered over one to four hours and the use of a pediatric microfilter is recommended. Blood is typically transfused whole in birds and collected from the same species of bird. The half-life of infused blood is about a week. Transfusing from other bird species is not generally indicated as transfused blood cells are rapidly destroyed.

Bandaging and Wound Management

Poultry have excellent wound healing capacity. Open wounds should be cleaned and bandaged until the patient is stable and can tolerate more extensive wound debridement or surgery. Immediate wound coverage decreases further tissue damage and desiccation. If immediate wound closure is not possible, packing the wound with moistened sterile gauze sponges or a water-soluble lubricating gel (K-Y Jelly, Johnson and Johnson Products, New Brunswick, NJ) limits desiccation. If surgical debridement is performed within 24 hours of a bird sustaining a severe injury, the patient may be placed at unnecessary risk. The level of tissue damage and surgical risk can usually be assessed within 24 hours post-injury. Initial wound cleaning, minor debridement, and temporary wound dressing may be preferable to aggressive surgical debridement to allow for patient stabilization. Severed tendons, major nerves, or ligaments should be re-anastomosed as soon as possible as tissue contraction can complicate repair. Coelomic penetration may require surgical exploration. Primary closure of wounds is indicated for stable birds presented within six to eight hours of trauma with minimal contamination and tissue trauma (Figure 19.10) [6]. Delayed primary closure is indicated for most acute wounds healthy enough for closure within three to five days of wound management with hydrophilic dressings (Figure 19.11). Use of water-based preparations is preferred in avian wounds. Honey is a water-soluble hydrophilic substance with antibacterial, antifungal, and antiviral properties that works well for wound healing and can be used in egg laying birds (Figures 19.12 and 19.13). Secondary closure or second-intention healing of wounds is indicated for extensive wounds requiring wound management for longer periods. These wounds can be closed once a healthy bed of granulation tissue is present or left to heal by second intention. Nonadherent bandaging materials are recommended to avoid disruption of the healing surface of the wound. Wound healing time is 10–14 days for skin healing in most avian patients.

Wing injuries distal to the elbow can be stabilized temporarily using figure-of-eight

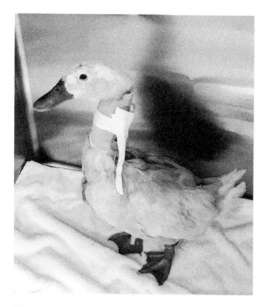

Figure 19.10 Primary closure was performed in this duck with a neck wound. In this case, a vacutainer tube and butterfly catheter are incorporated into the wound repair to act as a negative pressure drain.

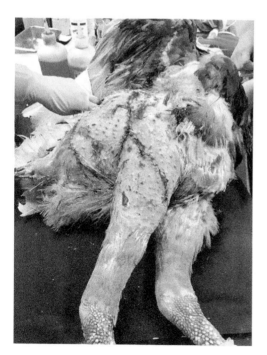

Figure 19.11 Example of delayed primary closure. This turkey was managed for several days with antibiotics and wound management before surgical closure.

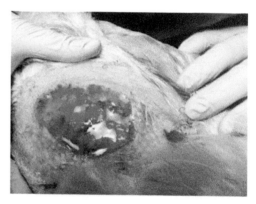

Figure 19.12 This dorsal wound on a chicken was unable to be surgically closed and was managed with a honey dressing.

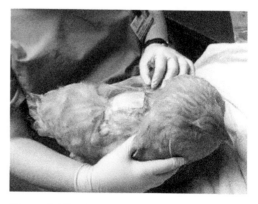

Figure 19.13 An adherent dressing was used over the wound shown in Figure 19.12 and was well tolerated by this hen.

bandages; shoulder and humeral fractures should be stabilized using a body wrap. Avoid excess pressure across the keel with body wraps that may compromise patient respiration. Cast padding covered with a layer of self-adherent bandage (Vetrap, 3M Health Care, St. Paul, MN) is ideal because it creates a soft padded bandage that is easily held in place and does not damage feathers. Self-adherent bandages can tighten when wet, so access of bandaged birds to open containers of water should be limited or monitored. Femoral fractures are managed with cage rest until the bird can withstand surgical fixation (Figures 19.14 and 19.15). Fractures involving the tibiotarsus can be managed with a Robert-Jones bandage. Tarsometatarsal fractures can be stabilized with a Robert-Jones bandage combined with a ball bandage or incorporated foot cast. Reviews of wound management, bumblefoot treatment, bandage types, and surgical and nonsurgical repair of fractures in avian species are available [6].

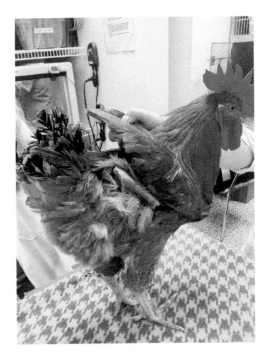

Figure 19.15 The rooster with the femoral fracture shown in Figure 19.14 at the time of recheck prior to fixator removal. Feathers have regrown, and the fixator was well tolerated.

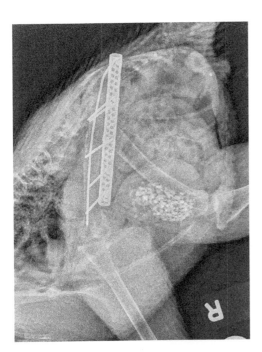

Figure 19.14 Post-operative radiograph of a rooster following Type 1a ESF (external skeletal fixator) for a femoral fracture repair.

Nutritional Support

Diets for stable hospitalized poultry should ideally be based around the natural diet and life-stage of the species. For example, laying hens require ~18.3% crude protein in the diet and protein requirements decrease with age. Replacement fluid therapy is critical before nutritional support is instituted in debilitated patients. Commercially available critical care feeding formulas, such as Emeraid Intensive Care Omnivore* (Lafeber Company, Cornell, IL), Hill's a/d diet (a/d® Canine/Feline, Hill's Pet Nutrition, Inc., Topeka, KS), or Critical Care Omnivore (Oxbow Animal Health, Omaha NE) can be used on a short-term basis. The authors generally feed up to 50 ml/kg PO via gavage tube several times daily in anorectic chickens that can tolerate assisted feedings. See Chapter 6 for detailed information on poultry nutrition.

Analgesia

Pain Recognition

Pain recognition can be more challenging in birds than mammals as pain assessment is highly subjective. Some signs of pain can include change in temperament, reduced mobility or perching, restlessness, decreased food consumption, lethargy, hunched body position, and lameness. Over-grooming and under-grooming can occur at painful sites. Heart rate and respiratory rate can vary with painful conditions, but blood pressure is generally elevated in birds experiencing pain. Any condition assumed to be painful to any other species should be assumed to be painful to avian patients.

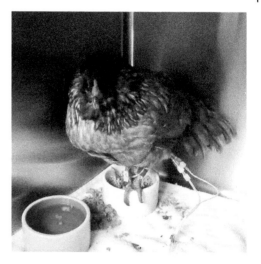

Figure 19.16 This hen is comfortable and eating immediately post-salpingohysterectomy with a fentanyl CRI.

Local Analgesia

Due to the tractable nature of most poultry species, the sole use of local analgesia can be considered to manage small wounds or focal pain. Toxicity to local anesthetics such as lidocaine and bupivacaine may be more of an issue with birds than mammals; lower dosages (2.7–3.3 mg/kg) have been associated with toxicity in birds. A dose of 1.33 and 1.96 mg/kg of IV bupivacaine was associated with a 50% probability of a clinically significant change in mean arterial pressure (MAP) in isoflurane-anesthetized chickens [20]. The ED50 of IV lidocaine is approximately 3 times greater than that of IV bupivacaine in chickens; 6 mg/kg of IV lidocaine was not associated with adverse cardiovascular effects [21]. Lidocaine, bupivacaine, and eutectic mixture of local anesthetic (EMLA) are commonly used in avian patients.

Opioids

Opioids should be considered in critical avian patients with moderate to severe pain, such as with trauma or surgery. Birds may not respond to μ agonists as κ and δ receptors are more common in the forebrain and midbrain of pigeons. A study in chickens showed some similarities to findings in the pigeon, but there were marked dissimilarities thought to be due either to species specific, or age related, differences [22]. Response to morphine is variable between different strains of chickens. A dose of 2 mg/kg intravenous butorphanol may be analgesic in chickens for up to two hours. Morphine used at 2 mg/kg caused sedation [23]. A single fentanyl bolus induced a dose-dependent and short-lasting reduction in isoflurane MAC (minimum anesthetic concentration) in chickens, but the clinical usefulness of a single fentanyl bolus is limited by its short duration of effect [24]. The authors have used fentanyl CRI (continuous rate infusion) in conjunction with general anesthesia and post-operatively for painful conditions in poultry (Figure 19.16).

Non-steroidal Anti-Inflammatory Drugs (NSAIDs)

Meloxicam administered at a dose of 1 mg/kg PO in chickens maintained plasma concentrations equivalent to those reported to be therapeutic for humans for 12 hours with no drug detected after four days in egg whites and eight days in egg yolks [25]. The walking ability of lame chickens was improved with the administration of the analgesic drug carprofen either orally [26] or subcutaneously [27]. The effect of various NSAIDs was also evaluated by

Hocking et al. in domestic fowl induced with acute pain by intra-articular injection of sodium urate crystals. Analgesic effects of carprofen, flunixin, ketoprofen, and sodium salicylate were observed at dose rates much higher than mammals [28]. Salicylic acid provided good analgesia at 50 mg/kg intravenous bolus dose rate, but the effects lasted only one hour in chickens [29].

Other Analgesics

Oral bioavailability of tramadol was higher in avian species compared to humans or dogs. Although this drug is used clinically in caged birds and shows great promise, further investigation is needed to determine appropriate dosing, efficacy, and safety among different species, including poultry. Gabapentin has been used as part of a multimodal plan for suspected neuropathic pain in birds. Self-mutilation has been reportedly decreased after the addition of gabapentin to the therapeutic regimen in avian species.

Common Emergency Presentations

Poultry Emergency Retrospective

The authors (JG, ER) recently published a retrospective documenting 78 poultry cases that presented on an emergent basis to their institution over a 3-year span [30]. The presenting complaints most frequently seen were trauma (n = 25) and reproductive disease (n = 17). The most common source of trauma was due to predators (n = 11), including raptors (n = 3), dogs/foxes (n = 6), and two chickens with traumatic wounds consistent with predation but with unwitnessed trauma. Although based on their initial presenting complaint, only 12.8% (10/78) chickens in this study were assumed to have reproductive disease, further assessment of chickens presenting to the ER revealed that 21.8% (17/78) had presumed or confirmed concurrent reproductive disease noted. Although

approximately half of the chickens presenting for an emergency were euthanized, the remainder were successfully discharged on medical management.

Trauma

Predator attack, fractures, wounds, gunshot trauma, head trauma, electrocution, and other injuries may cause emergent presentation of poultry (Figure 19.17). A thorough physical examination is essential to determine the extent of trauma and best approach for treatment. Prioritize therapy, cleanse wounds, and stabilize fractures initially, until patient stabilization allows surgical repair and more detailed treatment. Any animal with a bite wound should receive antibiotics after samples are collected for microbial culture and sensitivity. Head and neck wounds are common in poultry and may require surgical repair (Figures 19.18 and 19.19).

Fractures of the skull may occur and healing by second intention can occur if the animal is

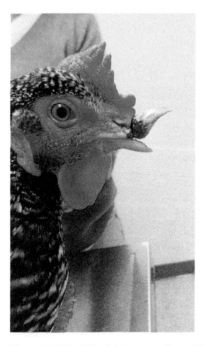

Figure 19.17 This chicken experienced traumatic injury to the beak.

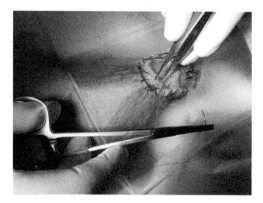

Figure 19.18 Primary closure was used to resolve the scalp wound in this hen.

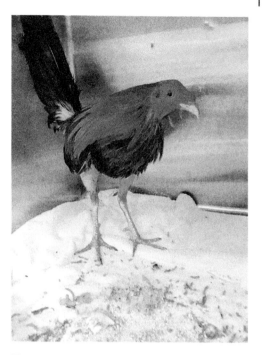

Figure 19.20 This rooster was confiscated from a cock fighting ring. Note the plucked feathers from the legs and absence of comb and full wattle.

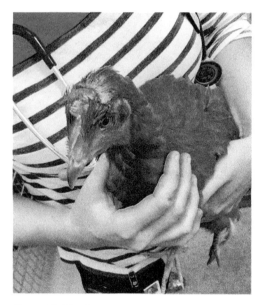

Figure 19.19 Post-operative appearance of the closed wound shown in Figure 19.18.

able to groom and eat [31]. Injuries over the coelomic cavity should be explored to rule out and manage penetrating wounds. Myiasis is commonly seen in older, untreated wounds in birds housed outdoors. Birds bruise green and a green appearance to the skin should not be mistaken for necrosis. Injured birds should be segregated, or any open wounds should be covered to prevent cannibalism from conspecifics. Practitioners should be aware of the appearance of roosters used in the illegal sport of cockfighting when birds present for wound

evaluation. Breeders often pluck the birds' feathers and cut off the roosters' wattles and/or combs to prevent other roosters from tearing them off in the ring (Figure 19.20). See Chapter 15 for more information on trauma and wound management.

The high mineral content of avian bones results in sharp fracture fragments that can easily damage adjacent vessels, nerves, skin, and muscle. Luxations should be reduced as soon as possible to have the best chance for joint mobility. See the Bandaging and Wound Management section for more specific information on wound management of fractures.

Head Trauma

Head trauma can be associated with physical examination findings of anisocoria, head tilt, depression or other neurologic signs, skull fractures, retinal detachment, or hemorrhage from the nares, oral cavity, ears, or anterior chamber of the eye. The most important neurological signs to monitor every 30 minutes are mentation and pupil symmetry, size, and pupillary light reflex. Changes in pupil size to dilated and loss of pupillary light reflex along with mentation progression to stuporous or coma are documentation of neurological deterioration. The chicken with head trauma may benefit from oxygen support. Intravenous fluid administration using isotonic saline and colloids are given in limited volumes (saline at 10 ml/kg and hydroxyethyl starch [HES] at 3 ml/kg) to maintain blood pressure at 80–90 mmHg systolic (hypotensive or limited volume resuscitation) to avoid increasing intracranial pressure. Administration of furosemide and/or mannitol should be considered in the case of minimal response to initial therapy or deterioration of the presenting neurological signs. The use of steroids with head trauma is not recommended. Ophthalmologic examination of both anterior and posterior segments should occur upon patient stabilization. Topical and/or systemic administration of antibiotics are indicated for corneal ulceration or perforation. Topical ophthalmic nonsteroidal anti-inflammatories can be used to treat uveitis in poultry without corneal ulceration.

Electrocution

Evidence of electrocution may not be evident for several days following injury. Clinical consequences of electrocution in birds include cardiac arrest, pericardial effusion, neurogenic pulmonary edema (causing acute respiratory distress), thermal burns particularly of the heat, feet, and carpi. Feather damage of the barbs and barbules, without damage to the rachis can be a classic sign of electrocution. If electrocution is suspected, treat symptoms manifested. Pericardial effusion is diagnosed with the help of an echocardiogram and treatment with pericardiocentesis. Neurogenic pulmonary edema causing acute respiratory distress may respond to one dose of furosamide (2 mg/kg) and supportive care with oxygen and sedation. Systemic administration of antibiotics, non-steroidal anti-inflammatories, and topical wound therapy may also be indicated. Prognosis for electrocution varies from fair to grave dependent upon the extent and severity of the damage.

Hypothermic Shock and Heat Stress

Adequate shelter should always be available for poultry, but debilitated and juvenile animals may not always seek shelter in poor weather conditions. Some chickens, particularly silkies and Polands, are particularly sensitive to hypothermia [32]. Frostbite may be seen more commonly in roosters because of their large comb and wattles. External heat support and warm fluids are indicated for rewarming hypothermic patients.

Poultry are most comfortable when housed in ambient temperatures ranging from 50 to 75 °F. High temperatures, particularly associated with high humidity, are associated with heat stress in chickens. As temperatures rise (82–95 °F), chickens increase peripheral blood flow and hold their wings away from their body to dissipate heat. As temperatures approach 105 °F, chickens display tachypnea and open-beak breathing. If body temperatures continue to rise, birds become listless and comatose and ultimately die of electrolyte, circulatory, or electrolyte imbalances [33]. Treatment for heat stress includes slowly reducing body temperature with spraying, cool water baths, or wrapping in cool wet towels (making sure not to induce hypothermia), fluid administration, and supportive care as needed.

Respiratory Emergencies

In cases of respiratory distress, the chicken patient should immediately be placed in an oxygen-enriched environment and observed for pattern of breathing. Because severely dyspneic birds do not tolerate handling, an oxygen cage with greater than 70% oxygen concentration is recommended. This can be accomplished with commercially available intensive care units with an oxygen flow rate of 5 L. Butorphanol (1 mg/kg) with midazolam (0.25–0.5 mg/kg), administered intramuscularly, may provide mild sedation and reduce anxiety associated with acute respiratory distress in the avian patient. Humidification of oxygenated air by bubbling through an isotonic solution is recommended to assist with clearance of respiratory secretions and foreign material in the trachea and bronchi [9].

Airway Obstruction

Airway obstruction is characterized by stridor and dyspnea that is exacerbated by exertion, and intervention is necessary to relieve obstruction. In severe cases, immediate placement of an air sac cannula is indicated. Following cannula placement, endoscopic examination of the trachea can allow removal of foreign bodies or identification of granulomas. A suction tube (urinary catheter) smaller than the diameter of the trachea may be passed to suction out foreign bodies. Tracheal surgery has been described to remove tracheal foreign bodies in birds. Membranous stenosis has been described in poultry following injury to the neck; this should be kept in mind when a bird that presents with evidence of airway obstruction with a history of recent predator attack.

Tracheal obstruction in chickens can be caused by obstructing respiratory secretions, food inhalation, and a variety of bacterial, viral, fungal (Figures 19.21–19.23), and parasitic

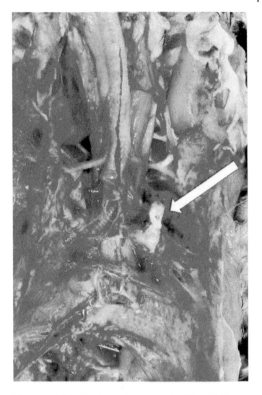

Figure 19.21 Post-mortem examination of the chicken shown in Figure 19.6. The arrow points to marked, segmental, fibrinoheterophilic bronchitis with intralesional fungal hyphae and pulmonary thrombosis obstructing the left bronchus.

causes. In emergency situations involving occlusion of the upper respiratory tract, such

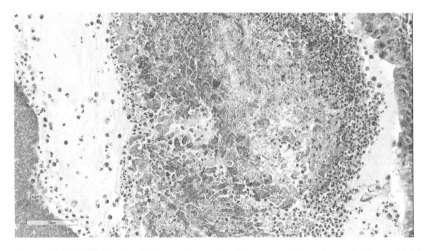

Figure 19.22 H&E stained photomicrograph of the gross lesion shown in Figure 19.21. Note the fibrinonecrotic material and heterophils in the bronchus.

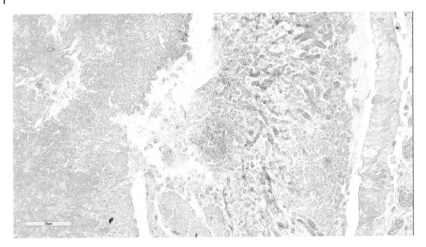

Figure 19.23 GMS stained photomicrograph of the gross lesion in Figures 19.21 and 19.22 demonstrating the presence of fungal hyphae consistent with aspergillosis.

as tracheal granulomas, foreign bodies, or severe head or facial trauma, air sac intubation may be necessary to ensure air flow through the respiratory tract; it is not indicated when significant lower respiratory tract disease is present. Sedation with a low dose of midazolam, local lidocaine block, or inhalant anesthesia may be necessary for placement of the air sac cannula. Specially made air sac cannulas are available or various types of tubing or standard endotracheal tubing can be modified; for example, a cuffed 3.0–4.0 mm inside diameter endotracheal tube can be used. The position for the tube is the same as for an endoscopic approach to the caudal thoracic and abdominal air sacs, with the caveat that there is reduced space in these air sacs compared to psittacine species due to the voluminous GI and reproductive tracts. A small skin incision is made over the triangle created by the cranial muscle mass of the femur, ventral to the synsacrum and caudal to the last rib. The body wall is penetrated with a pair of hemostats and the air sac cannula is inserted between the last two ribs or just caudal to the last rib. The bird should immediately begin to breathe through the tube if placed correctly. Inflating the cuff and suturing into place can secure the tube. A filter, such as the removed inner filter from a respirator

mask can be placed over the end of the tube to prevent entry of particulate matter [9].

Sinusitis

Poultry may present on an emergent basis for conjunctivitis or swelling of the periorbital sinuses (Figure 19.24). A variety of infectious organisms can cause sinusitis in chickens, including *Pasteurella* sp., *Escherichia coli, Pseudomonas* sp., *Mycoplasma* sp., *Mycobacterium* sp., *Chlamydia* sp., parasites, and many others [10]. Viral disease including

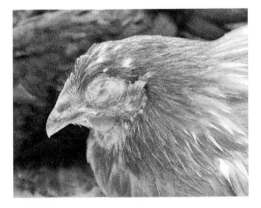

Figure 19.24 This hen presented with severe conjunctivitis. Note the presence of dried exudate on the side of the bird's head and neck. *Source:* Photograph courtesy of Yuko Sato.

avian influenza, Newcastle disease, and infectious laryngotracheitis can be associated with sinusitis in poultry, albeit rarely, so it behooves the practitioner to be aware of reportable diseases in poultry. A nasal flush can be performed on birds with sinusitis (general anesthesia and intubation may be required to protect the airway) to collect samples for diagnostic testing. Systemic and local treatment may be warranted depending on the etiology. Surgery may be needed to remove purulent material from the sinuses. More information can be found in Chapter 12.

Lower Airway Disease

Lower respiratory disease in chickens can occur in association with foreign body inhalation with subsequent aspiration pneumonia, inhaled toxins, respiratory system trauma, and a myriad of infectious etiologies. Coelomic pathology can also cause respiratory distress. Radiographs, respiratory washes, endoscopy, or other diagnostics may be needed to determine the type and extent of disease. In the case of aspiration pneumonia, initial radiographs may be normal, but evidence of local pneumonia or focal pulmonary abscesses can develop with time. Treatment may include hospitalization with oxygen therapy, nebulization, fluid therapy, and broad-spectrum antibiotics and antifungal medications. A full discussion of diagnosis and management of infectious causes of lower airway disease, including reportable diseases, is beyond the scope of this chapter; see Chapter 12 for more information.

Respiratory distress associated with inhaled toxic fumes and environmental pollutants can occur. Birds are sensitive to the effects of inhaled toxins, and clients should be educated about the risks of inhaled fumes such as overheating of nonstick coatings, self-cleaning ovens, bleach, ammonia, cigarette smoke, and others. Nonstick cookware, heat lamps, and other items with a nonstick coating can release polytetrafluoroethylene gas (PTFE) when cooking surfaces overheat or products are initially used. PTFE inhalation can cause pulmonary congestion, hemorrhage, and death. If a bird presents with a history of an inhaled toxin, immediate oxygen support is ideal. Saline nebulization can be beneficial. Bronchodilators such as terbutaline (Brethine, Novartis Pharmaceuticals Corporation, East Hanover, NJ) have been used parenterally and via nebulization in dyspneic birds suffering from inhaled toxins [9]. Prognosis of respiratory toxicosis may vary from good to grave dependent on the extent and severity of the toxins.

Chickens may suffer tracheal or air sac trauma from predator attack, a fall, or other trauma. The accumulation of subcutaneous air may result in respiratory compromise. Subcutaneous emphysema can be relieved by fine needle aspiration or by creation of a small skin incision that is sutured to the body wall and left open to allow healing of the air sac prior to healing of the skin.

Coelomic Disease

Ascites, masses, and dystocia may cause pronounced respiratory signs due to compression of the air sacs. If coelomic palpation reveals distention or the presence of a mass, ultrasound is useful to determine if free fluid is present. Ultrasound-guided coelomic aspiration can be performed on an emergency basis to remove fluid and provide immediate relief to the patient. Care should be taken to maintain the patient in an upright position during this procedure to prevent fluid from entering the lungs; oxygen provided via a facemask and mild sedation may be helpful for the procedure. Ultrasound can also help characterize any masses in the coelom (see Figure 19.5). Ascites is often associated with reproductive pathology and birds with coelomic fluid may have a guarded prognosis when carcinomatosis is associated with this presentation. See Reproductive Emergencies section for more information.

Gastrointestinal Emergencies

Crop Stasis and Ileus

Ingluvial hypomotility and ileus are relatively common GI emergency presentations and may be secondary to an underlying disease. Poultry may ingest poorly digestible items including grass, substrate, and feathers that could cause impaction. Historical findings may include crop distention, decreased fecal production, and sudden death. Crop distention, dehydration, respiratory distress, and weakness may be noted on examination. Causes of crop stasis and ileus include candidiasis and other infections (bacterial, viral, parasitic), atonic ingluvies (overstretched), gastrointestinal impactions, trauma, stricture, foreign bodies, metabolic disease, intussusception and volvulus, toxicosis (lead, zinc), and neoplasia. Helpful diagnostics can include CBC (complete blood count)/Chemistry, fecal or crop cytology, heavy metal (lead, zinc) levels, radiographs (empty crop if full prior to positioning), +/- advanced imaging. If possible, aspiration of crop contents and ingluvial flushing may help stabilize the patient until the primary cause can be addressed. Some cases of impaction may require surgical intervention. Treatment depends on etiology and supportive care measures including rehydration are warranted. See Chapter 17 for more information.

Diarrhea

Diarrhea is characterized by abnormally increased frequency, liquidity, and volume of fecal discharge. Birds with this condition may have abnormal stool (color, character), undigested food in the droppings, and soiled vent feathers. Causes of diarrhea may include bacterial infection (*E. coli, Salmonella sp.*, etc.), viral infection, parasitic infection, obstruction, metabolic disorders, dietary causes, maldigestion, and toxins. Fecal examinations including a direct observation, flotation, and Diff-Quik may be helpful, along with a fecal bacterial culture. Other diagnostics that can be helpful in determine the cause of diarrhea include CBC/

Chemistry (may be nonspecific or show signs of infection and dehydration), and radiographs, with or without additional imaging. Serum should be collected to rule out viral causes of diarrhea if indicated. Treatment is dependent on the cause and nursing care including fluids, warmth, and nutritional support can be beneficial.

Hepatic Lipidosis

Fat retention in the liver is common for all laying birds. In some cases, excessive amounts of fat can be deposited and lead to hepatic rupture, hemorrhage, and death. Caged layers are prone to this condition because of high caloric intake and minimal exercise. This condition can also be seen in obese backyard laying hens. Like other species, chickens with this condition have enlarged, friable, pale orange, soft, and easily fractured livers. Prevention of this condition involves feeding a diet with appropriate energy and protein levels and allowing exercise. In some situations, choline chloride, vitamin K, biotin, and vitamin E have been used to manage this condition with varying results.

Reproductive Emergencies

Other than trauma, reproductive emergencies are one of the more common emergencies seen in laying hens. Common presentations include egg binding and dystocia, coelomitis, oviductal prolapse, and reproductive neoplasia. See Chapter 16 for detailed information on reproductive disease.

Egg Binding and Dystocia

Chronic egg laying can result in weakness, osteopenia, egg binding, yolk peritonitis, oviductal obstruction, and pathologic fractures. Initial stabilization measures involve the administration of fluids, parenteral calcium, and possibly vitamin D if the diet is suboptimal (injectable vitamin A/D/E formulations are most often used). Diagnostics including CBC, chemistry (including ionized calcium), radiographs, ultrasound, and coelomocentesis can be helpful to determine the extent and type of disease. Care should be taken to remove any coelomic fluid before putting the bird in a non-vertical position. Options for egg removal can include lubricating the tissue and manual expression, hormonal therapy, ovocentesis to aspirate contents and implode the egg, or salpingohysterectomy. Ovocentesis runs the risk of coelomitis and is usually reserved for cases in which conservative therapy is unsuccessful. Salpingohysterectomy is recommended for birds with chronic recurring disease or when egg removal is otherwise unsuccessful.

Oviductal/Vent Prolapse

Oviductal prolapse can occur secondary to straining from a variety of conditions including egg laying or dystocia (Figure 19.25). Age, obesity, poor nutrition, and stress may predispose to this condition. It is common for conspecifics to traumatize prolapsed tissue. Prolapsed tissues should be cleaned and kept moistened to prevent desiccation. Temporary stay sutures on each side of the vent (avoid purse-string suture) may be warranted to keep prolapsed tissue in place but this is contraindicated if an egg is still within the reproductive tract. Salpingohysterectomy may be needed if conservative management is unsuccessful.

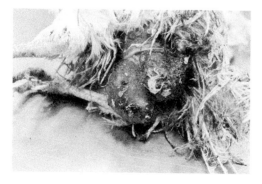

Figure 19.25 Severe vent prolapse involving the oviduct and colon was the cause of death in this hen.

Coelomitis

Inflammation related to free yolk in the coelomic cavity can occur in hens often without accompanying bacterial infection. Chickens with this condition may be off feed and depressed and the coelom may be distended. Although often diagnosed at necropsy, coelomocentesis can be performed to relieve dyspnea and to analyze fluid for yolk, inflammatory cells, and bacteria. Fluid therapy, analgesia, antimicrobials, and assisted feeding can be given to the individual hen if warranted. Salpingohysterectomy may be required to successfully manage this condition. Concurrent pathology including Marek's disease, salpingitis, and carcinomatosis may predispose to, and often accompany, coelomitis.

Cage-Layer Fatigue (Osteoporosis)

Chronic egg laying can result in hypocalcemia, leg weakness, osteoporosis, and death. Cage-layer fatigue is most common in caged birds and young hens in early egg production. Birds with this condition may have a history of decreased egg production and poor eggshell quality. Physical examination findings can include weakness, bone deformities such as bent ribs and curved keel bone, and inability to stand. Prevention of this condition involves feeding an appropriate laying ration, allowing access to sunlight, ensuring large particle calcium size, and preventing foraging of large amounts of inadequately balanced forage.

Phallus Prolapse

Phallus prolapse is occasionally seen in waterfowl and can occur secondary to infection or immunosuppression, trauma, and hypersexuality. Prolapsed healthy tissue should be cleaned, lubricated, and replaced. Analgesia, local or systemic antibiotics, and cold hypertonic solutions such as chilled dextrose can be helpful to reduce swelling and manage this condition. In cases of repeat prolapse or necrotic tissue phallus amputation may be necessary.

Musculoskeletal and Neurologic Emergencies

Pododermatitis

Pododermatitis, also known as bumblefoot, involves primary trauma at weight-bearing aspects of the feet followed by secondary bacterial infection. Swelling, ulceration, and erythema of the feet can be seen in this inflammatory condition. Obesity, inactivity, unequal weight bearing, trauma and inappropriate substrate can predispose to pododermatitis. Mild cases can be managed with substrate change, soaking, bandaging, and exercise while severe cases may require surgery (Figure 19.26). Aerobic and anaerobic culture should be performed at the time of surgery. Wound management, bandaging, and antibiotics can be used to address more severely affected birds. See Chapter 11 for more information on pododermatitis.

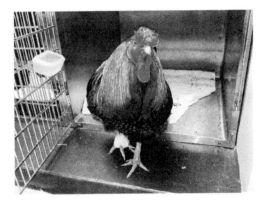

Figure 19.26 A bandage was used to manage mild pododermatitis in this Wyandotte rooster.

Lameness

Causes of lameness in poultry are varied and can include trauma, pododermatitis, Marek's disease, reproductive disorders, neurologic disease or general weakness, and others (Figure 19.27). History, and physical examination, including a neurologic examination, are important to determine the cause of lameness. Radiographs can help rule out fractures, osteomyelitis, and other pathology. Treatment is based on cause; see Chapter 11 for a complete description of lameness diagnosis and management.

Seizures

Seizures can occur secondary to trauma, heavy metal ingestion, hypoglycemia, cardiovascular disease, hypocalcemia, idiopathic epilepsy, and infectious disease including viral, bacterial, fungal, and parasitic causes. A neurologic examination is helpful to localize the lesion in

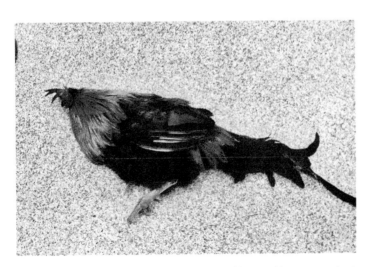

Figure 19.27 This rooster had a several days history of lameness prior to presenting non-ambulatory.

some cases. Diagnostics helpful to diagnose this condition may include radiographs, CBC, chemistry analysis including ionized calcium, heavy metal (lead and zinc) screening, and other testing as warranted. Treatment is based on suspected etiology. Intramuscular midazolam or intravenous diazepam can be used to control seizures. If the seizures cannot be controlled in this manner, additional therapies such as phenobarbital or levetiracetam can be considered.

Toxin Exposure

Chickens are susceptible to the toxic effects of heavy metal, pesticides including anticoagulant rodenticide, oil, and other environmental contaminants (Figure 19.28). General treatment of toxicity should include removal of the offending agent when feasible, supportive care, and treatment of clinical signs. When the toxicant is known, a specific antidote should also be given if possible. Prognosis of intoxication can vary from good to grave dependent upon amount and time of toxin exposure and type of intoxication.

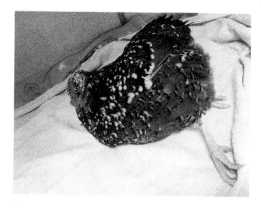

Figure 19.28 This chicken was non-ambulatory due to lead poisoning. Plasma lead levels were 51.5 ug/dl in this chicken. She was briefly ambulatory after initiation of chelation therapy but ultimately declined and was euthanized.

Euthanasia

Euthanasia may be necessary for disease with a poor prognosis, certain infectious disease, and if necropsy is needed to determine causes of morbidity or mortality in flock situations. Chickens can be euthanized by administration of intravenous euthanasia solution and sedation or general anesthesia prior to euthanasia may be warranted to reduce stress or pain.

References

1 Hopper, K., Epstein, S.E., Fletcher, D.J., and Boller, M., Authors the RECOVER Basic Life Support Domain Worksheet (2012). RECOVER evidence and knowledge gap analysis on veterinary CPR. Part 3: basic life support. *J. Vet. Emerg. Crit. Care (San Antonio)* 22 (S1): S26–S43.

2 Costello, M.F. (2004). Principles of cardiopulmonary cerebral resuscitation in special species. *Sem. Avian Exot. Pet Med.* 13 (2): 132–141.

3 Bowles, H., Lichtenberger, M., and Lennox, A. (2007). Emergency and critical care of pet birds. *Vet. Clin. N. Am. Exot. Anim. Pract.* 10 (2): 345–394.

4 Rozanski, E.A., Rush, J.E., Buckley, G.J. et al., Authors Recover Advanced Life Support Domain Worksheet (2012). RECOVER evidence and knowledge gap analysis on veterinary CPR. Part 4: advanced life support. *J. Vet. Emerg. Crit. Care (San Antonio)* 22 (Suppl 1): S44–S64.

5 King, A.S. and Payne, D.C. (1962). The maximum capacities of the lungs and air sacs of *Gallus domesticus. J. Anat.* 96: 495–503.

6 Graham, J. and Heatley, J. (2007). Emergency care of raptors. *Vet. Clin. N. Am.* 10 (2): 395–418.

7 Lichtenberger, M. and Lennox, A. (2016). Critical care. In: Current Therapy in Avian Medicine and Surgery (ed. B. Speer), 582–588. St. Louis, MI: Elsevier.

8 Lichtenberger, M. (2004). Principles of shock and fluid therapy in special species. *Sem. Avian Exot. Pet Med.* 13 (3): 142–153.

9 Graham, J. (2004). Approach to the dyspneic avian patient. *Sem. Avian Exot. Pet Med.* 13 (3): 154–159.

10 Gonzalez, M.S. and Carrasco, D.C. (2016). Emergencies and critical care of commonly kept fowl. *Vet. Clin. N. Am.* 19 (2): 543–565.

11 Ploucha, J.M., Scott, J.B., and Ringer, R.K. (1981). Vascular and hematologic effects of hemorrhage in the chicken. *Am. J. Physiol.* 240 (1): H9–H17.

12 Lichtenberger, M. (2005). Determination of indirect blood pressure in the companion bird. *Sem. Avian Exot. Pet Med.* 14 (2): 149–152.

13 Lumeij, J. and Ritchie, B. (1994). Cardiovascular system. In: Avian Medicine: Principles and Application (eds. B. Ritchie, G. Harrison and L. Harrison), 694–722. Lake Worth, FL: Winger's Publishing, Inc.

14 Pees, M., Krautwald-Junghanns, M., and Straub, J. (2006). Evaluating and treating the cardiovascular system. In: Clinical Avian Medicine, vol. 1 (eds. G. Harrison and T. Lightfoot), 379–394. Palm Beach, FL: Spix Publishing, Inc.

15 Naganobu, K., Fujisawa, Y., Ohde, H. et al. (2000). Determination of the minimum anesthetic concentration and cardiovascular dose response for sevoflurane in chickens during controlled ventilation. *Vet. Surg.* 29: 102–105.

16 Khamas, W., Rutllant-Labeaga, J., and Greenacre, C.B. (2015). Physical examination, anatomy, and physiology. In: Backyard Poultry Medicine and Surgery. A Guide for Veterinary Practitioners (eds. C.B. Greenacre and T.Y. Morishita), 95–117. Ames, IA: Wiley-Blackwell.

17 Edling, T. (2006). Updates in anesthesia and monitoring. In: Clinical Avian Medicine, vol. 2 (eds. G. Harrison and T. Lightfoot), 747–760. Palm Beach, FL: Spix Publishing.

18 Campbell, T. (1994). Hematology. In: Avian Medicine: Principles and Application (eds. B. Ritchie, G. Harrison and L. Harrison), 176–198. Lake Worth, FL: Wingers Publishing.

19 Beaufrère, H. Nutrition and fluid therapy in birds. In: Exotic Animal Emergency and Critical Care Medicine (eds. J. Graham, G. Doss, and H. Beaufrère), West Sussex (UK): Wiley-Blackwell. In press.

20 DiGeronimo, P.M., da Cunha, A.F., Pypendop, B. et al. (2017). Cardiovascular tolerance of intravenous bupivacaine in broiler chickens (*Gallus gallus domesticus*) anesthetized with isoflurane. *Vet. Anaesth. Analg.* 44 (2): 287–294.

21 Brandão, J., da Cunha, A.F., Pypendop, B. et al. (2015). Cardiovascular tolerance of intravenous lidocaine in broiler chickens (*Gallus gallus domesticus*) anesthetized with isoflurane. *Vet. Anaesth. Analg.* 42 (4): 442–448.

22 Csillag, A., Bourne, R.C., and Stewart, M.G. (1990). Distribution of mu, delta, and kappa opioid receptor binding sites in the brain of the one-day-old domestic chick (*Gallus domesticus*): an in vitro quantitative autoradiographic study. *J. Comp. Neuro.* 3: 543–551.

23 Singh, P.M., Johnson, C.B., Gartrell, B. et al. (2017). Analgesic effects of morphine and butorphanol in broiler chickens. *Vet. Anesth. Analg.* 44 (3): 538–545.

24 Da Rocha, R.W., Escobar, A., Pypendop, B.H. et al. (2017). Effects of a single intravenous bolus of fentanyl on the minimum anesthetic concentration of isoflurane in chickens (*Gallus gallus domesticus*). *Vet. Anaesth. Analg.* 44 (3): 546–554.

25 Souza, M.J., Bailey, J., White, M. et al. (2018). Pharmacokinetics and egg residues of meloxicam after multiple day oral dosing in domestic chickens. *J. Avian Med. Surg.* 32 (1): 8–12.

26 Danbury, T.C., Weeks, C.A., Chambers, J.P. et al. (2000). Self-selection of the analgesic drug carprofen by lame broiler chickens. *Vet. Rec.* 146 (11): 307–311.

27 McGeown, D., Danbury, T.C., Waterman-Pearson, A.E., and Kestin, S.C. (1999). Effect of carprofen on lameness in broiler chickens. *Vet. Rec.* 144 (24): 668–671.

28 Hocking, P.M., Robertson, G.W., and Gentle, M.J. (2005). Effects of non-steroidal anti-inflammatory drugs on pain-related behaviour in a model of articular pain in the domestic fowl. *Res. Vet. Sci.* 78 (1): 69–75.

29 Singh, P.M., Johnson, C., Gartrell, B. et al. (2013). Pharmacokinetics and Pharmacodynamics of Salicylates in Broiler Chickens. Singapore: Proceedings of AAVAC-UPAV Annual Conference.

30 Vaught, M.E., Gladden, J.N., Rozanski, E.A., and Graham, J.E. (2019). Reasons for evaluation on an emergency basis of and short-term outcomes for chickens from backyard flocks: 78 cases (2014–2017). *J. Am. Vet. Med. Assoc.* 254(10):1196–1203.

31 Waine, J.C. (1996). Head and neck problems. In: BSAVA Manual of Rapotors, Pigeon, and Waterfowl (eds. N.A. Forbes and N.H. Harcourt-Brown), 299–304. Cheltenham (UK): British Small Animal Veterinary Association.

32 Roberts, V. (2008). Galliform birds: health and husbandry. In: BSAVA Manual of Farm Pets (eds. V. Roberts and F. Scott-Park), 190–212. Gloucester, UK: BSAVA.

33 Crespo, R. and Shivaprasad, H.L. (2008). Developmental, metabolic, and other noninfectious disorders. In: Diseases of Poultry (ed. Y.M. Saif) (assoc. eds. A.M. Fadly, J.R. Glisson, L.R. McDougald, Nolan, L.K., Swayne, D.E. et al.), 12e, 1149–1196. Ames, IA: Blackwell Publishing.

20

Toxicology

Marieke H. Rosenbaum[1] and Cheryl B. Greenacre[2]

[1] *Infectious Disease and Global Health, Cummings School of Veterinary Medicine at Tufts University, Grafton, MA, USA*
[2] *Department of Small Animal Clinical Sciences, College of Veterinary Medicine, University of Tennessee, Knoxville, Knoxville, TN, USA*

Introduction

The most common cause of toxicosis in backyard poultry is heavy metal toxicosis due to ingestion of lead and/or zinc. Less common, but reported causes of toxicosis in poultry include aflatoxicosis, ionophore toxicosis, rodenticide exposure, botulism, excess selenium in the diet, or exposure to polytetrafluoroethylene (PTFE) fumes. Many plants have also been reported as toxic to poultry.

Lead Toxicosis

Lead (Pb) is a naturally occurring heavy metal in the environment that is associated with negative health outcomes across many species of animals, including poultry. Most lead exposure to humans and animals occurs secondary to industrialization and anthropogenic changes to the natural environment. In backyard poultry, the main documented sources of exposure include access to contaminated soil and to lead paint chips/dust associated with the home [1–3]. Lead exposure in farm animals can result from discarded manufactured materials that contain lead such as batteries, building materials,

lead shot, spent oil, lead paint, and leaded gasoline [4, 5]. Other sources of lead include contaminated grit, ground of shooting ranges, fishing weights, curtain weights, bullets, paint, and costume jewelry. Some soft plastics, such as coatings on electrical wires, have been shown to contain lead. Contaminated feed items are also a documented source of exposure for livestock [6]. Lead exposure poses a well-recognized public health risk and lead toxicosis in food animals including backyard poultry can contribute to the total burden of lead in the food supply chain of humans consuming milk, eggs, and meat from intoxicated animals [1, 5]. Given the increasing popularity of owning backyard chickens, it is important for veterinarians who treat them to understand the risk of lead exposure to both backyard chickens and to humans consuming their products.

Pathophysiology

Lead toxicosis in poultry can result from ingestion or inhalation of lead. Once ingested, lead is slowly absorbed into the bloodstream through the gastrointestinal tract. The physical form of lead, the size of the lead particle, the transit time of the gastrointestinal tract, and the nutritional status of the host all impact the quantity of lead that is absorbed. Birds tend to accumulate the heavy lead particles in the ventriculus to use as grit, and therefore increase the breakdown and absorption of lead into the bloodstream. Lead absorption across the gastrointestinal tract is enhanced when levels of calcium, zinc, and iron are deficient due to upregulation of transporters and receptors for these minerals that also have an affinity for binding lead. Once absorbed into the blood stream, lead is deposited in various organs with highest concentrations occurring in bone, liver, kidney, and eggs [7].

Lead is a potent neurotoxin although the exact mechanism of action is not well understood. It is thought that lead substitutes for calcium and interferes with neurotransmitter release, disrupting the function of GABA, dopamine and cholinergic receptors. Histopathologically, a segmental demyelination is observed.

Lead toxicosis also results in anemia through the inhibition of heme synthesis and through a reduction in the lifespan of red blood cells which is achieved through the inhibition of the enzyme delta-aminolevulinic acid dehydrogenase (ALAD). Lead inhibition of ALAD also causes an increased production of erythropoietin which results in inadequate maturation of red blood cells [8]. Limited information on the kinetics of lead in backyard poultry exists, and the half-life in poultry exposed to lead has not been determined [9]. In eggs, lead is preferentially deposited in the yolk and the shell and is virtually non-detectable in the albumin [7]. Young animals absorb higher quantities of ingested lead compared to adults. The non-absorbed fraction of ingested lead is excreted in the feces. Lead that has been absorbed into the blood stream is excreted primarily by the kidneys.

Clinical Signs

Lead toxicosis is associated with a wide range of nonspecific acute and chronic symptoms in poultry. Acute lead poisoning can present as loss of appetite, weight loss, ataxia, reduced egg production, crop stasis, lethargy, anemia, and death [10]. Chronic exposure is associated with more severe neurodegenerative processes including axonal loss in peripheral nerves, degeneration of motor nerves in the spinal cord, myodegeneration, and muscle atrophy [9, 11].

Chronic low-level lead toxicosis is likely underestimated among backyard poultry and is not always associated with recognizable signs and symptoms [7, 12]. Low levels of lead ingestion (e.g. 1 mg/kg feed) has been associated with decreased weight gains in poultry, however this is often too subtle a sign for owners to recognize [11].

Diagnosis

A bird suspected of having lead toxicosis based on the non-specific clinical signs stated above and a history of possible exposure to lead can be initially examined via a radiograph. This can be a "bird in the box" type radiograph where proper positioning is not necessary since the heavy metal will be easily visible (see Chapter 9). Radiographic abnormalities may include evidence of a metal dense foreign body, proventricular dilatation, and hepatomegaly. (Figure 20.1a,b) If no foreign body is present this does not rule-out a diagnosis of heavy metal toxicosis as the metal may have been completely absorbed, passed prior to the radiograph, inhaled as dust, or in fine particulate form (as is seen with soil contamination) which will not show up on radiographs. Antemortem diagnosis of lead toxicosis can be determined in minutes using ~5 μl of venous blood and a point of care blood lead analyzer. More sophisticated and precise methods to determine blood lead levels include inductively coupled plasma cell mass spectrometry, atomic absorption spectrometry, and anodic stripping voltammetry. The Louisiana Veterinary Medical Diagnostic Laboratory offers testing of blood lead, (using a minimum of 20 μl of blood) and serum zinc, copper, and mercury (using a

(a)

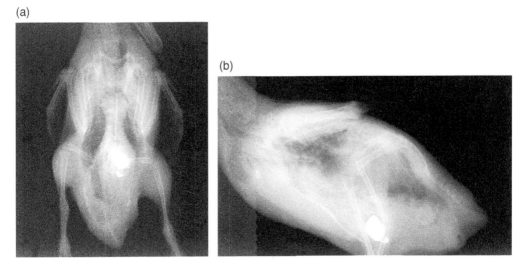

(b)

Figure 20.1 (a) Venrodorsal, and (b) lateral radiographs, of an adult Pekin duck hen that had elevated blood lead and serum zinc levels after ingesting 97 cents worth of coins (the pennies contained zinc), and costume jewelry (that had contained lead).

minimum of 20 μl of serum) using a flame atomic absorption assay. Lead levels >0.2 ppm are considered abnormal.

Postmortem diagnoses can be achieved by testing liver and/or kidney tissue. Tissue levels >6 mg/kg are often correlated with observable clinical signs; however, there is variability [13]. The symptomatic threshold for lead toxicosis in poultry is not established, and blood lead levels ranging up to 76 μg/dl are documented in poultry without clinical signs [7, 12]. On necropsy, lead shot or fragments of lead can sometimes be identified in the ventriculus (gizzard) or other segments of the gastrointestinal tract if large pieces were ingested. A common histopathologic finding in lead toxicosis is segmental demyelination, a result of Schwann cell degeneration leading to peripheral neuropathy.

Treatment

Acute cases of lead toxicosis in poultry can be treated using a three-pronged approach: (i) elimination of metal from the GI tract (where possible), (ii) chelation therapy to remove circulating lead from the blood stream and tissues, and (iii) supportive care. In extreme cases, blood transfusion may be indicated. The process of chelation enhances absorption of lead from the gastrointestinal tract; thus removal of lead from the GI tract will maximize the efficacy of chelation therapy. It is important to note that during chelation therapy, signs and symptoms of lead toxicosis may increase because treatment can result in transient increases in blood-lead levels from stress and as the metal is pulled out of bone and other tissues. Therefore, perform chelation and stabilization prior to performing procedures that would stress the bird.

To remove lead from the GI tract, emollient cathartics, gavage, endoscopy, and surgery can be performed (Figure 20.2a,b). Medical removal of small particles of the offending object(s) from the GI tract can be attempted with lubricants (emulsified corn oil, peanut butter), bulking agents (psyllium, mixed as per package directions) or proventricular flushing.

Chelators include calcium di-sodium EDTA, BAL (dimercaprol), DMSA (dimercaptosuccinic acid), and D-penicillamine (cupramine) (Table 20.1). The preferred method for chelation therapy is CaEDTA, which increases

(a)

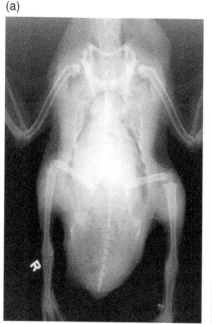

(b)

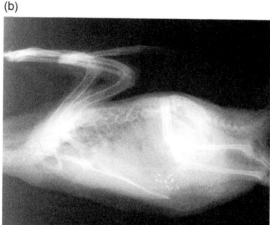

Figure 20.2   After stabilization, (a) ventrodorsal, and (b) lateral radiographs of the duck in Figure 20.1 after endoscopic removal of coins. The remaining particles were slowly removed via lubrication of GI tract by feeding corn oil in the diet.

urinary excretion by forming stable complexes with lead. CaEDTA must be given parenterally, as oral administration results in zero absorption of Ca EDTA into the bloodstream and it will increase lead absorption through the gastrointestinal tract. Treatment with CaEDTA should be given for three to five days, followed by two days off to allow for divalent cations that were chelated to replenish and for any nephrosis to subside. Blood lead levels should be checked three to four days after finishing chelation therapy. Several courses of treatment may be required as lead stored in bone and tissue can reenter the bloodstream, resulting in elevated blood lead levels and resurgence of acute signs. Combination therapy using CaEDTA and DMSA has been shown to improve clinical outcomes in humans and trumpeter swans. BAL (dimercarol) is a chelating agent that absorbs lead from red blood cells, however is painful to inject and is nephrotoxic, and therefore is not recommended.

Environmental remediation and removal of the source of exposure is paramount to successful treatment of lead toxicosis in poultry. Please refer to Table 20.2 for recommendations for environmental management and remediation.

Supportive care consists of fluid therapy and nutritional support. Supplementation with the antioxidant vitamin C can be used to counter free radical formation caused by lead, and vitamin B complex can be used to support recovery from injury to the nervous system. Proper calcium supplementation consistent with the life stage of the bird and treatment for anemia can reduce or prevent further absorption through the GI tract. Garlic supplementation has been shown to reduce tissue-lead concentrations in clinical trials with poultry, but the nutritional impact was not assessed [14, 15]. Selenium (Se) has also been found to reduce lead-induced apoptosis in the nervous tissue of chickens [16].

Table 20.1 Practical information regarding heavy metal chelators used in birds.

	Dose	Advantages	Disadvantages	Comment
Calcium disodium EDTA (Calcium versonate)	30–50 mg/kg IM or SQ q8-12h X 3–5 days ONLY, can be repeated3 (5 days on and 3–5 days off)	Inexpensive, acts quickly, known to chelate zinc extremely well.	Possible renal tubular damage due to renal excretion of large chelated molecule. Narrow therapeutic index. Does not penetrate the blood: brain barrier. Do not give orally as none is absorbed orally.	Not recommended to administer for longer periods since it chelates calcium. If patient does not have normal calcium levels then can be concurrently supplemented with calcium gluconate IM at 30 mg/kg q 12 – 24 h.
di-mercaptosuccinic acid (DMSA)	15–35 mg/kg PO q24h for 5 days of the week X 3–5 weeks.	Oral dosing, safer than calcium EDTA (not associated with renal damage), and it passes the blood–brain barrier.	Expensive, difficult to acquire, narrow therapeutic index, requires compounding for accurate dosing. Comes as 100 mg capsules that need to be compounded to small avian dosages.	Not recommended to administer for longer periods since it chelates calcium. If patient does not have normal calcium levels then can be concurrently supplemented with calcium gluconate IM at 30 mg/kg q 12 – 24 h. Developed for use in human children to treat lead toxicosis.
d-penicillamine	55 mg/kg PO q12h for 5 days, off 5 days (can mix with lactulose for better palatability)	Oral, passes the blood: brain barrier, soluble in water, used long term with Ca EDTA.	Tastes horrible! Possible teratogen - some cases have been documented in humans. May cause nausea and vomiting. The 125 mg capsules that need to be compounded to small avian dosages.	Do not use if the patient (or owner) has a known allergy to penicillin products. Known to chelate lead, iron, copper and mercury; unknown if it chelates zinc, although zinc is also a + 2 cation.

Table 20.2 Best practices for addressing and reducing lead exposure to backyard chickens and their owners.

- Test the soil on your property for lead in all areas the chickens can access, including their coop and any places they may range free.
- If you find lead, restrict birds' access to safe areas or bring in at least 2 ft of new clean soil to cover areas where lead was detected. Retest the soil annually, because rainfall and other factors can cause soil shifting and mixing.
- Inspect your house, garage (even cement-block structures can have lead paint on wooden windows), and other structures on your property for chipping paint – and keep your chickens and coop away from any such places. If you built your own coop, make sure any recycled wood and other materials are lead-free.
- Test the hose or spigot you use to provide the water for your chickens to rule out contamination from aging lead pipes or infrastructure.
- Provide chickens' feed and any supplements in feeders instead of scattering it on the ground.
- Have all family members, especially children, wash their hands after contact with soil and chickens – and consider wearing gloves. Change your shoes before going indoors.
- If you are concerned about possible exposure, have your veterinarian routinely screen your chickens for lead, which may be accumulating to above-normal levels even if they show no signs of illness.
- If your flock has had access to soil with elevated lead concentrations, or your veterinarian reports elevated levels, test eggs for lead to ensure they are safe for consumption. Wash any dust and soil off eggshells before preparing eggs.
- If you have a flock that has historically been exposed to lead, refrain from feeding the shells back to the birds and from using chicken feces and shells in compost meant for vegetable gardens. Lead is excreted in feces and deposited in shells.

The authors credit Genevieve Rajewski for this list, as she composed it after interviewing one author [MR] for a news piece.

One-Health Implications

Lead toxicosis in poultry poses a public health risk to families who consume the eggs, especially children. Numerous studies have detected lead in the edible fraction of eggs, primarily in the yolk [1–3, 7, 17]. Correlations between blood lead levels and yolk lead levels are documented [7], and studies have found strong correlations between soil lead levels and egg lead levels, indicating soil as a major exposure for backyard chickens [1–3]. Soil lead exposure in poultry is magnified by their behavioral characteristics, such as scratching, dust bathing, and feeding from the ground.

Pathways of lead exposure for poultry are understudied, but likely include a combination of factors (Figure 20.3). Poultry are exposed to lead in the soil, and may also be exposed by consuming worms and invertebrates, which have been shown to bioaccumulate lead [18]. Absorbed lead results in contaminated eggs, primarily the yolk and the shell. [7]. Many backyard poultry owners will crush and feed egg shells back to the flock as a source of calcium, or alternatively will compost the shells. The non-absorbed fraction of lead is excreted in the feces, which often end up in the compost, which is used to fertilized raised garden beds where food is grown. There is also the potential for feed and supplements such as calcium and bone meal to be contaminated with lead [19].

Veterinarians can act as an important source of information regarding the One Health implications of lead toxicosis in backyard poultry. Table 20.2 details recommendations for addressing lead contamination in the backyard environment in the context of backyard chicken keeping.

Zinc Toxicosis

Overview

Clinical signs of zinc (Zn) toxicosis can range from severe illness to subtle clinical abnormalities. Awareness of potential sources of zinc exposure and the wide range of clinical signs will facilitate recognition of this poorly understood disease. Zinc levels may increase

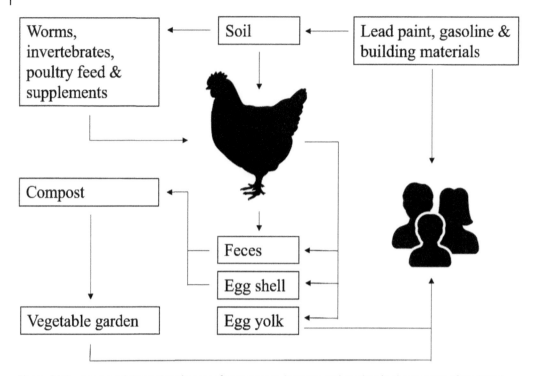

Figure 20.3 Lead cyclicity and pathways of exposure to humans and poultry in the context of backyard chicken keeping.

slowly over time, so the source of zinc in the environment may not necessarily be something "new," for example 2–3 years of exposure to an enclosure that is high in zinc may be a source. Although zinc is considered an essential trace element for survival, it can be toxic in excessive amounts. The recommended daily dietary intake of zinc for humans is 15 mg (USDA), and for chickens is considered to be 5.5 mg [20, 21]. Ingested toxic levels have been determined in cats, sheep, calves, chickens, ducklings and cockatiels. Toxic levels in cage paint is thought to be greater than 500 ppm [20, 22, 23].

Clinical Signs

Clinical signs of zinc toxicosis vary between species. In canines, zinc toxicosis causes primarily gastric ulceration. In birds, zinc toxicosis causes a myriad of signs including depression, anorexia, aggressiveness, agitation, regurgitation, vomiting, neurologic (seizures, lameness, head pressing), diarrhea, infertility,

and feather picking [24]. In one non–peer-reviewed study, 37/43 cockatoos with clinical signs of feather picking had elevated serum zinc levels. In addition, 97% (34/37) of these cockatoos ceased feather picking after chelation therapy [20].

Pathogenesis

The exact mechanism causing neurologic signs is unknown, but it is known that zinc is water soluble and is therefore stored in soft tissues, not bone like lead. High tissue zinc levels have been documented in the pancreas of affected cockatiels and ducklings. Affected cockatiels also had renal tubular degeneration and renal necrosis [20, 23, 24].

Diagnostic Tests

Radiographic abnormalities may include evidence of a metal dense foreign body, proventricular dilatation, and hepatomegaly.

A suggestion of zinc toxicosis can be made by identifying a metal dense foreign body in the GI system, but if no foreign body is present, that does not rule-out a diagnosis of heavy metal toxicosis. For example, if a bird was exposed to zinc oxide (white rust) powder, perhaps from licking the cage, there would be no radiographic evidence of metal.

Serum zinc levels have been shown to be effective in evaluating toxicosis in psittacine birds. The "cut-off" varies between species of bird, but generally levels greater than 2.0–2.5 ppm are considered toxic. Normal levels in humans are between 0.5 and 1.5 ppm. The Louisiana Veterinary Medical Diagnostic Laboratory uses a flame atomic absorption assay and can perform serum zinc levels on as little as 0.1 ml of serum. Do not submit the sample in tubes that may contain zinc such as those with rubber stoppers or with serum separator material, as this may falsely elevate the zinc levels. Note that some hematocrit clay may also contain zinc. Hard plastic "bullet"-shaped tubes are ideal. Post-mortem diagnosis of zinc toxicosis can be made by submitting fresh liver tissue for analysis to a diagnostic laboratory.

Treatment

Environmental correction is imperative in correcting this disease. Suspect objects should be removed and discarded or tested for zinc levels. Treatment of zinc toxicosis includes chelation therapy and supportive care. Chelators include calcium di-sodium EDTA, DMSA, and D-penicillamine (Cupramine). (Table 20.1) A study showed that DMSA worked well in treating a Hyacinth Macaw with zinc toxicosis [25]. Lactulose is often administered orally (0.5 mg/kg q12h) to help convert NH_3 to NH_4 to ease the burden on the liver during this time of toxicosis. Medical removal of small particles of the offending object(s) from the GI tract can be attempted with lubricants (emulsified corn oil, peanut butter), bulking agents (psyllium, mixed as per package directions), or proventricular flushing. The latter involves anesthetizing the bird, intubating, holding upside down while inserting a large sized red-rubber catheter through the oral cavity and on into the proventriculus and flushing with copious amounts of *warm* fluid. Care must be taken to not allow aspiration of fluid. If a large piece of metal has been ingested then endoscopic retrieval is possible (see video 20.1 on website of removing coins from a duck).

Potential Sources of Zinc

Common sources of zinc include ingestion of pennies minted after 1986, lead and/or zinc shot (common in waterfowl), galvinized (zinc coated to prevent rust) metal such as wire, bolts, links, and locks, Monopoly® game pieces, plastic twist-ties, some powder coating on cages, costume jewelry, glue on paper towel rolls, paints, and possibly human cereals with added zinc [20, 24, 26–28]. Powder coating of commercially available bird cages usually contains a safe (less than 250 ppm) amount of zinc, but there have been numerous cases where toxic levels (>500 ppm) have been identified. Birds drinking rain water run-off from a galvanized roof developed zinc toxicosis [27]. To test the level of zinc in a substance, submit to the Chemical Analysis Laboratory at University of Georgia or similar laboratory.

Most aviaries use wire that has been galvanized after welding, specifically Tinsley wire, known for its uniformity and smoothness. It is generally thought that excess surface zinc and zinc oxide (white rust) can be removed from newly purchased wire by rinsing with a vinegar solution.

An unusual source of zinc toxicosis can be from a retained piece of metal (such as 22-gauge pellets or lead shot). This has also been documented in humans (usually war veterans with shrapnel, or buckshot) and birds. A cockatoo presented with a history of falling off its perch. Radiographs showed proventricular dilatation, hepatomegaly, and a metal 22 pellet lodged in the skull at the nasofrontal joint (an acidic environment). The bird's zinc level was

19 ppm and lead was 0.4 ppm High levels can be tolerated in birds with chronic exposure. Treatment in this bird involved chelation therapy with calcium EDTA for five days prior to surgery to prevent a stress induced mobilization of lead and zinc to the bloodstream. Morbidity and mortality are higher in humans with lead toxicosis and dogs with zinc toxicosis if chelation therapy is not instituted prior to surgery. The pellet was surgically removed and the bird had an uneventful recovery. Apparently the 22-pellet had been in place for longer than three years [28].

Mycotoxicosis

Mycotoxins are natural toxins produced by fungi. There are hundreds of mycotoxins that can affect poultry. Aflatoxins are the most common and are potent and carcinogenic mycotoxins produced by the fungi *Aspergillus flavus*, *Aspergillus parasiticus*, and *Penicillium puberulum* [29]. All poultry are susceptible to aflatoxicosis, but ducklings, turkeys (especially poults) and pheasants are the most susceptible, whereas chickens, quail, and guinea fowl are considered less susceptible. [30, 31]. Aflatoxin B-1 is the most toxic and primarily effects the liver. In severe/acute cases neurologic and liver disease occur and a pale yellow liver can be seen at necropsy An insidious, chronic low level exposure is more common causing nonspecific signs of disease including unthriftiness, decreased egg production, decreased fertility and hatchability, anemia, hemorrhages, liver disease, paralysis/lameness, neurologic signs, increased susceptibility to infectious diseases, and death.

Diagnosis is sometimes difficult since definitive diagnosis requires testing for the specific toxin in the feed, and as stated above there are hundreds of different mycotoxins. One can submit the body and 1 kg of feed for necropsy and aflatoxin testing. Treatment includes removal of the contaminated feed, feeding uncontaminated feed, treatment of concurrent

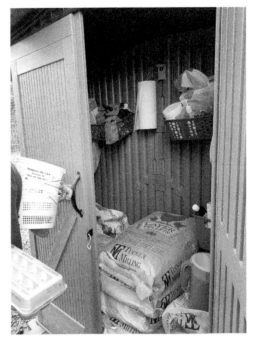

Figure 20.4 This inexpensive, plastic shed is keeping the poultry food clean and dry.

diseases, and supportive care. Proper storage of feeds to keep them clean, dry, and rodent free is imperative (Figure 20.4). Always check the smell of the feed before feeding. Also, proper ventilation is important since fungus likes to grow in high humidity environments.

Ionophore Toxicosis

Inophores, such as lasalocid, monensin, salinomycin, and narasin, have anticoccidial and antibacterial properties and are commonly used in poultry and ruminant feeds [30, 32]. Toxic levels, due to mixing errors or concomitant use of sulfonamides, can cause potassium to leave and the calcium to enter cells causing cell rupture and the clinical signs of toxicosis including stunting, lameness, and paralysis. There may be no histopathological signs of disease. Naïve turkeys switched suddenly to monensin-containing feed can receive toxic levels and show paralysis with both feet extending backward [30].

Rodenticide Exposure

Anticoagulent rodenticide exposure can cause severe clinical signs in poultry. First-generation anticoagulant rodenticides include warfarin, chlorophacinone, diphacinone, and coumatetralyl, and require continual ingestion by rodents to induce toxic effects. Second-generation anticoagulants, include brodifacoum, bromadiolone, difenacoum, and difethialone and are fatal to rodents after one meal [30].

Clinical signs in poultry include sudden death with hemorrhage, especially in cases of exposure to the second generation anticoagulants. Hemorrhage is most often observed in the lung, intestine, and peritoneal cavity. Definitive diagnosis of anticoagulant toxicosis involves as anticoagulant screen on the liver of dead birds [30].

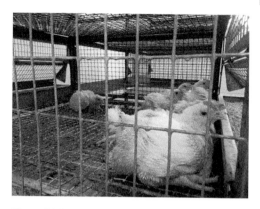

Figure 20.5 Note the bird in the foreground with visible coelomic distension. Also note the bird in the left background that is not with the others, stunted and is lethargic. This group of young birds was mistakenly given a diet with too much selenium resulting in coelomic effusion, stunting, and unthriftiness.

Botulism

The most common presentation of botulism to veterinary hospitals is ducks or geese in the summer that have been feeding on maggots with the botulinum toxin from the bacteria *Clostridium botulinum*. Clinical signs include an ascending paralysis, developing into "limberneck" and then drowning. Chickens can also get botulism. Other birds ingesting carcasses of dead birds can be an additional source of the toxin. Definitive diagnosis involves examining intestinal contents and blood for botulism toxin (mouse inoculation assay), diagnosis is suspected by finding no other cause of death at necropsy [30].

Excess Selenium in the Diet

Selenium toxicosis is not common but can occur in younger animals exposed to high, about 10 times physiological needs, amounts

of the selenium in the diet, usually due to feed mixing errors. Decreased hatchability of eggs occurs at selenium levels in feed >5 ppm, while levels of >10 ppm are associated with complete cessation of egg laying. Young birds are more susceptible than adults, as 8 ppm in starter rations resulted in reduced growth [30]. Rations containing as little as 2.5 ppm resulted in meat in eggs having in excess of suggested tolerance limit levels of selenium in food for human consumption [30]. A group of chicks was mistakenly fed a diet with excess selenium and they exhibited stunting, lethargy, ascites, and at necropsy also had heart and liver abnormalities (Figure 20.5) [33]. These chicks may also have received an excess of salt in their diet.

Non-stick Cookware Toxicosis

Non-stick cookware, such as Teflon*, is made with polytetrafluoroethylene (PTFE). Some red heat lamps are also coated in PTFE and have caused death in chickens [34]. If burned or heated to over 536 °F (280 °C), the PTFE fumes are released, which causes immediate pulmonary hemorrhage and death in birds anywhere in the household. Rarely immediately supplied fresh air, oxygen, and steroids will prevent death. At necropsy edematous and hemorrhagic lungs area seen.

Plant Toxins

Exposure to plant toxins is unusual in backyard poultry, but a list of plant toxins reported to cause illness in poultry is listed in Table 20.3. Refer to Diseases of Poultry (ed. Swayne DE) for more detailed information [32].

Table 20.3   Plants reported to be toxic to poultry.

Common name	Scientific name	Active toxin	Toxic part of plant
Avocado	*Persea americana*	—	Fruit
Black locust	*Robinia pseudoacacia*	—	Leaf
Bladder pod	*Sesbania [Glottidium] vesicaria*	—	Seed
Cacao	*Theobroma cacao*	theobromine	Bean waste from processing
Cassava	*Manihot* spp.	cyanide, polyphenols	Root
Carolina jessamine	*Geisemium sempervirens*	—	All parts
Castor bean	*Ricinus communis*	—	Bean
Coffee senna, Sickle pod	*Cassia occidentalis, C. obtusifolia, Senna occidentalis*	—	Seeds
Corn cockle	*Agrostemma githago*	githagenin	Seed
Cotton seed meal	*Gossypium* spp.	gossypol	Seed
Coyatillo	*Karwinskia humboldtiana*	—	Fruit and seed
Crotalaria spp.	*Crotalaria* spp.	pyrrolizidine alkaloid, monocrotaline	Seed, leaf, stem
Daubentonia spp.	*D. longifolia, Sesbania drummondii, S. macrocarpa*	—	Seed
Death camas	*Zygadenus* spp.	—	Leaf, stem, root
Eucalyptus cladocalyx	*Eucalyptus cladocalyx*	cyanide or prussic acid	Leaf
Galenium pubescens	*Galenium pubescens*	nitrate	All parts
Hemlock	*Conium maculatum*	conine	Seed
Jimsonweed	*Datura stramonium, D. ferox*	Scopolamine, hyoscyamine	Seed
Leucaena leucocephala	*Leucaena leucocephala*	mimosine	Leaves
Lily of the Valley	*Convallaria majalis*	—	Flowers, leaves, stems
Milkweed	*Asclepias* spp.	asclepidin	All parts
Nightshade	*Solanum nigram*	belladonna	Immature fruit
Oak	*Quercus* spp.	tannin	Leaf
Oleander	*Nerium oleander*	glycoside	All parts
Onions, green	*Allium ascalonicum*	—	All parts

Table 20.3 (Continued)

Common name	Scientific name	Active toxin	Toxic part of plant
Oxalate	Many plants including *Galenium pubescens*	Oxalic acid	Leaf, stem
Parsley	*Ammi majus*	photosensitizing	All parts
Pokeberry	*Phytolacca americana*	—	Fruit
Potato	*Solanum tuberosum*	solanine	Green or spoiled potatoes, peelings, sprouts
Ragwort	Senecio jacobea	pyrrolizidine alkaloid	All parts
Rapeseed meal	*Brassica napus*	erucic acid, glucosinolate, sinapine, tannin, phytic acid	Seed
Sweet pea	*Lathyrus* spp.	—	Seed (pea)
Tobacco	*Nicotiana tabacum*	nicotine sulfate	Leaf, stem
Velvetweed	*Malvacea* spp.	cyclopenoid fatty acids	Seed
Vetch	*Vicia* spp.	Cyanogenic glycoside	Seed (pea)
Yellow jessamine	*Gelsemium sempervirens*	—	All parts
Yew	*Taxus* spp.	taxine	All parts

Source: Adapted from, Fulton RM. Toxins and Poisons. In: Swayne DE, Glisson JR, McDougald, et al. (eds.), Diseases of Poultry, 13th ed., 2013, 1287–1315.

References

1 Leibler, J.H., Basra, K., Ireland, T. et al. (2018). Lead exposure to children from consumption of backyard chicken eggs. *Environ. Res.* 167.

2 Spliethoff, H.M., Mitchell, R.G., Ribaudo, L.N. et al. (2014). Lead in New York city community garden chicken eggs: influential factors and health implications. *Environ. Geochem. Health.*

3 Grace, E.J. and MacFarlane, G.R. (2016). Assessment of the bioaccumulation of metals to chicken eggs from residential backyards. *Sci. Total Environ.*

4 Humphreys, D.J. (1991). Effects of exposure to excessive quantities of lead on animals. *Br. Vet. J.*

5 Puschner, B., Roegner, A., Giannitti, F. et al. (2013). Public health implications of lead poisoning in backyard chickens and cattle: four cases. *Vet. Med. Res. Rep.*

6 Schlerka, G., Tataruch, F., Högler, S. et al. (2004). Acute lead poisoning in cows due to feeding of lead contaminated ash residue. *Berl. Munch Tierarztl. Wochenschr.*

7 Trampel, D.W., Imerman, P.M., Carson, T.L. et al. (2003). Lead contamination of chicken eggs and tissues from a small farm flock. *J. Vet. Diagn. Investig.*

8 Agency for Toxic Substances and Disease Registry (ATSDR). (2020). Toxicological profile for Lead. Atlanta, GA: U.S. Department of Health and Human Services, Public Health Service.

9 Mazliah, J., Barron, S., Bental, E. et al. (1989). The effects of long-term lead intoxication on the nervous system of the chicken. *Neurosci. Lett.*

10 Salisbury, R.M., Staples, E.L.J., and Sutton, M. (1958). Lead poisoning of chickens. *N. Z. Vet. J.*

11 Bakalli, R.I., Pesti, G.M., and Ragland, W.L. (1995). The magnitude of lead toxicity in broiler chickens. *Vet. Hum. Toxicol.*

12 Mordarski, D.C., Leibler, J.H., Talmadge, C.C. et al. (2018). Subclinical lead exposure among backyard chicken flocks in Massachusetts. *J. Avian Med. Surg.*

13 Franson, J. (1996). Interpretation of tissue lead residues in birds other than waterfowl. In: Environmental Contaminants in Wildlife: Interpreting Tissue Concentrations, 265–279. Boca Raton, FL: CRC Press.

14 Hossain, M., Akanda, M., Mostofa, M., and Awal, M. (2014). Therapeutic competence of dried garlic powder (*Allium sativum*) on biochemical parameters in lead (Pb) exposed broiler chickens. *J. Adv. Vet. Anim. Res.*

15 Hanafy, M.S., Shalaby, S.M., el-Fouly, M.A. et al. (1994). Effect of garlic on lead contents in chicken tissues. *Dtsch Tierarztl. Wochenschr.*

16 Zhu, Y., Jiao, X., An, Y. et al. (2017). Selenium against lead-induced apoptosis in chicken nervous tissues via mitochondrial pathway. *Oncotarget.*

17 Bautista, A.C., Puschner, B., and Poppenga, R.H. (2014). Lead exposure from backyard chicken eggs: a public health risk? *J. Med. Toxicol.*

18 Darling, C.T.R. and Thomas, V.G. (2005). Lead bioaccumulation in earthworms, *Lumbricus terrestris*, from exposure to lead compounds of differing solubility. *Sci. Total Environ.*

19 Scelfo, G.M. and Flegal, A.R. (2000). Lead in calcium supplements. *Environ. Health Perspect.*

20 Van Sant, F. (1998). Zinc and parrots: more than you ever wanted to know. *Proc. Assoc. Avian Vet.*: 305–312.

21 National Research Council (NRC). (1994). Nutrient Requirements of Poultry: 9e. Washington, DC: The National Academies Press. https://doi.org/10.17226/2114.

22 Dewar, W.A., Wight, P.A.L., Pearson, R.A., and Gentle, M.J. (1983). Toxic effects of high concentrations of zinc oxide in the diet of chick and laying hen. *Br. Poult. Sci.* 24: 397–404.

23 Kazacos, E.A. and Van Vlect, J.T. (1989). Sequential ultrastructural changes of the pancreas in zinc toxicosis in ducklings. *Am. J. Pathol.* 134: 511–522.

24 Dumonceaux, G. and Harrison, G.J. (1994). Toxins. In: Avian Medicine: Principles and Application (eds. B.W. Ritchie, G.J. Harrison and L.R. Harrison), 1030–1052. Lake Worth, FL: Wingers Publishing.

25 Romagnano, A., Grinden, C.B., Degernes, L., and Mautino, M. (1995). Treatment of a hyacinth macaw with zinc toxicity. *J. Avian Med. Surg.* 9 (3): 185–189.

26 Howard, B.R. (1992). Health risks of housing small psittacines in galvinized wire mesh cages. *J. Am. Vet. Med. Assoc.* 200: 1667–1674.

27 Smith, A. (1995). Zinc toxicosis in a flock of hispaniolan amazons. *Proc. Assoc. Avian Vet.*: 447–453.

28 Greenacre, C.B. and Ritchie, B.W. (1999). Lead and zinc Toxicosis from a retained projectile in a bird. *Compendium* 21 (5): 381–383.

29 Hoerr, F.J. (2019). Aflatoxicosis in poultry. https://www.merckvetmanual.com/poultry/mycotoxicoses/aflatoxicosis-in-poultry (accessed 1 January 2021)

30 Porter, R.E. (2019). Poisonings in poultry. https://www.merckvetmanual.com/poultry/poisonings/poisonings-in-poultry (accessed 1 January 2021)

31 Hoerr, F.J. (2019). Mycotoxicoses in Poultry. https://www.merckvetmanual.com/poultry/mycotoxicoses/mycotoxicoses-in-poultry (accessed 1 January 2021)

32 Fulton, R.M. (2013). Toxins and poisons. In: Diseases of Poultry, 13e (eds. D.E. Swayne, J.R. Glisson, L.R. McDougald, et al.), 1287–1315. Wiley-Blackwell.

33 Surai, P.F. (2002). Selenium in poultry nutrition 1. Antioxidant properties, deficiency and toxicity. *World's Poult. Sci. J.* 58: 333–347.

34 Boucher, M., Ehmler, T.J., and Bermudez, A.J. (1999). Polytetrafluorethylene gas intoxication in broiler chickens. *Avian Dis.* 44: 449–453.

21

Soft Tissue Surgery

M. Scott Echols

Echols Veterinary Services, Salt Lake City, UT, 84121, USA

Introduction

In contrast to production practice, pet poultry and waterfowl commonly require surgical correction of various disorders. The popularity of backyard poultry and waterfowl, which are sometimes kept as indoor companions, means that more requests than ever are being made for advanced veterinary care. Clinicians treating these animals should at least be aware that surgical options for a large variety of soft tissue disorders are available. While not exhaustive, this chapter provides clinicians information on a large variety of soft tissue surgical procedures that may be encountered in poultry and waterfowl.

A basic understanding of general surgical principles should be understood prior to performing avian surgery. Although there are many anatomical and physiological differences between birds and mammals, surgical techniques are similar. Due to small patient size and anatomical differences (avian air sacs, for example), microsurgical instrumentation with magnification and focused light is often necessary for efficient avian surgery. For larger poultry and waterfowl, standard surgical instruments are often used. Because of physiologic variations (compared to mammals, birds

exchange oxygen on inspiration and expiration and can frequently go into cardiac arrest following relatively brief apnea), anesthetic techniques in avian species differ and are discussed elsewhere in the literature.

Doolen listed several principles that hold true to maximize avian surgical success and are listed as follows [1]:

1) Minimize hemorrhage.
2) Minimize tissue trauma.
3) Minimize anesthetic time.
4) Minimize anesthetic and metabolic complications.
5) Provide postsurgical support and analgesia.

These principles are simple enough but are important to understand and practice during all avian surgical procedures. Other than brief mention, the following are not covered in this chapter but are essential to patient surgical success: pre-surgical patient evaluation, appropriate anesthetic techniques, perioperative support (including fluid therapy, thermal support, antimicrobials, and pain control as needed) and longer-term pain management (Figure 21.1a–d). The reader is encouraged to pursue education related to these topics prior to performing avian surgery.

· · ·

Backyard Poultry Medicine and Surgery: A Guide for Veterinary Practitioners, Second Edition.
Edited by Cheryl B. Greenacre and Teresa Y. Morishita.
© 2021 John Wiley & Sons, Inc. Published 2021 by John Wiley & Sons, Inc.
Companion website: www.wiley.com/go/greenacre/medicine

(a)

(b)

(c)

(d)

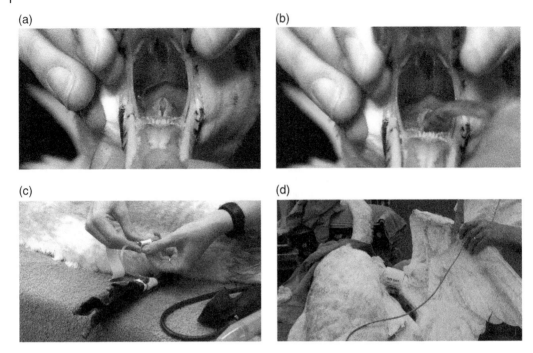

Figure 21.1 Poultry and waterfowl deserve perioperative supportive measures as with other animals. Perioperative support includes, but is not limited to, (a-b) intubation as with this Pekin duck (*Anas platyrhnchos*), (c) intravenous fluid support and (d) indirect blood pressure evaluation as with this mute swan (*Cygnus olor*) and peri-operative pain relief, thermal, hydration, and antimicrobial management as dictated by the needs of the patient.

If interested in avian surgery, actively pursue continuing education. One of the best continuing education courses is at one's own hospital in the form of a necropsy. If permitted by the caretakers, perform as many necropsies on animals as possible to gain experience and exposure to avian anatomy, tissue handling, and instrument use. Also attend continuing education courses that teach avian medicine and surgery. Publications in refereed journals that focus on avian topics provide numerous well-referenced papers on surgical techniques, in addition to medical topics. Some of these journals are referenced herein.

Also familiarize yourself with the numerous potential surgical "tools." These "tools" include radiosurgery, microsurgical instruments, endoscopes, high powered microsurgical loupes with light, operating microscopes, laser units, and other items that have become commonplace with avian surgery. Advanced diagnostics including digital radiographs, ultrasound, and high resolution computed tomography (CT) and magnetic resonance imaging (MRI) may be used to help better define the scope of the disease being addressed to better guide surgery. Consult with surgical instrument companies, colleagues, and avian continuing education resources to stay current.

Throughout this chapter, case report examples are used to demonstrate certain points. Some of these case reports involve non-poultry or waterfowl birds and are intended to give the reader a greater depth and understanding of potential surgical techniques that may be used and complications that may be encountered.

Suture Material

Suture material has been poorly studied in living avian species. There are, however, numerous studies describing various suture materials and patterns in mostly poultry tendons conducted on deceased animals. In one study, either nylon, polyglyconate, or polybutester was used for long digital flexor tenorrhaphy in live chickens using. The trial was carried out to eight weeks before euthanasia. The results showed that all three suture materials had insignificant differences in maximum load to failure, scar maturity, and tissue reactivity at four and eight weeks [2]. Various chicken organs have been used as models of human tissues. Again, most of these studies are focused on deceased animals and offer little long-term outcome information as to tensile strength, tissue reactivity, infection rates, and other clinical factors that determine the efficacy of a given suture material or pattern in living avian tissue.

Chromic catgut, polyglactin 910, polydioxanone (PDS), monofilament nylon, and monofilament stainless steel have been evaluated in rock doves (*Columba livia*) [3]. The authors concluded that PDS was slowly absorbed and strong and caused minimal tissue reaction making it most suitable for closing body wall incisions [3].

In a separate study of polygalactin-910, chromic catgut, and PDS used in cloacopexy surgery in pigeons, the authors concluded that inflammation and fibrosis were most prominent with polygalactin-910 [4]. Because of the degree of inflammation and fibrosis, the authors felt that polygalactin-910 would be more appropriate for cloacopexy as a means to promote adhesion formation at the surgical site [4]. Based on clinical experience and limited studies, PDS is used as the author's primary monofilament, absorbable suture in bird surgeries and is implied throughout this chapter when no specific details are given.

Upper Respiratory Tract and Trachea

Infraorbital Sinus Surgery

Diseases of the sinus, especially related to infections, trauma, and cancer, are occasionally noted in waterfowl and poultry. Some of these require surgical intervention. The classic but non-specific signs of sinus disease include swelling of infraorbital sinuses, ocular and nare discharge, and head shaking (Figure 21.2). Solid masses, such as with cancer and walled off granulomas, may present with infraorbital sinus swelling only (Figure 21.3 a and b).

Especially among Galliformes, there are a number of viral and bacterial diseases that result in significant upper respiratory infections and may be reportable. These diseases include, but are not limited to, *Mycoplasma gallisepticum*, Newcastle disease virus, and infectious bronchitis virus. Especially in flock situations, birds showing upper respiratory disease have significance for more than just the individual (Figure 21.4a–c). Properly characterizing and addressing infectious sinusitis in poultry species is important for more than just the individual and is discussed in the Respiratory Diseases chapter of this book.

Because of the cavernous anatomy of the infraorbital sinus and its many diverticuli and chambers, fluid, soft tissue, and inflammatory debris can build up unnoticed. Once the debris fills one portion of the infraorbital sinus it either spills over into an adjacent chamber or diverticulum (which may continue to go unnoticed) or reaches a point where a swelling is evident externally. Oculonasal discharge,

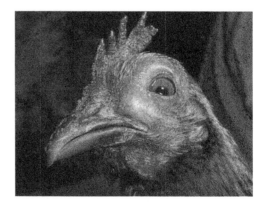

Figure 21.2 Typical signs of avian sinus infections include a distended infraorbital sinus, ocular, and nare discharge and head shaking which were all present in this chicken.

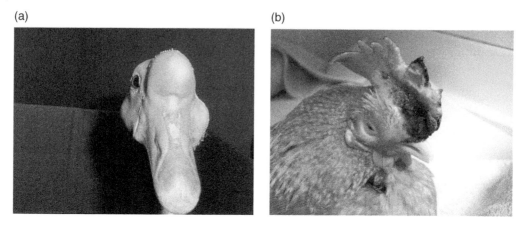

Figure 21.3 (a) Birds with non-infectious sinus disease often display a mass or distension of the sinus with minimal or no ocular and nare discharge as with this post-biopsy white Chinese goose (*Anser cygnoides*) with a sarcoma originating from the left infraorbital sinus, or (b) this chicken with a sarcoma involving the comb and sinus. *Source:* Photograph courtesy of Dr. Cheryl B. Greenacre.

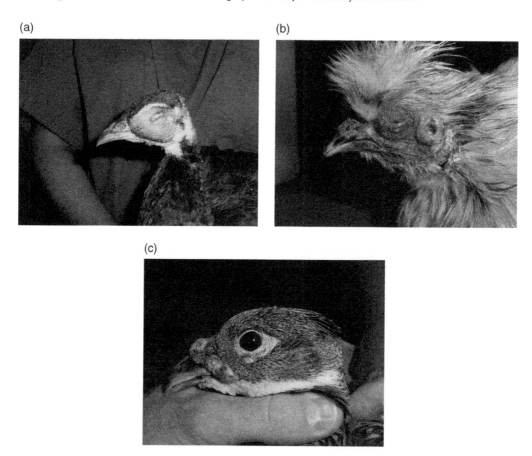

Figure 21.4 Poultry species with sinusitis or solid sinus masses should be evaluated for infectious disease that may have flock and/or regulatory importance such as (a) with *Mycoplasma gallisepticum* noted in this Indian peacock (*Pavo cristatus*), (b) lymphoma due to avian sarcoma leukosis virus in this chicken and (c) pox virus infection in this Impeyan pheasant (*Lophophorus impejanus*).

conjunctivitis, and/or head shaking may or may not be present before a physical swelling is noticed by the owner or attending veterinarian. By the time a bird is identified as having a sinus mass or supportive clinical signs, it may have advanced disease that affects many regions of the infraorbital sinus(es).

Diagnostics such as skull radiography, choanal or nares inspection via magnified light or endoscopy, CT, MRI, infectious disease testing (PCR, culture and sensitivity, etc.), sinus aspiration (with or without flushing small amounts of sterile saline), and cytology can be used to better characterize the cause and distribution of the swelling (Figure 21.5). While early cases of infectious sinusitis (before the debris becomes caseated) may respond to appropriate antibiotic therapy, most cases involve at least partially solidified masses that require surgical removal.

Unless guided differently by advanced diagnostics, incisions are best made directly over swollen sinus tissue and away from the eye (Figure 21.6a–b). Skin overlying inflamed sinus tissue is often very vascular and hemostasis is generally needed. Conversely, once inside the sinus the tissue is generally poorly vascular unless a mass is attached to the sinus wall or surrounding bone and muscle as sometimes occurs with cancer. The beak may be opened to increase potential sinus space to improve visualization.

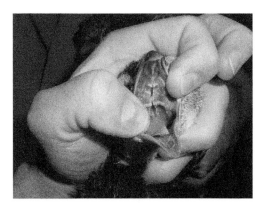

Figure 21.5 Indian peacock (*Pavo cristatus*) with a choanal granuloma associated with *Mycoplasma gallisepticum* sinusitis.

Magnification with light is essential to adequately inspect the infraorbital sinus. Microsurgical and miniaturized instruments are also beneficial when retrieving debris from deep recesses within the sinus (Figure 21.7a–d). The normal sinus space should be clear with no visible debris or discharge. Any discharge, foreign bodies or debris are removed. Solid tissue may come out as an impression mold of the sinus space. Neoplastic tissue may form extension to and through the sinus spaces requiring either partial removal or more radical resection of surrounding tissues. Submit collected tissue for culture and sensitivity, other infectious disease testing, and/or histopathological evaluation if not done so previously.

The sinus space can hold a surprising amount of material, and every attempt to remove debris should be made. Additionally, invasive material may extend into the beak diverticuli and opposite side of the head. Occasionally multiple surgical entries are required to reach visible debris. Trephination, as described for psittacine birds, into the beak or skull is rarely needed for addressing sinus disease in poultry and waterfowl but may be considered if necessary [5].

Once the bulk of the fluid, debris, and abnormal tissue is removed, the surgical site can be left open to drain (if infectious disease is suspected) or closed if the sinus was clean such as with an excised encapsulated mass (Figure 21.8). Post-operative care may include daily or twice-daily flushing the open wound with an appropriate antiseptic solution (such as dilute chlorhexidine) until the wound closes. Use caution with any flush solution that is highly tissue reactive such as hydrogen peroxide as this may cause more inflammation and inflammatory fluid and debris accumulation. Open sinusotomy wounds generally heal rapidly and make flushing difficult within three to five days. If appropriate, sinusotomy closure is standard, and any sutures placed can generally be removed in 10–14 days. Systemic antibiotics and analgesics are given as needed.

(a)

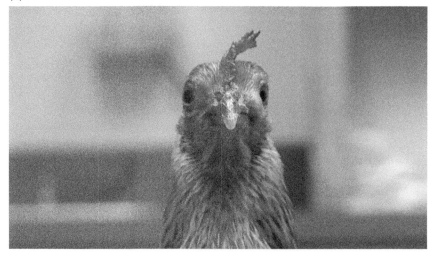

(b)

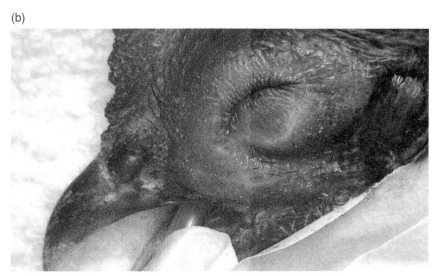

Figure 21.6 (a) A chicken with bacterial sinusitus presents with mild infraorbital sinus swelling. (b) The area is prepped for surgery and the incision is made over the swollen sinus (rostral diverticulum of the infraorbital sinus in this case).

Tracheal Surgery

Numerous cases describing tracheal surgery in birds have been reported [6–13]. Tracheal surgery in poultry and waterfowl is sometimes required to resolve traumatic injuries, avulsions, intraluminal foreign bodies, parasites, or other mass obstructions and strictures. As with sinusitis, some tracheitis cases in poultry and waterfowl are caused from or associated with

infectious diseases that affect other animals (Figure 21.9).

Partial tracheotomies can be used to access the tracheal lumen to remove foreign bodies non-retrievable via less invasive techniques (endoscopy, suction, etc.) [12]. Palpation, tracheal endoscopy, radiography, and/or transillumination can be used to identify the general location of the tracheal lesion. Endoscopic

(a)

(b)

(c)

(d)

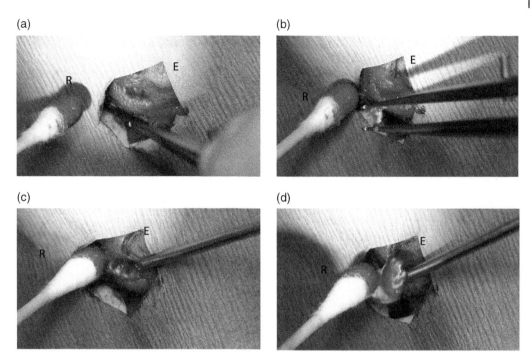

Figure 21.7 (a) The same chicken in Figure 21.6 is covered with a drape and the rostral diverticulum of the infraorbital sinus has been incised and granulomatous tissue can be seen deep within the sinus. (b) Microsurgical ring tipped forceps are used to retrieve a small granuloma. (c and d) A small ear loop curette is used to retrieve a large granuloma from deep within the sinus. R = Rostral, E = Eye.

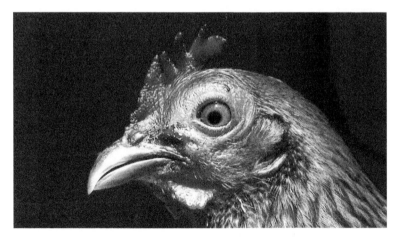

Figure 21.8 Post sinusotomy in the chicken featured in Figures 21.6 and 21.7, the wound is left open to heal by second intention.

intraluminal tracheal examination is preferred as the other methods are less dependable to both identify and determine the extent of tracheal luminal lesions [14]. An air sac breathing canula is often required during tracheal surgery to provide adequate ventilation and gas anesthetic delivery. If concerned about distal migration of the foreign body, temporarily place a 25-gauge needle (or two) through the center of the trachea just distal to the object.

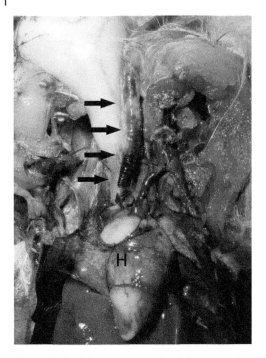

Figure 21.9 Inflammatory tracheal disease, such as hemorrhagic tracheitis (arrows) associated with avian sarcoma leukosis virus infection in this chicken, may be infectious and have implications that affect multiple animals. A definitive diagnosis of such cases should be determined. H = Heart.

With the patient in dorsal recumbency, the ventral neck skin is incised over the general location of the foreign body. The trachea is readily found beneath the skin. Perform a transverse tracheotomy just proximal to the foreign body on the ventral half of the trachea between the tracheal rings. Handle the tissue with care and make precise incisions so as to limit trauma to the trachea. If possible, avoid cutting the recurrent laryngeal nerves running alongside the trachea and preserve adhering and local blood vessels. Stay sutures may help to both retract the trachea out the incision and guide closure. Retrieve the foreign body being careful not to damage the tracheal luminal tissue. Pre-place small size simple interrupted sutures (4–0' and smaller depending on the size of the bird) along the incised trachea and bring tissue edges back to normal apposition [9]. Tie knots on the serosal tracheal surface. Generally at least one tracheal ring is incorporated on each side of the incision. Subcutaneous and skin closure is routine.

The crop may need to be reflected laterally and the thoracic inlet approached if the foreign body is located distally within the trachea. Incise the skin over the thoracic inlet and distal crop [15]. Bluntly dissect the skin from the crop. Bluntly dissect the crop from the surrounding tissues keeping local blood vessels intact. Once freed, the crop can be reflected to the bird's left. The distal trachea and sternotracheal muscles (which traverse obliquely and are attached proximally at the caudal lateral distal trachea) are identified. Transect the sternotracheal muscles near the tracheal attachments and coagulate or ligate bleeding vessels within the muscle bellies. Bluntly dissect the interclavicular air sac. Using a small blunt hook, latch the distal syrinx at the tracheal bifurcation and gently retract cranially. As a note, some ducks (especially *Anas* genus) have a well-developed asymmetrical osseous bulla at the distal end of the trachea. This structure is easily seen radiographically and should not be misinterpreted as an abnormality (Figure 21.10a–b). This normal structure should be carefully preserved. A tracheotomy is performed as above.

Tracheal resection and anastomosis is reserved for tracheal necrosis, avulsions, severe trauma, neoplasia, tracheal collapse, tracheal strictures, and other fixed obstructive masses that cannot be resolved non-invasively and significantly affect respiration. As a note, some tracheal strictures can be adequately treated with endoscopic debulking. One common reported cause of tracheal stricture is the result of trauma from endotracheal intubation [8, 9]. The cause of the stricture may be due to chemical disinfectant residues on improperly cleaned tubes, inflated cuffed endotracheal tubes, and/or simple trauma resulting from tube movement, advancing the tube distally into the narrowing trachea or other undue pressure within the tracheal lumen resulting in mucosal inflammation and subsequent fibrosis [9].

(a)

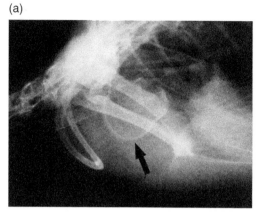

(b)

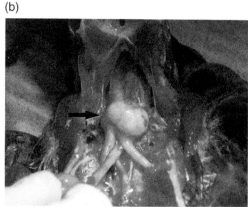

Figure 21.10 The osseous syringeal bulla (arrow) is a normal structure found at the distal end of the trachea in male ducks of some species and can be seen (a) on radiographs, as with this lesser scaup (*Aythya affinis*), during surgery of the distal trachea or (b) at necropsy as with this cinnamon teal (*Anas cyanoptera*).

These iatrogenic tracheal strictures typically result in severe dyspnea one to three weeks after the offending intubation. Birds may exhibit dyspnea once 50% or more of the tracheal lumen is blocked.

Tracheal collapse has been reported in waterfowl following animal bite trauma to the bird's neck [10, 11]. Tracheal resection and anastomosis with good outcomes were reported [10, 11]. Similarly, an acute, 4-cm displaced tracheal avulsion was reported in a mallard duck (*Anas platyrhynchos*) with severe rapidly progressive dyspnea presumably resulting from some type of trauma [13]. The trachea was successfully anastomosed restoring respiration 30 minutes following surgery. The bird was found dead three weeks later and the cause of death was not determined [13]. While only reported in one ostrich, a 2.5-cm section of 0.75-cm-wide polypropylene rings constructed from a 12-ml syringe case was used to support six collapsed tracheal rings that were transected as a result of blunt trauma and neck laceration [16]. The polypropylene rings were sutured to the tracheal cartilages and submucosa (without perforating the lumen) using 2–0 PDS. Surgery was successful and the ostrich was doing well at least six-months post-surgery [16].

The approaches are as described above. The damaged tissue is resected leaving as much viable trachea as possible in effort to reduce tension along the anastomosis site. Either the tracheal rings are bisected ("split ring technique") or the annular ligaments between the rings are cut [11]. The split ring technique allows for better anatomical alignment during the anastomosis, however both methods have been successfully used with birds [11]. As with a partial tracheotomy, pre-placing sutures helps with tracheal anastomosis. Both simple interrupted and near-near-far-far patterns have been successfully used with tracheal anastomoses in birds [7–11].

With all invasive tracheal procedures, granulation tissue formation, and subsequent additional luminal stenosis may be seen within 5–14 days of surgery [10]. Anti-inflammatory medications and often antibiotics and antifungals are indicated perioperatively as the trachea is not sterile [9]. Patients should be rested for at least two to three weeks following tracheal surgery with regular follow-ups to check for the presence of stricture formation.

Celiotomy Approaches

A celiotomy is used to access the coelom in birds. The specific approach is determined by access needed, surgeon preference, and individual bird anatomy and physical condition as each entry point has distinct advantages and disadvantages. The approaches generally require the bird to be in dorsal or lateral recumbency. If ascites or significant organomegaly is present, elevating the proximal half of the body may help reduce pressure on the heart, lungs, and more cranial air sacs improving ventilation. Regardless, most birds do not ventilate well while in dorsal or lateral recumbency, and positive pressure ventilation is often required throughout the procedure (even if the bird appears to respire normally).

Left Lateral Celiotomy

The left lateral celiotomy provides good exposure to the proventriculus, ventriculus, spleen, colon, left male and female reproductive tracts, hepatic lobe, lung, heart apex, kidney, and ureter [17]. Place the anesthetized patient in right lateral recumbency with the wings pulled dorsally, right leg caudally and left leg cranially. In some cases, the left leg is best pulled caudally, especially when a more cranial approach to the lateral coelom is required. Tape the extremities in place with masking tape, Durapore™ (3M, St Paul, MN) or any other tape that is easily removed. Make a longitudinal incision from cranial to caudal in the left paralumbar fossa. The incision may extend from the cranial extent of the pubis to the uncinate process of the last rib. If needed, the incision can be further extended cranially by incising through the last rib(s) at the costochondral junction(s). Use radiosurgery, laser, sutures or simple hemostasis (digital pressure) to control hemorrhage.

Once through the skin, bluntly dissect through the lateral coelomic muscles including the external oblique, internal oblique, and transversus abduminus mm. It is best to dissect the muscles in the direction of their fibers to reduce excessive tearing. At this point the abdominal air sac is visible dorsally. The air sac is commonly punctured to approach more dorsal structures but is preserved if possible. Palpebral, Gelpi, or similar retractors are very

useful to better expose the underlying structures. The muscles are closed individually, if clearly defined, via a simple interrupted pattern. Thin, stretched or indistinguishable muscles may be closed in one layer. Skin may be closed via multiple patterns (simple interrupted, simple continuous, everting, Ford interlocking, etc.) and is based on surgeon preference. Monitor for subcutaneous emphysema and air leakage through the skin incision. Re-suture as needed to reduce emphysema and stop air movement through the skin incision.

Right Lateral Celiotomy

A right lateral celiotomy provides good exposure to the duodenum and pancreas and right male and female (if present) reproductive tracts, lung, heart apex, kidney, ureter, and hepatic lobe. This approach is far less commonly performed given the more frequent need to access the ventriculus and female reproductive tract via a left lateral celiotomy. The approach is otherwise reversed from a left lateral celiotomy and closure is routine.

Ventral Celiotomy

A ventral midline, transverse or combination celiotomy is used to expose the middle and/or both sides of the coelomic cavity gaining access to the liver, intestines, pancreas, kidneys, ureters, cloaca, and the oviduct. The testes and ovaries can also be accessed via a ventral approach but does require manipulating surrounding tissues to improve exposure. The incision is made on the ventral midline from just caudal to the sternum extending caudally to the interpubic space. The supraduodenal loop (ileum) lies relatively ventral along the midline of the caudal coelom and can be easily transected if not careful. For this reason, the midline incision should be made as cranial as possible unless the caudal ventral coelom must be explored as with some cloacal surgeries. After the skin incision is made, the linea alba is tented upward and carefully transected being careful not to damage underlying organs. The air sacs are preserved using ventral approaches.

The transverse and combination ventral celiotomy can be used to increase exposure to the coelomic cavity in birds. A transverse incision is made just caudal to the sternum. If needed, a ventral midline incision is used in conjunction with the transverse incision ("T" incision) to increase exposure. Alternatively, a transverse incision can be made on the left or right half of the midline, combined with a ventral midline incision, creating a "L" incision. The "T" or "L" incision is only made if increased exposure is needed. As discussed above, underlying structures should be carefully avoided when incising through the underlying coelomic wall.

The linea alba and other transected muscle is closed in a simple interrupted pattern. As found in some overweight poultry and waterfowl, the subcutaneous tissue may need to be closed (commonly a simply continuous pattern). Skin closure is routine.

Gastrointestinal Tract

The gastrointestinal tract, from oral cavity to vent, may require surgical corrective procedures in pet poultry and waterfowl. The beak, while technically the starting point of the gastrointestinal tract, is highly specialized and variable between species. Surgery of the beak, most commonly trauma related, will not be covered here. Additionally, "debeaking" procedures performed in some production facilities as a behavior management practice are not recommended for pet animals.

The approaches and closure methods for the avian gastrointestinal tract have not been critically evaluated, controlled, and reported in scientific journals as most such surgeries are based on anecdotal experience [18]. While there is a belief that avian gastrointestinal tract surgery carries an "unacceptably high incidence of postoperative complications," the author feels these procedures can be performed safely and effectively in many circumstances [18].

Because of the potential for leakage of food or intestinal contents and dehiscence, careful attention should be paid to aseptic technique and meticulous closure. Antibiotics may be required for many gastrointestinal surgeries and should be determined based on the surgeon's evaluation.

Oral Cavity Surgery

Diseases of the oral cavity are infrequently reported in poultry and waterfowl. Most simple trauma and infections can be medically managed. Larger lacerations and removal of small masses may require surgical debridement or excision and closure. Occasionally oral parasites such as flukes and others may be found in waterfowl and can usually be mechanically removed. Disruptions of the hyoid apparatus, may result in difficulty swallowing, breathing, and vocalizations [19]. A fractured ceratobranchial bone (of the hyoid) resulted in difficulty swallowing, localized soft tissue swelling, and ipsilateral epiphora in a black African goose. Except for intermittent epiphora, all clinical signs resolved with antibiotics and supportive therapy [19].

Oral masses, especially neoplastic, may interfere with breathing and deglutition and should always be investigated. Oral squamous cell carcinoma has been reported in several chickens and, as with other neoplasms, should be considered along with abscesses, granulomas, and cysts when oropharyngeal masses are noted [20]. Oral pox lesions (see Figure 21.4c) rarely require surgical removal and are usually treated conservatively. Successful treatment of oral neoplasia in poultry and waterfowl has not been described likely because reported cases describe large masses that either resulted in euthanasia or are found on necropsy. If small, oral masses may be removed. Otherwise, biopsy oral masses in at least 2 locations. Abscesses, granulomas, and cysts may be drained or debrided. Consider more radical removal, cryotherapy, radiation, chemotherapy, or other modalities for neoplastic lesions.

Sublingual entrapment (impactions) are occasionally seen in herbivorous waterfowl and some require surgical correction. Common presenting signs include difficulty swallowing, ventral intermandibular swelling and rarely debilitation with chronic and severe impactions (Figure 21.11). Although risk factors have only been suggested, ingesting dry fibrous foods may be a major predisposition to sublingual impactions[21]. With impactions, the food accumulates lateral to the frenulum beneath the tongue. In early cases, the beak can be opened and the material simply pulled out. Brown recommends preventing birds from grazing for 7–10 days following removal of simple impactions [21]. This time off coarser food hopefully gives the sublingual "pouch" time to return to normal size.

With chronic cases, an intermandibular pocket forms requiring removal of the food and surgical resection of the stretched tissue (Figure 21.12 a–c). The bulk of the impaction can be removed per os. If the mass is large and chronic, it may cause local oral mucosal necrosis and subcutaneous food invasion. A ventral intermandibular approach is made and all remaining food and necrotic tissue is removed. With or without subcutaneous food invasion, the excess sublingual "pouch" is resected on either side of the frenulum (one or both sides may be stretched) and sutured closed in a simple interrupted or continuous pattern. The goal is to decrease the potential space to prevent additional impactions. If the subcutaneous tissue is infected and cannot be completely removed, marsupialize the ventral intermandibular skin and allow healing by second intention. Otherwise, the author tacks the partially resected oral mucosa to the subcutaneous tissue and overlying skin, to further reduce any potential space. Skin closure is routine. Antibiotics may be required.

Post-surgery, dry fibrous foods are avoided. Options for feeding include access to natural pond grasses (swans), access to green watered grass (geese), short cut commercially available grasses (using a food processor), or pellets. The latter two are intended to be short-term options. The owners should periodically inspect the oral cavity for signs of impaction for up to three weeks post-surgery and when dry and coarse food sources may increase risk of re-impaction.

Esophageal Surgery

There are few discussions on esophageal surgical procedures in birds. Most center on pharyngeal lacerations, crop burns (that extend up into the cervical esophagus), esophageal foreign bodies, and simple trauma. For the most part, the avian cervical esophagus is expansible and is easily closed in a simple interrupted or continuous inverting pattern. The overlying skin is preferably closed in a separate layer or with the esophagus incorporated into the closure. One more common reason for esophageal surgery is to place an esophagostomy feeding tube.

Mostafa et al. describes laceration of the upper third of the esophagus in a male ostrich (*Struthio camelus*) [22]. A 10-cm skin laceration resulted in underlying damage to the cervical esophagus. The esophagus was closed in a simple continuous pattern using 3-0′ polyglycolic acid. The skin was closed using nonabsorbable suture material in a simple interrupted pattern.

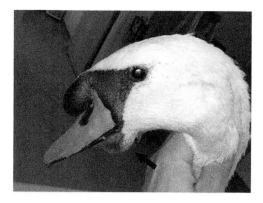

Figure 21.11 Sublingual food intrapment and impactions (arrow) are occasionally seen in herbivorous waterfowl, such as this mute swan (*Cygnus olor*).

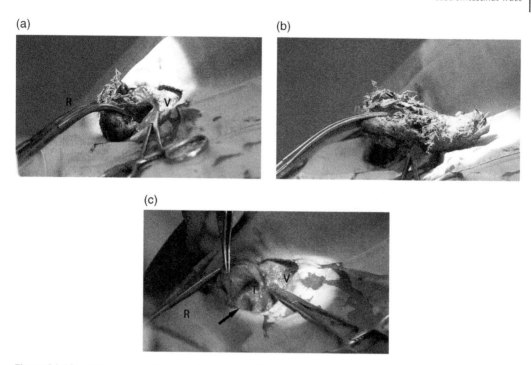

Figure 21.12 Using a ventral approach to the caudal intermandibular space of the mute swan in Figure 21.11, (a) the impacted food mass is being retracted from the ventral oral cavity out the incision until (b) the entire mass is removed. Once the mass and remaining debris are removed, the ventral oral cavity and frenulum (arrow) are visible. R = Rostral, T = Tongue Base, V = Ventral.

The wound healed uneventfully, and sutures were removed 10 days after surgery [22].

An esophagotomy was successfully performed on a Canada goose (*Branta canadensis*) to remove an esophageal impaction consisting of legumes, grass, and fishing line [23]. The esophageal incision was closed with 4-0′ polyglactin 910 in a simple interrupted pattern and then oversewn in a simple continuous pattern and skin closed in a simple interrupted pattern. The authors noted that if an esophageal foreign body is stuck and cannot be retrieved per os, it should be lubricated and pushed into the crop (if possible) for an ingluviotomy [23].

Crop Surgery

Ingluviotomy may be indicated for determination of crop masses (neoplasia, food impaction, and foreign bodies), repair damaged tissue (especially from predator bite wounds and infection) and to gain access to the thoracic esophagus, proventriculus, and ventriculus via intraluminal endoscopy. As a note, some chickens infected with Marek's disease virus have crop distention and should be considered as a differential as the infection may have implications for other birds (Figure 21.13 a and b).

Incise the skin over the bird's right side or middle of the crop near the thoracic inlet. Bluntly separate the skin and crop until you can pull the crop partly out of the incision. Remove abnormal tissue, masses, impacted food, or foreign bodies if present. A two-layer closure works best with crop incisions. The first layer is closed with an inverting suture. One author notes that the skin and crop should not be closed together as a single layer as this may increase the risk of dehiscence [15]. However, the author closes the skin and crop together as the second layer and has not noted

(a)　　　　　　　　　　　　　　　　(b)

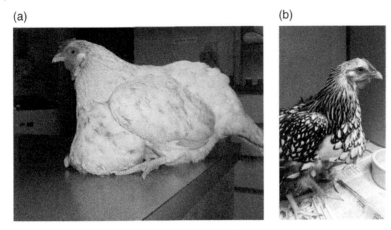

Figure 21.13 (a) As shown here, chickens infected with Marek's disease virus may develop a distended crop due to lymphoma of the innervating ingluvial nerves. (b) As shown here, a crop bra can be fashioned to provide temporary support. *Source:* Photograph courtesy of Dr. Cheryl B. Greenacre.

problems in clinical cases. Realize that the crop does have peristaltic movements separate from the overlying skin and closing the two together may affect motility.

The same approach is used to perform thoracic esophageal, proventricular, and ventricular endoscopy. One report noted using endoscopy and an endoscopic wire basket retrieval device to snare a ventricular foreign body (rubber tube) via an ingluviotomy in a gray parrot (*Psittacus erithacus*) [24]. Another report described use of multiple ingluviotomies and ventricular endoscopic retrievals to remove artificial grass fibers from a gyr falcon (*Falco rusticolus*) [25]. Due to the density of the artificial grass mass, only small pieces of the mass could be removed during each surgery (which totaled 5). Once the bulk of the mass was removed, the bird was offered feathered quail acting as casting material. The bird casted up the remaining foreign material two days later [25]. The same principles of ingluviotomy and endoscopy apply to poultry and waterfowl.

Crop repair is most often indicated following trauma. After the traumatic incident and prior to surgery, wait until the margins of the necrotic tissue are clearly visible (usually four to seven days after burn trauma). Acute crop,

non-thermal, trauma can usually be immediately surgically addressed. Remove all necrotic tissue and close as described above. The crop has an incredible ability to stretch and even large crop resections seem to be well tolerated by most birds. Subsequent feedings will obviously need to be reduced depending on the post-operative size of the crop. Rarely, a proventricular feeding tube may be required if crop resection is extensive and this area needs to be bypassed during the healing process.

While a total ingluviectomy would be rare, it can be performed if the crop must be resected as with severe trauma, cancer limited to the ingluvies, necrosis, and infection. A resection and anastomosis is performed with an attempt to limit as much tension as possible on the cervical-thoracic esophageal suture line. One study showed that using a stent (straight macaroni) to guide esophageal closure dramatically reduced six week post-operative mortality (due to surgical site stricture) from 50% to 0–3% in cropectomized chickens [26]. The anastomosis site may be closed in two layers (simple interrupted followed by continuous inverting) or as best determined by the surgeon. Skin closure is routine. Interestingly, some cropectomized birds may regenerate a new "out-pouching" soon after removal of the crop [26].

One obvious complication of ingluviectomy is reduced feeding post-operatively. One serious potential cause of reduced feed intake (aside from the absent crop) is incision site stricture which may be reduced by a stent as described above. However, studied laying chickens showed lowered serum calcium, egg specific gravity, and overall egg production post-ingluviectomy compared to non-ingluviectomized controls. The authors postulated that the crop serves as an important storage depot of feed providing nutrients necessary for egg shell quality during non-feeding periods [27]. Ready access to food, and possibly calcium supplementation, should be considered if a laying hen is ingluviectomized.

Proventricular and Ventricular Surgery

The "stomach" of birds consists, from orad to aborad, of the proventiculus, isthmus, and ventriculus, respectively. In general, the proventiculus and isthmus are soft muscular organs and the ventriculus is composed of strong contractile muscles and a tough inner lining (koilin layer) designed to crush food, sometimes with the aid of ingested stones. The proventiculus secretes digestive enzymes that help prepare the food for mechanical digestion in the ventriculus. The isthmus is the short region between the proventriculus and the ventriculus.

Birds that eat a coarse diet such as granivores, like Galliformes, have well-developed paired thick and thin muscles with a thick koilin layer on the mucosal surface [28]. Birds that consume a soft diet such as planktivores (plankton and crustacean), pisciovores (fish), and carnivores have a relatively thin-walled ventriculus and koilin layer [28]. Depending on the type of waterfowl and its diet, the ventriculus may range from poorly to well developed.

Proventriculotomy and ventriculotomy are reserved primarily for the removal of foreign bodies not eliminated via conservative therapy or non-retrievable using endoscopy or other less invasive techniques. Although not reported in poultry or waterfowl, ventricular diverticula were found in parakeet auklets (*Aethia psittacula*) kept on loose stone substrate. It was postulated that stones left in the soft ventriculus of these fish, krill, and copepod eating birds could result in diverticula formation and ventriculotomy should be considered if the foreign bodies are present in this species [28]. However, most reported cases involve gastrointestinal impactions in ratites, but have also been described in kiwis (*Apteryx australis*), umbrella cockatoos (*Cacatua alba*), Micronesian kingfishers (*Halcyon cinnamomina cinnamomina*) and sarus cranes (*Grus antigone*) [29–32]. Ventricular foreign bodies and subsequent obstruction and perforation have been reported as an important cause of mortality in bustards [33]. Food, fiber, and sand proventicular impactions are reported in waterfowl with lead toxicosis [28]. While seemingly absent from the refereed literature, poultry, and waterfowl also develop proventricular and ventricular foreign bodies that require surgical extraction.

The same approaches to the proventriculus and ventriculus are also used to obtain biopsies (neoplasia, etc.), address perforating ulcers and diverticula and to explore the serosal surface of the proventriculus, isthmus, and ventriculus. Prior to surgery, conservative therapy using bulking agents, fluid therapy, and basic support should be attempted.

The ventriculus consists of two opposing muscle pairs: the cranial and caudal thin muscles and the lateral and medial thick muscles [34]. The alternating contractions of the thin muscles, duodenum, thick muscles, and proventriculus make up the gastroduodenal motility sequence in poultry [28]. Contrast fluoroscopy can be used to view organ shape and ventricular contraction sequence [28].

The myenteric nerves cover the entire surface of the thin ventricular muscles and isthmus. Studies in domestic fowl have shown that in order for proper gastroduodenal motility to occur, the myenteric plexus associated with the isthmus must remain intact. It is also suspected that initiation and regulation of the thick muscles also acts via the nerves covering the isthmus. Specifically, isthmus denervation reduces the frequency of duodenal and muscular "stomach" (ventricular) contractions by 50% and abolishes glandular "stomach" (proventricular) contractions (in turkeys) [35]. The nerves encircling the isthmus do not appear important in regulating thin muscle contractions [34]. These findings support the need for atraumatic and precise surgery when incising the isthmus as discussed below.

For adult birds undergoing proventriculotomy or ventriculotomy, fast the patient for at least 12 hours to help "clean" the gastrointestinal tract. If possible, use handfeeding formula 1–2 days prior to surgery as these easily digestible foods tend to leave little residue in the ventriculus. Discontinue feeding formula food 6–12 hours prior to surgery. Pre- and post-operative antibiotics should be considered as with other animals undergoing enterotomies.

A left lateral or ventral midline combined with transverse celiotomy may be used to approach the ventriculus. If the ventriculus is displaced medially (as supported by contrast study radiographs), the ventral midline approach is more appropriate. Some surgeons prefer a ventral midline approach to enter the ventriculus through the caudoventral sac (see below). The proventriculus and isthmus are approached via a left lateral celiotomy.

With either a lateral or ventral approach, place stay sutures in the white tendinous portion of the ventriculus to help retract the organ(s) out of the coelomic cavity and improve exposure [36]. Due to its location, the proventriculus cannot be exteriorized but visualization is improved by retracting the ventriculus. It is best to pack moist sponges around the retracted organs to help prevent coelomic contamination.

Via a left lateral celiotomy, incise into the relatively avascular isthmus and extend the incision orad into the proventriculus or aborad to the ventriculus as needed. At this point, both the proventriculus and ventriculus can be explored. Due to the massive mobile muscular tunic and high tensile strain on the tendinous centers, the ventriculus does not have a good site for incisional entry [18]. Additionally, an endoscope may be introduced to improve visualization and help retrieve foreign bodies when present. The caudal thoracic (cranial coelomic) esophagus can be partially evaluated via this approach. Additional ribs may need to be transected to better view the lower esophagus. Irrigation and suction are often needed; be careful not to contaminate the coelomic cavity. Use fine monofilament, absorbable suture in a simple continuous pattern to close the wound. If possible, oversew with a continuous inverting pattern. Meticulous closure is required to help prevent dehiscence.

Using the ventral midline approach, the ventriculus may also be approached via the caudoventral sac [36]. The ventriculus has two blind sacs (craniodorsal and caudoventral) covered with relatively thin muscles. The ventriculus is slightly rotated clockwise to help expose the caudoventral sac. Incise through the muscle fibers to enter the ventricular lumen. Again, use meticulous closure. This tissue does not invert, so use interrupted sutures placed close together. In a study of Coturnix quail undergoing caudoventral sac ventriculotomy, ventricular mucosal healing was not complete until 21 days post-surgery [18].

While collagen patches have been suggested in mammals to help intestinal wounds heal, they may be detrimental to birds. Porcine submucosal collagen patches placed over the serosal surface of the ventricular suture line in Cortunix quail that underwent ventriculotomies resulted in a statistically significant increase in gross or microscopic perforations [18]. The authors of the study suggested that the collagen patch generated a lymphocytic xenograft rejection response [18].

In one study of proventriculotomies performed in ostriches, 6 of 18 died immediately post-operatively and 4 of the 12 surviving birds died within 30 days of the procedure [30]. The authors noted that many of the birds were debilitated prior to surgery and recommended an esophagotomy be performed in all young or debilitated birds at the same time as surgery to provide post-operative nutrition as many birds are anorectic for several days after surgery. The authors also made note that no adverse sequelae were noted from the esophagotomy [30]. In a separate report involving phytobezoars in 3 Micronesian kingfishers (*Halcyon cinnamomina*), the authors noted that one 1 bird died during ventriculotomy via a ventral midline approach [37]. The other two birds were treated medically. When medical therapy failed to resolve the phytobezoar in one, ventricular endoscopy was unsuccessful and the bird died during preparation for ventriculotomy. Although the success rate was poor in this group, the authors recommended brief medical management followed by surgical extraction in non-resolving cases [37]. Despite these reported surgical mortalities, the author feels that proventriculotomy and ventriculotomy can be safely performed in poultry and waterfowl and should be considered if conservative measures fail.

Lower Intestinal Surgery

With the exception of research studies on cecal surgery and colostomies in poultry, lower intestinal surgery is rarely reported in avian medicine. However, both metallic and non-metallic intestinal foreign bodies are described in multiple bird species [38]. Non-metallic lower gastrointestinal foreign bodies are most frequently linear, occasionally form a nidus or enterolith and diagnosed based on palpation or necropsy. Radiographs, with or without barium or iodine (especially if gastrointestinal perforation is suspected) and ultrasound may also aid in diagnosis. One case report describes a 14 month female Eclectus parrot (*Eclectus roratus*) with a mineralized intestinal foreign body. The foreign body and proximal part of the duodenum were removed and the bird recovered uneventfully. The details of the actual surgery were not included other than the foreign body was brittle upon removal and had a central fiber like structure [38]. One paper briefly notes

that an ostrich died of complications associated with small intestinal resection and anastomosis performed because of a perforating intestinal foreign body. The same ostrich underwent a proventriculotomy two months previously [30]. In a separate ostrich case, a 7.5-month castrated male died suddenly 4 months after castration. A segment of intestines was herniated and entrapped within the right pulmonary ostium, was dilated, and underwent ischemic necrosis. The cause of the entrapment was believed to be due to disrupting the air sac walls separating the right caudal thoracic and abdominal air sacs. Eventually the intestine found its way through the opening resulting in the herniation. The author noted that care should be taken to not disrupt this air sac integrity (at least in ostriches) [39].

Intestinal resection, repair and anastomosis are delicate procedures in birds. Use microsurgical instruments to remove necrotic or damaged bowel and spare healthy tissue and the surrounding vascular supply. Use 6-0' to 10-0' absorbable monofilament suture on quarter circle atraumatic needles for intestinal anastomosis and enterotomy closures [15]. Six to eight simple interrupted sutures are often necessary for end to end anastomosis. Enterotomy closures should be performed so as to limit intestinal stricture.

Duodenal feeding tubes may be needed to bypass a diseased proventriculus, ventriculus, or other upper intestinal area. Via a midline or transverse celiotomy, an indwelling jugular catheter no less than 1/3 the small intestine diameter is placed through the left coelomic wall and into the descending duodenal loop [15]. Advance the catheter through the descending and ascending duodenal loop and remove the catheter's needle. Use 5-0' monofilament suture to attach the duodenum to the coelomic body wall and provide a tight seal. Test the catheter patency and duodenostomy seal by injecting sterile saline and then close the body wall. Secure the external portion of the catheter using monofilament suture. Coil the external catheter and secure it to the bird's leg and wing. Divide the liquid diet into small frequent feedings. Flush the catheter with warm isotonic fluids before and after each use to prevent catheter obstruction. Closely monitor the incision site and patient for signs of coelomitis, leakage and catheter damage. When done, cut the sutures and pull the catheter leaving the incision to heal by second intention [15]. The intestine is at least temporarily adhered to the body wall.

Duodenal aspiration may be helpful in identifying occult parasitic (*Giardia* spp. and other protozoa) and *Mycobacteria* spp. infections and small intestinal bacterial overgrowth [40] (Figure 21.14). Via a ventral midline surgical approach, the duodenal loop is isolated [41]. Using a 25 gauge or smaller needle, aspirate the duodenal contents for culture and cytology. Additionally, use another needle with the bevel side up to aspirate the mucosal surface of the duodenum. Oftentimes, occult mycobacterial organisms can be recovered cytologically by aspirating affected thickened duodenal mucosa. Closure is standard and the collected samples should be processed and evaluated as soon as possible.

During percutaneous implosion and subsequent collapse of a soft shelled egg in an eclectus parrot (*Eclectus roratus solomonensis*), a tear in the cloacal mucosa developed requiring closure and ultimately a duodenal serosal patch [42]. The iatrogenic 5 mm cloacal tear, located between the opening into corprodeum and uterine opening into the urodeum, was approached via a ventral midline cloacotomy and sutured closed. The bird did not produce feces for over 36 hours after surgery. A barium series supported a terminal colonic-rectal obstruction. Ventral midline coeliotomy revealed that the entire intestinal tract was severely distended and suture material surrounded the distal colon near its junction with the cloaca (causing the obstruction). Upon manipulation, the colon ruptured in two places. The fecal material was removed and the colonic defects were closed with 5–0′ polydioxanone in a simple interrupted pattern. The serosa of the adjacent duodenum was sutured circumferentially over the repaired colonic defects using 8–0′ nylon in a simple interrupted pattern at 2-mm intervals without penetrating the lumen of the colon or duodenum. The sutures were placed approximately 2 mm from the sutured colonic defects. The sutures placed during the original surgery were removed allowing feces to enter the cloaca. The cloacal wall defect was closed with 5–0′ polydioxanone in a simple continuous pattern. A salpingohysterectomy was also performed.

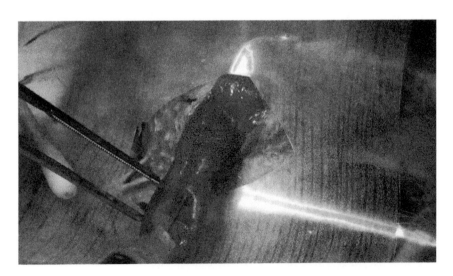

Figure 21.14 Duodenal aspiration using a 25 gauge needle in a blue headed pionus (*Pionus menstruus*).

The bird recovered uneventfully and was followed up to three years post-surgery and doing fine [42].

Cecal surgery has been described but only under experimental conditions and cecectomized or cecal ligated chickens, ducks, geese, and turkeys are used in digesta analysis and other studies [43–47]. In many avian species, ureteral urine flows aborad (via peristalsis) into the colon and ceca where water absorption occurs. At least in chickens and turkeys, when the ceca are ligated total water excretion is increased [45–48]. Cecostomized chickens show increased water intake and reduced transit time of digesta in the ceca [49]. Cecal ligation alters nitrogen metabolism in adult and young chickens [46, 47]. Also, both cecal ligation and colostomy in turkeys significantly alters cecal (colostomy only), ileal and rectal motility possibly due to changes in lower intestinal water content [45]. Current studies show the importance of avian ceca in water balance, and other metabolic functions, and should be considered if this organ is surgically manipulated.

While described primarily for research purposes, cecectomy is a fairly simple procedure. Clinically, cecectomy would be indicated to address diseases that could not be medically managed such as cancer, necrosis, etc. The bird is placed in right lateral recumbency with the left leg pulled cranially for a paralumbar approach [44]. A 3–4 cm paralumbar fossa incision is made, being careful to avoid penetrating the air sacs, and the ceca are retracted. Each cecum is then separated from the ileum via blunt dissection of the ileocecal ligament. Vessels running within the ligament are ligated. Ligate each ceca 1.0 cm distal to the ileal junction with absorbable suture. Remove the ceca. Carefully lavage the coelom and cecal stumps to ensure no free ingesta is present. Closure is routine [44].

Colostomy, while not reported in clinical cases, has been frequently described in chickens and turkeys for experimental purposes (in studies that require separation of urine from feces) [50, 51].

This procedure might conceivably be used as a temporary or permanent solution to address distal colonic and/or proximal cloacal disease (such as cancer) where the affected tissue must be removed and a continuous colonic-cloacal segment would not be possible.

The technique in chickens starts with exteriorizing the colon via a distal ventral midline incision and milking the feces from the distal colon into the cloaca and/or proximally. Next, transect the distal colon approximately 1.5–2.0 cm proximal to the cloaca and ligate both ends of the colon. Atruamatic intestinal forceps can be used to gently clamp the distal colon during manipulation instead of ligation. Using 4–0′ silk, ligate the seromuscular coat of the colon to the peritoneal tissue, lateral to the cloaca and vent, at three points in a triangular shape. Ligate the distal most aspect of the colonic mesentery to prevent bleeding out the stoma. Next place three sutures forming a triangle with the seromuscular aspect of the proximal transected colonic segment and the skin, again lateral to the cloaca and vent. Last, suture the everted colonic mucosal tissue (remove colon ligation sutures if placed) to the skin in a simple interrupted pattern to complete the stoma. The authors recommended antibiotics for three to five days post-surgery and frequent monitoring of the stoma for closure, infection or other complications and showed that chickens did quite well for months following this procedure [50]. A similar procedure, with some variation, has been reported to be successful in turkeys [51].

The cloaca of birds consists of three main compartments (from orad to aborad): the coprodeum, the urodeum, and proctodeum. The distal colon enters the coprodeum which is separated from the urodeum via a coprourodeal fold. The ureters enter the urodeum through a sphincter muscle and an opening that is covered by transitional epithelium preventing ureteral reflux [52]. Further, the urodeum is separated from the proctodeum via the uroproctodeal fold. Feces combine with urine and urates form the complete dropping which is eliminated through the proctodeum and out the external vent. In young birds the bursa of Fabricius can be found in the dorsal wall of the proctodeum and is the site of B-cell production. This structure reaches maximum size at 8–10 weeks of age and then involutes as the bird ages. By 7–10 months of age the bursa is considerably involuted.

The most common cloacal abnormalities seen in Galliformes and waterfowl result from trauma (animal attacks, dystocia, "vent pecking," etc.), but prolapse, infections, neoplasia, and other disorders may be encountered. When performing cloacal surgery, careful attention must be paid to the normal anatomic features especially the colon-coprodeal and ureter-urodeal junctions. The goal of cloacal surgery is to restore as much of the normal anatomy and function as possible.

A 7-year-old female umbrella cockatoo (*C. alba*) was evaluated after an incisional cloacopexy that incorporated the pubis [53]. The bird had a chronic history of cloacal prolapse. Six days post-cloacopexy, the bird's coelomic cavity was explored because of a recent history of anorexia, regurgitation, elevated creatine kinase, hyperuricemia, and decreased intraceolomic detail on screening radiographs. Midline celiotomy revealed yellow serous fluid throughout the coelom, a 2–3 cm section of colon trapped between the cloaca and body wall and adhesions between the colon and cloacopexy site. Adhesions were removed revealing 2 mm colonic and cloacal tears which were repaired with 4-0'PDS in a simple interrupted inverting pattern. Cloacopexy sutures were removed to further free the entrapped colon. The bird passed feces the next day but died 3-days post-surgery. Upon necropsy, an adhesion incorporating the cloaca, colon and body wall at the level of the caudal margin of the keel blocking the passage of fecal material was found. The gastrointestinal tract was distended with greenish fluid proximal to the adhesion. The authors noted that this and another bird (sulfur-crested cockatoo, *Cacatua galerita*) had a segment of large intestine trapped in the potential space between the cloacopexy sites and ventral body wall ultimately leading to the death of both [53].

A 2.0-cm-diameter cloacalith was found and subsequently removed from within the coprodeum of a four-year-old blue-fronted Amazon parrot (*Amazona aestiva*) [54]. The parrot was evaluated for acute onset of respiratory noises and straining. A cloacal mass was palpable on physical examination and saline infusion cloacoscopy was used to visualize the mass. The cloacolith was fragmented using 3-Fr biopsy forceps and larger pieces lavaged out. The remaining small pieces of the cloacolith passed shortly after recovery from anesthesia. Stone analysis revealed the cloacolith was composed of 100% urates. The bird was found to be normal at one week and nine months post-surgery. The cause of the cloacolith was not determined [54].

An infiltrative lipoma of the cloacal serosa was successfully removed from a 14-year-old blue-crowned conure (*Aratinga acuticaudata*) with a three-week history of straining and vocalizing during defecation [55]. Physical examination revealed a 2.5 cm soft tissue swelling on the mid-caudoventral coelom. Ventral midline celiotomy was used to identify a subcutaneous soft tissue mass extending through the body wall musculature into the coelom and adhered to the cloacal serosa. The mass was causing the cloaca to deviate caudally and ventrally. The mass was removed via blunt dissection without penetrating the cloaca. Histopathologic evaluation determined the mass was an infiltrative lipoma with adipose tissue at the surgical margins. The bird was clinically normal with no evidence of tumor recurrence one and seven months post-surgery [55].

Ventplasty

Ventplasty is reserved for chronic cloacal prolapse. In the author's experience, chronic cloacal prolapses are most commonly associated with prolonged egg laying. However, intestinal parasites, chronic masturbation (ducks), coelomic masses, and more may all result in a cloacal prolapse. The cause of the cloacal prolapse should be determined and resolved if possible. If the prolapse is chronic, the cloacal muscles and supporting structures may be permanently stretched and non-functional. The goal of ventplasty is to reduce the vent size such that cloacal prolapse does not recur. It should be understood that ventplasty will likely fail if the underlying cause of the prolapse is not resolved and the bird continues to strain post-operatively.

The extent of the dilated vent will determine how much tissue must be resected. For mild to moderate distension, usually one section of the vent is resected. For more severe distension, two areas of vent resection may be required. The basic incision is the same, but one versus two resections is based on surgeon preference in relation to the animal's needs. Pre- and post-operative antibiotics should be considered and based on culture and sensitivity results of a cloacal swab or cloacal tissue culture.

Prior to making the incision(s), estimate how much tissue needs to be resected in order to make a normal vent diameter. Triangular incisions work best with the "base" of the triangle on the leading edge of the vent and the "point" away from the vent. A single incision works best over the cranial ventral side of the vent while two opposing incisions can be performed at the right and left lateral sides.

Once the resection site(s) is(are) determined, excise the desired triangular area(s) taking epidermis and dermis. Save excised tissue in formalin if needed. If the sphincter and transverse cloacal muscles are visible, spare these muscles. The dermis can usually be bluntly resected from the underlying muscular and submucosal tissue layers. When apposed, the new epidermal edges should form the desired vent diameter. If needed, more epidermal/dermal tissue is removed.

With the appropriate "new" vent margins, close the surgery site. First close the submucosa with the dermis. Place simple interrupted absorbable sutures medial (which represents the new vent wall) to lateral for all tissue layers. Next, close the dermis in the same fashion. Finally, the overlying epidermis is closed. The distal cloacal mucosa should extend distally to the vent epithelial margins without additional measures. If not, simply suture the mucosa in place as needed. The end result should be one suture line extending cranially (single vent resection) or one suture line extending laterally on the left and right sides of the vent (double vent resection). The new vent diameter should be just large enough to allow passage of droppings. Use lubricated cotton tipped applicators to test the patency of the vent. Sutures are absorbable but can be removed in two weeks if needed.

If this patient is female, egg laying must be controlled either via a salpingohysterecomy, behvaviorally, and/or chemically. Otherwise dystocia or rupture of the ventplasty sutures may result.

Liver

Liver surgery is generally limited to partial hepatectomy to remove solitary masses and liver biopsy. Numerous non-invasive diagnostics such as serum biochemistries, radiographs, high detail CT and MRI and more, can be performed to help determine if liver surgery is necessary.

Liver biopsy is a fairly common procedure and is very useful in determining hepatic pathology. Liver biopsy is obviously indicated when hepatic disease is suspected, but is also used to evaluate environmental toxins and in determining response to therapy. A thrombocyte estimate and capillary clot time (normal is less than five minutes) can be performed prior to surgery [56]. With that stated, avian platelets can only be estimated as they tend to clump in birds [57]. If a coagulopathy is suspected, give vitamin K_1 (0.2–2.5 mg/kg IM) 24–48 hours pre-operatively [57]. If ascites is present, as much fluid as possible should be drained via coelomocentesis prior to surgery.

Minimally invasive endoscopic and ultrasound-guided and blind percutaneous biopsies are also described [56, 58, 59]. One study showed that ultrasound guided liver biopsies resulted in 96.7% and 63.3% recovery of hepatic tissue in pigeons and quail (*Corturnix coturnix*) respectively [57]. While only a small amount of liver tissue was recovered using a Tru-Cut biopsy needle and biopsy aid in the study, the authors noted the sample size was sufficient for histopathological evaluation. In the study, one of 19 quails died under anesthesia due to hemopericardium. While no pigeons died during the procedure, 6 of 15 necropsied pigeons (40%) had right liver lobe hematomas one week post-surgery. The authors concluded that "ultrasound guided liver biopsy without a biopsy aid [such as endoscopy] is too risky considering the size of the avian liver" [57].

A cranial ventral midline coelomic (just caudal to the sternum) approach works well for most hepatic surgeries and is the author's preferred method over endoscopic liver sampling. Incise through the midline skin and linea alba to gain access to the cranial coelom and ventral hepatic peritoneal cavities. With hepatomegaly, the liver is readily visible and the right lobe is usually larger. With microhepatica, the liver is tucked under the sternum. Use cup-end biopsy forceps or curved hemostat to collect as large a piece of liver as possible without undue risk of hemorrhage. As an example, 3×10 mm liver biopsies (mean biopsy sample was 62.4 mg) were safely collected from 36 captive and 157 free ranging harlequin ducks (*Histrionicus histrionicus*) [60]. In another study, 0.5 and 1.2 g (6% and 18% hepatectomies, respectively) liver biopsies were safely collected from a total of 16 galahs (*Eolophus roseicapillus*) [61].

Typically the edge of the liver is biopsied using either instrument while the cup-end forceps are more appropriate for selecting specific lesions and with microhepatica. When biopsying the liver's edge, bleeding is often minimal and sutures are rarely required. If hemorrhage is persistent, use hemostats to clamp on the bleeding area until hemostasis is established. Absorbable gelatin foam (Gelfoam˚, Pharmacia and Upjohn Company, Kalamazoo, Michigan)

may also be placed along the cut liver's edge to further reduce bleeding. If possible, collect extra tissue for culture and electron microscopy. Close the muscle and skin layers as with other coelomic surgeries.

Although complications such as uncontrolled hemorrhage, perforation of intestines and other underlying organs and introduction of ascitic fluid into the air sacs are reported, these problems are fairly uncommon with the coelomic approach discussed above [56]. Even with severe liver disease, complications such as clinically evident coagulopathies are uncommon in the author's experience.

Selected laboratory values will likely change following a liver biopsy. In pigeons and quails undergoing ultrasound guided Tru-Cut liver biopsies, aspartate aminotransferase (AST), creatinine kinase (CK), lactate dehydrogenase (LDH), alkaline phosphatase (ALP), total protein (TP), and albumin were measured before and one week after surgery. In pigeons the AST and albumin both significantly increased post-surgically while only AST increased in the quails [57]. In a study of mixed wild raptors, "liver and kidney" values increased within five days after liver biopsy [62]. With the exception of mildly elevated alanine aminotransferase immediately following (18% liver weight) biopsies, galahs that underwent 6% and 18% hepatectomies had normal serum bile acids and elevated AST, CK, and ALP values that were statistically no different from sham operated birds immediately following, four and seven days post-surgery. This last report suggests that these "liver enzymes" elevated as a result of celiotomy and not liver trauma [61].

In chickens, if both bile ducts are ligated, severe fibrosing cholehepatitis results within 28 days [63]. The typical lesions that result from extrahepatic bile duct ligation in poultry include cholestasis, fibrosis, proliferated biliary ductules and increased Ito (fat storing) cells within the liver [64]. While not jaundiced, chickens with both bile ducts ligated also developed intensely yellow stained droppings 6–7 days post-surgery [63]. Bile duct ligation results in jaundiced skin, diarrhea, low serum testosterone and atrophic and sclerotic testes 10 weeks post-surgery in one-year-old chickens likely as a result of the hepatic fibrosis and obstructive cholestasis [65].

The left and right bile ducts are located on the caudal visceral surface of the respective liver lobe and typically unite on the right hepatic lobe then branch (hepatocystic duct) to enter the gall bladder (if present) or the duodenum (common hepatoenteric duct) [66]. Bile ducts are easily avoided during liver biopsy but should be considered a potential issue with extensive hepatectomies, cholecystectomy, distorted anatomy (especially with neoplasia) and proximal duodenal surgery.

In one study involving 8 Pekin ducks infected with duck hepatitis B virus that underwent serial surgical liver biopsies at four to five week intervals (34 surgical procedures total), there was only one perioperative death with no evidence of wound complications or intra-abdominal sepsis [67]. Seven of 157 (4.5%) free-ranging and 0 of 36 captive harlequin ducks died during recovery from anesthesia following liver biopsy and radio transmitter implantation. It was determined that none of the deaths were attributable to the liver biopsies [60]. With a little experience, surgical liver biopsies can be easily and safely performed in poultry, waterfowl, and other birds.

Pancreas

Birds, and their pancreas, seem to tolerate pancreatic surgery well. Following 99% pancreatectomy in chickens, the splenic pancreatic lobe undergoes a rapid enlargement (400% increase) over 16 days [68]. Partially depancreatomized chickens, with splenic lobe intact, also seem to maintain metabolic parameters remarkably well although a post-surgical transitory hyperglycemia may be noted. One conclusion drawn is that the avian splenic lobe appears to be "extremely competent following removal of the major avian pancreatic lobes in adjusting to the demands placed on it for adequate nutrient absorption and distribution" [68].

Total pancreatectomy is fatal, but subtotal pancreatectomy (leaving the splenic lobe intact) results in transient "diabetes" that resolves in 12 days in Peking ducks [69]. Based on the author's experience and published studies, pancreatic biopsies and partial debulking is well tolerated in birds.

Pancreatic duct ligation results in severe damage to the pancreas [70]. Most of the pancreas lies within the duodenal loop and has 1–3 draining ducts that enter the terminal duodenum in close proximity to the bile and hepatic ducts. The potential complications of bile duct ligation are listed above. Pancreatic duct ligation results in atrophic pancreatic acini and interstitial fibrosis in chicks. Pancreatic duct obstruction has been a proposed cause of stunting syndrome in chickens [70].

A high grade pancreatic exocrine adenocarcinoma was removed from a five-year-old male cockatiel (*Nymphicus hollandicus*) via celiotomy [71]. The report describes a "large, firm, white multinodular pedunculated mass (2.5 cm in diameter) that originated between the distal portion of the pancreas and ascending loop of the duodenum." The authors also reported they removed the distal tip of the pancreas adjacent to the mass at the same time. Neoplastic cells were surgically evident at the biopsy margins. Six weeks after surgery, the bird was doing well and celecoxib (10 mg/kg PO SID) was administered for three months. One hundred forty-two days post-surgery the bird presented with dyspnea and died during diagnostic sample collection. The bird had diffuse metastatic pancreatic adenocarcinoma. Of note, the bird had acute diffuse renal tubular necrosis (possibly due to the celecoxib) [71].

Pancreatic Biopsy

Pancreatic biopsy is indicated when pancreatic disease, such as pancreatitis and neoplasia, is suspected and accurate diagnosis is needed for individual case management (Figure 21.15).

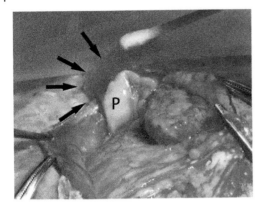

Figure 21.15 Diseases of the pancreas (P), such as these benign cysts (outlined by arrows) in a Pekin duck (*Anas platyrhnchos*) with sterile coelomitis, may require biopsy or partial pancreatectomy.

A cranial ventral midline approach is used similar as with liver biopsy. The dorsal and ventral pancreatic lobes rest between the ascending and descending duodenal loop. The duodenum is located to the right of midline and is often covered by a thin coelomic membrane. Incise through the thin membrane and gently retract the duodenal loop. After examining the pancreas and duodenum for gross abnormalities, select the distal (free) end of the dorsal pancreatic lobe (unless another site is clearly abnormal). Using hemostats, clamp the pancreas just distal to its distal-most vessel coming off the duodenum. Remove the distal pancreatic fragment and submit for histopathologic evaluation. Usually, a 3–8 mm section of pancreas is harvested. Remove the hemostats, but re-apply if bleeding occurs. Sutures to control hemostasis are rarely indicated. Close the coelom in standard fashion.

Urinary Tract

Renal Surgery

Because of the dorsal coelomic location within the renal fossae and complex vascular system, kidney surgery is often limited to focal procedures such as biopsy and superficial mass removal. The close associations with the lumbar and sacral plexuses and extensive vascular network surrounding the kidneys lead to the high probability of significant hemorrhage and possible neurologic damage expected during surgery.

Most cases of avian renal disease can be managed conservatively. However, some require additional diagnostics to better guide diagnosis and therapy. The only means to definitively diagnose avian renal disease and specific pathologic patterns is with a kidney biopsy and histopathologic evaluation. A renal biopsy is most frequently performed during endoscopic examination of the coelomic cavity and specifically, kidneys. However, a renal biopsy can be easily performed using 5-French cup biopsy forceps during exploratory coeliotomy.

Using a left lateral paralumbar fossa (most common with endoscopy) or ventral midline approach (celiotomy), the kidney is identified dorsal to the abdominal air sac. A right lateral approach may be used if disease is suspected to be limited to that side. The kidney is visualized and examined as much as possible. A small incision is made through the abdominal air sac and any other overlying membranes to expose the serosal surface of the kidney. Generally, one to three 5-Fr cup biopsy samples are collected from the cranial renal division in effort to avoid the large vessels coursing through and around the kidneys. The middle renal division may also be biopsied especially if the cranial division is atrophied or covered by vascular tissue (such as with an active ovary or neoplasia) (Figure 21.16). Once the tissue is collected, the site is monitored for excessive bleeding. Direct pressure using a cotton tip applicator or hemostatic agent (such as Gelfoam) may be used if needed. Kidney biopsy samples are immediately placed in formalin and body wall closure is standard.

In a study of 89 free living birds of prey, 126 endoscopic renal biopsy samples (2 biopsies from 37 birds) using 1.8 mm biopsy cup forceps were taken [72]. Post-biopsy hemorrhage

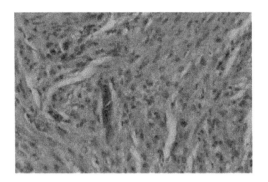

Figure 21.16 Renal neoplasia, such as this hematoxylin and eosin stained histopathologic section of an undifferentiated sarcoma in a Toulouse goose (*Anser anser domesticus*), may significantly alter the appearance of renal tissue during exploratory surgery.

averaged 67 seconds (10–172 seconds). The average biopsy was 2.2 mm long, 1.3 wide and 1.0 mm deep. All samples contained proximal and distal tubuli and 1 to 89 glomeruli, with most having 25–29 gomeruli per histologic slide. One hundred thirteen of 126 samples could be evaluated well or very well. Sixty six samples revealed lesions including subcapsular bleeding (19/66), inflammation (16/66), cell casts (12/66), periodic acid Schiff positive reactions (8/66), and protein casts (6/66). Correlation between endoscopically visible change and histologic disease was 76.1% (96/126). The cranial division was considered the best site to collect biopsy samples due to its size and visibility. The authors noted it was possible to obtain specimens from the middle and caudal renal divisions in larger birds [72].

A separate study examined the effects of intramuscular meloxicam on kidney tissue in Japanese quail (*Coturnix japonica*). Fifteen birds underwent 5-french endoscopic biopsy cup biopsies from two sites in the cranial division of the left kidney with minimal complications [73]. In the author's experience, 1 to 3 3 or 5-French cup biopsies can be safely collected from the cranial and/or middle renal divisions in birds.

Renal histologic lesions are rarely pathognomonic for a specific disease process as many different diseases cause similar kidney changes.

The author encourages veterinarians to work with a pathologist familiar with normal and abnormal avian histology. Oftentimes, it is the pathologist's interpretation of a renal biopsy combined with the attending veterinarian's case familiarity that enables both parties to make a definitive diagnosis or build a reasonable differential diagnoses list compatible with the kidney lesions noted.

Urolithiasis and Ureteral Obstructive Disease

Urolithiasis refers to the "formation of large urate 'stones' in the ureters," is primarily seen in pullets and caged laying hens and can result in increased mortality and decreased egg production [74]. Urolithiasis appears to be a primarily poultry disorder but has been rarely described in other avian species.

Birds affected with uroliths may show no or vague clinical signs. In the author's experience, many are initially suspected radiographically by finding small radiodense objects in the dorsal caudal coelom with no associated physical or other laboratory abnormalities. Some birds may exhibit excessive straining when producing a dropping which is also consistent with egg laying, diarrhea, intra-coelomic masses and more. A contrast pyelogram may be used to further support ureteral obstruction. Ultimately, the stone will need to be visualized with endoscopy or celiotomy or, less commonly, with advanced high resolution CT.

Common intracoelomic findings include a dilated ureter obstructed with one or more urate stones (that may be visible on radiographs), atrophic ispsilateral renal tissue and a normal to hypertrophic (compensatory) contralateral kidney. Renal histologic lesions noted with urolithiasis have included glomerular nephritis, tubular nephrosis, ureteritis and interstitial mononuclear infiltrates. In birds, ureteral obstruction (as may occur with ureteroliths, cloacal masses, urodeal fold thickening, etc.) may cause a post-obstructive form of renal disease.

Based on studies in chickens, it may take significant renal loss before uric acid levels become persistently elevated. Uric acid values elevated within 1–2 days of ligating one ureter at its junction with the cloaca and the other, along with caudal renal vein occlusion, at the midpoint of the opposite kidney in chickens. However, the uric acid values returned to normal within 12–14 days after surgery which was attributed to the hypertrophy of the unobstructed remaining kidney tissue [75]. With the exception of a small island of tissue adjacent to the left adrenal gland, both kidneys atrophied significantly cranial to the ligated ureters. In studied chickens, the total kidney weights birds with urolithiasis do not differ significantly to those without uroliths [75]. This demonstrates the tremendous compensatory capacity of the healthy remaining kidney tissue and may explain why urolithiasis affected birds seem otherwise normal.

Simple ligation of a bird's ureter results in ipsilateral renal atrophy and this result is similarly expected with urolithiasis. Naturally occurring ureteroliths in chickens are known to contain uric acid, urates, calcium, and ammonia.

The cause of urolithiasis in poultry flocks is not completely understood. However, coronavirus-associated nephritis in pheasants can induce interstitial nephritis, ureteral impaction, tubular dilatation, and subsequent visceral gout. In addition to infectious bronchitis virus infection (IBV, a coronavirus), other proposed causes or urolithiasis in poultry include water deprivation, excess dietary calcium and nutritional electrolyte imbalances. By adding additional phosphorous, changing the form of calcium from small particle size to flakes and modifying the IBV vaccination protocol, investigators have been able to significantly reduce the incidence of urolithiasis in a previously affected layer flock. However, it has not been determined which management change results in the beneficial effect.

Treatment of urolithiasis in birds is rare. A 21-year-old male double-yellow headed Amazon parrot (*Amazona ochracephala*) with a history of lifelong straining to void and chronic intermittent vomiting for a "few years" was diagnosed with septic ureterolithiasis [76]. Dorsocaudal coelomic radiodense opacities were found on screening whole body radiographs. Urolithiasis was diagnosed via exploratory coeliotomy. Multiple surgeries were required to remove the stones. A kidney biopsy was not collected and a relationship to renal disease could not be made. The ureteroliths were composed of "monosodium uric acid crystals and proteinaceous material mixed randomly or forming irregular laminae." Although the bird had dry flaky skin, a urate pasted vent, dull feathers and heterophilic (28 840 cells/µl) leukocytosis (32 000 cells/µl), the authors concluded that the clinical signs associated with ureterolithiasis in this bird were non-specific and may result in delayed diagnosis with other birds. The cause was not determined [76].

For those birds in which the urolithiasis appears to be causing pain, renal compromise or other associated problems, surgical removal may be the best option. While lithotripsy has been reported to manage renal stones in a Magellanic penguin (*Spheniscus magellanicus*), there are no other such reports for managing uroliths in birds [77].

The patient is placed in dorsal recumbency and a ventral midline incision is made. The intestines are gently moved medially or laterally in effort to visualize both kidneys. The ureters are located on the ventral medial surface of the kidneys. Affected ureters are often significantly dilated making visualization easier. If the ureters are clear, the stone may be visualized. Otherwise, follow the dilated ureter distally until the obstruction can be felt or seen. A small and precise longitudinal incision is made on the ventral surface of the dilated ureter over the obstructed area. Remove the stone(s) and any debris present. Using a lacrimal duct cannula, small ball tipped or standard red rubber feeding tube or an appropriately sized IV catheter without the stylet, flush the ureter proximally and distally to ensure patency. Close the ureterotomy site with fine (5-0′ to 8-0′)

absorbable suture material in a simple inter-rupted pattern being careful to minimally reduce the lumen size. Any fluid and debris leaked from the surgery site should be removed prior to closure. Coelomic closure is routine.

Female Reproductive Tract Surgery

Reproductive tract disease is very common in poultry and waterfowl, especially in female birds. These domesticated birds have been selectively bred, in many cases, over centuries and have a high reproductive drive. This trans-lates into prolonged egg laying seasons and complications resulting from this physically and energetically demanding process. In addi-tion, the physiologic changes associated with egg laying (such as weight gain, medullary hyperostosis, etc.) can result in unwanted con-sequences (fatty liver disease, fractures, etc.) when the process becomes more continuous with shortened rest periods.

Emergency surgery of the avian reproduc-tive tract is rarely indicated. However, pre-sur-gical conditioning is recommended for all stable birds with reproductive tract diseases to improve the chance of a positive surgical out-come. To correct obesity and any nutritional imbalances and possibly reduce reproductive drive, the diet is modified to reduce caloric intake and increase foraging opportunities. For pet poultry and waterfowl, this often means reducing diets high in simple sugars (such as corn and flour based foods and treats) and allowing the birds to forage for food naturally outside (if possible). Caloric restriction may also be considered, especially if the hen is over-weight. Pre-surgical conditioning may occur over several weeks to months and depends on the problem(s) and health status of the bird.

The drive to produce eggs is very strong in poultry and domestic waterfowl (especially ducks). However, attempts are still made to reduce reproductive stimulation in hens with reproductive disease. With poultry, affected hens may need to be removed from the presence of a rooster and separated from other actively laying hens until the reproductive disease is resolved. If possible, place the hen with other non-cycling birds or non-predatory animals. With waterfowl, the problem is more commonly associated with owners petting, stroking, and cuddling the pet. This activity should be dis-couraged. However, the owner can still interact with the bird, just with minimal handling. Separating a waterfowl hen from her bonded mate may result in significant stress. Unmated ducks, which are being kept with other egg lay-ing ducks, may be placed with non-cycling birds or non-predatory animals as with chickens. Decreasing the photoperiod to 8–10 hours of light a day may be beneficial. As noted above, getting hens engaged in other activities such as foraging, swimming (waterfowl) and trick train-ing (best with ducks) can help minimize repro-ductive stimulation (Figure 21.17a-g).

Leuprolide acetate (Lupron Depot, TAP Pharmaceuticals, Inc., Deerfield, IL, USA) has been used clinically to suppress reproductive activity in many birds. Lueprolide acetate depot is a long-acting GnRH analog that (in women) results in an initial stimulation fol-lowed by prolonged suppression of pituitary gonadotropins. Repeated monthly injections are intended to result in receptor down-regula-tion and decreased secretion of gonadal steroid hormones. From the author's experiences and reported information, recommended doses vary but have been safely used from 100 μg/kg up to 1000 μg/kg IM q 14–28 days to help sup-press reproductive activity in birds. Attia et al. showed that a single IM injection of leuprolide acetate providing 10 μg/kg BW per day for 30 days in broiler hens caused marked reduc-tion in egg production [78]. The authors also reported a linear decline in oviduct, but not ovary, weight with an increasing dose of leu-prolide acetate [78].

When extrapolated to other bird species, these findings suggest that leuprolide acetate may decrease egg production and have value to decrease oviduct size in preparation for

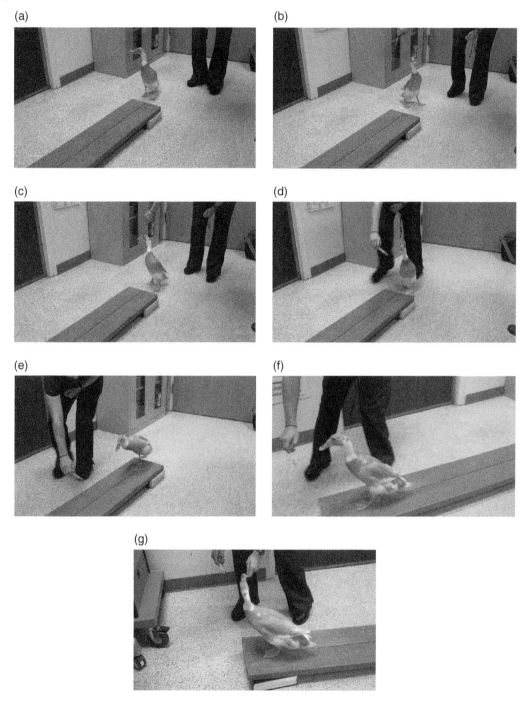

(a)

(b)

(c)

(d)

(e)

(f)

(g)

Figure 21.17 A mixed breed domestic duck (*Anas platyrhnchos*) is clicker trained to perform productive, and discourage reproductive, behaviors. The duck twirls while following the owner's clicker (right hand). Then the duck continues to follow the clicker while walking 2 planks of wood. Finally, the duck is rewarded with a treat. Clicker training and numerous other methods can be used to allow owners to positively interact with their birds and encourage productive activity without reinforcing reproductive behaviors.

salpingohysterectomy. Per the author's experience, some reproductively active female waterfowl and poultry can override the effects of leuprolide acetate with continued stimulation. For that reason, GnRH agonists are rarely used as a sole "treatment" to stop egg laying or prepare for surgery. Behavior and dietary modification are often combined with GnRH agonists to prepare reproductively active birds for surgery.

Deslorelin (Suprelorin®, Peptech Animal Health/Virbac, Australia) implants have also been recommended for the same purpose but are typically implanted every 3–12 months as needed. Noonan, et al. studied the effects of 4.7 and 9.4 mg deslorelin subcutaneous implants (versus placebo) in two-year-old egg laying chickens over a one year period of time [79]. One hundred percent of deslorelin implanted birds stopped laying eggs and had an ultrasound determined "inactive ovary" by two weeks post-implantation. All placebo birds continued egg laying. Egg laying in the deslorelin groups was suppressed a mean of 180 days (range 125–237) and 319 days (range 229–357 [with 2 birds still suppressed beyond this time]) with the 4.7 mg and 9.4 mg implants, respectively [79].

In contrast to chickens, Japanese quail decreased egg laying for only 70 days when given 4.7 mg deslorelin acetate implants [80]. Additionally, of the 10 experimental group quail, only 6 ceased egg production. The other 4 birds, and the control group animals, continued to lay throughout the 180 day study. Interestingly, several of the experimental birds laid eggs with atypical color patterns two days after receiving the implant [80]. Although only representing two species, these studies demonstrate the potential wide variation of effects of deslorelin acetate on egg laying suppression in poultry species.

Both of these GnRH agonists, over time, pose significant expenditure outlay, and should not be considered a "first choice" maintenance treatment modality for controlling reproductive activity, unless all environmental, nutritional and behavioral factors involved have been evaluated and deficits addressed. The author uses leuprolide acetate or deslorelin acetate as a means to help "condition" the bird in preparation for surgery. The goal of GnRH agonist use being to help reduce reproductive activity and subsequently reproductive organ size and vasculature. Editor's note: The Food and Drug Administration (FDA) may consider ducks a food animal species and therefore GnRH agonists would be a prohibited drug. In addition, deslorelin is a scheduled drug labeled for use in ferrets only.

The author strongly feels that environmental, dietary and behavioral modifications are often needed for long-term successful management of reproductive tract diseases in hens, even after surgery. Occasionally long-term GnRH agonist use is needed, especially if the owners are non-compliant with other recommended modifications or used as a form of chemotherapy for some reproductive tract neoplasia (not well founded at the time of writing). Even if the oviduct and most of the ovary are surgically removed, the reproductive drive remains high in domestic poultry and waterfowl. Continued stimulation can result in internal ovulation and other problems. These issues should be discussed with owners prior to considering surgery.

Anatomy of the Avian Oviduct

The oviduct, or salpinx, develops from the left Mullerian duct and can be divided into 5 regions. The cranial-most region is the infundibulum, which is the site of fertilization and engulfs the ovulated ovum (Figure 21.18). The ovum next moves into the largest region, the magnum, which produces albumin that surrounds the developing egg. The inner and outer shell membranes are then formed in the isthmus. The egg is then "plumped" with water and solutes, calcified to form a shell and pigments deposited during the prolonged stay in the shell gland or "uterus." The shell gland transfers the complete egg through the

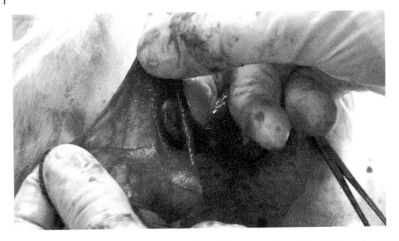

Figure 21.18 The proximal most portion of the oviduct, or infundibulum featured in this chicken during celiotomy, serves to engulf or "catch" the mature follicle as it is released from the ovary.

uterovaginal sphincter into the vagina. The uterovaginal area contains sperm-storage tubules allowing many species to store viable spermatozoa for prolonged periods of time (greater than 21 days in turkey hens) [81]. The vagina terminates at the cloaca and coordinates with the shell gland to ultimately expel the egg.

In adults, there is normally a left ovary and oviduct as any embryological right tissue typically regresses. However, there are numerous reports of right ovaries and/or oviducts in poultry, birds of prey and parrots. There is even a double oviduct line of Rhode Island Red chickens that commonly have right oviducts [82]. While some eggs may be produced in a right oviduct, these are rarely fully functional [82].

The oviduct is suspended within the coelomic cavity via a dorsal and ventral ligament. Blood is supplied to the oviduct by the cranial, middle and caudal oviductal arteries running in the dorsal mesentery. Only generalizations can be made as the origins of each vessel vary between species. The cranial oviductal artery arises from the left cranial renal artery, aorta or external iliac artery. The middle oviductal artery comes from the left ischiadic artery or its branch, the medial renal artery. The caudal oviductal artery arises from the left internal iliac artery or the pudendal artery. The veins draining the cranial oviduct empty into the caudal vena cava (via the common iliac vein), while those draining the caudal oviduct enter the renal portal or hepatic systems.

Diseases of the Oviduct

Oviductal disorders may be incidental findings or clinically relevant and are surgically addressed as needed. Birds with oviductal disease may present with non-specific clinical signs. The most commonly recognized abnormalities with oviductal disease are related to a space occupying coelomic mass including compression of surround organs, coelomic distension, coelomitis and ascites. Generally, abnormal oviductal tissue is removed at the time of exploratory surgery.

Common congenital defects recognized in birds include a right oviduct ranging from rudimentary, discontinuous and atretic up to full size and functional of which many are cystic (Figure 21.19). The author has noted a direct correlation between the presence of right oviducts and non-specific reproductive tract problems in hens (including cystic ovarian follicles, excessive egg laying, etc.). However, the cause and effect, if any, of this relationship is not clear. Cystic oviductal tissue

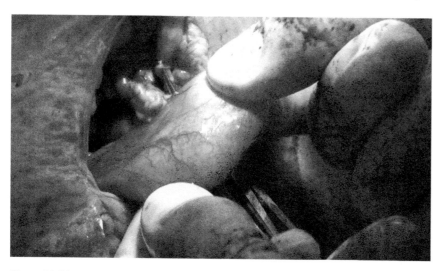

Figure 21.19 A right oviduct from a chicken is exteriorized out the ventral midline incision during exploratory celiotomy.

can be substantial, may be associated with cancer and is always removed by the author when identified. Persistent right oviducts typically have a limited blood supply but are removed in a similar fashion as the more normal left counterpart.

Ectopic ovulation occurs when the infundibulum fails to engulf an ovum or fails to retain the ovum because of oviductal rupture or reverse peristalsis. The ectopic ovum is often found in various stages of development from yolk to a shelled egg. Potential causes include infundibulum failure from oviductal fat, trauma, or disease, exuberant reverse peristalsis and oviductal disease. Ectopic ovulation is thought to occur frequently and has been reported in 28.6% of necropsied birds from nine orders [83]. The author has also seen ectopic ovulation associated with a persistent right oviduct in several avian species. Ectopic ovulation of yolk commonly results in mild, self-resolving, sterile yolk coelomitis and requires no or minimal supportive therapy (fluid therapy, anti-inflammatories, etc.).

Partially and completely shelled ectopic eggs result when a developing egg goes into the ceolomic cavity through an oviductal rupture or via reverse peristalsis from oviductal or even

cloacal disease. Any disruption in the oviduct function such as cloacal or oviductal masses (including egg binding, impactions, and neoplasia), salpingitis, cystic hyperplasia and oddly shaped or large eggs can potentially result in ectopic eggs. A large ectopic egg can cause a penguin-like stance in small birds and is often associated with ascites and varying degrees of depression. Ectopic eggs can often rest within the coelom unnoticed in larger hens. Diagnosis can often be suspected using radiography, ultrasonography, and sometimes endoscopy (depending on how much debris is in the coelom), but celiotomy is often required for definitive diagnosis. Ectopic eggs should always be considered when conservative therapy for egg binding fails. Partially and fully formed ectopic eggs should be surgically removed after stabilizing the patient and determining the underlying cause(s).

Severe sterile and life threatening septic egg yolk coelomitis may result from ectopic ovulation or eggs, systemic sepsis and oophoritis. Acute egg yolk coelomitis may result in significant depression, anorexia and ascites and rarely, respiratory distress and death. Depending on the degree of inflammation associated with egg yolk coelomitis, coelomic adhesions may result and be found days to more than a year after the episode during coeliotomy. Coliforms such as *Escherichia coli*, *Yersinia pseudotuberculosis* and *Staphylococcus spp* are commonly identified in septic yolk coelomitis [84]. *Salmonella sp.* may also be found with septic oophoritis and should be considered with bacterial coelomitis. Coelomocentesis and cytologic fluid analysis and culture are used for definitive diagnosis. Treatment of severe egg yolk coelomitis, especially when associated with bacteria, includes aggressive supportive care, antimicrobials, identifying and resolving causative factors if possible and occasionally may require coeliotomy to removed infected tissue.

Egg Binding and Dystocia

Egg binding and dystocia are commonly described problems in pet bird medicine. However, these are uncommonly seen in poultry and waterfowl except with small birds. Oviposition is the expulsion of the egg from the oviduct and is conducted by vigorous contractionof the oviductal muscles and peristalsis of the vagina. Egg binding is simply defined as prolonged oviposition (egg is arrested in oviduct longer than normal for the given species) while dystocia implies the developing egg is within the distal oviduct either obstructing the cloaca or prolapsed through the oviduct-cloacal opening. Dystocia is often more advanced than egg binding alone, has many potential causes and is commonly associated with functional (malformed eggs, cloacal masses, and obesity), metabolic (calcium imbalance and nutritional deficiencies), environmental (temperature changes, lack of exercise, and other stressors) and hereditary diseases.

Most cases of egg binding and dystocia are managed medically and are discussed elsewhere. Surgical intervention (primarily exploratory celiotomy) is rarely required in poultry and waterfowl.

Oviduct Cystic Hyperplasia

Cystic oviductal hyperplasia or dilatation has been reported in many bird species including poultry. Although little etiologic information is forwarded, cysts may occur secondary to improper formation of the oviduct. Hyperplastic oviducts are often thickened with white to beige masses and distended with brown or white mucoid fluid. Affected birds often show no signs (and the disease is discovered incidentally) or occasionally signs typical of reproductive tract disease (especially if the oviduct is significantly enlarged). Antimicrobials may be tried if organisms are recovered from aspirated samples, otherwise salpingohysterectomy is indicated.

Oviduct Impaction

An impacted oviduct is usually distended and simply contains caseated material and misshapen, ruptured, soft-shelled, partially or fully formed eggs. Potential causes include excess mucin and albumin secretion secondary to inspissated egg material and cystic hyperplasia. Salpingitis is often found concomitantly, especially in older birds. Metritis, salpingitis, egg binding, dystocia, and neoplasia commonly precede oviductal impactions. Oviductal impactions are described in many bird species and, in the author's experience, common in prolific egg layers (Figure 21.20a–b).

Typical of most reproductive tract diseases, vague clinical signs with or without coelomic swelling and ascites are common with oviductal impaction (Figure 21.21a–g). Affected birds may show persistent "broodiness" with recent cessation of egg laying. Definitive diagnosis is made at celiotomy or sometimes via ultrasound and endoscopy with aspiration of the oviductal contents. Chronic oviductal impactions may be found incidentally during exploratory celiotomy and are often associated with a history of sudden cessation of egg laying several months or years prior to presentation. Acute impactions may be treated by salpingotomy, culture, and appropriate antibiotic use and oviductal flushing while severe or chronic disease are best treated with salpingohysterectomy.

Oviduct Prolapse

Powerful coelomic contractions combined with the process of oviposition can result in oviductal prolapse which is often secondary to

(a)

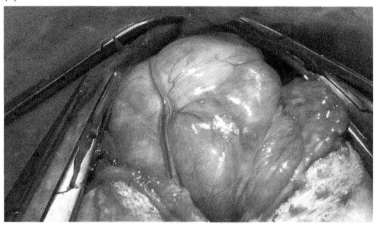

(b)

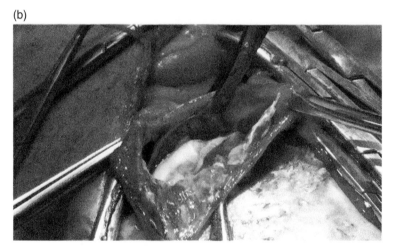

Figure 21.20 A Pekin duck (*Anas platyrhnchos*) has a severely impacted oviduct and sterile salpingitis. While the mass was hot to the touch, no organisms could be found on culture or cytologic and histopathologic evaluation. (a) The distended and vascular oviduct completely fills the ventral midline incision obscuring view of all other coelomic tissue. (b) Because it was too large to exteriorize, the oviduct was incised and fluid and debris were removed (a sterile spoon shown here is scooping out solid granulomatous debris) to better facilitate salpingohysterectomy.

dystocia. A temporary prolapse is normal immediately after laying an egg (oviposition). Predisposing factors may include large or abnormally shaped eggs, general debilitation, malnutrition, systemic illness, disease of the oviduct and sometimes, normal egg laying. In turkeys selected for high meat yield, decreased vaginal collagen has been associated with uterine prolapse [85, 86]. The uterus is most commonly prolapsed but vagina and other portions of the oviduct may also prolapse. The cloaca,

and rarely colon, may also prolapse and should be distinguished from the oviduct.

Because the exposed tissue can rapidly become devitalized and infected, aggressive treatment with warm saline flushes, antibiotics and replacement of the prolapsed oviduct is warranted. If the prolapsed oviduct is edematous, topical dextrose, dimethyl sulfoxide (DMSO) and/or steroids may be needed to reduce the swelling. If an egg is present in the prolapsed or oviductal tissue, ovocentesis and

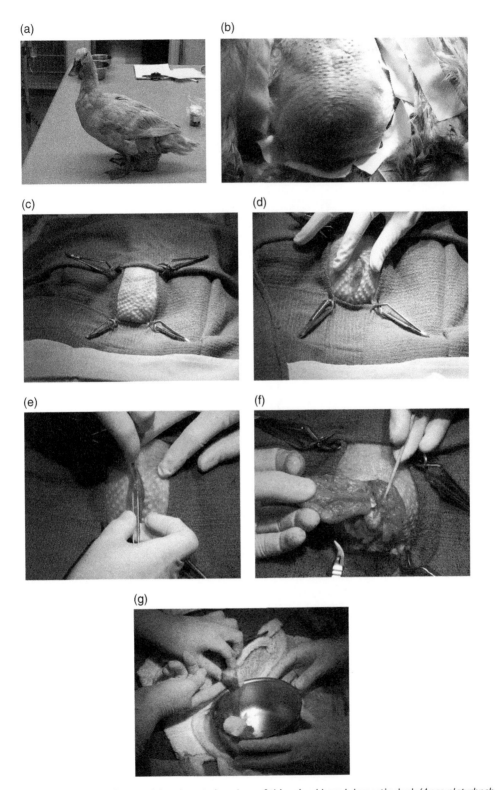

Figure 21.21 (a) The caudal and ventral coelom of this mixed breed domestic duck (*Anas platyrhnchos*) is severely distended. (b) Once the feathers have been plucked and the site surgically prepared, the ventral coelom is noticeably distended. (c) Shown on chicken, after tape is used to control the feathers, (c) a sterile drape is secured with towel clamps, (d) the skin is incised for a ventral celiotomy, and (e) the coelomic wall is incised revealing (f) egg-related coelomitis and (g) removal of inspissated eggs from the oviduct. Birds with severe oviductal disease commonly present for non-specific coelomic distension. *Source:* Photographs c-g courtesy of Dr. Cheryl B. Greenacre.

implosion of the egg is often needed to reduce associated pressure and aid in egg shell removal. It is best to only aspirate the egg by inserting the needle directly through the shell and not through the oviductal tissue which can easily tear and potentially lead to problems later. After stabilizing the bird, remove the egg medically if possible and replace the prolapsed tissue. Two transcloacal sutures may be required to prevent the immediate recurrence of prolapsed tissue.

Salpingohysterectomy is indicated when the oviduct is necrotic and/or the egg (or its fragmented shell) cannot be removed medically or pass on its own. If an oviductal torsion is present distal to the egg (within the oviduct), attempting to force deliver the egg will often result in further damage. Oviductal torsion, neoplasia, adhesions, and other anatomic disorders should be considered if a bound egg cannot be delivered without forceful techniques and surgical options should be pursued.

Oviduct Torsion

Oviductal torsion has been infrequently reported in birds. Torsion of the oviduct may occur following a tear of the dorsal, and possibly ventral, oviductal ligament(s) or associated with oviductal cysts [87, 88]. In four parrots, all birds presented with signs of egg binding and/or general lethargy and had a history of previously laying "many eggs" prior the oviductal torsion. One thin cockatiel presented with lethargy, depression and coelomic distension and died despite emergency therapy. Of the three other parrots, two cockatiels were treated with salpingohysterectomy and one eclectus parrot (*Eclectus roratus vosmaeri*) was treated with a salpingotomy, egg removal, torsion correction, and subsequent closure of the oviductal ligament tear. All birds recovered uneventfully from surgery. The eclectus successfully laid normal clutches after surgery [88]. An 11-month-old chicken was found to have a 360° oviductal torsion and cyst twisted around the dorsal ligament on necropsy. Severe oviductal congestion, hyperemia, devitalization and dilatation were noted [87].

Salpingitis and Metritis

Salpingitis, inflammation of the oviduct, is common in birds (Figure 21.22). In poultry, salpingitis has been listed as the most prevalent form of reproductive tract disease [89]. *E. coli* infections are fairly common in poultry and can cause salpingitis, but *Streptococcus* sp., *M. gallisepticum*, *Acinetobacter* sp., *Corynebacterium* sp., *Salmonella* sp. and *Pasteurella multocida* have all been implicated from various species. Some ground-nesting species, such as Anseriformes and emus, may develop non-lactose fermenting, gram negative (*Pseudomonas aeruginosa*, *Proteus mirabilis*, *Proteus vulgaris*) salpingitis [90]. Non-infectious salpingitis can also be seen, especially with chronic sterile oviductal impactions, and is fairly common per the author's observations.

Metritis is inflammation within the shell gland portion of the oviduct and may result from or cause egg binding, chronic oviductal impaction and rupture, coelomitis and septicemia. *Prosthogonimus ovatus* and other related trematodes (flukes) can inhabit the oviduct of poultry and waterfowl and result in salpingitis with heavy infestations [91]. Other infectious agents ascending from the vagina or cloaca or systemic infections can also cause salpingitis. Specifically in poultry, vent cannibalism has been implicated as a precursor to salpingitis [89] (see Reproductive Diseases chapter.).

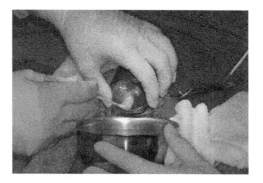

Figure 21.22 Introperative photograph of removing an ectopic egg from the coelomic cavity of a chicken. The bird also had a bacterial salpingitis and an impacted oviduct. Bacteria were observed microscopically on cytology but the organism was not cultured or speciated. *Source:* Photograph courtesy of Dr. Cheryl B. Greenacre.

Birds with non-septic salpingitis or metritis often show vague signs of illness, while septic birds are usually clinically ill. Egg shell deformities and embryonic and neonatal infections are often secondary to metritis. Definitive diagnosis is made at celiotomy or endoscopy with aspiration of oviductal fluid for cytologic and microbiologic analysis or if the oviduct has no liquid contents, biopsy with culture. Use antibiotics based on culture and sensitivity results. If trying to spare the oviduct, repeated endoscopic evaluation, direct and indirect oviductal flushing and long-term antimicrobials are recommended. Salpingohysterectomy is indicated for most cases.

Salpingohysterectomy

Salpingohysterectomy is the surgical removal of the oviduct, infundibulum to uterus, and is indicated for chronic egg laying and any oviduct disease that cannot be medically managed (Figure 21.23). Every attempt should be made to understand the bird's overall health status prior to surgery, as the patient should ideally be stable. Athough rare compared to sterile inflammation, birds with septic yolk

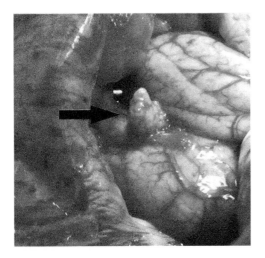

Figure 21.23 An oviductal mass (focal adenocarcinoma) is found on the magnum region of the oviduct in this chicken and is an indication for salpingohysterectomy.

peritonitis generally carry a poor prognosis. Patients with underlying health problems such as various lung, liver and kidney diseases, can also complicate surgery. Otherwise healthy salpingohysterectomy candidates typically do well with the procedure.

Oviductal hypertrophy occurs secondary to elevated estrogen levels during sexual activity and can take up most of the left side of the intestinal-peritoneal portion of the coelomic cavivity. This oviductal hypertrophy includes increased vascularity and risk of bleeding during surgery [92]. If the patient is stable, time permits, and increased reproductive tract vascularity is suspected, the author conditions the bird prior to surgery as described previously in this chapter.

In the author's experience, a left lateral approach offers the best exposure to the left female avian reproductive tract. However, a ventral midline approach is better for exploratory celiotomy, especially when the degree of coelomic disease and/or presence of right sided reproductive tract components are unknown.

Perform a left lateral celiotomy. After incising through the left abdominal air sac, the ovary and oviduct are readily visible. Gently retract the cranial oviduct (infundibulum area) out the incision and ligate using a surgical clip or cauterize suspensory ligament vessels as needed. The closer the bird is to laying, the larger the vessels present. Depending on the size, the cranial, middle and/or caudal oviductal artery(ies) may need to be ligated with a surgical clipped or cauterized. Once visualized, a surgical clip is placed at the base of the oviduct just proximal to its junction with the cloaca. Suture material can be used in larger poultry and waterfowl. Excise the oviduct.

When performing a ventral midline celiotomy, the air sacs do not need to be breached. A careful evaluation of the caudal coelom is made and right oviductal tissue, in addition to the more normal left, is identified and removed as described above. With a little more difficulty, right oviductal tissue can also be accessed from a left lateral approach.

Well-developed preovulatory follicles (F1 and F2 +/− F3 and F4) may pose a risk for intra-coelomic ovulation and can usually be easily removed. Use cotton tip applicators to rotate the follicle in one direction continuously until it separates from its pedicle (Figure 21.24a–b). This may require 15–30 full rotations until the follicle is free. Once free, simply remove the follicle. If concerned about a well-developed vascular pedicle, use surgical clips and then excise the follicle. One study in domestic chickens demonstrated a pause in laying that increased with the number of follicles removed compared to sham operated hens [93].

Cystic follicles should either be aspirated (drained) or ideally removed. If a follicle is accidentally incised, yolk will leak into the coelom. Simply "mop up" excess yolk and other fluid if present. Collect culture and samples for histopathologic evaluation as needed.

Endoscopic salpingohysterectomy of juvenile cockatiels has been described and may potentially be applied to young poultry or waterfowl [94]. A left lateral coelomic endoscopic approach (left leg pulled caudally) was

(a)

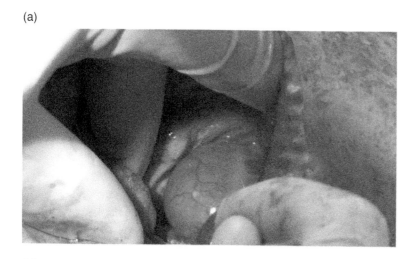

(b)

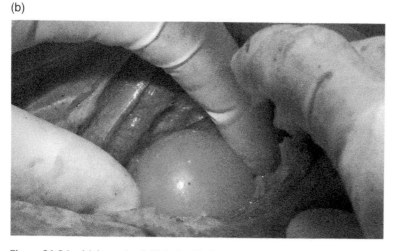

Figure 21.24 (a) An active follicle in this Pekin duck (*Anas platyrhnchos*) is being rotated with the aid of a cotton tipped applicator. (b) After 15–30 full rotations, the blood supply to the follicle diminishes (seen here) and the follicle can be simply pulled out with minimal risk of hemorrhage.

performed on 3–11-month-old cockatiels. Once visualized, the supporting ligament of the infundibulum was carefully pulled laterally toward the coelomic entry site using flexible endoscopic grasping forceps (Karl Storz Veterinary Endoscopy, Inc., Goleta, CA, USA). This action broke down the supporting structures (ventral and dorsal suspensory ligaments of the cranial oviduct and uterus) and separated the oviduct from the overlying kidney, caudal vena cava and left ureter. Next, a cotton-tipped applicator was placed in the cloaca and was used to better visualize the cloacal-uteral junction and ensure the oviduct was "peeled" from the surrounding tissues. The oviduct was exteriorized and then crushed and cut with microsurgical forceps and scissors, respectively, at the point of exit from the coelomic cavity, just cranial to the uterovaginal sphincter. The endoscope was replaced to check for hemorrhage and closure was routine [94].

Multiport endoscopic salpingohysterectomy has also been performed and studied in 14 white Carneau pigeons (*C. livia*) [95]. Mean surgery time was 34 minutes. While the procedures were generally considered effective (complete removal of the oviduct) and safe, minor complications were noted. Mild damage or hematoma formation was found post-surgery in 28% of test subjects. Also one bird had remnant distal oviductal tissue post-surgery. No ovarian follicles were removed during endosurgery. Ovarian activity, including pre-ovulatory follicles, was noted up to 90 days post-surgery in some of the birds. The authors reported that standard salpingohysterectomy (via celiotomy) and endosurgical salpingohysterectomy can result in serious yolk ceolomitis in ducks, quail, and chickens, respectively [95]. Details of a "standard salpingohysterectomy" were not given. As explained above, the author recommends removing active ovarian follicles when performing salpingohysterectomy.

Endoscopic salpingohysterectomy has several distinct limitations and benefits. As indicated in the first study, this procedure was acceptable in the juvenile birds due to a poorly developed blood supply of the oviduct and that if attempted in mature, egg producing cockatiels, may result in fatal hemorrhage [94]. Additionally, this procedure required an endoscope and two surgeons. The author has worked with parrots that were endoscopically "salpingohysterectomized" only to find incomplete oviductal removal and subsequent active tissue remnants that resulted in various forms of reproductive related coelomic disease. All birds required exploratory celiotomy to correct the problems.

On the positive side, a properly done endoscopic procedure results in minimal hemorrhage, can be performed safely and offers an option for juvenile salpingohysterectomy. Endoscopic salpingohysterectomy does not preclude behavioral and dietary management as these birds can still internally ovulate and develop ovarian disease if reproductively stimulated. However, this is an option to consider for juvenile birds, especially domestic ducks, that have a high risk of chronic egg laying and no need for egg production by the owner.

Caesarian Section and Reproductive Tract Sparing

Caesarian section is indicated when the bird's reproductive capabilities need to be spared and is typically limited to egg binding with an otherwise normal, or minimally diseased oviduct. Depending on the location of the egg, a caudal left lateral or ventral midline approach is used. The oviduct should be incised directly over the bound egg and away from prominent blood vessels. After removing the egg, inspect the oviduct for other abnormalities and collect biopsies and cultures as needed. Close the oviduct in a single simple interrupted or continuous layer using fine (4–0' or smaller) absorbable suture material. Ceolomic closure is standard. The author recommends resting the hen from reproductive stimuli for at least two to four weeks as dictated by culture and/or histopathologic results.

Anatomy of the Avian Ovary

A right and left ovary and oviduct are present in the embryologic stages of all chicks, but the right half regresses due to the action of Mullerian inhibiting substance prior to hatch [81]. Although a persistent right oviduct with or without a functional right ovary is present in some birds, most birds only have a left female reproductive system. The brown kiwi is an exception and normally has a functional left and right ovary. About 480 000 oocytes develop by hatching in the chicken. Of these, about 2000 can be seen as a mass of small ova and approximately 500 reach maturity and ovulate within the lifespan of domestic species and even fewer mature in wild species. By 2.5 years of age, chicken hens ovulate approximately 500 times which is equivalent to a woman entering menopause [96]. Ovarian follicles are arranged hierarchically. The largest follicle (F1) will ovulate on the next day, the second largest (F2) the following day and so on (Figure 21.25).

The ovary is attached to the cranial renal division and dorsal body wall by the mesovarian ligament and receives its blood supply from the ovarian artery, which originates off the left cranial renal artery or directly off the aorta. Baumel notes that accessory ovarian arteries may also arise from other adjacent arteries [97].

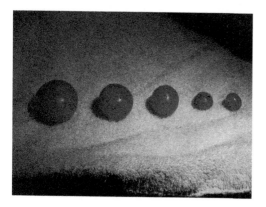

Figure 21.25 Active F1-F5 follicles were removed from a Pekin duck (*Anas platyrhnchos*) with salpingitis. The F1 follicle is the largest.

The ovarian artery will further divide into many branches with the greatest blood flow directed to any large preovulatory follicles present. Ovarian veins unite into main anterior and posterior veins that drain into the overlying vena cava. As more specifically described by Baumel, multiple left ovarian veins may exist and drain into the cranial oviductal vein, which then enters the common iliac vein and finally the caudal vena cava [97].

The author has noted the cranial oviductal vein is too short or poorly developed to recognize grossly. Instead, multiple short veins seem to enter the common iliac vein over the length of its contact with the dorsum (base) of the ovary. This, in part, makes ovariectomy in adult birds difficult as there is not a single artery and vein to ligate.

Surgery of Avian Ovary

Partial and "Complete" Ovariectomy

Ovariectomy in hens is a challenging and oftentimes high-risk procedure. Ovariectomy has been used in many poultry studies and mention of this procedure can be found throughout the literature [98–102]. Unfortunately, most papers poorly describe the specific details of ovariectomy or its complications. In one chicken study, it was noted that ovariectomized birds "lost considerably more blood than sham-operated hens" [102]. Terada et al. described ovariectomy by "destroying ovarian tissue by local application of small pieces of dry ice" [101].

Although it has been stated that the short stalk of the cranial renal artery or proximity to the aorta are what make ovariectomy difficult, the author suggests that the intimate and lengthy attachment to the overlying common iliac vein is what makes this procedure risky [80, 92]. As mentioned above, multiple small ovarian veins often connect directly into the common iliac vein. It is often venous, and not arterial, bleeding from a lacerated common iliac vein that usually causes life-threatening hemorrhage during ovariectomy. As with the oviduct, the ovary can dramatically change in size and vascularity with reproductive activity. As with salpingohysterectomy, the bird is ideally conditioned (described earlier) to reduce ovarian vascularity. Some diseases requiring ovariectomy do not allow attending clinicians the time to "condition" the avian patient prior to surgery.

Ovariectomy is reserved for ovarian diseases such as cancer, chronic recurring cysts, persistent follicular activity, oophoritis and other diseases that cannot be managed medically and are life-threatening without further treatment. A true complete ovariectomy is very difficult to achieve in adult birds. Most "ovariectomies" are partial with the goal to debulk abnormal tissue.

A cranial left lateral celiotomy often provides the best exposure to the left ovary. However, a ventral midline approach can also be used successfully, especially if access is needed to a right cystic oviduct present. It is important to clean the surgical field of fluid and debris to best visualize the ovary and its vasculature. Surrounding organs may need to be gently pushed aside using moistened cotton-tip applicators or other non-traumatic instruments.

The first step of ovariectomy is to debulk its mass. The goal of this first step is to be able to visualize the ovarian attachment to the overlying common iliac vein and any other vessels present. If the ovary is inactive or juvenile, very little debulking is needed. If present, remove large preovulatory follicles as discussed under "Salpingohysterectomy." Aspirate and drain any cystic follicles present being careful not to spill contents into the coelomic cavity, especially if there is concern of oophoritis. When aspirating follicles, guide a small gauge (23–25 g) needle into the most visibly avascular portion (stigma) and aspirate contents. Butterfly catheters are useful for this procedure. Using this aspiration technique, a significant amount of an active and/or cystic follicle can be removed improving visualization of and around the ovary. As a note, blood filled follicles may represent previously ruptured blood vessels from an invasive mass and warrants caution when attempting debulking.

Once the fluid component is minimized, progressively clamp or surgically clip the ovarian mass closer to its dorsal base. When used properly, angled Debakey neonatal vascular clamps are atraumatic, will rest in the surgical site without obstructing view and seem to provide some hemostasis to the ovarian mass. Once a section of the mass is surgically clipped or clamped, surgically excise or cauterize and remove the ventral-most ovarian segment. Reassess the mass and move the clamp (or place new surgical clips) closer to the ovarian base and repeat the excision process. This process is repeated until the surrounding vasculature is identified and the course of the common iliac vein can be seen.

Once the mass has been debulked, several options exists for complete or partial ovariectomy. Altman reports using an electrocautery ball electrode to coagulate ovarian follicles in immature females [103]. The same procedure can result in ovarian regeneration and subsequent ovulatory activity in mature hens [103]. The author has noted some juvenile bird ovaries can be gently "peeled" in toto from caudal to cranial off its dorsal attachments with no or minimal bleeding. In these cases, the caudal edge of the ovary is grasped with angled hemostats and pulled in a cranial direction with a clear separation, and minimal effort, from the dorsally located common iliac vein. If attempting this procedure, stop if any resistance is noted to prevent tearing the overlying vein.

Another technique with juvenile or sufficiently debulked ovaries is to place surgical clips in the potential space between the dorsal ovarian base and the common iliac vein. Gently lift the caudal pole of the ovary and place a small to medium surgical clip from caudal to cranial across the ovarian vascular supply. Although difficult without good exposure, a last surgical clip can be placed from cranial to caudal in the same manner in an attempt to ligate the more cranially located ovarian artery. This is generally only possible via a cranial left lateral approach. With the blood supply adequately clamped, the ovary can be gently shaved off with precise radiosurgery using an Ellman B "loop" series or blade electrode (Ellman International, Inc., New York, NY, USA), precise cold excision or left to die without a blood supply. Altman describes this method as "a difficult, high-risk procedure" but the author has successfully performed ovariectomies in adult hens using this technique [103]. Obvious complications include hemorrhage when trying to remove the surgically clipped ovary and inadequate, blind, placement of the surgical clips.

The author has used another approach when the ovarian attachment to the overlying common iliac vein is indistinguishable or there is erosion into the overlying vessel and the entire ovary must be removed for the bird's survival (as with otherwise untreatable cancer). Debulk the ovarian mass as described above. Once clearly identified, using a surgical clip ligate the common iliac vein just caudal to the ovary and cranial to its junction with the caudal renal vein. Next, using a surgical clip ligate the common iliac vein just cranial to the ovary and caudal to its junction with the caudal vena cava. If done properly, the ovarian artery and common iliac veins are effectively clamped allowing one to carefully dissect the entire ovary from the overlying vessel(s). If needed, the ventral wall of the common iliac vessel can be safely removed. There is the real potential of damaging the left adrenal gland, significantly altering blood flow through the renal portal system and the cranial renal division and causing physical damage to the overlying kidney and lumbar and/or sacral nerve plexus(es). The author has noted that once the common iliac vein is ligated, the cranial renal division rapidly changes colors but returns to normal within a few minutes.

As has been shown in young chickens and Japanese quail, transplanted ovarian tissue (from other birds of the same species) may grow and become functional [104, 105]. These studies were conducted in young (one-day-old chickens and one-week-old quail) birds and transplantation was more often successful when immunosuppressive therapy was given [104, 105]. However, these studies support the concern that dislodged ovarian tissue may remain viable, implant and become functional if left in the coelom, especially as an autologous "transplant." While this statement has not been proven in adult birds, the author recommends removing any free ovarian tissue that becomes dislodged during surgery.

With all of the above described ovariectomy procedures, it should be understood that none have been satisfactorily studied in pet birds and that each caries a significant risk to the patient. Partial ovariectomy (at least active follicle removal) is commonly performed alongside salpingohysterectomy (Figure 21.26). With each procedure, closure is routine.

Diseases of the Ovary

Cystic Ovarian Disease

Although the cause is often unknown, cystic ovarian disease has been reported in numerous bird species [90, 106]. Cystic ovaries are sometimes

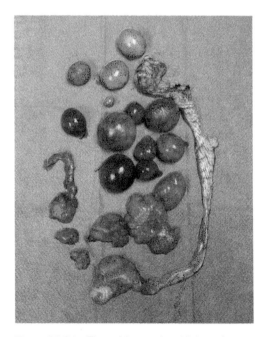

Figure 21.26 The oviduct and multiple active ovarian follicles were removed in a domestic duck (*Anas platyrhnchos*). *Source:* Courtesy of Dr. Brian Speer.

secondary to neoplasia. Depending on their size, ovarian cysts may be found incidentally if small or may cause coelomic distension when large and/or numerous and can be associated with ascites. Large or numerous cysts can often be diagnosed non-invasively using ultrasound. Cysts can be treated by ultrasound guided transcoelomic aspiration or more directly via celiotomy or endoscopy. If collected, evaluate the fluid for evidence of infection, neoplasia, or other abnormalities. Severe cystic disease may require partial or complete ovariectomy and should include biopsy for histopathological evaluation. Leuprolide acetate has also been suggested to reduce or resolve ovarian cysts in birds. Deslorelin has also been recommended anecdotally. However in the author's experience, aspiration or physical removal is the only means to remove ovarian cysts.

Oophoritis

Ovarian infections can be life-threatening and are often associated with septicemia especially in poultry. *Salmonella pullorum* is the etiologic agent of pullorum disease of poultry and most frequently affects the ovary [107]. Clinically affected birds usually show more severe, but non-specific signs of illness and if not treated quickly, septic coelomitis and death may result. Abnormally shaped or colored follicles identified during celiotomy or endoscopy should be either removed (celiotomy) or carefully aspirated for cytologic and microbiologic analysis and broad spectrum antibiotics initiated pending culture results. An injection needle with Teflon guide (Karl Storz Veterinary Endoscopy America, Goleta, CA) is particularly useful as an endoscopic means to aspirate ovarian follicles. If possible, completely drain the abscessed follicle(s) being careful to not contaminate the coelom. Partial or complete ovariectomy may be required for chronically infected and caseated follicles.

Reproductive Tract Neoplasia (Ovary and Oviduct)

Ovarian cancer is reported with some frequency in birds and can be associated with egg retention, ascites, cystic ovarian disease, medullary hyperostosis, coelomic hernias, oviductal impaction and general malaise [90, 108]. One study noted that 38% of USDA Inspection Service mature fowl condemnation is the result of neoplastic disease, most of which are from the genital tract. Fredrickson states "there is indeed a unique propensity for hens (poultry) to develop cancer of the reproductive system in the almost total absence of tumors at other sites" [109]. Ansenberger et al. reports that the incidence of ovarian cancer in 2.5–3.5-year-old hens is 4–20% [96]. Granulosa cell tumors and ovarian adenocarcinomas are most frequently reported but carcinomas, leiomyosarcomas/leiomyomas, adenomas, teratomas, dysgerminomas, fibrosarcomas, lipomas, and lymphomatosis have all been identified in bird ovaries [90, 91, 109, 110]. Oviductal tumors are less common than ovarian neoplasia and include adenocarcinomas/adenomas, adenomatous hyperplasia, carcinoma and carcinomatosis [108, 110].

Granulosa cell tumors and possibly other reproductive tract neoplasms may be functional and cause increased plasma hormone levels [109].

Polyostotic (medullary) hyperostosis may also result in a paraneoplastic syndrome with functional ovarian and oviductal neoplasms [108, 110]. Interestingly, one study found that hyperestrogenism did not cause polysostotic hyperostosis in several species of birds with various neoplastic and non-neoplastic reproductive tract diseases [111]. Regardless, the author has frequently observed significant medullary hyperostosis in many waterfowl and poultry with reproductive tract diseases including cancer.

Clinical signs of ovarian and oviductal cancer vary and are non-specific for most reproductive tract diseases including coelomic swelling, dyspnea, ascites, poor or altered reproductive performance and lethargy. If a mass compresses the overlying lumbar or sacral nerve plexus, lameness (usually left sided) may be seen. Diagnosis can be further supported using radiography, ultrasonography, CT, MRI, exploratory celiotomy, endoscopy, and biopsy. Once a definitive diagnosis is made, options for therapy include chemotherapy, radiation therapy and partial or complete ovariectomy. All carry a guarded to poor prognosis unless the neoplastic tissue is completely removed.

Male Reproductive Tract Surgery

Anatomy of the Avian Testicle

Avian male reproductive anatomy of most birds consists of three main gross structures, the testes, epididymis, and ductus deferens. Some birds also possess a phallus (discussed below). The paired testes are located ventral to their respective left or right cranial renal division. The mesorchium connects the testes to the dorsal body wall. The left testicle is typically larger than the right in most young birds, but this relationship can change as the bird ages. In seasonal breeders, such as some passerines, the testes can increase 300–500 times in size and should not be interpreted as neoplasia. Large active testes can also be readily evident radiographically (Figure 21.27). In addition to size, the color of the testicles can also change with fluctuating hormone levels ranging from black in the sexually immature or inactive cockatoos to white or yellow in the chicken.

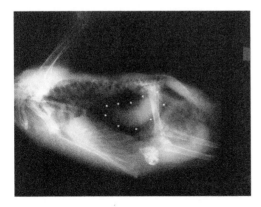

Figure 21.27 Lateral radiographic view of a crested duck (*Anas platyrhnchos*) with normal but enlarged testes. The approximate silhouette of the superimposed left and right testes is outlined with "*".

The epididymis is located at the testicular hilus, or dorsomedial aspect of the testes. The ductus deferens continue from the epididymis as highly convoluted tubes running lateral to and alongside the ureters and then terminate at the urodeum as a papillae ventral to the ureteral ostium.

The testicular artery arises from the cranial renal artery and provides most of the arterial blood supply to the testes. An accessory testicular artery may arise directly from the aorta. The venous drainage is returned either directly to the caudal vena cava or forms a common stem with the adrenal veins. Kremer and Budras found that two testicular veins empty directly into the caudal vena cava of Pekin drakes (*A. platyrhynchos*) [112]. Given the diversity within the class Aves, it is likely that multiple variations of the testicular vasculature exist.

Although most birds lack a copulatory organ, some birds possess a non-protrusible (Galliformes) or protrusible (ratites and Anseriformes) phallus. Domestic chickens and turkeys have a non-intromittent phallus, consisting of a median and two lateral phallic bodies, on the floor of the lip of the vent. Lymphatic flow through the phallic bodies and their laterally associated lymphatic folds result in tumescence. Because the lymphatic folds and lateral phallic bodies accumulate more fluid than the median body, the phallus everts during tumescence producing a groove for semen to travel. Semen is deposited when the phallus contacts the everted oviduct opening in the hen.

Surgery of the Male Avian Reproductive System

Castration

Clinical avian castration is infrequently discussed, especially in comparison to salpingohysterectomy, suggesting that male reproductive tract diseases are relatively uncommon. Although caponization is common in the poultry industry (performed between one to two weeks or up to six weeks of age), routine castration is rare in pet birds. As a result, there is little information regarding the behavior and physiologic altering effects of castration in pet birds.

It is known that caponized chickens (capons) have increased coelomic fat weight, total hepatic lipid content and saturated fatty acid percentage compared to intact birds [113]. The medical consequences, if any, of this body change are not known.

Castrated Gambel's (*Callipepla gambelii*) and scaled (*C. Squamata*) quail have reduced or eliminated courtship behaviors and lower rates of male-male threats. However, the castrates maintained ornate plumage, exhibited overt aggression and frequently won contests when actually engaged [114]. Yearling European starlings (*Sturnus vulgaris*) castrated when non-reproductively active were shown to be significantly more aggressive than non-castrated controls [115]. The authors concluded that "nonreproductive aggression in yearling male starlings is independent of gonadal sex steroids and suggests it even increases following castration" [115].

These limited results suggest that persistent "male" behaviors are either already learned at the time of castration, result from hormones other than testosterone or another source of testicular hormones is still present post-castration. It is known that some species have an appendix epididymis extending from the epididymis into the adrenal gland that may secrete androgens following castration. The author has performed castration in roosters in effort to stop crowing. While castrated roosters did exhibit reduced crowing behavior, it did not stop. The author concluded that castration was not appropriate or effective to eliminate crowing behavior in roosters.

Until further studies are available, castration should be used judiciously to alter avian behaviors, especially in adult birds and should always be considered secondary to more conservative methods of behavior management. However, castration has real benefit with testicular cancer, abscesses/granulomas, cysts and other conditions that may not respond to medical management alone.

Several methods of castration have been forwarded and include simple extraction (caponization), laser ablation, intracapsular suction, en bloc surgical excision and endoscopic orchidectomy. Even with early age caponization, testicular regrowth is well documented. This supports the need for complete testicular removal, which is why the author prefers en bloc surgical excision.

Caponization is typically performed in young male chickens to create meat that is believed to be more tender, juicier and tastier than that of an intact rooster [116]. Heavy chicken breeds are caponized at two to four weeks while some slow-growing meat-type birds are done after six weeks old. As the bird ages, the tunica albugenea of the testes becomes hard making caponization more difficult and time consuming. The procedure is typically done without anesthesia with the bird held or strapped to a table. A sterile preparation is given to the appropriate side and an incision made between the last two ribs through the lateral body wall which is then spread with a "spreader." Done correctly, specialized caponizing forceps are used to enter the incision, delicately hold the entire testes and pull with a twisting motion until the testicle is free and removed. The wound is disinfected and left to close by second intention. Incompletely caponized birds may regrow the testes and the birds tend to develop secondary sex characteristics unlike true capons [116]. A similar technique using standard curved forceps is described in 9–10-week-old Japanese quail (*Coturnix coturnix japonica*) [117].

Use a cranial left lateral approach or ventral midline incision with transverse flap to evaluate the testes. Due to the cranial location, the lateral celiotomy is often extended cranially by cutting the last two ribs to improve exposure to the testes. With a left lateral approach, puncture through the caudal thoracic and/or the abdominal air sac(s) to expose the left testis. The right testis may be exposed through the same incision by cutting through the midline junction of the corresponding air sacs or the process may be repeated with a right lateral celiotomy. With gentle traction, pull the testis ventrally and surgically clip the dorsal blood supply. Use of a right angle surgical clip often makes the approach easier. If two can be placed, then incise between the surgical clips and remove the testis. Otherwise, use electrocautery to carefully free the testis from the surgical clip and vascular cord. The cautery should destroy any remaining testicular cells attached to the surgical clip but be careful to not damage the overlying blood vessels, kidney, or adrenal gland.

Alternatively, if the testicular blood supply is small, a hemostat can be temporarily used in place of asurgical clip and the testis pulled free. Leave the hemostat on the vascular stump for one to two minutes prior to release. Use direct pressure hemostasis as needed. Diode laser excision can also be used through this approach and may be performed without the need for direct hemostasis. Closure is routine.

Multiport endoscopic orchidectomy has been described in Carneau pigeons [95]. While the details of the procedure are described in the paper, endoscopic orchidectomy produced good results in 10 of 11 pigeons with mean surgical time of 39 minutes. Mild hemorrhage and partial necrosis of the cranial renal pole was noted in 27% of the tested birds and represented the most common complication of surgery. The one surgical failure (regrowth of the testes) was considered due to surgeon inexperience. When performed using appropriate equipment and techniques, the authors concluded that endoscopic orchidectomy was successful and safe in pigeons [95]. The technique could potentially be used in poultry and waterfowl. As is expected and mentioned in the study, large testes are more difficult to remove endoscopically. In the author's experience orchidectomy is more often needed for clinically abnormal (cancer, cysts, etc.) and often large testes requiring celiotomy.

Vasectomy

Vasectomy is a useful to produce "teaser males" and aid in population control and has been described in small passerines and budgerigars. In anesthetized budgerigars, a 3 mm incision, 7 mm lateral to the cloacal sphincter (vent), was used for the initial approach [118]. Careful dissection was made through the coelomic musculature and fat. An operating microscope was used to find and aid in the removal of a 5 mm section of the vas deferens. Only the skin incision was closed. The authors recommended performing left and right vasectomy two weeks apart. Two of 12 birds died post-operatively and one was found to have pre-existing disease. The only other complications were post-operative tenesmus for two days and accumulation of droppings around the vent in 3 of the remaining 10 birds. The procedure was successful (no semen upon collection attempts) in 9 of the 10 surviving birds [118].

Anesthetized Bengalese (*Lonchura striata*) and zebra (Taeniopygia guttata) finches have been vasectomized similarly to the procedure described above [119]. In the anesthetized finches, a 3 mm incision 5 mm lateral to the cloaca was made using an operating microscope. The muscle and fat were incised to locate the seminal glomera (glomus). It was noted that the seminal glomera of the Bengalese finch was "obvious and highly accessible," and that of the zebra finch was "less obvious and in some cases difficult to locate." The vas deferens was carefully separated from the ureter and "one or more pieces" were removed with no ligature. The skin was closed. The authors performed single (14 days apart) and bilateral vasectomies successfully. The procedure was successful in 12 of 12 Bengalese and 14 of 15 zebra finches [119].

In larger species, the vas deferens zig zags lateral to the ureter and can be transected endoscopically or via celiotomy. A left, and sometimes right, lateral coelomic approach is(are) used. The ureter is avoided to prevent damage. In roosters vasectomized just distal to the epididymus, spermatogenesis ceased within five to seven days [120].

The author prefers endoscopic vasectomy in large birds, most commonly as a means of population control in gallinaceous birds.

As described by Samour, the ductus deferens is identified endoscopically (as if evaluating the kidney) and grasped just distal to the epididymis and approximately 5–8 mm is removed with simple traction [121].

At this location, the ductus deferens is usually not closely associated with the ureter. Depending on the species, both ductus deferens may be approached through one endoscopic portal. Alternatively, two endoscopic entry points (left and right) can be used. Vasectomy does not stop courtship and copulation [121].

Diseases of the Male Avian Reproductive System

Orchitis

Inflammation of the testicle, or orchitis, is usually due to bacterial infections and may originate from septicemia, renal obstruction, cloacitis or even prolapsed or ulcerated phalli. Affected birds may show signs of septicemia. However, the author has seen cases of focal orchitis with no associated clinical signs or reduced fertility only. Orchitis may be diagnosed via cytology and/or microbiologic analysis via aspiration through endoscopy or celiotomy when the whole testicle appears abnormal or, biopsy when focal lesions are seen.

Initial treatment for bacterial orchitis should include antibiotics based on culture and sensitivity results. If a focal granulomatous lesion is seen and appropriate antimicrobials have proven ineffective, the testicle can be partially ablated. Clamp with hemostats or surgically clip the testicular tissue dorsal (toward the blood supply) to the lesion(s) and remove using cold excision, laser or electrocautery. Avian testicular tissue has great regenerative capabilities and may redevelop following partial ablation. En bloc surgical removal of the affected testicle is indicated for diffuse, non-medically-responsive orchitis.

Testicular Neoplasia

Avian testicular neoplasia most commonly includes sertoli and interstitial cell tumors,

seminomas, teratomas and lymphoproliferative diseases. Sertoli cell tumors seem to be the more prevalent testicular neoplasm in birds. Reported neoplasms of the epididymis and ductus deferens include leiomyosarcoma and carcinoma. Chronic weight loss, coelomic swelling and unilateral paresis are most commonly associated with testicular cancer. Surgical removal of the affected testicle is the treatment of choice and carries a good prognosis as long as metastasis is not present. As noted in the literature and in the author's experience, many testicular tumors are cystic. Cystic testicular masses can be aspirated and drained during surgery to reduce their mass and facilitate removal. Some testicular tumors may metastasize as has been reported in a guinea fowl (*Numida meleagris*) with malignant seminoma [122].

Cystic Testicular Disease

Non-neoplastic cystic testicular disease is very infrequently reported and its significance is unknown. Cystic dilatation of the seminiferous tubules (and testes), has been produced in fowl fed a diet high in sodium [123]. Cystic testicles have also been noted in chickens fed egg albumen as a source of protein [123]. Dilatation of the seminiferous tubules, but not gross cystic testicular change, has been noted in roosters affected with epididymal cysts and stones of unknown origin [120]. As mentioned above, consider cancer first when cystic testicles are found. Cystic testicles should be drained, biopsied and ideally removed.

Disorders of the Phallus

Male waterfowl have a protrusible phallus, which is highly variable and particularly long and corkscrewed in the Muscovy duck (*Cairina moschata*). Partial and complete phallic prolapses are possible in waterfowl with large phalli and are usually secondary to trauma, local infection, and masturbation. Over exuberant vent sexing and mating, *Neisseria* spp. (suspected to be sexually transmitted in geese and the cause of "goose gonorrhea") and

(a)

(b)

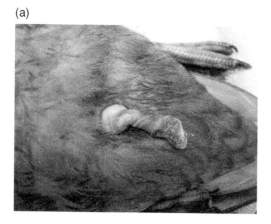

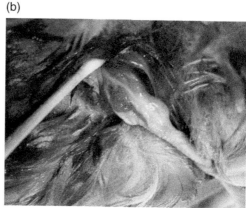

Figure 21.28 A Prolapsed phallus of a domestic duck (*Anas platyrhnchos*) is readily apparent. (a) The distal end of the phallus is necrotic requiring amputation. (b) Examine the full extent of the exteriorized phallus for additional lesions prior to considering simple replacement versus amputation. *Source:* Courtesy of Dr. Laura Wade.

contamination have all been implicated causes of phallic infections. A prolapsed phallus may become enlarged, ulcerated and/or necrotic compounding the problem (Figure 21.28a–b). Frostbite and resultant necrotizing dermatitis of a prolapsed phallus has been noted in ostriches [124]. Birds with severe prolapse and infection may be significantly depressed and often lose interest in copulation.

Clean exposed phalli and carefully debride abnormal tissue prior to replacement. Topical antibiotic creams, DMSO and systemic antibiotics may be beneficial and their use is based on clinical findings. The cloaca may need partial closure (via transcloacal sutures) to prevent recurring prolapses. If the prolapse is prolonged and will not stay when replaced, use 4–0′ monofilament absorbable suture to gently tack the phallus to its resting position within the cloacal mucosa. Severely necrotic phalli often need surgical debridement (Figure 21.29). Using absorbable suture in an encircling

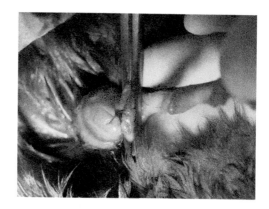

Figure 21.29 The phallus of the same duck in Figure 21.28 is ligated at its proximal base. The hemostat is distal to the ligature and will be the site of amputation. *Source:* Courtesy of Dr. Laura Wade.

pattern, ligate the phallus proximal to necrotic tissue. It is best if there is a clear demarcation from healthy tissue. Amputate the tissue distal to the ligature ensuring that all necrotic tissue is removed.

References

1 Doolen, M. (1997). Avian soft tissue surgery. In: *Association of Avian Veterinarians Annual Conference*, 499–506. Reno, NV.

2 Jann, H.W., Stein, L.E., Good, J.K. et al. (1992). Comparison of nylon, polybutester and polyglyconate suture materials for long digital flexor tennorrhapy in chickens. *Vet. Surg.* 21: 234–237.

3 Bennett, R.A., Yaeger, M.J., Trapp, A., and Cambre, R.C. (1997). Histologic evaluation of the tissue reaction to five suture materials in the body wall of rock doves (*Columba livia*). *J. Am. Med. Surg.* 11 (3): 175–182.

4 Pollock, C., Wolf, K., Wight-Carter, M., and Nietfeld, J. (2006). Comparison of suture material for cloacopexy. In: *Association of Avian Veterinarians Annual Conference*, 31–32. San Antonio, TX.

5 Speer, B. (2012). Surgical procedures of the psittacine skull. In: *Proc. AAV Annu. Conf*, 181–191.

6 Achar, R.A.N., Lozana, P.A.M., Achar, B.A. et al. (2001). Experimental model for learning in vascular surgery and microsurgery: esophagus and trachea of chicken. *Acta Cirurg. Bras.* 26: 101–106.

7 Aguilar, R.F. and Redig, P.T. (1997). What is your diagnosis? *J. Am. Med. Surg.* 11: 121–124.

8 Evans, A., Atkins, A., and Citino, S.B. (2009). Tracheal stenosis in a blue-billed currasow (*Crax alberti*). *J. Zoo Wildl. Med.* 40: 373–377.

9 de Matos, R.E.C., Morrisey, J.K., and Steffey, M. (2006). Postintubation tracheal stenosis in a blue and gold macaw (*Ara araruana*) resolved with tracheal resection and anastomosis. *J. Am. Med. Surg.* 20: 167–174.

10 Clippinger, T.L. and Bennett, R.A. (1998). Successful treatment of a traumatic tracheal stenosis in a goose by surgical resection and anastomosis. *J. Am. Med. Surg.* 12: 243–247.

11 Guzman, D.S.-M., Mitchell, M., Hedlund, C.S. et al. (2007). Tracheal resection and anastomosis in a mallard duck (*Anas platyryhnchos*) with traumatic segmental tracheal collapse. *J. Am. Med. Surg.* 21: 150–157.

12 Howard, P.E., Dein, F.J., Langenberg, J.A. et al. (1991). Surgical removal of a tracheal foreign body from a whooping crane (*Grus americana*). *J. Zoo Wildl. Med.* 22: 359–363.

13 Crystal, M.A. and Clark, G. (1992). What is your diagnosis? *J. Am. Ved. Med. Assoc.* 200: 1547–1548.

14 Diaz-Figueroa, O. and Mitchell, M.A. (2003). What is your diagnosis? *J. Am. Med. Surg.* 17: 239–241.

15 Bowles, H.L. et al. (2006). Surgical resolution of soft tissue disorders. In: *Clinical Avian Medicine*, vol. II (eds. G.J. Harrison and T.L. Lightfoot), 775–830.

16 McClure, S.R. et al. (1995). Surgical repair of traumatically induced collapsing trachea in an ostrich. *J. Am. Ved. Med. Assoc.* 207: 479–480.

17 Dennis, P.M. and Bennett, R.A. (1999). Ureterolithiasis in a double-yellowheaded Amazon parrot (*Amazona ochracephala*). In: *Association of Avian Veterinarians Annual Conference*, 161–162. New Orleans, LA.

18 Ferrell, S., Werner, J., Kyles, A. et al. (2003). Evaluation of a collagen patch as a method of enhancing ventriculotomy healing in Japanese quail (*Coturnix coturnix japonica*). *Vet. Surg.* 32: 103–112.

19 Kasaback, C.M. and Holland, M. (1998). What is your diagnosis? *J. Am. Ved. Med. Assoc.* 213: 27–28.

20 Vãsquez, S., Quiroga, M.I., Alemañ, N. et al. (2003). Squamous cell carcinoma of the oropharynx and esophagus in a Japanese bantam rooster. *Avian Dis.* 47: 215–217.

21 Brown, D. (2006). Possible etiology of submandibular lingual entrapment in herbivorous waterfowl. *Exotic DVM* 8: 7–9.

22 Mostafa, M.B. and Galiwango, B. (2004). Traumatic oesophageal perforation in a male ostrich (*Struthio camelus australis*). *Vet. Rec.* 154: 669.

23 Muscatello, G. (1998). Oesophageal impaction in a Canada goose (*Branta Canadensis*). *Aust. Vet. J.* 76: 537–540.

24 Hernandez, S.J., Blasier, M., Wilson, H. et al. (2006). Endoscopic removal of (pro)ventricular foreign bodies in parrots. In: *Association of Avian Veterinarians Annual Conference 2006 Proceedings*, 359–361. San Antonio, TX.

25 Lloyd, C. (2009). Stage endoscopic ventricular foreign body removal in a gyr falcon (*Falco rusticolus*). *J. Am. Med. Surg.* 23: 314–319.

26 Voitle, R.A., Roland, D.A., and Stonerock, R.H. (1974). A rapid and effective technique for cropectomy in mature or maturing chickens. *Poult. Sci.* 53: 1247–1250.

27 Stonerock, R.H., Roland, D.A., and Voitle, R.A. (1975). The effect of cropectomy on selective reproductive and physiological characteristics of laying hens. *Poult. Sci.* 54: 288–294.

28 Degernes, L.A., Wolf, K.N., Zombeck, D.J. et al. (2012). Ventricular diverticula formation in captive parakeet auklets (*Aethia psittacula*) secondary to foreign body ingestion. *J. Zoo Wildl. Med.* 43: 889–897.

29 Speer, B.L. (1998). Chronic parital proventricular obstruction caused by multiple gastrointestinal foreign bodies in a juvenile umbrella cockatoo (*Cacatua alba*). *J. Am. Med. Surg.* 12 (4): 271–275.

30 Honnas, C.M., Blue-McLendon, A., Zamos, D.T. et al. (1993). Proventriculotomy in ostriches: 18 cases (1990-1992). *J. Am. Ved. Med. Assoc.* 202 (12): 1989–1992.

31 Honnas, C.M., Jensen, J., Cornick, J.L. et al. (1991). Proventriculotomy to relieve foreign body impaction in ostriches. *J. Am. Ved. Med. Assoc.* 199 (4): 461–465.

32 Kinsel, M.J. et al. (2004). Ventricular phytobezoar impaction in three micronesian kingfishers (*Halcyon cinnamomina cinnamomina*). *J. Zoo Wildl. Med.* 35: 525–529.

33 Bailey, T.A. et al. (2001). Two cases of ventricular foreign bodies in the kori bustard (*Ardeotis kori*). *Vet. Rec.* 149: 187–188.

34 Hall, A.J. and Duke, G.E. (2000). Effect of selective gastic intrinsic denervation on gastric motility in turkeys. *Poult. Sci.* 79: 240–244.

35 Chaplin, S.B. and Duke, G.E. (1990). Effect of denervation of the myenteric plexus on gastroduodenal motility in turkeys. *Am. J. Phys* 259: G481–G489.

36 Bennett, R.A. (1994). Techniques in avian thoracoabdominal surgery. In: *Association of Avian Veterinarians Core Seminar Proceedings*, 45–57. Reno, NV.

37 Kinsel, M.J., Briggs, M.B., Crang, R.F. et al. (2004). Ventricular phytobezoar impaction in three micronesian kingfishers (*Halcyon cinnamomina cinnamomina*). *J. Zoo Wildl. Med.* 35: 525–529.

38 Wagner, W.M. (2005). Small intestinal foreign body in an adult Eclectus parrot (*Eclectus roratus*). *J. S. Afr. Vet. Assoc.* 76: 46–48.

39 Pye, G.W. (2007). Intestinal entrapment in the right pulmonary ostium after castration in a juvenile ostrich (*Struthio camelus*). *J. Am. Med. Surg.* 21: 290–293.

40 Baron, E.J. and Finegold, S.M. (1990). Microorganisms encountered in the gastrointestinal tract. In: *Diagnostic Microbiology*, 8e (eds. E.J. Baron and S.M. Finegold), 246. The CV Mosby Company: St. Louis.

41 Speer, B.L. (1998). A clinical look at the avian pancreas in health and disease. In: *Proceedings Association Avian Veterinarians Annual Conference*, 57. St Paul, MN.

42 Briscoe, J.A. and Bennett, R.A. (2011). Use of a duodenal serosal patch in the repair of a colon rupture in a female Solomon Island eclectus parrot. *J. Am. Ved. Med. Assoc.* 238: 922–926.

43 Adedokun, S.A., Utterback, P., Parsons, C.M. et al. (2009). Comparison of endogenous amino acid flow in broilers, laying hens and caecectomized roosters. *Br. Poult. Sci.* 50: 359–365.

44 Wang, Z.Y., Shi, S.R., Zhou, Q.Y. et al. (2008). The influence of caecectomy on amino acid availability of three feedstuffs for ganders. *Br. Poult. Sci.* 49: 181–185.

45 Karasawa, Y. and Duke, G.E. (1995). Effects of cecal ligation and colostomy on motility of the rectum, ileum and cecum in turkeys. *Poult. Sci.* 74: 2029–2034.

46 Son, J.H. and Karasawa, Y. (2000). Effect of removal of cecal contents on nitrogen utilitzation and nitrogen excretion in caecally ligated chickens fed on a low protein diet supplemented with urea. *Br. Poult. Sci.* 41: 69–71.

47 Son, J.H., Karasawa, Y., and Nahm, K.M. (2000). Effect of caecectomy on growth, moisture in excreta, gastrointestinal passage time and uric acid excretion in growing chicks. *Br. Poult. Sci.* 41: 72–74.

48 Son, J.H. and Karasawa, Y. (2001). Effects of caecal ligation and colostomy on water intake and excretion in chickens. *Br. Poult. Sci.* 42: 130–133.

49 Son, J.H., Ragland, D., and Adeola, O. (2002). Quantification of digesta flow into the caeca. *Br. Poult. Sci.* 43: 322–324.

50 Manangi, M.K., Clark, F.D., and Coon, C.N. (2007). Improved colostomy technique and excrement (urine) collection for broilers and broiler breeder hens. *Poult. Sci.* 86: 698–704.

51 Jirjis, F.F., Waibel, P.E., Duke, G.E. et al. (1997). An improved colostomy technique in turkeys. *Br. Poult. Sci.* 38: 603–606.

52 Gumus, E. et al. (2004). The relationship between uretero-cloacal structure in birds and sigmoidalrectal pouch surgery in humans. *Aktuel. Urol.* 35: 228–232.

53 Radlinksy, M.G., Mutus, R., Daglioglu, S. et al. (2004). Colonic entrapment after cloacopexy in two psittacine birds. *J. Am. Med. Surg.* 18: 175–182.

54 Beaufrere, H., Nevarez, J., and Tully, T.N. (2010). Cloacolith in a blue-fronted amazon parrot (*Amazona aestiva*). *J. Am. Med. Surg.* 24: 142–145.

55 Mehler, S.J., Briscoe, J.A., Hendrick, M.J. et al. (2007). Infiltrative lipoma in a blue-crowned conure (*Aratinga acuticaudata*). *J. Am. Med. Surg.* 21: 146–149.

56 Jaensch, S. (2000). Diagnosis of avian hepatic disorders. *Sem. Avian Exotic Pet Med.* 9 (3): 126–135.

57 Zebisch, K., Krautwald-Junghanns, M.E., and Willuhn, J. (2004). Ultrasound-guided liver biopsy in birds. *Vet. Rad. Ultrasound* 45: 241–246.

58 Nordberg, C., O, Brien, R.T., Paul-Murphy, J. et al. (2000). Ultrasound examination and guided fine-needle aspiration of the liver in Amazon parrots (*Amazona* species). *J. Am. Med. Surg.* 14 (3): 180–184.

59 Taylor, M. (1994). Endoscopic examination and biopsy techniques. In: *Avian Medicine: Principles and Applications* (eds. B.W. Ritchie, G.J. Harrison and L.R. Harrison), 327–354. Lake Worth, FL: Wingers Publishing.

60 Mulcahy, D.M. and Esler, D. (2010). Survival of captive and free-ranging harlequin ducks (*Histrionicus histrionicus*). *J. Wildl. Dis.* 46: 1325–1329.

61 Jaensch, S.M., Cullen, L., and Raidal, S.R. (2000). Assessment of liver function in galahs (*Eolophus roseicapillus*) after partial hepatectomy: a comparison of plasma enzyme concentrations, serum bile acid levels and galactose clearance tests. *J. Am. Med. Surg.* 14: 164–171.

62 Lierz, M., Ewringmann, A., and Göbel, T. (1998). Blood chemistry values in wild raptors and their changes after liver biopsy. *Berl. Münch Tierärztl.* 111: 295–301.

63 Onderka, D.K., Langevin, C.C., and Hanson, J.A. (1990). Fibrosing cholehepatitis in broiler chickens induced by bile duct ligations or inoculation of *Clostridium perfringens*. *Can. J. Vet. Res.* 54: 285–290.

64 Handharyani, E., Ochiai, K., Iwata, N. et al. (2001). Immunohistochemical and ultrastructural study of Ito cells (fat-storing cells) in response to extrahepatic bile duct ligation in broiler chickens. *J. Vet. Med. Sci.* 63: 547–552.

65 Yoshioka, K., Sasaki, M., Imai, S. et al. (2004). Testicular atrophy after bile duct ligation in chickens. *Vet. Pathol.* 41: 68–72.

66 McLelland, J. (1993). Apparatus digestorius (*Systema alimentarium*). In: *Handbook of Avian Anatomy*, 2e (eds. J.J. Baumel et al.), 301–327. The Nuttall Ornithological Club.

67 Carp, N.Z., Saputelli, J., Halbherr, T.C. et al. (1991). A technique for liver biopsy performed in Pekin ducks using anesthesia with Telazol. *Lab. Anim. Sci.* 41: 474–475.

68 Hazelwood, R.L. and Cieslak, S.R. (1989). *In vitro* release of pancreatic hormones following 99% pancreatectomy in the chicken. *Gen. Com.p Endocr.* 73: 308–317.

69 Laurent, F., Karmann, H., and Mialhe, P. (1987). Insulin, glucagon and somatostatin content in normal and diabetic duck pancreas. *Horm. Metabol. Res.* 19: 134–135.

70 Martland, M.F. (1986). Histopathology of the chick pancreas following pancreatic duct ligation. *Vet. Rec.* 118: 526–530.

71 Chen, S. and Bartrick, T. (2006). Resection and use of a cyclooxygenase-2 inhibitor for treatment of pancreatic adenocarcinoma in a cockatiel. *J. Am. Vet. Med. Assoc.* 228: 69–73.

72 Müller, K., Göbel, T., Müller, S. et al. (2004). Use of endoscopy and renal biopsy for the diagnosis of kidney disease in free-living birds of prey and owls. *Vet. Rec.* 155: 326–329.

73 Sinclair, K.M., Church, M.E., Farver, T.B. et al. (2012). Effects of meloxicam on hematologic and biochemical analysis variables and results of histologic examination of tissue specimens of Japanese quail (*Corturnix japonica*). *Am. J. Vet. Res.* 73: 1720–1727.

74 Echols, M.S. (2006). Evaluating and treating the kidneys. In: *Clinical Avian Medicine Volume I* (eds. G.J. Harrison and T.L. Lightfoot), 451–492. Palm Beach, FL: Spix Publishing.

75 Wideman, R.F. and Laverty, G. (1986). Kidney function in domestic fowl with chronic occlusion of the ureter and caudal renal vein. *Poult. Sci.* 65: 2148–2155.

76 Dennis, P.M. and Bennett, R.A. (2000). Ureterotomy for removal of two ureteroliths in a parrot. *J. Am. Vet. Med. Assoc.* 217: 865–868.

77 Machado, C. et al. (1987). Disintegration of kidney stones by extracorporeal shock wave lithotripsy in a penguin. In: *Proc 1st International Conf Zoo Avian Med*, 343–349.

78 Attia, Y.A., Burke, W.H., and Yamani, K.A. (1994). Response of broiler hens to forced molting by hormonal and dietary manipulations. *Poult. Sci.* 73 (2): 245–258.

79 Noonan, B., Johnson, P., and de Matos, R. (2012). Evaluation of egg-laying suppression effects of the GnRH agonist deslorelin in domestic chickens. *Proc. Assoc. Avian Vet. Assoc.*: 321.

80 Petritz, O.A., Sanchez-Migallon Guzman, D., Paul-Murphy, J. et al. (2013). Evaluation of the efficacy and safety of single administration of 4.7 mg deslorelin acetate implants on egg production and plasma sex hormones in Japanese quail (*Corturnix coturnix japonica*). *Am. J. Ved. Res.* 74: 316–323.

81 Johnson, A.L. (2000). Reproduction in the female. In: *Sturkie's Avian Physiology*, 5e (ed. G.C. Whittow), 569–596. San Diego, CA: Academic Press.

82 Wentworth, B.C. and Bitgood, J.J. (1988). Function of bilateral oviducts in double oviduct hens following surgery. *Poult. Sci.* 67: 1465–1468.

83 Keymer, I.F. (1980). Disorders of the avian female reproductive system. *Avian Pathol.* 9: 405–419.

84 Romagnano, A. (1996). Avian obstetrics. *Sem. Avian Exotic Pet Med.* 5: 180–188.

85 Buchanan, S., Robertson, G.W., and Hocking, P.M. (1999). The relationship between vaginal collagen, plasma oestradiol and uterine prolapse in turkeys. *Res. Vet. Sci.* 67: 153–157.

86 Buchanan, S., Robertson, G.W., and Hocking, P.M. (2000). Development of the reproductive system in turkeys with a high or low susceptibility to prolapse of the oviduct. *Poult. Sci.* 70: 1491–1498.

87 Ajayi, O.L., Antia, R.E., and Omotainse, S.O. (2008). Oviductal volvulus in a Nera black chicken (*Gallus gallus domesticus*) in Nigeria. *Avian Pathol.* 37: 139–140.

88 Harcourt-Brown, N.H. (1996). Torsion and displacement of the oviduct as a cause of egg-binding in four psittacine birds. *J. Avian Med. Surg.* 10 (4): 262–267.

89 Reid, G.G., Grimes, T.M., and Eaves, F.W. (1984). A survey of disease in five commercial flocks of meat breeder chickens. *Aust. Vet. J.* 61 (1): 13–16.

90 Speer, B.L. (1997). Diseases of the urogenital system. In: *Avian Medicine and Surgery* (eds. R.B. Altman, S.L. Clubb, G.M. Dorrestein and K. Quesenberry), 625–644. Philadelphia, PA: WB Saunders.

91 Joyner, K.L. (1994). Theriogenology. In: *Avian Medicine: Principles and Application* (eds. B.W. Ritchie, G.J. Harrison and L.R. Harrison), 748–804. Lake Worth, FL: Wingers Publishing.

92 Orosz, S. (1997). Anatomy of the urogenital system. In: *Avian Medicine and Surgery* (eds. R.B. Altman, S.L. Clubb, G.M. Dorrestein and K. Quesenberry), 614–622. Philadelphia, PA: WB Saunders.

93 Johnson, P.A., Brooks, C., and Wang, S.Y. (1993). Plasma concentrations of immunoreactive inhibin and gonadotropins following removal of ovarian follicles in the domestic hen. *Biol. Reprod.* 49: 1026–1031.

94 Pye, G.W., Bennett, R.A., and Plunske, R. (2001). Endoscopic salpingoysterectomy of juvenile cockatiels (*Nymphicus hollandicus*). *J. Avian Med. Surg.* 15 (2): 90–94.

95 Hernandez-Divers, S. et al. (2007). Endoscopic orchidectomy and salpingohysterectomy of pigeons (*Columba livia*): an avian model for minimally invasive endosurgery. *J. Avian Med. Surg.* 21: 22–37.

96 Ansenberger, K., Richards, C., Zhuge, Y. et al. (2010). Decreased severity of ovarian cancer and increased survival in hens fed a flaxseed-enriched diet for 1 year. *Gyneco. Oncol.* 117: 341–347.

97 Baumel, J.L. (1993). Systema Cardiovasculare. In: *Handbook of Avian Anatomy: Nomina Anatomica Avium*, 2e (eds. J.L. Baumal, A.S. King and J.E. Breazile), 407–475. Cambridge, M: Nuttall Ornithological Club.

98 Lea, R.W., Richard-Yris, M.A., and Sharp, P.J. (1996). The effect of ovariectomy on concentrations of plasma prolactin and LH and parental behavior in the domestic fowl. *Gen. Comp. Endocrinol.* 101: 115–121.

99 Petrowski, M.L., Wong, E.A., and Ishii, S. (1993). Influence of ovariectomy and photostimulation on luteinizing hormone in the domestic Turkey: evidence for differential regulation of gene expression and hormone secretion. *Biol. Reprod.* 49: 295–299.

100 Proudman, J.A. and Opel, H. (1989). Daily changes in plasma prolactin, corticosterone, and luteinizing hormone in the unrestrained, ovariectomized hen. *Poult. Sci.* 68: 177–184.

101 Terada, O., Shimada, K., and Saito, N. (1997). Effect of oestradiol replacement in ovariectomized chickens on pituitary LH concentrations and concentrations of mRNAs encoding LH β and α subunits. *J. Reprod. Fertil.* 111: 59–64.

102 Zadworny, D. and Etches, R.J. (1987). Effects of ovariectomy or force feeding on the plasma concentrations of prolactin and luteinizing hormone in incubating Turkey hens. *Biol. Reprod.* 36: 81–88.

103 Altman, R.B. (1997). Soft tissue surgical procedures. In: *Avian Medicine and Surgery* (eds. R.B. Altman, S.L. Clubb, G.M. Dorrestein and K. Quesenberry), 704–732. Philadelphia, PA: WB Saunders.

104 Sony, Y. and Silversides, F.G. (2008). Transplantation of ovaries in Japanese quail (*Coturnix japonica*). *Anim. Reprod. Sci.* 105: 430–437.

105 Sony, Y. and Silversides, F.G. (2007). Offspring produced from orthotopic transplantation of chicken ovaries. *Poult. Sci.* 86: 107–111.

106 Vegad, J.L. and Kolte, G.N. (1979). An ovarian condition with multiple cystic follicles in a hen. *Vet. Rec.* 105: 446.

107 Randall, C.J. (1987). *A Colour Atlas of Diseases of the Domestic Fowl and Turkey*. England: Wolfe Medical Publications Ltd.

108 Stauber, E., Papageorges, M., and Sande, R. (1990). Polyostotic hyperostosis associated with oviductal tumor in a cockatiel. *J. Am. Ved. Med. Assoc.* 196 (6): 939–940.

109 Fredrickson, T.N. (1987). Ovarian tumors of the hen. *Environ. Health Perspect.* 73: 35–51.

110 Latimer, K.S. (1994). Oncology. In: *Avian Medicine: Principles and Application* (eds. B.W. Ritchie, G.J. Harrison and L.R. Harrison), 640–672. Lake Worth, FL: Wingers Publishing.

111 Baumgartner, R., Hatt, J.-M., Dobeli, M., and Hauser, B. (1995). Endocrinologic and pathologic findings in birds with polyostotic hyperostosis. *J. Am. Med. Surg.* 9: 251–254.

112 Kremer, V.A. and Budras, K.D. (1990). The blood vascular system in the testis of Peking drakes (*Anas platyrhynchos* L.). macroscopic, lightmicroscopic, and scanning electron microscopic investigations. *Anat. Anz. Jena* 171: 73–87.

113 Chen, K.L. et al. (2009). Effect of caponization and different exogenous androgen on hepatic lipid and β-oxidase of male chickens. *Poult. Sci.* 88: 1033–1039.

114 Hagelin, J.C. (2001). Castration in Gambel's and scaled quail: ornate plumage and dominance persist, but courtship and threat behaviors do not. *Horm. Behav.* 39 (1): 1–10.

115 Pinxten, R., De Ridder, E., De Cock, M. et al. (2003). Castration does not decrease nonreproductive aggression in yearling male European starlings (*Sturnis vulgaris*). *Horm. Behav.* 43: 394–401.

116 Rikimaru, K., Takahashi, H., and Nichols, M.A. (2011). An efficient method of early caponization in slow-growing meat-type chickens. *Poult. Sci.* 90: 1852–1857.

117 Busso, J.M., Satterlee, D.G., Roberts, M.L. et al. (2010). Testosterone manipulation postcastration does not alter cloacal gland growth differences in male quail selected for divergent plasma corticosterone stress response. *Poult. Sci.* 89: 2191–2698.

118 Samour, J.H. and Markham, J.A. (1987). Vasectomy in budgerigars (*Melopsittacus undulatus*). *Vet. Rec.* 120: 115.

119 Birkhead, T.R. and Pellatt, J.E. (1989). Vasectomy in small passerine birds. *Vet. Rec.* 125: 646.

120 Janssen, S.J., Kirby, J.D., and Hess, R.A. (2000). Identification of epididymal stones in diverse rooster populations. *Poult. Sci.* 79: 568–574.

121 Samour, J. (2010). Vasectomy in birds: a review. *J. Am. Med. Surg.* 24: 169–173.

122 Golbar, H.M., Izawa, T., Kuwamura, M. et al. (2009). Malignant seminoma with multiple visceral metastasis in a guinea fowl (*Numida meleagris*) kept in a zoo. *Avian Dis.* 53: 143–145.

123 Siller, W.G., Dewar, W.A., and Whitehead, C.C. (1972). Cystic dilatation of the seminiferous tubules in the fowl: a sequel of sodium intoxication. *J. Pathol.* 107: 191–197.

124 Stewart, J. (1994). Ratites. In: *Avian Medicine: Principles and Application*, vol. 128 (eds. B.W. Ritchie, G.J. Harrison and L.R. Harrison). Lake Worth, FL: Wingers Publishing.

22

Chicken Behavior

Christine Calder[1] and Julia Albright[2]

[1] *Behavior Department, Midcoast Humane, Brunswick, ME, USA*
[2] *Department of Small Animal Clinical Sciences, College of Veterinary Medicine, University of Tennessee, Knoxville, TN, USA*

Introduction

The popularity of backyard chickens has grown exponentially over the past decade due to their wide variety of uses, such as a food source (eggs, meat, or both), pest control, garden fertilization, and companionship [1]. Suburban and urban chicken flocks are often small (less than 20 birds) and consist primarily of hens [1] (Figure 22.1–22.3). A recent survey indicated flock keepers are interested in allowing their chickens to perform species-specific behaviors like foraging, nesting, and roosting and therefore provide open access to their yard every day [1]. According to the same survey, the majority of respondents (76.6%) did not observe abnormal behaviors such as aggression and self-mutilation that can plague large commercial farms and even other domestic animals. However, behavioral issues can still arise in backyard chicken populations and few behavioral resources are available to advise flock keepers and veterinarians. Some veterinarians are gaining a better knowledge on other areas of poultry health, but unfortunately, many still lack expertise in a chicken's fundamental behavioral needs [2]. In

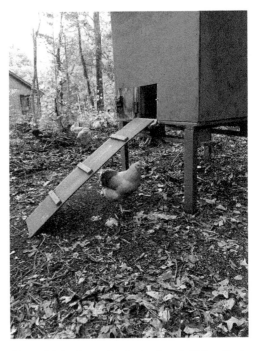

Figure 22.1 Example of a backyard chicken flock.

order to optimize the health and wellbeing of backyard chickens, this chapter serves to provide information on basic normal and abnormal behaviors, as well as their behavioral and environmental needs.

Backyard Poultry Medicine and Surgery: A Guide for Veterinary Practitioners, Second Edition.
Edited by Cheryl B. Greenacre and Teresa Y. Morishita.
© 2021 John Wiley & Sons, Inc. Published 2021 by John Wiley & Sons, Inc.
Companion website: www.wiley.com/go/greenacre/medicine

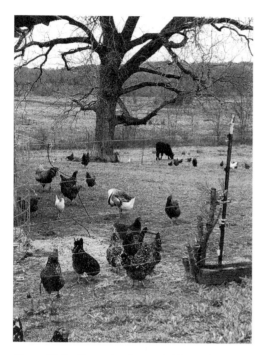

Figure 22.2   Example of a rural chicken flock.

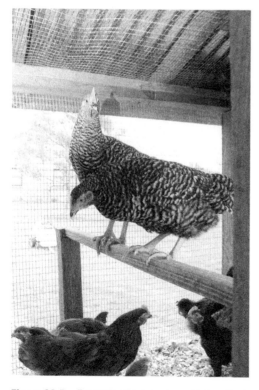

Figure 22.3   Example of a suburban chicken flock.

Origins and Domestication

The modern-day chicken is a domesticated species that evolved primarily from the Red Junglefowl (*Gallus gallus*) and Gray Junglefowl (*Gallus sonneratti*) over 8000 years ago in South and Southeast Asia [3–5]. Today, several species of junglefowl can still be found living wild in Southeast Asia in groups of one male and several females, single males living alone, or several males living together in contrast to most domesticated chicken flocks [3, 4]. Compared to its domestic relatives, the Junglefowl tends to live in forests and semi-open areas and spends more daylight time foraging for food, even when a food source is readily available [3, 4, 6]. Domestic chicken breeds tend to be larger in size as well as have larger eggs, clutches (300 eggs per year compared to 10–15 per year in Junglefowl), and offspring, and are less fearful of humans compared to their Junglefowl ancestors [4, 7]. Junglefowl frequently move their perching roosts to avoid predators and reduce crowding at dawn, whereas domesticated chickens tend to choose the same general roosting areas every night [4]. In addition to reproductive behaviors, Junglefowl also display less conspe-

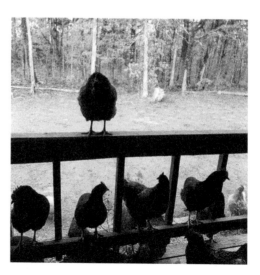

Figure 22.4   Chickens are highly social and often perch together. These chickens are waiting to be fed.

cific agonistic behaviors than their domesticated counterparts, most likely due to avoid injury or even death from fighting; however, domesticated chickens tend to be more sociable and tolerant of a higher density with their conspecifics [4, 8] (Figure 22.4).

Sensory Perception

Vision

Understanding species-specific behavior and cognition first requires insight into that species' unique sensory perception. Evolutionary history causes each species to develop vastly different perceptual systems and interpretations of environmental sensory input. For instance, vision plays an important role in foraging and communication in chickens [9]. A chicken's retina contains rods, cones, and double cone photoreceptors that allow a chicken to see red, blue, and green, in addition to light frequencies on the ultraviolet spectrum [10]. The double-cone photoreceptor, a specialized receptor found in birds, reptiles, and most fish species, provides exquisitely sensitive motion detection and allows chickens to be adept hunters of small prey items [11]. In fact, when given the opportunity, chickens are known to be efficient and ruthless predators of insects, lizards, mice, and snakes [12].

Auditory

Compared to other bird species and humans, chickens tend to be more sensitive to lower-frequency sounds, reflecting the significant role low frequency vocalizations in their social communication [13]. Chicks develop audition by day 12 of incubation and by day 19 they start using clicking sounds to communicate with other chicks in the clutch and the hen, presumably to synchronize hatching [13–15]. This synchronization is a critical aspect of chick survival and allows the hen and the chicks to leave the nest sooner in search of food and water [13].

Taste and Olfaction

Taste and olfaction are often collectively referred to as chemoreception. Genetic and behavioral studies suggest chemoreception is salient to chickens but to a lesser extent than other sensory systems [9]. Chickens show preferences and aversions to a wide range of odors, but visual cues such as shape, color, and texture appear to be the strongest motivators in food selection [9, 12]. However, chemoreception is critical in the detection of predators as well as social recognition. Odors derived from the preen gland are believed to be the main source of an individual chicken's body odor [12, 16].

Touch

Similar to other birds and mammals, chicken skin contains many specialized sensory nerve cells allowing for the perception of pressure, touch, pain, heat, cold, and limb position. However, the most highly innervated organ in

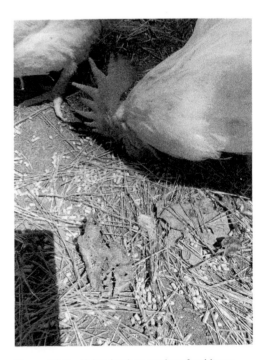

Figure 22.5 Using beak to explore food items scattered on the ground.

the bird is the multifunctional beak [17]. A chicken, like most birds, uses its beak to explore the environment, manipulate food items, build nests, drink, preen feathers, and inflict injury during agonistic encounters [17] (Figure 22.5). The beak tip, also called the bill tip organ, contains many pressure responsive mechanoreceptors, allowing the chicken to peck, manipulate, and respond to very small objects with high precision [18]. Damage or injuries to the beak can be very painful and result in neuromas and chronic pain [19]. Clinical signs of beak damage include guarding behavior (tucking the bill under the wing) and a decrease in preening and pecking [20].

Behavioral Development

Species-specific behaviors start to develop during the embryonic state [12]. Chicks often hatch in ground nests, a location highly

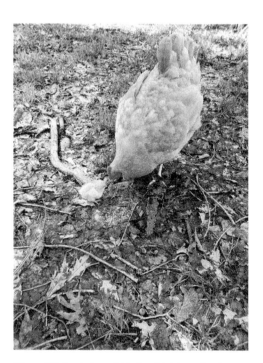

Figure 22.6 A day-old baby chick learning how to find food.

vulnerable to many predators. Chickens are a precocial species – hatching with mature traits such as open eyes, down feathers, and a relatively well-developed brain – to increase ability to find food and avoid predators [15]. Almost immediately after hatching chickens can walk, find food and water, make independent decisions, learn from past experiences, and effectively communicate [12, 15] (Figure 22.6).

Even though chickens do not have an established socialization developmental stage, within 48 hours of hatching, chicks can quickly learn to identify, approach, and follow stimuli that are most indicative of their mother under natural conditions [12, 15, 21]. Chicks that are hatched artificially may not learn appropriate feeding behavior (i.e. suitable food items, best locations for these items, and correct pecking technique) and if raised with other species, including humans, can have difficulty recognizing conspecific breeding partners in the future [4, 9, 12, 15].

Social Behaviors

Just as with other domesticated species, chickens are innately social animals [22, 23]. The evolutionary benefit to group living is "safety in numbers," but existing in close proximity to conspecifics inevitably leads to conflict over resources [24]. Behaviors such as aggression, courtship, breeding, parental care, appeasement, and synchronized behaviors such as eating, preening, and dust bathing evolved to minimize injury from aggression and predation and maximize reproductive success [4, 12, 23, 25, 26, 27] (Figure 22.7). Chickens often form strong social bonds with some, but not all, of the chickens in their flock [8]. A backyard flock should consist minimally of two chickens because chickens are natural flock animals and can become very distressed if kept in isolation [12]. However, encounters with unfamiliar birds are often stressful [28, 29].

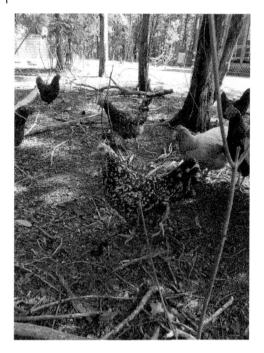

Figure 22.7 Group of social hens.

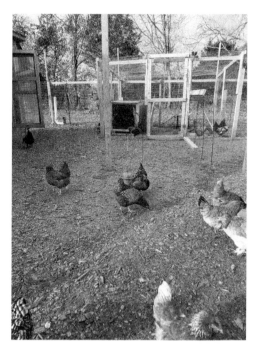

Figure 22.8 Rooster housed in a separate cage within the hen cage.

Less conflict occurs in small flocks composed of only hens compared to a combination of males and females [8, 27]. For those choosing to include males in their backyard flock, optimal interactions are associated with a minimum of two or three hens per rooster and limiting the flock to three to 10 birds per yard area for most backyard flock owners [8, 27].

It is the rooster's responsibility to guard, breed, and find tasty traces of food that attracts females [8, 9]. In a rooster-less flock or a flock with too few males per female, a female may assume these responsibilities. One of her ovaries starts to produce male hormones and this "man hen" can display male characteristics such as aggression, crowing, and developing spurs [23].

It is not uncommon for some roosters to display aggressive behavior to people who enter their perceived territories. This issue can be handled through avoidance, such as removal from the flock, placing the rooster in a separate cage or pen within the larger chicken yard (Figure 22.8), or reducing any injury from

spurs by applying methylmethacrolate covering over the end of the spur (C. Greenacre, personal communication). Chickens are very easy to train, and more chicken owners are using reward-based techniques common in zoo and companion animal behavior modification. For example, one of the authors (CC) uses target training to teach the rooster to move on cue to a specific location across the pen. This cue can then be used to encourage the bird to engage in an appropriate behavior away from the person entering the yard. Other references can be consulted for additional details [24].

Aggression to Determine Social Order

Despite common sentiment about the "pecking order," chicken social hierarchies are not often linear or stable [4]. In a linear hierarchy, Bird A consistently gains resources over Birds B and C, and Bird B over Bird C. Nonlinear hierarchies, such as the triangular example of Bird A is dominant over Bird B, and Bird B over Bird C, but Bird C consistently gaining resources over Bird A, are also common [12]. Stability refers to the consistency in relationships, regardless of the type of hierarchical structure. Smaller flocks tend to have more stable, linear hierarchies, whereas the social dynamics of larger flocks may be in constant flux without any recognizable dominance structure [8, 12, 23, 25]. The establishment of territories along with the availability and distribution of resources also plays an important role in the stability of the flock [8]. Abundant and widely distributed resources lead to diminished competition and conflict [23, 25]. Research suggests chickens are able to recognize and remember approximately 40 different individual chickens, and this may be one determinant of the natural flock size of 25–40 birds [4]. Placing chickens in larger flocks means a bird may be constantly coming into contact with new birds, or perceived new birds within the flock, resulting in stress, antagonistic, and potentially injurious behaviors [4, 27]. Roosters tend to form separate social hierarchies from the hens within the flock and during mating season, aggression between males is more likely to occur due to an increase in testosterone and competition for mating opportunities [8].

Bullying in the form of pecking and posturing is common if food, perches, and nesting areas are limited [8, 23]. Posturing, or the threat of aggression, is less energetically costly for the bird because these behaviors often result in one bird displaying appeasement postures or moving away to avoid conflict. However, not all pecking is motivated by one chicken's intention to harm another [23]. While gentle allopreening or picking of another birds' feathers can be normal behaviors, excessive feather picking among birds often indicates underlying social instability in the flock and can be a welfare concern due to the associated stress, injury, and pain [25]. Excessive self-directed preening or feather-picking can also be a sign of social or environmental welfare concerns and is discussed in the following section. Normal molting should also be ruled out as a reason for feather loss (Figures 22.9 and 22.10).

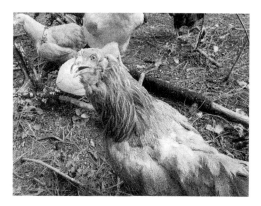

Figure 22.9 Molting chicken. Note area of feather loss.

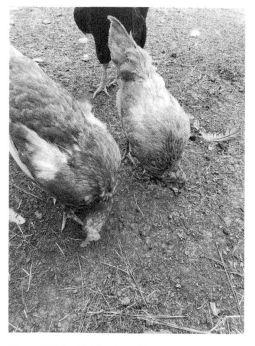

Figure 22.10 Molting hens. Note area of feather loss.

Comfort and Grooming Behaviors

Self-maintenance behaviors in chickens include grooming behaviors (e.g. dust bathing and preening) along with comfort behaviors (e.g. roosting and perching) [12, 23, 25]. These behaviors appear to be socially facilitated and are often displayed almost simultaneously as a group [12, 23, 25]. Participation in these species-specific behaviors are measurements of good welfare and reduced stress level in the flock [12, 23, 25].

Dust Bathing

Dust bathing and preening (Figure 22.11) remove stale preen oil and ectoparasites from the plumage [25, 30]. Removing the stale preen oil allows the feathers to stay fluffy and insulate the chicken. There are several stages of dust bathing [12, 23, 25] (Table 22.1). Tossing, scratching, and rubbing can happen in any

Table 22.1 Stages of dust bathing.

Dust Bathing (approximately 10 min/day)
Find a suitable substrate
Scratch a depression to sit in
Bird leans to one side and uses its top leg to scratch at the substrate
Roll back sternal and use wings to spread substrate over feathers
Rub into the substrate
Stand up
Shake
Preening ends the behavior

order but preening is always the final stage [12, 23, 25]. A low resilience behavior, chickens allot time to this behavior when the opportunity arises [12]. Chickens typically find any type of fine-grained substances that can penetrate the feathers and then be shaken off acceptable for dust bathing [12, 23, 25]. The behavior is reduced if the birds are stressed or ill and consistent dust bathing is considered one measure of good welfare in a flock [25].

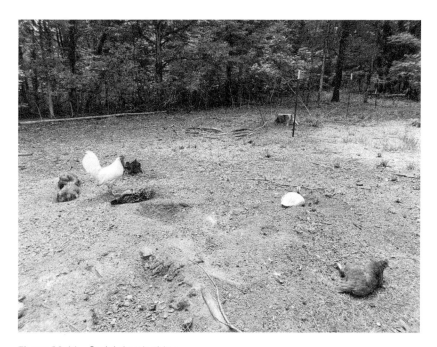

Figure 22.11 Social dust bathing.

Preening

Preening maintains plumage condition by cleaning, keeping the feather barbs and barbules aligned, and distributing preen oil from the uropygial gland over the feathers. Preen oil provides waterproofing and improves wind resistance during flight [12, 23, 24] (Table 22.2). Preening tends to be very soothing for the birds but can become excessive under certain circumstances, resulting in extreme feather loss or mutilation of the adjacent soft tissue (i.e. feather plucking) [12, 23, 25]. Short, frequent bouts of preening may be associated with stress [12]. Preening is an important social and maintenance behavior to chickens and in limited-space production facilities (i.e. battery cages), this behavior is often the last behavior to drop off in times of high stress, and first behavior to return when environmental circumstances change for the bird (Figure 22.12).

Table 22.2   Stages of preening.

Preening
First: Nibble deep down in plumage (at the base of the feathers) with their beak.
Second: Perform a combing motion as they run feathers through her beak to keep the vein portion together and intact.
Third (self-pecking): The bird gently pecks at the surface of the plumage to remove small fine particles.

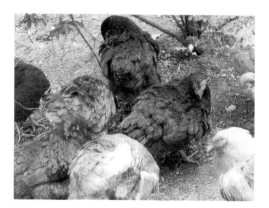

Figure 22.12   Example of preening.

Roosting or Perching

Chickens are also highly motivated to perform roosting, or perching, and the behavior is first seen in very young chicks [12, 31, 32] (Figures 22.13 and 22.14). This behavior allows

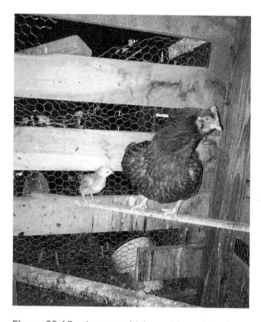

Figure 22.13   A young chick perching with a hen.

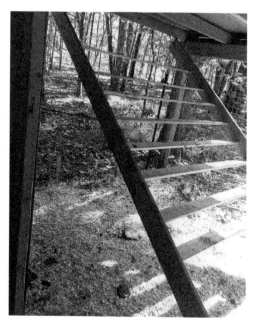

Figure 22.14   Handmade perching ladder.

chickens to escape predators, unwanted conspecific interactions, and to strengthen leg bones [12, 23, 31, 32] (Figures 22.15 and 22.16). This is a socially facilitated behavior and adequate space is needed for all chickens to roost or perch at the same time (minimum 15 cm of perch space per bird) [12, 31]. Studies have shown chickens prefer large, round perching areas over small, square, or triangular spaces [32]. Adequate perching space also helps reduce floor egg laying by encourage the use of nesting boxes [12, 23, 25, 31, 32] (Figures 22.17 and 22.18).

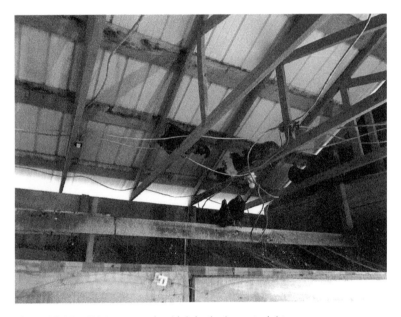

Figure 22.15 Chickens roosting high in the barn at night.

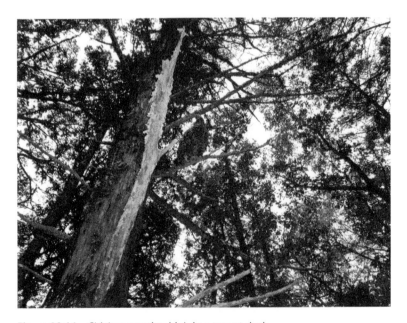

Figure 22.16 Chicken roosting high in a tree at dusk.

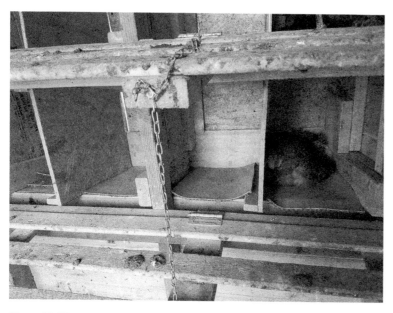

Figure 22.17 Adequate perching areas encourage use of nest boxes.

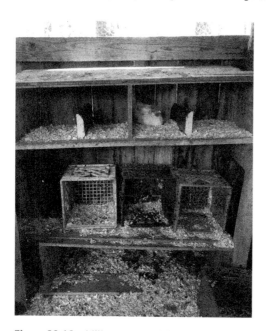

Figure 22.18 Milk crates used for nest boxes.

Reproductive Behaviors

Chickens are a sexually dimorphic species with roosters and hens varying greatly in size and appearance (Figure 22.19). They tend to be polygynous, although it is not unusual for certain males and females to selectively mate at each breeding cycle [4, 33, 34]. A ratio of one male to 10 females is considered ideal to increase fertility and social stability in the flock [23]. Mating often follows a diurnal

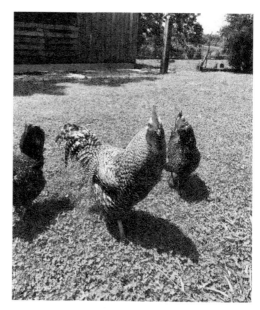

Figure 22.19 Sexual dimorphism shown with male rooster in foreground and smaller females in background.

pattern, occurring early in morning and later in the afternoon. Due to morning egg laying, peak copulation and successful fertilization often occur in late afternoon [35].

Mating

In stable flocks, mating can be initiated by either the female or male. The rooster initiates mating by exhibiting a courtship dance: circling the hen while hopping, ruffling feathers, and dropping his head and wing toward the hen [36]. If a hen is receptive to mating, she may remain motionless while squatting with her wings held out slightly from her body. This is called lordosis [23]. The rooster then mounts the hen and grabs her comb, neck feathers, or the skin on the back of her head or neck followed by the tread (walking quickly in place on the hen's back). This treading can cause feather loss over the base of the hen's wings. Mating is complete when the rooster dips his tail to the side of the hen's tail and spreads his tail feathers so that their cloacae come into contact. The rooster's ejaculate is released directly into the hen's vagina via her cloaca. Copulation sequence ends with the hen standing, shaking, and fluffing her feathers [34]. A rooster may mate anywhere from 10 to 30 or more times per day, depending on the availability of hens and competition from other roosters [34]. Young hens are less discriminatory and may show receptive behavior to a variety of males (and even humans) [23]. Conversely, some females show a strong general avoidance to specific males and thus rarely mate with those males [33]. Rooster-specific behaviors such as aggression and vocalization are not desirable in most urban settings. Furthermore, females do not require the presence of a male to complete sexual maturity or produce eggs [12]. The relative ease of maintaining an egg-producing hen flock is a major factor in the skyrocketing popularity of backyard chickens.

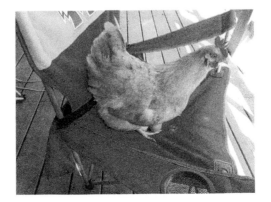

Figure 22.20 Egg laying hens are highly motivated to find a nest.

Egg Laying

The hormonal regulation of sexually dimorphic nesting and egg laying in hens is first triggered by light [12, 25]. In response to direct light stimulation to the pineal gland, the hypothalamus brain structure releases gonadotrophin-releasing hormones (GnRHs) that, in turn, triggers the release of two types of gonadotrophin hormones from the anterior pituitary gland: luteinizing hormone (LH) and follicle-stimulating hormone (FSH). A surge of plasma LH occurs four to six hours before ovulation [35]. Ovulation occurs 24 hours after estrogen and progesterone are released from the post-ovulation follicle, triggering nest site selection and building [12]. Hens are highly motivated to search for an appropriate site and build nests (Figure 22.20). In addition to abnormal repetitive behaviors, sham nest building, and vocalizations, the lack of access to suitable nesting sites can lead to egg retention, an extra calcium layer on the shell, resulting in a welfare issue [25].

Nesting

Wild Junglefowl lay individual eggs at 24- to 48-hour intervals [12]. The hen often leaves the nest after each egg is laid to eat, drink, eliminate, and sometimes preen and dustbathe [12]. This behavior is very similar in our domesticated chickens, especially those given the opportunity to incubate their own eggs. In production situations, although they prefer enclosed nests, domestic hens display similar nesting behaviors if provided deep litter [36] (Figure 22.21). There are four key nesting phases and total time from restlessness to laying egg is 1–2 hours [25] (Table 22.3). If the hen is interrupted during the nesting process, or if there is limited access to nesting boxes or material,

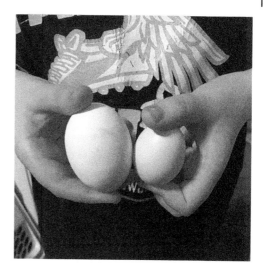

Figure 22.22   Example of a jumbo egg.

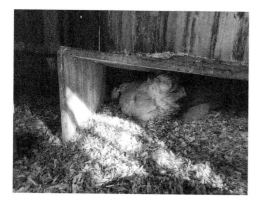

Figure 22.21   Hens will nest on the floor if the litter is deep enough.

Table 22.3   Phases of nesting.

Egg Laying (1–2 h to complete)
Phase I: The hen is restless showing a lot of movement and pacing. She will give a pre-laying or "gackel"-call as she separates herself from the flock and positions herself in a way that her keel is raised.
Phase 2: Starts with nest site examinations. The hen will enter a nest sites then crouch. During this phase, she may enter and exit several nest sites before choosing one.
Phase 3: The hen enters the nest and begins nest building.
Phase 4: The hen squats in the nest, oviposition or actual laying of the egg followed finally by sitting on the egg.

she displays increased locomotion, exploratory activities, and vocalizations, and an increase in the gackel-call, a vocalization specific to periods of egg-laying [25, 36].

Limited access to preferred nesting sites can also cause egg size and texture changes to occur [25, 37, 38].

Larger or "jumbo-sized" eggs (Figure 22.22) occur with delayed oviposition because yolk is retained longer and more albumin is deposited, both of which result in increased egg mass [37]. Other egg shell abnormalities indicating delayed oviposition include calcium dusting (extra calcium on surface), leading to bumpy or roughly textured eggs; white banding or equatorial bulge that develops when contraction of the egg shell gland (uterus) occurs before shell is hardened; and flat-sided eggs resulting from two eggs developing in a single eggshell gland and the additional pressure creating a flattening effect [37]. These size and shape egg abnormalities can be an indicator of poor environmental conditions and bird welfare [25].

Broodiness

Broodiness is a natural behavior in which birds temporarily cease the egg laying cycle to incubate a clutch of eggs. It is also associated with defensive behaviors when the nest is approached or the hen hears distress calls from the unhatched chicks [9, 23, 39] (Figure 22.23). Broody behavior is regulated by the pituitary gland hormone prolactin. In cases where broodiness is desired (e.g. foster incubation), the behavior can be induced by exogenous prolactin administration, or through the more natural means of prolonged exposure to chicks or uncollected eggs left in the nest [40]. Broody behavior has many physiological effects such as a decrease in metabolic rate, food consumption, and heart rate, even when frightened [23, 40]. Broody hens do leave the nest daily to eat, drink, and defecate [23]. They may also engage in social grooming behaviors such as dust bathing and preening during this time [23].

As domestic chickens are genetically selected for increased egg laying production, broodiness behavior tends to be less prevalent compared to wild counterparts [4, 12, 23]. Broodiness is inversely related to egg production and,

therefore, low broody behavior in domestic species has been selected, although this behavior can vary between breeds [23]. Leghorns tends to lack broodiness and show little maternal attachment toward chicks, whereas Silkies are known for their strong maternal and broody behaviors. Silky hens will even incubate and hatch a clutch of eggs she did not lay [23]. Removing eggs daily helps reduce broodiness since the presence of eggs in the nest stimulates broody behaviors [23]. Some hens display broody behavior without the presence of eggs or if her eggs did not hatch successfully. In this situation, the hen can be removed from the nest and caged on the floor of the coop with food and water for 1–2 days to break the egg laying cycle before introducing her back to the flock [23].

Feeding Behavior

Foraging, Pecking, and Scratching

Foraging and its relating behaviors of beak pecking and foot scratching of the ground are critical species-specific behaviors for chickens, as evidenced by the amount of time spent engaged in these behaviors [3, 25]. Red Junglefowl spend approximately 60% of the active part of the day ground pecking and 34% ground scratching in search of food in the wild [3]. When given the same opportunity, domestic chickens spend less of their daily time budget (approximately 40%) ground pecking and scratching, however [3]. A peak in foraging and feeding occurs early and late in the light period, with juveniles searching and eating more protein (insects) and adults eating a more herbivorous diet [41]. When foraging for food, chickens peck the ground with their eyes closed [12]. Pecking is interspersed with rapid scratching movement of the feet [12, 25]. The purpose of scratching is to detect and uncover high quality food items that might be hidden in the environment [25]. Chickens show headshaking and side-to-side beak

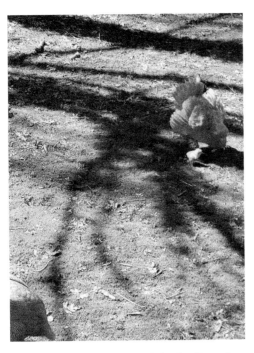

Figure 22.23 Defensive hen behavior. Note wing posture.

wiping motion to clean the beak of sticky residues if unpalatable foods are ingested [25].

Social Influence on Feeding and Foraging (Social Facilitation)

Pecking is an exploratory behavior that can be enhanced through social learning [22, 25]. This behavior may help the bird identify and avoid poisonous foods [26]. It also can help chickens accept new items [26]. Adult domestic hens showing high rates of pecking and scratching often attracts other birds to the area [22]. Hens may use this behavior to entice their chicks away from unpalatable foods [22]. An interesting behavior displayed by chickens of all ages is food running, or a bird grabbing a large piece of food or prey item in its beak and swiftly running with the item. Although its exact purpose is unclear, some have postulated it is to prevent others from stealing the food item, or conversely, to attract other birds to help break it apart [12].

Drinking behavior develops in first few days of life and is closely associated with feeding throughout the day (Figure 22.24). Chickens drink with their eyes open and they use a scooping movement with their head, neck, and beak [12]. There are several common water delivery systems for backyard flocks. The flow rate is limited in a nipple system, causing chickens to make more frequent visits to nipple drinkers and spend more time at the drinker compared to the same amount of water ingested from a bell drinker [42] (Figure 22.25). Droppings tend to be dryer in chickens drinking from the nipple system [12]. However, the bell drinker tends to be more unstable resulting in spillage and soiled litter than the nipple system [42].

Fear, Distress, Frustration

As prey species, chickens are commonly wary of new stimuli or stimuli that could indicate the threat of predation. A normal fear response to perceived threat involves a transient motionless state followed by walking, running, or flying away [23, 25]. The response can be quite frantic and dramatic to confuse a predator. Any noise, bright light, or sudden movement can induce startle and fear, and the degree of the fear response depends on a myriad of factors such as species, environment, housing, previous learning experiences, and health status. The degree of fearfulness tends

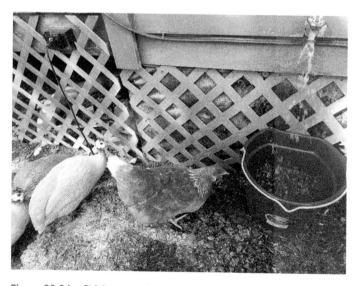

Figure 22.24 Chickens need access to fresh water sources.

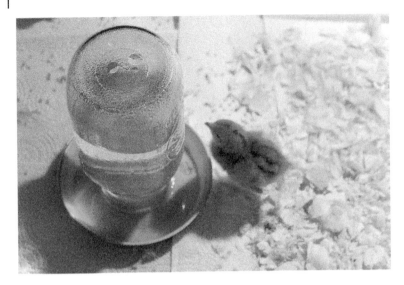

Figure 22.25 Example of a bell drinker.

to vary by breed. For instance, the domestic brown egg layers tend to be relatively docile while White Leghorn chickens are known to be "flightier" or more easily triggered by fear-producing stimuli [23].

Abnormal Behaviors

Abnormal behaviors can result from any deviation from homeostasis. This may mean physical discomfort or disease, but it also refers to emotional distress. Backyard chickens do not suffer behavioral issues to the same extent as industry poultry or even companion birds, due to the prevalence to suitable environments for natural behaviors. Genetic selection may also be a factor [1]. Confined and/or environmentally deprived chickens are more likely to experience frustrations leading to increased aggression, displacement preening, stereotyped pacing, and other undesirable behaviors [1, 12, 23, 25]. Nevertheless, abnormal behaviors can occur in any flock and environmental and social factors that influence the emotional state of the chickens should be considered as part of any medical or behavioral treatment plan.

Behavioral Indicators of Illness

When assessing the health of a flock or individual chicken, the first step is to visually assess the birds. Healthy poultry stand with head up high, wings folded close to the body, and legs extended directly under their body [23] (Figure 22.26). Sick chickens often sit in the crouched position with their head drawn close to their body, eyes closed, and feathers appear ruffled or soiled. Healthy birds often readily respond to external stimuli by freezing with their head high, avoiding, or running away, whereas severely diseased birds are often unresponsive to external stimuli and do not attempt to run away [23]. Chickens have anywhere from 24 to 30 distinct calls or vocalizations that communicate a wide range of information from mating and nesting to distress and alarm [9, 22, 43]. There are calls to signal to intruders approaching a territory, as well as food locations and content emotional state [9, 22, 43]. Silence in a flock is concerning and often an indicator of illness or emotional distress (i.e. danger is perceived) [23].

Temperature regulation can induce specific behaviors. If hot, young chicks will avoid the heat source and pile in the corner of the pen or brooder [23] (Figure 22.27 and 22.28).

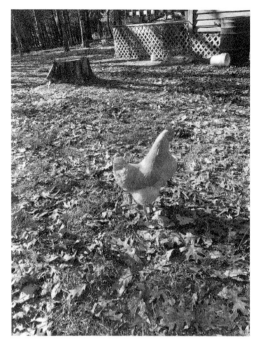

Figure 22.26 Normal healthy chicken posture.

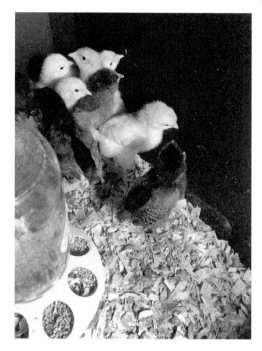

Figure 22.28 Week old chicks piled in the corner indicating they may be too warm.

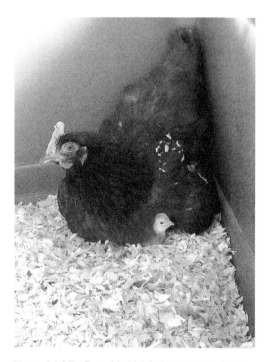

Figure 22.27 Day old chick being protected and kept warm by hen.

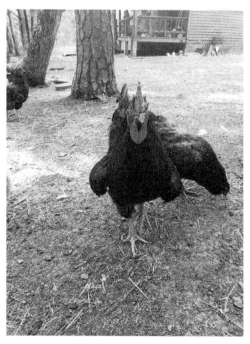

Figure 22.29 Wings drooping and panting indicating the bird is hot.

Conversely, if cold, chicks will huddle under the heat source. Adult chickens open-mouth breathe when hot, while holding drooped wings down and away from their body in an attempt to dissipate heat [23] (Figure 22.29). When hot, chickens may eat less and drink more water leading to watery stool [23]. Heat tolerance may vary by breed [23]. In cold temperatures, chickens may tuck their beak under their wing to keep warm [12].

Displacement Preening or Pecking

Feather pecking is an undesirable behavior that always indicates some suboptimal condition in the flock [23, 25, 44]. Additionally, feather pecking seems to "spread" through a flock either by social facilitation or observational learning. There may also be a genetic component to the behavior and evidence indicates feather peckers are more fearful than non-feather pecking birds [43]. A high density of birds can increase the incidence of this behavior along with lack of foraging opportunities or lack of foraging success (hard ground) [23, 44]. Considered a displacement behavior, excessive feather pecking is redirected ground pecking or preening behavior [23, 44]. Pecking trauma among chickens can result in fresh or dried blood on feathers, feather loss, abrasions, and lacerations [23, 44]. Young chicks may even peck at their own or flock mate's traumatized toes, or another chick's cloaca [23]. The location of trauma can be indicative of cause [23]. For instance, head and facial trauma in roosters often indicates fighting or male aggression, whereas feather loss and trauma to the nape of the neck and back can indicate excessive male mating behavior [23]. Mating behavior could be overt male aggression or damage inflected on the hen by the rooster during receptive lordosis posture [23].

Chickens often peck at individuals that look and/or act differently and this can be socially facilitated [23]. Often starting at the tail base, pecking, and feather loss can progress to the head and neck [23]. This type of pecking is eas-

ily learned from other birds and can be distressing to the targeted birds, especially if they are housed in such a way that they cannot escape [23]. Bright lights can stimulate feather picking therefore a reduction in the intensity of lights can decrease feather picking and cannibalism [23, 45]. Using red lighting has also been shown to reduce allo-pecking in layer facilitates, but the mechanism (e.g. masking sight of blood or general reduction in visual stimulation) has never been tested [45, 46]. In addition to changing the lighting, reducing the number of chickens in the flock, separation of birds, and increasing foraging and enrichment opportunities may reduce this behavior.

Vent Picking or Pecking

Vent picking or pecking, is pecking the vent, or cloacal area, of hens lying in the nest box with the head facing into the box and the tail or caudal area exposed [23]. When laying an egg, part of the cloaca can prolapse, especially in diseased or obese chickens [23]. The cloaca will usually invert almost immediately post-laying, but other birds may be attracted to the red color and peck at it [23]. This behavior may become habitual and spread in the flock [23]. It can also lead to cannibalism, which is a severe form of pecking that results in very damaging soft tissue injury and sometimes death. Just as with feather pecking, low light and reduced density can reduce the incidence of this behavior [23, 46, 47].

Floor Eggs and Egg Eating

Floor Eggs
Floor eggs, as the name suggests, are those eggs lain outside of the nest box and on the ground or litter. They are considered undesirable for human consumption because they appear dirty, broken, and are more susceptible to bacterial infections such as *Salmonella* [47]. Floor eggs result from inadequate number of boxes or perches [48]. Chicks reared without perches

may not know how to climb up to the nesting boxes [31].

Egg Eating

Chickens are omnivores and their normal diet consists of protein from a variety of sources, including their own eggs. Although egg eating is not a natural behavior per se, a bird may inadvertently break and open a conspecific egg, resulting in a good taste and positive reinforcement of subsequent egg consumption [47, 48]. Egg eating is best managed by preventing accidental breakage through collecting eggs as soon as they are laid and providing adequate nest space and litter [48, 49].

Chicken Welfare and Prevention of Problem Behaviors

Enrichment

Enrichment provides an animal the opportunity to perform species-specific behaviors to improve welfare and reduce stress. Outlets for prevalent normal behaviors such as foraging and dust bathing, as well as other activities that are mentally and physically stimulating should be considered. It may be necessary to add or subtract certain objects or interactions with humans, other species, and the same species to reduce stress but improve appropriate mental stimulation. For poultry, categories include social, environmental opportunities and resources, and sensory enrichment. Often all five senses are targeted to encourage exploration of the environment and provide choice of interactions.

Social Enrichment

Since chickens are flock animals and innately social, a flock of at least two (hens) is necessary. As discussed above, the optimal group size depends on the size of the area, distribution of resources, and sometimes temperament of the birds. Regular gentle handling by humans can facilitate future handling and

care [4]. Furthermore, positive reinforcement training can aid in cooperative care for husbandry procedures and be a great source of mental stimulation [50].

Sensory Enrichment

Providing any animal with objects to explore and manipulate can be an outlet for natural foraging behavior, reduce fearfulness, and provides the animal with behavioral choice in interacting with the environment. All of these can improve welfare. For chickens, great forms of mental enrichment include providing novel types of foods for pecking and consuming, along with swings and ladders for manipulation (Figures 22.30 and 22.31). Foods (e.g. corn on the cob, lettuce, squash, popcorn) hung on strings from the coop roof encourages foraging, exploration, and pecking, and can reduce stereotypical, agonistic, and other undesirable behaviors. Scattering food under bedding and substrate will encourage scratching, pecking, and other normal food seeking behaviors. In

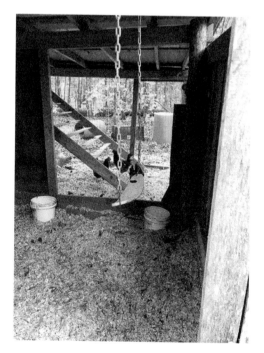

Figure 22.30 A child's swing as enrichment for chickens.

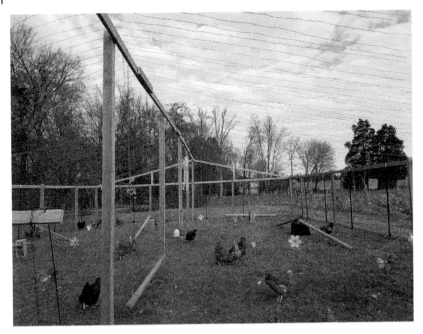

Figure 22.31 Examples of enrichment opportunities provided in this enclosure include swing perches, angled perches, elevated areas, colorful flowers, and multiple food and water dispensers.

addition, classical music has been shown to decrease fear and increase production in layer birds although not broiler chickens [51].

Conclusion

Chickens raised in a "backyard" setting often have few behavioral and welfare problems associated with industry raised chickens. However, it is critical for backyard flock owners and veterinarians to have a good understanding of normal chicken behavior and recognize abnormal behavioral issues in order to maintain the best health, production, and welfare for these birds.

References

1 Elkhoraibi, C., Blatchford, R.A., Pitesky, M.E. et al. (2014). Backyard chickens in the United States: a survey of flock owners. *Poult. Sci.* 93 (11): 2920–2931.

2 Crespo, R., Faux, C., Dhillon, S.A. et al. (2010). Pet poultry training for veterinary practitioners. *J. Vet. Med. Educ.* 37 (4): 383–387.

3 Dawkins, M.S. (1989). Time budgets in red junglefowl as a baseline for the assessment of welfare in domestic fowl. *Appl. Anim. Behav. Sci.* 24 (1): 77–80.

4 Eklund, B. and Jensen, P. (2011). Domestication effects on behavioural synchronization and individual distances in chickens (*Gallus gallus*). *Behav. Proc.* 86 (2): 250–256.

5 Eriksson, J., Larson, G., Gunnarsson, U. et al. (2008). Identification of the yellow skin gene reveals a hybrid origin of the domestic chicken. *PLos Genet.* 4 (2): e1000010.

6 Jensen, P., Schütz, K., and Lindqvist, C. (2002). Red jungle fowl have more

contrafreeloading than white leghorn layers: effect of food deprivation and consequences for information gain. *Behaviour* 139 (9): 1195–1209.

7 Katajamaa, R., Larsson, L.H., Lundberg, P. et al. (2018). Activity, social and sexual behaviour in Red Junglefowl selected for divergent levels of fear of humans. *PLoS One* 13 (9): e0204303.

8 Queiroz, S.A. and Cromberg, V.U. (2006). Aggressive behavior in the genus *Gallus* sp. *Braz. J. Poult. Sci.* 8 (1): 1–4.

9 Wood-Gush, D.G. (1955). The behaviour of the domestic chicken: a review of the literature. *Br. J. Anim. Behav.* 3 (3): 81–110.

10 Lewis, P.D. and Gous, R.M. (2009). Responses of poultry to ultraviolet radiation. *World's Poult. Sci. J.* 65 (3): 499–510.

11 Kram, Y.A., Mantey, S., and Corbo, J.C. (2010). Avian cone photoreceptors tile the retina as five independent, self-organizing mosaics. *PLoS One* 5 (2): e8992.

12 Nicol, C.J. (2015). The Behavioural Biology of Chickens. Boston: *C.A.B.* International.

13 Grier, J.B., Counter, S.A., and Shearer, W.M. (1967). Prenatal auditory imprinting in chickens. *Science* 155 (3770): 1692–1693.

14 Rumpf, M. and Tzschentke, B. (2010). Perinatal acoustic communication in birds: why do birds vocalize in the egg? *Open Ornithol. J.* 3 (1): 141–149.

15 Di Giorgio, E., Loveland, J.L., Mayer, U. et al. (2017). Filial responses as predisposed and learned preferences: early attachment in chicks and babies. *Behav. Brain Res.* 325: 90–104.

16 Karlsson, A.C., Jensen, P., Elgland, M. et al. (2010). Red junglefowl have individual body odors. *J. Exp. Biol.* 213 (10): 1619–1624.

17 Gentle, M.J., Waddington, D., Hunter, L.N. et al. (1990). Behavioural evidence for persistent pain following partial beak amputation in chickens. *Appl. Anim. Behav. Sci.* 27 (1): 149–157.

18 Freire, R., Eastwood, M.A., and Joyce, M. (2011). Minor beak trimming in chickens leads to loss of mechanoreception and

magnetoreception. *J. Anim. Sci.* 89 (4): 1201–1206.

19 Gentle, M.J. (2011). Pain issues in poultry. *Appl. Anim. Behav. Sci.* 135 (3): 252–258.

20 Marino, L. (2017). Thinking chickens: a review of cognition, emotion, and behavior in the domestic chicken. *Anim. Cogn.* 20 (2): 127–147.

21 Jaynes, J. (1957). Imprinting: The interaction of learned and innate behavior: II. The critical period. *J. Comp. Physiol. Psychol.* 50 (1): 6.

22 Nicol, C.J. (2004). Development, direction, and damage limitation: social learning in domestic fowl. *Anim. Learn. Behav.* 32 (1): 72–81.

23 Linares, J.A. and Martin, M. (2010). Poultry: Behavior and Welfare Assessment. In: *Encyclopedia of Animal Behavior*, M.J. Breed and J. Moore (eds.), 2: 750–756. Oxford: Academic Press.

24 Video showing clicker training of chickens. https://youtube/iZ-JnjBTkBw (accessed 19 June 2019).

25 Costa, L.S., Pereira, D.F., Bueno, L.G. et al. (2012). Some aspects of chicken behavior and welfare. *Braz. J. Poult. Sci.* 14 (3): 159–164.

26 Sherwin, C.M., Heyes, C.M., and Nicol, C.J. (2002). Social learning influences the preferences of domestic hens for novel food. *Anim. Behav.* 63 (5): 933–942.

27 Al-Rawi, B. and Craig, J.V. (1975). Agonistic behavior of caged chickens related to group size and area per bird. *Appl. Anim. Ethol.* 2 (1): 69–80.

28 Nicol, C. (2006). How animals learn from each other. *Appl. Anim. Behav. Sci.* 100 (1–2): 58–63.

29 Craig, J.V. and Bhagwat, A.L. (1974). Agonistic and mating behavior of adult chickens modified by social and physical environments. *Appl. Anim. Ethol.* 1 (1): 57–65.

30 Martin, C.D. and Mullens, B.A. (2012). Housing and dustbathing effects on northern fowl mites (*Ornithonyssus sylviarum*) and chicken body lice (*Menacanthus stramineus*) on hens. *Med. Vet. Entomol.* 26 (3): 323–333.

31 Barnett, J.L., Tauson, R., Downing, J.A. et al. (2009). The effects of a perch, dust bath, and nest box, either alone or in combination as used in furnished cages, on the welfare of laying hens. *Poult. Sci.* 88 (3): 456–470.

32 Muiruri, H.K., Harrison, P.C., and Gonyou, H.W. (1990). Preferences of hens for shape and size of roosts. *Appl. Anim. Behav. Sci.* 27 (1): 141–147.

33 Siegel, P.B. (1984). The role of behavior in poultry production: a review of research. *Appl. Anim. Ethol.* 11 (4): 299–316.

34 https://thepoultrysite.com/articles/natural-mating-and-breeding. (accessed 27 May 2019).

35 Knight, P.G., Wilson, S.C., Gladwell, R.T. et al. (1984). Hypothalamic contents of LHRH and catecholamines during the ovulatory cycle of the hen (*Gallus domesticus*). *J. Reprod. Fertil.* 71 (1): 289–295.

36 Zimmerman, P.H., Koene, P., and van Hooff, J.A. (2000). Thwarting of behaviour in different contexts and the gakel-call in the laying hen. *Appl. Anim. Behav. Sci.* 69 (4): 255–264.

37 Ahn, D.U., Kim, S.M., and Shu, H. (1997). Effect of egg size and strain and age of hens on the solids content of chicken eggs. *Poult. Sci.* 76 (6): 914–919.

38 Appleby, M.C. and McRae, H.E. (1986). The individual nest box as a super-stimulus for domestic hens. *Appl. Anim. Behav. Sci.* 15 (2): 169–176.

39 Edgar, J.L., Paul, E.S., and Nicol, C.J. (2013). Protective mother hens: cognitive influences on the avian maternal response. *Anim. Behav.* 86 (2): 223–229.

40 Sharp, P.J., Macnamee, M.C., Sterling, R.J. et al. (1988). Relationships between prolactin, LH and broody behaviour in bantam hens. *J. Endocrinol.* 118 (2): 279–286.

41 Savory, C.J., Wood-Gush, D.G., and Duncan, I.J. (1978). Feeding behaviour in a population of domestic fowls in the wild. *Appl. Anim. Ethol.* 4 (1): 13–27.

42 Bruno, L.D., Maiorka, A., Macari, M. et al. (2011). Water intake behavior of broiler chickens exposed to heat stress and drinking from bell or and nipple drinkers. *Braz. J. Poult. Sci.* 13 (2): 147–152.

43 Collias, N.E. (1987). The vocal repertoire of the red junglefowl: a spectrographic classification and the code of communication. *Condor* 89: 510–524.

44 Wysocki, M., Bessei, W., Kjaer, J.B. et al. (2010). Genetic and physiological factors influencing feather pecking in chickens. *World's Poult. Sci. J.* 66 (4): 659–672.

45 D'eath, R.B. and Stone, R.J. (1999). Chickens use visual cues in social discrimination: an experiment with coloured lighting. *Appl. Anim. Behav. Sci.* 62 (2–3): 233–242.

46 Broom, D.M. and Fraser, A.F. (2015). Domestic Animal Behaviour and Welfare, 5e, 260. Boston, MA: CAB International.

47 Cepero, R. and Hernándiz, A. (2015). Effects of housing systems for laying hens on egg quality and safety. In: 16th European Symposium on the Quality of Eggs and Egg Products, 1–18. Nantes, France.

48 https://extension.psu.edu/prevention-of-egg-eating-in-chickens. (accessed 27 May 2019).

49 https://poultry.extension.org/articles/poultry-behavior/egg-eating-by-chickens-in-small-and-backyard-flocks/. (accessed 27 May 2019).

50 Hazel, S.J., O'Dwyer, L., and Ryan, T. (2015). "Chickens are a lot smarter than I originally thought": changes in student attitudes to chickens following a chicken training class. *Animals* 5 (3): 821–837.

51 Dávila, S.G., Campo, J.L., Gil, M.G. et al. (2011). Effects of auditory and physical enrichment on 3 measurements of fear and stress (tonic immobility duration, heterophil to lymphocyte ratio, and fluctuating asymmetry) in several breeds of layer chicks. *Poult. Sci.* 90 (11): 2459–2466.

Section 5

Diagnosis of Disease

23

Euthanasia
Cheryl B. Greenacre

Avian and Zoological Medicine Service, Department of Small Animal Clinical Sciences, College of Veterinary Medicine, University of Tennessee, Knoxville, TN, USA

Introduction

The American Veterinary Medical Association publishes guidelines titled "AVMA Guidelines for the Euthanasia of Animals" that veterinarians should follow and consult for any activity that involves euthanasia. The guidelines can be accessed at https://www.avma.org/KB/Policies/Documents/euthanasia.pdf [1]. The most recent version was published in 2013 and is updated on a regular basis. This new, expanded version is 102 pages long and includes sections on species that were not addressed in earlier versions, such as how to handle animals before and during euthanasia, veterinary medical ethics, pre-euthanasia techniques, human behavior during euthanasia of an animal, and disposal of carcasses. It also includes an avian section pertaining to pet birds, aviary birds, and birds used in falconry, racing, zoos, and educational facilities. The new guidelines emphasize evidence-based medicine and research, but unfortunately in the area of euthanasia of birds, there is little, if any, research or evidence-based medicine published compared to that for mammals. What scientific literature is available pertains to chickens in a commercial environment, otherwise it is anecdotal information [2–17].

There are separate sections in the guidelines for wild birds under "Captive and Free-ranging Nondomestic Animals."

Another document offering guidelines for euthanasia of poultry is from the Canadian Poultry Industry Council, titled "Practical Guidelines for On-Farm Euthanasia of Poultry, 2nd edition, 2016." This can be found at https://www.poultryindustrycouncil.ca/wp-content/uploads/2016/08/PIC-Practical-Guidelines-for-On-Farm-Euthanasia-of-Poultry.pdf. It has very detailed photographs for step-by-step demonstration of euthanasia techniques and follows the "AVMA Guidelines for the Euthanasia of Animals."

For birds raised for food, there is a separate document, titled "AVMA Guidelines for the Humane Slaughter of Animals: 2016 Edition." For birds that need to be depopulated rapidly to protect animals and/or humans in extraordinary circumstances such as a natural disaster, hazardous zoonotic disease outbreak, terrorist activity, or radiological incident, there is a separate document, titled "AVMA Guidelines for the Depopulation of Animals: 2019 Edition." These last two documents are completely separate from the euthanasia document and can be accessed, respectively, at https://www.avma.

Backyard Poultry Medicine and Surgery: A Guide for Veterinary Practitioners, Second Edition.
Edited by Cheryl B. Greenacre and Teresa Y. Morishita.
© 2021 John Wiley & Sons, Inc. Published 2021 by John Wiley & Sons, Inc.
Companion website: www.wiley.com/go/greenacre/medicine

org/KB/Resources/Reference/AnimalWelfare/Documents/Humane-Slaughter-Guidelines.pdf, and https://www.avma.org/KB/Policies/documents/AVMA-Guidelines-for-the-Depopulation-of-Animals.pdf

Some peer-reviewed reports are available in the literature regarding euthanasia of individual or small groups of birds, but most of the information consists of anecdotal reports in book chapters, guidelines from various associations, journal roundtable discussions, and editorials. The method of euthanasia depends on species, size, anatomic and physiologic characteristics, environment, degree of domestication, clinical state, and anticipated and actual response to restraint. People performing the euthanasia should be knowledgeable about what is normal behavior for a bird compared to what is considered a stressed or fearful bird and handle the bird appropriately to reduce stress before and during euthanasia.

According to the 2013 AVMA Guidelines for Euthanasia, acceptable methods of euthanasia of birds include injection of a sodium pentobarbital euthanasia solution IV with or without the bird being unconscious or under anesthesia, or intracoelomic, intracardiac, or intraosseous injection of a sodium pentobarbital euthanasia solution while unconscious or under anesthesia. Anesthesia is defined as either halothane, isoflurane, or sevoflurane with or without nitrous oxide. Acceptable methods of euthanasia of birds with conditions include inhalant anesthetics alone at high concentrations (isoflurane, sevoflurane, halothane with or without nitrous oxide), carbon dioxide (>40%), carbon monoxide, nitrogen, argon, and the physical methods including cervical dislocation (preferably <200 g), decapitation (preferably <200 g), gunshot (field conditions), and the following only as a secondary methods if unconscious or under anesthesia: potassium chloride, exsanguination, and thoracic compression. Realize that barbiturate salts are alkaline and irritating and that intracoelomic injections are irritating, especially if they inadvertently get into an air sac. Also realize that intraosseous injections should not be given in pneumatic bones such as the femur or humerus because these are lined with respiratory epithelium and connect to the respiratory tract.

What I Do in Practice

Some poultry owners consider their birds as part of the family, while others consider them production animals (Figure 23.1). No matter the use of the animal, in practice I always render the bird unconscious prior to euthanasia, usually by mask induction with isoflurane gas anesthesia while holding it gently wrapped in a towel. One could also use sevoflurane gas anesthesia or an injectable anesthetic such as ketamine/xylazine or ketamine/dexmedetomidine. Sometimes, a pre-anesthetic agent is given 15–30 min prior to anesthetic induction using butorphanol or midazolam. Once the bird is unconscious, I draw at least 3 ml of blood from the right jugular vein and place in a serum separator tube to store for later serological testing. Then an overdose of sodium

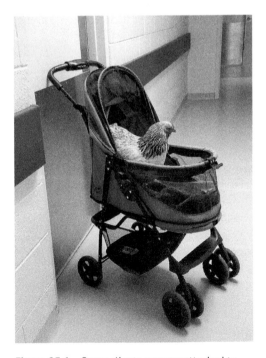

Figure 23.1 Some clients are very attached to their backyard poultry and consider them part of the family. It is not uncommon for poultry to arrive at our hospital in strollers.

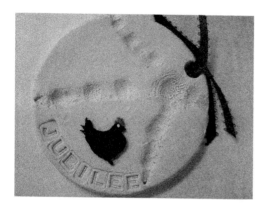

Figure 23.2 A claw paw made for the owner by imprinting the foot of the bird in the clay material, which is later baked and then sent to the owner along with a sympathy card.

pentobarbital is given intravenously in the right jugular vein. Check for cessation of heartbeat with a stethoscope. We offer a clay paw imprint of the foot for the owner, and if the owner allows, we strongly encourage a full necropsy with histopathology (Figure 23.2). Commonly we send a sympathy card.

Overview of Methods

Acceptable

Intravenous (IV) injection with an injectable euthanasia agent (such as sodium pentobarbital) is the quickest and most reliable means of euthanizing birds when it can be performed without causing undue stress. Most birds get stressed with handling so I personally prefer to gently restrain them in a towel while mask inducing with isoflurane or sevoflurane with or without prior sedation with midazolam given intramuscularly (IM) or intranasally (IN) 15–30 minutes prior to induction. Other sedatives can be used.

Acceptable with Conditions

The guidelines are clear to state that "Methods acceptable with conditions are equivalent to acceptable methods when all criteria for application of a method are met."

Inhaled Anesthetics

Birds given high concentrations of inhaled gas anesthetics lose consciousness rapidly and then death occurs after they are rendered unconscious. The condition is that a high concentration of gas be used and the restraint cause little to no stress. This method usually induces minimal tissue damage in case a necropsy is needed.

Carbon Dioxide

Birds require comparatively high (>40%) concentrations of carbon dioxide to induce anesthesia followed by loss of consciousness. There is much scientific literature available on the use of carbon dioxide for the use of euthanasia of chickens, ducks, and turkeys. It is important that the application rate of carbon dioxide is just right so that the increase in carbon dioxide is rapid enough to have a short time to loss of posture and unconsciousness, but slow enough that there is less aversion or reaction to the gas. Even though birds are unconscious, they tend to flap with carbon dioxide and this can damage (bruise) tissue if needed for necropsy (Figure 23.3).

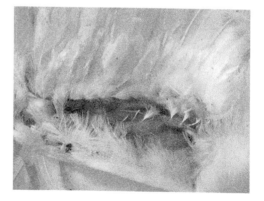

Figure 23.3 Subcutaneous bruising on the ventral surface of the left wing (antebrachium) of a white Leghorn chicken euthanized with carbon dioxide. The elbow is on the right and the carpus is on the left. Performed properly, carbon dioxide euthanasia renders the birds unconscious prior to death and therefore not feeling pain, although they flap, which is disconcerting to the observer and can cause tissue damage.

Carbon Monoxide

Not generally used in clinical settings due to risk to personnel.

Argon and Nitrogen

Not generally used in clinical settings due to availability.

Cervical Dislocation

Sometimes the cervical dislocation is needed in a field situation, say an emergency at an aviary or flock setting. Cervical dislocation is typically performed in birds that are <200 g but has been described in birds as large as 2.3 kg. Acceptable with the condition that the person performing the cervical dislocation is experienced in performing the procedure. Experience in technique can be gained by practicing on birds that have been freshly euthanized by another humane method for other purposes. Cervical dislocation must result in luxation at the first cervical vertebra from the skull and must not result in primary crushing of the vertebrae or spinal cord [1] (Figure 23.4).

Decapitation

Again, sometimes in a field situation, may need to use this method. Again, decapitation is typically done in birds that are <200 g but has been described in birds as large as 3.5 kg. Acceptable

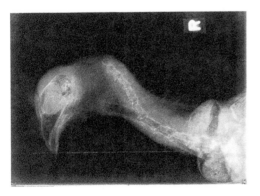

Figure 23.4 Radiograph of an 18-week-old culled production chicken that had cervical dislocation performed by mechanical, rather than manual, means. Cervical dislocation should result in luxation between the first cervical vertebra and the skull.

with the condition that the person performing the decapitation is experienced in performing the procedure and the device used is very sharp and kept in good working order. One study showed that visual evoked responses were present up to 30 seconds after decapitation.

Gunshot

Not used in a clinical setting due to obvious dangers to personnel, and other, better methods are available.

Adjunctive Methods

Adjunctive methods are those methods that can be used *only* if the bird is unconscious and anesthetized prior to their use, and include IV or intracardiac potassium chloride, exsanguination, or thoracic compression. These methods are unacceptable if performed in a conscious bird. Exsanguination is useful if the blood is needed for further testing in the bird.

Unacceptable

In the conscious bird. it is unacceptable to perform thoracic compression, exsanguinate, or administer potassium chloride.

Eggs

Bird embryos that are >80% through incubation should be euthanized by above acceptable methods or acceptable with conditions methods including anesthetic overdose, decapitation, or prolonged (>20 minutes) exposure to carbon dioxide. Eggs that are less than 80% through incubation can be destroyed by prolonged (>20 minutes) exposure to carbon dioxide, cooling (< 4° C for 4 hours), freezing, or egg addling.

Disposal of Body/Carcass

Ensure proper disposal of an animal's remains to avoid environmental contamination and human and animal exposure to disease or drug residues. Disposal of remains must be conducted in accord with all federal, state, and local regulations.

References

1 AVMA Guidelines for the Euthanasia of Animals: 2020 Edition. https://www.avma.org/KB/Policies/Documents/euthanasia.pdf (accessed 1 January 2021).

2 Bennett, R.A. (2001). AAV opposes thoracic compression. *J. Am. Vet. Med. Assoc.* 218 (8): 1262.

3 Blackshaw, J.K., Fenwick, D.C., Beattie, A.W., and Allan, D.J. (1998). The behavior of chickens, mice and rats during euthanasia with chloroform, carbon dioxide and ether. *Lab. Anim.* 22 (1): 67–75.

4 Close, B., Banister, K., Baumans, V. et al. (1996). Recommendations for euthanasia of experimental animals: part 1. *Lab. Anim.* 30: 293–316.

5 Close, B., Banister, K., Baumans, V. et al. (1997). Recommendations for euthanasia of experimental animals: part 2. *Lab. Anim.* 31: 1–32.

6 Coenen, A.M.L., Lankhaar, J., Lowe, J.C., and McKeegan, D.E.F. (2009). Remote monitoring of electroencephalogram, electrocardiogram, and behavior during controlled atmosphere stunning in broilers: implications for welfare. *Poult. Sci.* 88 (1): 10–19.

7 Erasmus, M.A., Lawlis, P., Duncan, I.J., and Widowski, T.M. (2010). Using time to insensibility and estimated time of death to evaluate a nonpenetrating captive bolt, cervical dislocation, and blunt trauma for on-farm killing of turkeys. *Poult. Sci.* 89 (7): 1345–1354.

8 Franson, J.C. (1999). Euthanasia. In: Field Manual of Wildlife Diseases. General Field Procedures and diseases of birds (eds. M. Friend and J.C. Franson), 49–51. Washington, D.C., BRD Information and Technology Report: US Geological Survey, Biological Resources Division.

9 Gregory, N.G. and Wotton, S.B. (1990). Comparison of neck dislocation and percussion of the head on visual evoked responses in the chicken's brain. *Vet. Rec.* 126 (23): 570–572.

10 Hess, L. (Assoc ed.) (2005). Euthanasia techniques in birds – roundtable discussion. *J. Avian Med. Surg.* 19 (3): 242–245.

11 Ludders, J.W. (2001). Another reader opposing thoracic compression for avian euthanasia. *J. Am. Vet. Med. Assoc.* 218 (11): 1721.

12 Mason, C., Spence, J., Bilbe, L. et al. (2009). Methods for dispatching backyard poultry. *Vet. Rec.* 164 (7): 220.

13 Miller, E.A. (ed.) (2000). Minimum Standards for Wildlife Rehabilitation, 3e. St. Cloud, MN: National Wildlife Rehabilitators Association, (Sec.7.3), 77 pages. 4. Euthanasia of nonconventional species: zoo, wild, aquatic, and ectothermic animals.

14 Fair, J.E. (ed.). (2010). Guidelines to the Use of Wild Birds in Research. Washington, D.C., Ornithological Council.

15 Orosz, S.B. (2006). Guidelines for Euthanasia of Nondomestic Animals, 46–49. American Association of Zoo Veterinarians.

16 Raj, A.B.M. (1996). Aversive reactions to argon, carbon dioxide and a mixture of carbon dioxide and argon. *Vet. Rec.* 138 (24): 592–593.

17 Raj, A.B.M. (2006). Recent developments in stunning and slaughter of poultry. *World's Poult. Sci. J.* 62: 462–484.

24

Egg Diagnostics

Teresa Y. Morishita[1], Josep Rutllant-Labeaga[1] and Darrin Karcher[2]

[1]*College of Veterinary Medicine, Western University of Health Sciences, Pomona, CA, USA*
[2]*Department of Animal Science, Purdue University, West Lafayette, IN, USA*

The most common reason for backyard flock owners to seek assistance on egg diagnostics is the egg's failure to hatch to a viable chick. Another reason could be that the egg appears unaesthetic and is deemed inedible by the flock owner.

Failure to Hatch

The egg can fail to hatch as a result of internal factors, such as poor hen nutrition; or external factors, such as incorrect incubation temperature and humidity [1]. In these cases, the egg is fertile but is unable to hatch as a result of internal or external factors. Hence, the first step in investigating why an egg does not hatch is determining if it was a fertile egg to begin with.

Egg Formation

Formation of an egg has been extensively documented and in-depth reviews for further reading include King and McLelland (1984), Burley and Vadehra (1989), or Whittow (2000) [2–4]. The egg is a complete source of nutrients for the developing chick. It takes approximately 24–28 hours to produce an egg. In the chicken, egg production is initiated when a mature ovum is released into the infundibulum, the first portion of the hen's oviduct [5] (Figure 24.1a). This process starts at the ovary. The mature avian ovary is composed of finger-like stalked projections or follicles (Figure 17.1b), each one of which has a single layer of granulosa cells surrounding the primary oocyte. The structure of the ovary resembles a bunch of grapes, with each individual grape being a follicle. The primary oocyte of the chicken can expand its cytoplasm considerably, reaching approximately 30 mm diameter, to accumulate the proteins and lipids that form the yolk. The surrounding stromal tissues of the follicles, the well-vascularized theca interna and theca externa, rearrange toward the time of ovulation to leave a vascular-free area called the stigma (Figure 24.1b). The stigma ruptures during ovulation, and the oocyte with the surrounding granulose cells leaves the follicle. If some vessels are still present and rupture at the time of ovulation, blood spots can be observed on the yolk. The remaining thecal cells of the follicle do not transform into a corpus hemorrhagicum or corpus luteum as in mammals.

In the process of forming an egg, the egg spends approximately 15–30 minutes in the

Backyard Poultry Medicine and Surgery: A Guide for Veterinary Practitioners, Second Edition.
Edited by Cheryl B. Greenacre and Teresa Y. Morishita.
© 2021 John Wiley & Sons, Inc. Published 2021 by John Wiley & Sons, Inc.
Companion website: www.wiley.com/go/greenacre/medicine

infundibulum (Figure 24.1a), a short period of time to synthesize and incorporate a significant number of layers. External layers of the yolk membrane and the chalaziferous layer are produced primarily in the caudal portion of the infundibulum. In addition, the ovum is fertilized in this portion of the oviduct if viable sperm is present in the sperm glands.

After leaving the infundibulum, the ovum then enters the portion of the oviduct known as the magnum (Figure 24.1a), which has an abundance of mucus-secreting glandular cells. The transit time in the magnum is about three hours. During this time, approximately 50% of the total albumen is produced and appears homogeneous and dense in nature, although both dense and thin albumen are formed. Hence, differentiation between dense (thick) and thin albumen results from the addition of water occurring after the egg leaves the magnum. The thick portion is added first

and is the closest to the yolk [5]. It provides most of the protein for the developing embryo. In addition, white rope-like structures known as chalazae form at both poles of the egg (Figure 24.2). Diseases such as infectious bronchitis can make the dense albumen thin. In chickens that are affected, the thick egg white becomes thin and runny, so the lack of a thick egg white is noticeable [6–8].

The main function of the next segment of the oviduct, the isthmus (Figure 24.1a), is the synthesis and addition of the shell membranes. Before the shell membranes are completed more water is added "plumping" the already existing albumen and further differentiating the two albumen types, thick and thin. The whole process takes approximately one to two hours to be completed.

The egg remains in the uterus, where the eggshell is formed, for most of the time (around 20 hours) (Figure 24.1a). During the first three

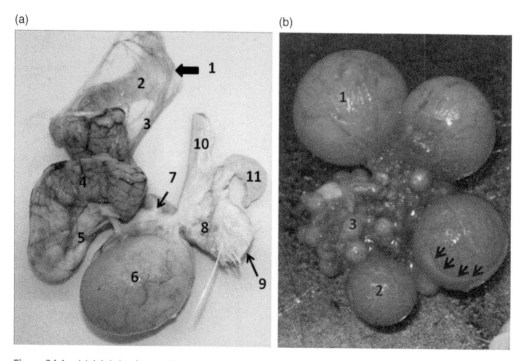

(a)　　　　　　　　　　　　　(b)

Figure 24.1 (a) Adult hen's reproductive tract: 1. infundibular openning (ostium abdominale); 2. infundibulum; 3. ventral suspensory ligament; 4. magnum; 5. isthmus; 6. uterus (shell gland) containing a calcified egg; 7. vagina; 8. cloaca; 9. vent; 10. colorectum; 11. regressed right ovary. (b). Adult hen's ovary with follicles at different stages of development (1: mature - 3: immature). Notice the area (arrows) without vascular blood supply corresponding to the stigma. *Source:* Pictures courtesy of Drs. Wael Khamas and Josep Rutllant.

to five hours, the organic matrix is formed and in the following 15–16 hour phase, calcium is deposited to form the inorganic substance consisting of more than 95% of crystallized calcium carbonate. The most common source of the calcium for eggshell production is intestinal absorption when dietary calcium levels are adequate. Alternative sources may come from mobilization of bone calcium stores and renal reabsorption. If there is inadequate calcium in the diet, hens may lay shell-less eggs or no eggs. Often, hens that are unable to obtain calcium from the diet extract calcium from their own bones, leading to disorders such as cage layer fatigue or osteomalacia. The color of the eggshell depends on the breed of chicken. It is interesting to note that, in general, chickens with red earlobes tend to lay brown eggs and those with white earlobes tend to lay white eggs [5]. The exceptions are those breeds such as the Araucana that lay greenish-colored eggs. The eggshell coloration depends on the presence of pigments (brown-red) such as porphyrins, a byproduct of hemoglobin.

Finally, the egg's transit through the vagina takes seconds to a few minutes and the secretions produced in this segment of the oviduct may contribute to the formation of the cuticle. The cuticle can be easily rubbed off, so gentle egg handling is necessary to avoid its removal. Finally, the egg passes through the cloaca and is laid (Figure 24.1a).

Normal Egg Anatomy

The fully formed chicken egg consists of four main parts: *Germinal disc, yolk, albumen with chalaza, and shell* [9–11]. The germinal disk (also known as the blastodisc, or, if fertilized, the blastoderm) is a circular structure of approximately 3–4 mm in diameter located on the surface to the yolk and is white-gray in color (Figures 24.2 and 24.3a–b). It contains the remnant of the oocyte nucleus while the cytoplasm is an extremely thin layer that covers the rest of the surface of the yolk. The yolk is suspended in the center of the egg by the chalaza. The yolk (vitellus) consists mainly of lipoproteins and phosphoproteins arranged in concentric layers (Figure 24.2). Depending on the content of protein and lipids, it can be distinguished into alternating yellow and white layers of the yolk but cannot be visually

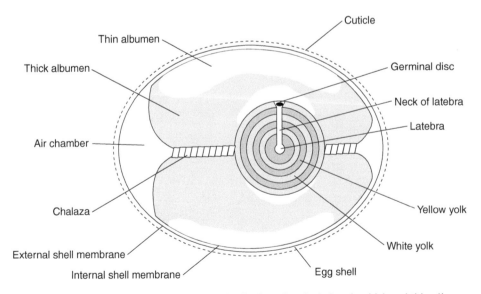

Figure 24.2 Diagram of a hen's egg in a longitudinal section depicting the thick and thin albumen surrounding the yolk, with the chalzae rope-like structures at both ends of the yolk.

(a)

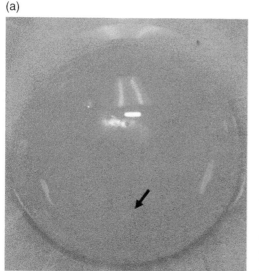

(b)

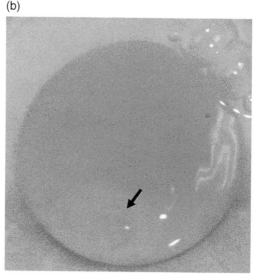

Figure 24.3 (a) Egg yolks from non-fertilized and (b) fertilized eggs. The arrows show the germinal disc or blastodisc (a) and blastoderm (b).

observed. The innermost central nucleus of white vitellus is known as the latebra and is connected to the germinal disk through the neck of the latebra. The main function of the yolk is to nurture the developing embryo.

The yolk membrane is the thinnest of all egg layers but could present the principal barrier for fertilization. It is composed of four different layers that can only be distinguished with electron microscopy: (i) plasma membrane (plasmalemma) of the oocyte; (ii) perivitelline membrane or lamina (also known as inner layer of vitelline membrane); (iii) continuous membrane or lamina; and (iv) extravitelline membrane or lamina (also known as the outer layer of vitelline membrane) [12]. The first two layers are produced by the oocyte and the granulosa cells while still in the ovary as a follicle. The last two layers are produced as the eggs pass through the infundibulum. The yolk membrane is the barrier between the yolk and the albumen but allows for the movement of water and electrolytes.

The albumen (or egg white) is the main component surrounding the yolk. Although it is described as having less structure than the yolk, two different regions can be identified;

thick (dense) and thin (liquid) albumen (Figure 24.2), depending on the proportion of water and protein (ovomucin) [2]. Thick albumen has a higher quantity of ovomucin than thin albumen and consequently has more internal structure. The chalazae are parts of the dense albumen that fix the yolk to the egg poles. They are made of twisted strands of ovomucin fibers arranged in a spiral as a result of the rotation of the egg while it descends in the oviduct. The thin albumen contains mucin with less fibrous arrangement, and consequently less structural scaffold, giving an appearance of higher fluidity. The inner layer of the thin albumen is attached to the yolk and the outer layer is in contact with the shell membrane, but only at the egg poles. The main functions of the albumen are to mechanically protect the embryo with a soft environment and nurture the embryo with a good source of protein.

The shell membranes are two thin, pliable but strong membranes, composed mainly of several layers of protein fibers (Figure 24.2). It is only at the egg poles that the inner shell membrane is fused with the dense albumen. In the other regions of the egg, the inner shell membrane is in contact with the thin albumen. The inner shell membrane is firmly attached to the outer shell membrane, which in turn is also tightly attached to the eggshell. A few minutes after the egg is laid, and as it cools down, the internal and external membranes detach at the blunt pole creating the air cell. During the process of embryo development, the head of the embryo lies adjacent to this air cell (Figure 24.2). Being aware of egg anatomy will assist in egg culture techniques.

Finally, the eggshell is mainly composed of two basic parts: The organic matrix and the inorganic interstitial substance, which is composed of inorganic salts. Both parts are interrelated and intermingled. The organic matrix is the primary biological layer and is composed of a meshwork of fine fibers of different arrangements infiltrated with calcite crystals. The eggshell has microscopic pores all over the surface, which open into pore canals that end at the level of the outer surface of the outer shell membrane. This passageway from external surface to shell membrane is the reason why egg membranes may need to be cultured, as it may provide clues as to the hygienic condition of egg management. These pores are covered and plugged by the cuticle, the outermost organic layer of the egg (Figure 24.2). The cuticle is an extremely thin proteinaceous layer, which is permeable to gases [13]. It is generally recommended to only lightly brush off any organic debris from eggs, rather than washing them, to prevent damage to the cuticle. If eggs are to be cleaned then it is recommended to use water that is warmer, specifically 20 °F (11 °C) warmer, than the egg so that contaminants are not drawn into the egg via vacuum action through the pores in the shell [14].

Fertile and Nonfertile Eggs

From external appearances, one cannot tell if an egg is infertile or fertile. Chickens lay eggs whether they are fertile or infertile. The only way to determine whether a newly laid egg is fertile is to crack it open. An infertile egg only has a white-gray dot on the surface of the egg yolk (Figure 24.3a). This area is called the blastoderm. A fertile egg has a white donut-like structure with a white-gray dot in the center on the yolk surface (Figure 24.3a). This structure is the blastoderm, the developing chick. Fertility rates are normally deemed to be the number of fertile eggs laid over a period of time when compared to all eggs laid during that same time period. It is not practical to determine the fertility rate of backyard poultry, as the only way to determine this is to open eggs up. This practice contradicts the backyard owner's goal of hatching new chicks [15]. Hence, for veterinarians faced with questions of hen fertility, the best recommendation is to incubate all potentially hatchable eggs. If fertility determination is needed, flock owners need to know that eggs will need to be sacrificed and opened.

Maximizing Egg Fertility

Backyard flock owners may want to develop their own genetic lines or breeds and they can use artificial insemination to breed their chickens. As mentioned previously, chickens have the ability to store viable sperm in the sperm glands that line the infundibulum. While sperm can live for prolonged periods in this gland, specifically 7–14 days in chickens and 40–50 days in turkeys, the probability of hens laying fertile eggs declines after five to seven days [16]. To guarantee a high percentage of fertile eggs, it would be better to allow hens and roosters to mate naturally. This is more commonly seen in backyard flocks in which the sexes are mixed. The ideal ratio of roosters to hens is one rooster to five to seven hens [15]. This ensures a high rate of fertile eggs. Although this is an ideal ratio in a backyard flock, one additional factor that should be considered is if the flock only has only one rooster. Flocks that have a single rooster have more behavioral problems. A single rooster in a flock tends to be more aggressive to its human caretakers and this may be a problem for owners with young children, as the rooster may attack its human caretakers [15]. Hence, in small flock situations where fertile eggs are needed, it is highly recommended that two roosters are added to the flock with some additional hens so that the roosters can establish a pecking order of their own rather than with their human caretakers.

Hatching Fertile Eggs

If potentially fertile eggs are laid, the next step is to incubate the eggs. Eggs are unique in that they can be laid fertile and the developing chick can remain in suspended animation until incubation, during which time the developing chick can continue its development. Once development starts, it must continue until hatching or the developing embryo will die. The only time that chick development can be delayed is the point at which the fertile egg is laid but has not yet been incubated [15]. Poultry breeders have utilized this unique feature of chick development to hold newly laid eggs under refrigerated temperatures until a batch is laid, at which time all eggs are incubated to ensure synchronous hatching of a large batch of chicks. If you are storing hatching eggs, they should be held at 55–65 °F (13–18 °C) and at a humidity ranging from 80 to 90% with the large end of the egg facing upwards. Hatchability will decrease if eggs are stored longer than seven days [15]. Depending on the type of incubator and the number of eggs, if the goal is to hatch as many as possible, then the eggs should probably be incubated soon after laying. When eggs are placed in an incubator, it is ideal to mark the date of lay or the expected day of hatch in pencil on the eggshell to ensure that it is incubated for the appropriate time period for that species [15].

Incubation of Eggs

When incubating hatching eggs, four factors need to be in alignment in order to successfully hatch a chick. These four factors include temperature, humidity, ventilation, and egg position [15]. The temperature for incubation can vary depending on the type of incubator: "Still" air versus "forced" air. A "still" air incubator does not have an internal fan to circulate the air; therefore, a temperature of 102 °F (39 °C) is required. A "forced" air incubator contains an internal fan to circulate the air and the ideal temperature is 99.5 °F (37.5 °C). In either type of incubator, the temperature should be constant and uniform. Humidity at 60% for the first 18 days of life is ideal, increasing to 70% for the last three days of hatch [17, 18]. Humidity is very important because if there is not enough humidity, chicks can become entrapped in the dehydrated shell membranes and cannot hatch out of the egg. If they are able to hatch out, the chick will be very exhausted and stressed. Ventilation is required as the embryo develops because oxygen is needed for the developing chick. For this factor, it is recommended that flock owners follow the manufacturers' recommendation for the particular incubator used. Eggs are usually rotated at least five times a day to prevent the yolk from sticking to the shell and hindering chick development. The incubation time varies per poultry species (Table 24.1) [17, 18]. It should be noted that waterfowl require a higher level of humidity compared to chickens.

Table 24.1 Incubation times of common poultry species.

Species	Incubation period
Chickens	21 d
Turkeys	26–28 d
Pheasant	22–23 d
Quail	23–24 d
Peafowl	27–28 d
Guinea Fowl	26–30 d
Duck	28 d
Muscovy Duck	33–35 d
Goose	29–31 d
Swan	42 d

Source: Hayes, C. [17], Schwartz, D.L. [18].

Chick Embryo Development

Normal chicken development inside the egg is a complex process that needs to be understood in order to identify possible causes of malformations, lack of development, or embryo mortality during incubation. Historically, the chicken embryo was one of the first embryos studied and described because the eggs were easily available, and the incubation conditions were not difficult to mimic [19]. By cutting a small window in the eggshell and covering it with glass, the formation of an embryo could be directly observed. Under normal conditions, it takes 21–22 days to develop a live chick (1 day in the oviduct and 20–21 days in the nest or incubator). The first step occurs in the infundibulum with the fertilization of the ovum or germinal disk (haploid) by the sperm (haploid), which forms the zygote (single diploid cell) [20]. The zygote undergoes a series of cell divisions at the level of the isthmus and becomes the blastoderm or embryo. The process of cell division or embryonic development is temporarily interrupted during the laying process and is resumed to completion once the temperature increases again during natural brooding or artificial incubation. When the temperature of the egg is below 68 °F(20 °C), the embryo becomes quiescent and development stops. However, if temperature reaches 68 °F (20 °C) or above, embryonic activity starts again. The best time to store viable fertilized eggs that are placed in cool storage below 68 °F (20 °C) is as soon as possible after collection. Once in the incubator, the temperature must be controlled within very close parameters (optimal temperature 99.5 °F [37.5 °C]) and oscillations should be avoided for normal embryo development and maximum viability results.

All the cells in the blastoderm divide in a single monolayer on top of the yolk and create a central zone known as the *area pellucida* (clear area) and a marginal area known as the *area opaca*. The cells in the *area pellucida* divide faster, creating a superimposed number of layers that become the ectoderm (outer or upper-most), mesoderm (middle), and endoderm (deeper or inner-most) [21, 22]. The major body parts that are formed from these three initial embryonic layers are

1) **ectoderm:** Nervous system, epidermis, and its derivates (feathers, beak, claws) and some of the skeletal and connective tissue of the head;
2) **mesoderm:** Muscles and skeletal tissues, reproductive, urinary, and circulatory (heart and vessels) systems;
3) **endoderm:** Lining of digestive tract and associated organs (liver and pancreas) and respiratory system.

While the chick embryo is growing, four associated membranes can be distinguished (Figure 24.4) [21, 22]. Although they are similar to those described in mammals, the chick embryo must develop independently and outside of the hen's body, which makes these membranes especially important for accessing the nutrients present in the egg and acting on essential living functions (respiration, excretion, and mechanical protection). These four membranes and their major functions are

1) **yolk sac:** Although initially the embryo is a flat structure, it progressively folds cranio-caudally and laterally, leaving an aperture at the ventral aspect of the coelomic cavity and creating the yolk stalk. The yolk sac is the membranous sac that is attached to the embryo at the yolk stalk and mainly provides nourishment. After Day 6 of incubation, the yolk sac surrounds all of the yolk and is the site of primary vessel growth, blood cell formation, and germ cell differentiation before these cells migrate into their respective organs. Around Day 19 of incubation, the yolk sac is drawn into the abdominal/coelomic cavity. Sometimes, the yolk sac may not be fully regressed and a remnant of the yolk stalk can be found at Meckel's diverticulum (see Chapter 7);

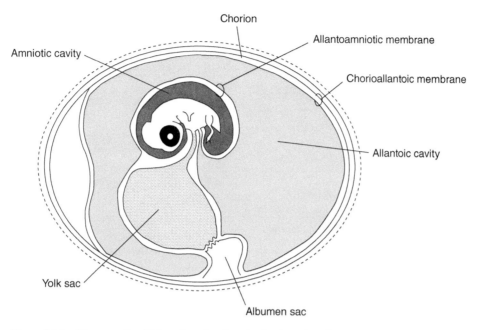

Figure 24.4 Diagram of a chick embryo in a longitudinal section showing the different membranes and sacs formed around the embryo for protection, nourishment, and basic life functions.

2) **amnion:** When the most peripheral membranes in the egg (future chorion) grow dorsally as two different folds (one cranial and one caudal), the embryo sinks and allow the folds to join dorsally, covering, and completely surrounding the embryo and thus forming the amnion and the amniotic cavity. This cavity is filled with watery fluid (amniotic fluid) in which the embryo floats and is protected from external forces or impacts;

3) **allantois:** The allantois arises during Day 3 of incubation as an outgrowth of the hindgut, which passes through the umbilicus close to the yolk stalk. It grows rapidly and occupies the space between the amnion and the chorion by Day 10 of incubation. Vessels from and to the heart (umbilical or allantoic arteries and veins) rapidly colonize this membrane and occupy the space between the allantois and the chorion. When the chorioallantoic membrane is completely apposed to the shell membrane, the exchange of respiratory gases can occur (respiratory function). The allantoic sac also has an important excretory function in collecting urinary and digestive waste that precipitates as uric acid components. As uric acid is a solid nitrogenous waste product, it does not diffuse across the allantoic membrane, which allows it to remain in close proximity without toxic effects;

4) **Chorion:** The chorion is the most peripheral membrane and fuses externally with the inner shell membrane and internally with the allantois. As mentioned previously, the chorion, together with the allantois (chorioallantoic membrane), serves to mediate gas and water exchange.

In order to identify the developmental stage of chick embryos, a simplified table describing the formation of the major organs or structures is presented in Table 24.2 [19, 23].

During this process the position of the chick changes progressively so that the anterior part of the body lies toward the large end of the egg by day 14, the head is covered by the right wing by day 18, and the feet are in contact with the head when the egg is ready to hatch (see video on website showing chick hatching).

Table 24.2 Simplified table describing the developmental stage of chick embryos and the formation of major organs or structures.

Day	Organs or anatomical structures present
0	Small germinal disc not fertilized
1	Blastoderm, embryonic tissue
2	Formation of blood vessels on top of yolk
3	Leg and wing buds, heart formation and beats can be observed
4	Formation of eyeball (pigmented area)
5	Identification of limb joints (elbow and knee), digits and toes
6	Beak and feather tracts
7	Web between toes and, egg tooth
8	Initial appearance of feathers, nictitating membrane
9	Phalanges in toes
10	Primordium of comb
11	Allantois has the maximum size, embryo looks like a chick
12	First complete feathers
13	Claws
14	Whole body covered by feathers
15	Vitellus (yolk) shrinks
16	Egg white disappear
17	Urates appear
18	Total growth near completion
19	Yolk sac attached to body cavity
20	No presence or minimal yolk sac
21	Newly hatched chick

Sources: Hamburger, V. and Hamilton, H. [19], Warin, S. [23].

Monitoring Chick Development

As the chick develops in the egg, development can be monitored by using the process known as candling. Anyone who incubates eggs should have a candler, and these are available for purchase through poultry supply companies. Candling is the use of a strong external light source to view the developing egg through its thin shell. Dark-shelled eggs or the thicker eggs of waterfowl are not candled as easily as those of chickens. While candling is useful for monitoring chick development, its frequent use can also disrupt chick development if performed excessively or if eggs are handled roughly. As the chick develops, the branching of pulsating blood vessels can be observed through the eggshell. When the egg is candled and no visible branching blood vessels are observed but rather replaced by a static blood ring, this is an indication of early embryonic mortality during the early incubation period.

If there is no branching of blood vessels after a few days of incubation, this indicates that the egg may have been infertile or that there was early embryonic mortality. Most mortality in hatching eggs occurs in the early or late period of incubation. If there are no signs of life in the egg, then egg diagnostics could be employed to help determine the cause of death. Eggs should immediately be removed if there is no branching of blood vessels or if a static blood ring is present after five to seven days of incubation.

Egg Diagnostics

In the early stages of incubation, the primary diagnostic tools used are egg visualization, egg pathology, and egg culture [24, 25]. Hatching eggs that do not show visible signs of life should be cracked open and emptied into a sterilized glass petri dish or bowl to observe for the remnants of the blastoderm or blastodisc. Depending on the degree of work-up required by the owner, this area can be clipped out of the yolk with sterile ophthalmic surgical scissors and forceps and placed in formalin for further histologic examination to determine if it was fertile. In addition, as bacteria play an important role in egg infections, the egg can also be cultured and plated in blood agar and MacConkey's media to check for aerobic bacteria [24, 25]. Some of the common isolated bacteria that are found in eggs and ill chicks are *Escherichia coli*, *Klebsiella* species,

Staphylococcus aureus, *Steptococcus* species, *Pseudomonas aeruginosa*, *Salmonella* species, and *Proteus mirabilis* [6, 24, 25].

Bacterial Culture of Eggs

There are many sites where eggs can be cultured, depending on the questions that need to be answered. These include the egg roll, egg membranes, and yolk [24, 25]. Positive determination of bacterial presence in the egg usually indicates problems with nest sanitation, egg storage, hen infection, and/or hatchery sanitation [24, 25]. These bacteria, which can result in a decrease in hatchability, can also cause weak chicks to hatch with subsequent omphalitis (yolk sac infection) [6, 24, 25]. The basic tools needed to perform egg culture include an incubator, and bacterial media such as sheep blood agar and MacConkey's media plates. These two solid plate media are the basic culture medium necessary for egg microbiology techniques, as the major bacteria associated with egg infections can be isolated from these media. These media should be incubated at 98.5 °F (37 °C) in air for 24 hours. If there is no growth, then these media plates should be incubated for an additional 24 hours.

Egg Roll Culture

On occasion, the external surface of the egg needs to be cultured to determine the bacterial load to which it is exposed in the nest environment. For this procedure, with sterile gloves pick the newly laid egg from its nest environment and gently roll the surface of the egg on two blood agar and two MacConkey's media agar plates. The egg can then be placed in a sterile Whirlpak bag and incubated in brain-heart infusion broth for 18 hours [24, 25]. After incubation, the suspension should be centrifuged and the resulting pellet should be plated on blood agar and MacConkey's media. This will determine if there are nest management sanitation problems. Nest material should be frequently cleaned to ensure that there is minimal fecal debris on the surface of hatching eggs. Bacteria enter the egg through the eggshell pores, so a clean nest environment and timely collection of eggs minimizes bacterial contamination.

Egg Membrane Culture

It is sometimes necessary for the shell membranes to be cultured, especially when there is suspected contamination resulting from improper storage and handling of the egg [24, 25]. When an egg is laid, sometimes it can be stored at varying temperatures and this may cause sweating/condensation on the surface of the egg. The moisture on the surface of the egg can facilitate bacteria to enter the egg via the eggshell pores. The shell membranes can serve as a partial mechanical barrier to hinder bacteria from reaching the nutrient-rich yolk. To determine bacterial presence at the level of the shell membrane, take an egg carton, or a similar alternative container, and place the egg that is to be cultured in one of the egg slots to hold the egg upright with the large end up. Be careful not to come into contact with the egg carton as it is not sterile. Pour 70% alcohol over the top of the egg and let it air dry. Using a sterile forcep, gently break and remove the shell. This provides access to the air cell. Take a sterile cotton-tipped swab that has been moistened with brain-heart infusion broth and place it in the air cell. Gently work the swab between the layers of shell membrane so that at least the top half of the egg is swabbed. You can pick up the egg from the egg carton if it facilitates culturing. Place the swab in a tube of brain-heart infusion broth and incubate for 18 hours at 98.5 °F (37 °C) in air. At this point, Salmonella-selective media can also be used if needed. After incubation, plate on blood agar and MacConkey's media for 48 hours and incubate at 98.5 °F (37 °C) in air. The presence of bacteria can usually be noted after 24 hours of incubation.

Egg Yolk Culture

Culturing the egg yolk is one of the most important diagnostic tools in egg diagnostics [24, 25]. The yolk is nutrient rich and can enhance and support bacterial growth. The presence of bacteria in this region of the egg indicates contamination from the external outer shell to the yolk or may indicate infection from the hen. Because the yolk is nutrient rich, bacteria, upon reaching the yolk, can multiply rapidly; therefore, the timing of infection can be estimated. If there are bacteria present as a result of unsanitary nesting or egg storage conditions, early infection would probably have occurred, with early embryonic mortality. Bacterial infection of the yolk at hatching usually results in a weak chick that has omphalitis. This would most likely occur as a result of contamination caused by unsanitary and improper hatching conditions. Yolk that is contaminated with bacteria is often dark and sometimes brown in color [24, 25]. There may be an odor to the egg. Sometimes both the egg white and yolk are cultured together as a pooled sample. However, the egg white has antibacterial properties and this may hinder the culture of low numbers of bacteria unless they are placed in an enrichment broth, such as brain-heart infusion broth, rather than plating directly on bacterial media plates.

Exploding Eggs

Eggs have been reported to explode in incubators. The exploding eggs are usually the result of an infected egg. The egg yolk can become contaminated with bacteria and provides a good nutrient source for them. As the bacteria multiply, they also produce gas and this causes the egg to explode in the incubator. *Pseudomonas aeruginosa* is the most common bacteria that is associated with exploding eggs [6, 24, 25]. Unfortunately, if there are other eggs within the incubator, an exploding egg can spread its contaminated debris onto other eggs and contaminate them. This can lead to more exploding eggs. Eggs can become contaminated when the bacteria from the contaminated debris enters a new egg via the eggshell pores. Under the appropriate conditions, additional eggs can become infected. If an exploding egg occurs, be aware that additional eggs may explode and the chicks, if they hatch, may not flourish. They may potentially have omphalitis. The incubators should be thoroughly disinfected after an exploding egg incident, based on recommended disinfectant protocols, as soon as feasibly possible [26–28].

Egg Breakouts

An egg breakout can be performed on eggs that do not hatch. An egg breakout provides clues as to why the developing chick did not successfully hatch into a viable chick. As mentioned previously, there internal and external factors can influence the hatch of a viable chick. Internal factors are inherent to the developing chick and include nutrition of the hen. For example, if the hens are not provided with adequate nutrition, the hatching chick is weak. A lack of vitamin E can result in a weak hatching muscle, which results in the chick being unable to use its neck (hatching) muscle to break open the shell. The inability to break open the shell results in a dead-in-shell chick. External factors affect a chick from hatching, given it is a fully capable chick. These external factors include temperature, humidity, and ventilation of the incubator environment [29, 30]. For example, if humidity is too low the shell membranes dry out. The chick may have pipped (broken through the shell membrane and shell), but because of the low humidity, the shell membranes become dried out. These dried-out membranes then harden and become adhered to the chick. The chick is not able to break free and uses its energy in attempting to do so. If it becomes exhausted, the chick will

Table 24.3 Common egg breakout findings and potential internal or external causes.

Egg breakout finding	Potential causes
Cracks in shell	Improper or rough handling of eggs
Moldy contents	Hatchery sanitation issues
Abnormal body parts (brain, eye, beak); hemorrhage	Too high incubation temperatures
Chicks with red hocks	Hen nutrition or high incubation temperatures
Chicks that have pipped but dead-in-shell and shell membranes not dried out	Hen nutrition or humidity too high during the incubation period
Chicks that have pipped but dead-in-shell and shell membranes dried out	Too low humidity
Unhealed navels	Bacterial contamination

Sources: Morishita, T.Y. [15], Ande, T.B. and Wilson, H.R. [29], Stephenson, A.B. [30].

die in its shell. Table 24.3 provides information about egg breakout and its possible causes (Table 24.3). It should be noted that even under normal conditions not all eggs will hatch. Normally, for any given batch that is incubated, 2–4% may be infertile; 2–3% die early in the incubation period (up to day 7); 1% die during the middle phase of incubation (Day 7–14); and 3–4% die during the late phase of incubation (Day 14–21). All dead-in-shell chicks can be placed in formalin and submitted for necropsy.

Unaesthetic Eggs

The other reason why flock owners ask for egg diagnostics is that the egg may be deemed inedible because it appears unaesthetic and unappetizing. Egg quality and appearance issues can stem from nutrition, environmental hazards and egg mishandling [31].

Abnormalities of the Yolk

Color

Yolk color is influenced by diet. Hens that are fed commercial diets tend to have pale yellow yolks when compared to the darker yellowish orange yolks from hens that are allowed access to grass [15]. Some backyard flock owners have been known to feed marigold flower petals, which are naturally high in carotenoids, to impart a darker orange color to their hens' egg yolks [15]. Yolk color that is green, platinum, olive or mottled are derived from hens consuming seeds, cottonseed meal or anticoccidial drugs. In all instances, hens should not have access to these types of items in their diet [31].

Taste

Yolk flavor can be influenced by the hen's diet. While not commonly fed to hens, fish by-products can impart a fishy flavor to the eggs [15]. Additionally, storage of eggs near pungent items can impart an off-flavor to the eggs [31].

Blood Spots

On occasion, fresh blood can be found on the egg yolk's surface (Figure 24.5). A common misconception is that it may be a developing embryo. The red blood is often referred to as

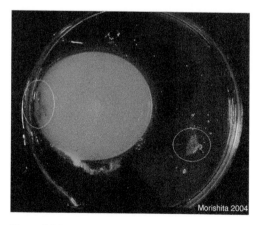

Figure 24.5 An egg with both blood spots (left circle) and meat spots (right circle).

blood spots and represents the blood from the rupture of ovarian blood vessels when the yolk was released from the ovaries. Some hens are more nervous than others and blood spots are noted in some genetic lines [15]. The blood should not be part of embryonic development unless the egg was previously incubated. However, eggs destined for human consumption should be collected immediately after they are laid rather than incubated.

Meat Spots

The other debris that can be found in the egg white takes the form of light beige debris, often referred to as meat spots (Figure 24.5). Meat spots are the sloughed inner lining of the oviduct and are usually noted in hens that have been laying eggs for a long period of time without a molt. It is more often observed in hens that have not had a natural molt [15]. Molting is a period of time during which the hen needs to rest its reproductive system. The oviduct regresses until the hen begins a new lay cycle. Brown egg layers may have pigmented protein inclusions that can be misrepresented as meat spots although there is nothing wrong with the egg [31].

Thin Egg White

When an egg is cracked out, the yolk is surrounded by an inner thick egg white (albumen) and an outer thin albumen. Infectious bronchitis is a disease that can affect the magnum and can result in eggs of poor internal egg quality, which have runny egg whites [6–8, 32].

Worms in Eggs

In hens with severe roundworm infections, there can be occasions when a worm becomes encased in the egg. This can occur when an adult worm exits the gastrointestinal tract and happens to migrate up the reproductive tract. If it migrates up to the magnum, it is incorporated within the egg [33].

Egg within an Egg

An egg within an egg is a rarity that can occur. While in the oviduct, reverse peristalsis can happen resulting in the reproductive system creating a new egg around the existing egg. This reverse peristalsis occurs in the presence of an acute stressor to the hen [31].

Ruptured Shell Membranes

On occasion, the outer shell membrane can break or form incompletely, leaving an opening in the calcified shell from which the disrupted shell membranes form a tuft [34].

Misshapen Eggs

Besides affecting internal egg quality, infectious bronchitis can also impact external egg quality. The infectious bronchitis virus can affect the uterus (shell gland), resulting in eggs that are wrinkled (Figure 24.6) [6, 7].

Yolkless and Double-Yolked Eggs

On occasion, in hens that are beginning to lay, there is an incoordination within the reproductive tract. A yolk may not be released, but some egg white is made, moves down the

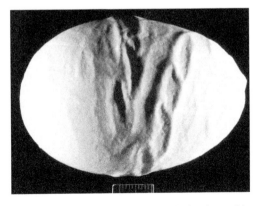

Figure 24.6 Wrinkled egg from a laying hen with infectious bronchitis.

reproductive tract, and become encased in shell membranes and a calcified shell. These yolkless eggs are normal in appearance and are usually less than one half the size of a normal egg.

Double-yolked eggs are formed when two yolks are released at the same time and become encased within the egg. Some genetic lines of chickens have a tendency to form double-yolked eggs. Double-yolked eggs can be 1.5 times larger than normal eggs.

In conclusion, egg laying complaints usually result in eggs not hatching out or the production of abnormal eggs. It is important to identify the causes of these abnormal hatches or abnormal eggs, so that any future problems can be prevented for the flock owner.

References

1 Morishita, T.Y. (1999). Clinical assessment of chickens and waterfowl in backyard flocks. *Vet. Clin. N. Am. Exot. Anim. Pract.* 2: 383–404.

2 King, A.S. and McLelland, J. (1984). *Birds: Their Structure and Function, Volume 1*, 239–257. England: Bailliere Tindall.

3 Burley, R.W. and Vadehra, D.V. (1989). *The Avian Egg.* New York: Wiley.

4 Whittow, G.C. (2000). *Sturkie's Avian Physiology*, 5e, 584–596. San Diego: Academic Press.

5 Spiegle, S.J., Ison, A.J., and Morishita, T.Y. (2004). Making of an Egg. In: *Poultry Health Resources* (ed. T.Y. Morishita), Factsheet 2019-11. Pomona, CA: Western University of Health Sciences.

6 Morishita, T.Y. (1990). Establishing a differential diagnosis for backyard poultry flocks. In: *Proceedings of the 1990 Annual Conference of the Association of Avian Veterinarians*, 136–146. Phoenix, AZ: Association of Avian Veterinarians.

7 Morishita, T.Y. (1994). *Respiratory syndromes in backyard poultry.* In: , 35–44. Reno, Nevada: Association of Avian Veterinarians Annual Conference.

8 Morishita, T.Y. (1995). Common reproductive problems in the backyard chicken. In: *Section 11: Topics in Clinical Medicine, Main Conference Proceedings*, 465–467. Philadelphia: Association of Avian Veterinarians Annual Conference.

9 King, A.S. (1975). Chapter 65: urogenital system. In: *The Anatomy of the Domestic Animals*, 5e, vol. II (ed. R. Getty), 1919–1961. Philadelphia: Saunders Company.

10 Nickel, R., Schummer, A., and Seiferle, E. (translated by Siller, W.G. and Wight, P.A.L.) (1977). *Anatomy of the Domestic Bird*, 81–83. Berlin: Paul Parey.

11 Pollock, C.G. and Orosz, S.E. (2002). Avian reproductive anatomy, physiology and endocrinology. *Vet. Clin. N. Am. Exot. Anim. Pract.* 5: 441–474.

12 Bakst, M.R. and Howarth, B. (1977). The fine structure of the hen's ovum at ovulation. *Biol. Reprod.* 17: 361–369.

13 Mortola, J.P. (2009). Gas exchange in avian embryos and hatchlings. *Comp. Biochem. Physiol. Part A* 153: 359–377.

14 Damerov, G. (1994). Food borne bacteria. In: *Chicken Health Handbook* (ed. G. Damerov), 231–243. Pownal, VT: Storey Communications, Inc.

15 Morishita, T.Y. (1995). Poultry management 101: poultry management topics for avian veterinarian. In: *Section 7: Practice Management. Main Conference Proceedings*, 327–331. Philadelphia, PA: Association of Avian Veterinarians Annual Conference.

16 Joyner, K.L. (1994). *Theriogenology, in Avian Medicine: Principles and Application*, 748–804. Lake Worth, FL: Winger's Publishing.

17 Hayes, C. (1995). *Raising Turkeys, Ducks, Geese, Pigeons, and Guineas.* Blue Ridge Summit, PA: TAB Books Inc.

18 Schwartz, D.L. (1995). *Grower's Reference on Gamebird Health*, 357. Okemos, MI: AVION, Inc.

19 Hamburger, V. and Hamilton, H. (1992). A series of normal stages in the development of the chick embryo. *Dev. Dynam.* 195: 231–272. (reprinted from *Journal of Morphology* 1951; **88**, 49–92).

20 Romanoff, A.L. (1960). *The Avian Embryo: Structural and Functional Development*. New York: Macmillan.

21 Noden, D.M. and De Lahunta, A. (1985). *The Embryology of Domestic Animals. Developmental Mechanisms and Malformations*, 1e. Baltimore: Williams & Wilkins.

22 McGeady, T.A., Quinn, P.J., Fitzpatrick, E.S., and Ryan, M.T. (2006). *Veterinary Embryology*, 1e. Ames, Iowa: Blackwell Publishing.

23 Warin, S. (2013) The poultry site: embryonic development, day by day. http://www.thepoultrysite.com/articles/1459/embryonic-development-day-by-day (accessed 1 October 2013).

24 Morishita, T.Y. (1995) Egg diagnostic techniques. *The Ohio State University, Veterinary Extension Newsletter*, (January–March), **23**, 2–3.

25 Morishita, T.Y. (1998). Egg diagnostic techniques. In: *114th Annual Convention, Ohio Veterinary Medical Association Annual Conference Proceedings*, vol. 3. Columbus, Ohio, Session (Small Ruminant), 391 (5 pp).

26 Morishita, T.Y. (1990) A word about . . . disinfectants, in *California Poultry Letter, Cooperative Extension*, August, University of California-Davis, Davis, California.

27 Mejia, A., Morishita, T.Y., and Lam, K.M. (1994). The effect of seven hatchery disinfectants on a *Staphylococcus aureus* strain. *Prevent. Vet. Med.* 18: 193–201.

28 Morishita, T.Y. and Gordon, J.C. (2002). Cleaning and disinfection of poultry facilities. In: *Poultry Health Resources* (ed. T.Y. Morishita), Factsheet 2019-05. Pomona, CA: Western University of Health Sciences.

29 Ande, T.B. and Wilson, H.R. (1981). Hatchability of chicken embryos exposed to acute high temperature stress at various ages. *Poult. Sci.* 60: 1561–1566.

30 Stephenson, A.B. (1985). Position and turning of turkey eggs prior to incubation. *Poult. Sci.* 64: 1279–1284.

31 Anderson, K.A., Karcher, D.M., and Jones, D.R. (2017). Identifying and responding to factors that can affect egg quality and appearance. North Carolina State University Extension, AG-169, 1–8. https://content.ces.ncsu.edu/factors-that-can-affect-egg-quality-and-appearance

32 Morishita, T.Y. (1996). Common infectious diseases in backyard chickens and turkeys (from a private practice perspective). *J. Avian Med. Surg.* 10: 2–11.

33 Morishita, T.Y. and Schaul, J.C. (2007). Parasites of birds. In: *Flynn's Parasites of Laboratory Animals* (ed. D.G. Baker), 217–302. Ames, IA: Blackwell Publishing Professional.

34 Morishita, T.Y., Aye, P.P., Harr, B.S., and Clevenger, B. (1998). Egg shell deformation due to outer shell membrane anomaly. *J. Avian Med. Surg.* 12: 268–270.

25

How to Perform a Necropsy

Jarra Jagne[1] and Elizabeth Buckles[2]

[1] *Department of Population Medicine and Diagnostic Sciences, Cornell University, College of Veterinary Medicine, Ithaca, NY, USA*
[2] *Department of Biomedical Sciences, Cornell University, College of Veterinary Medicine, Ithaca, NY, USA*

Introduction

Postmortem examination of the avian patient is an important part of health monitoring and surveillance of regulatory diseases. For the owner of the individual chicken and the practicing veterinarian, it can provide important information regarding the efficacy of premortem diagnostics and treatments of the pet. For the owner of a backyard flock, the post mortem provides information regarding the overall health of the flock, including the presence of communicable diseases. Diagnosis of disease in poultry, whether a pet or a production flock, is also essential due to the economic significance of poultry. Backyard and pet poultry are susceptible to the same economically significant and sometimes reportable diseases as commercial flocks and often are not vaccinated for common diseases. Thus, these birds can be important sentinels for the emergence of diseases in an area or act as portals of entry for disease in commercial birds. Another reason for conducting necropsies is obtaining forensic or legal information in the investigation of hoarding cases, as seen increasingly in backyard poultry production.

With practice, an avian post mortem examination can be performed in a relatively short period of time. It is important for the prosector to always conduct necropsies in a systematic manner, following a standard procedure. This will allow for detection of subtle abnormalities as well as provide information on the normal organs. Diagnostic laboratories and pathologists appreciate a detailed clinical history and descriptions of post mortem findings; both are essential for proper interpretation of test results. Clinical history should include the breed, age, and sex of the bird as well as a detailed description of any clinical signs involving the various organ systems. It is always important to collect management information from the owner. Details on housing, nutrition, source of birds, treatments, production type, and any vaccinations will assist in the diagnostic process. Additional flock information should include the size of the flock and morbidity and mortality rates. The prosector should take detailed notes on the findings and/or take digital images of the necropsy findings.

A complete post mortem includes collection of appropriate samples for bacterial culture, viral testing and histopathology using aseptic techniques. The prosector should avoid

Backyard Poultry Medicine and Surgery: A Guide for Veterinary Practitioners, Second Edition.
Edited by Cheryl B. Greenacre and Teresa Y. Morishita.
© 2021 John Wiley & Sons, Inc. Published 2021 by John Wiley & Sons, Inc.
Companion website: www.wiley.com/go/greenacre/medicine

contamination of organs with intestinal contents, feed material, etc. to improve the chances of detecting disease organisms. In the case of bacterial cultures, multiple organisms can overgrow in a plate and prevent the growth of organisms in pure culture. In cases of suspected toxicities or nutrient imbalances submission of feed samples will assist in diagnosis.

Tissues for histopathology should be fixed in 10% neutral buffered formalin with a tissue:formalin volume ratio of 1:10. To save on shipping costs, the tissues can be fixed for 24 hours and then sealed in a thick plastic "seal-a-meal"–type bag with a small amount of formalin, prior to shipping. Diagnostic laboratories will provide detailed information on shipping of samples to the facility, and familiarity with these procedures will greatly expedite testing. A list of poultry necropsy laboratories by state is available online [1].

The practitioner should be familiar with the lesions of common diseases discussed elsewhere in this publication, as well as diseases that are reportable at the state or federal level [2]. Most diagnostic laboratories are happy to answer any questions that may arise with regard to these issues.

Finally, an appropriate area for necropsy should be identified based on whether the necropsy is done out in the field on a farm or in the veterinarian's office. Biosecurity is paramount when performing avian necropsies. On the farm, it is advisable to perform necropsies outside the farm perimeter or a distance away from the poultry coops, especially if the veterinarian suspects an infectious disease. At the clinic, a room designated for necropsies should have appropriate tables, sinks, cleaning supplies, and disinfectants. Avian necropsies result in shedding of many feathers and feather dust; thus, cleanup can be challenging. Care should be taken to minimize aerosolization of avian biologic materials, and the necropsy should be performed in an area not accessible by living patients. The prosector is advised to wear appropriate personal protective equipment, at the minimum gloves, designated clothing such as surgical scrubs, lab coat or coveralls, and a surgical mask. The remains of the avian patient can generally be disposed of similarly to the mammalian patient, and cremation seems to be the method of choice in many laboratories. In the case of regulatory diseases, specialized disposal may be necessary and is usually conducted by federal and state officials.

External Exam and Skin Removal

Before beginning the necropsy, collect all the materials needed for dissection and sample collection. Figure 25.1 shows a variety of instruments that will be used as the post mortem progresses. These include a sharp knife (a), nitrile gloves (b), scalpel blades (c), scalpel handle (d), forceps (e), poultry shears (f), scissors (g), aerobic culture media and swab (h), viral/mycoplasma transport media (i), plastic bags (j), formalin in a container that can be tightly sealed (k), plastic tissue cassette (l), specimen cups (m), tongue depressor (n), ruler (o), and rongeurs (p).

Before opening the bird, proper identification by species, breed, sex, given name, wing band, or leg band numbers is done. It is important to record the bird's weight and the body condition scored before a thorough external examination is performed.

Overall Evaluation and Body Condition

The Gregory and Robins scoring system from 0 to 3 is one of the more popular scoring systems: a score of "0" indicates a protruding keel bone and depressed contour to the breast muscles, and a score of "3" indicates plump breast muscles, which provide a smooth contour with the keel [3]. Post-mortem changes should be taken into consideration at this stage. These include levels of decomposition, presence of rigor mortis, and oral and vent discharges. Palpate the wings, legs, and body and examine

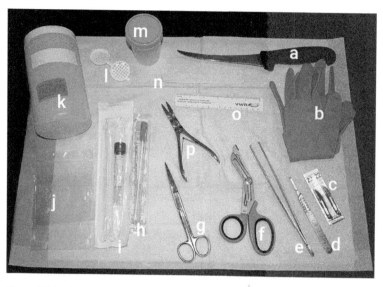

Figure 25.1 Instruments used as the post mortem progresses. These include a sharp knife (a), nitrile gloves (b), scalpel blades (c), scalpel handle (d), forceps (e), poultry shears (f), scissors (g), aerobic culture media and swab (h), viral/mycoplasma transport media (i), plastic bags (j), formalin in a container that can be tightly sealed (k), plastic tissue cassette (l), specimen cups (m), tongue depressor (n), ruler (o) and rongeurs (p).

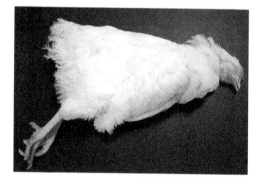

Figure 25.2 Perform a thorough external evaluation including the head and feet.

the feathers for stress lines, irregularities, and ectoparasites. Palpate the keel to assess body condition. Perform a thorough examination of the structures of the head and of the feet (Figure 25.2).

Head

External examination of the head (Figure 25.3) includes assessment of several features including the nares (a), comb (b), eyes, and mouth, The inset shows the features of a male bird

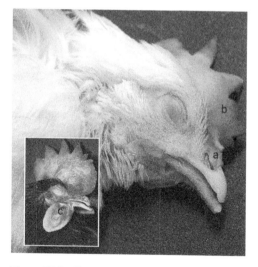

Figure 25.3 External examination of the head includes assessment of several features including the nares (a), comb (b), eyes and mouth. The inset shows the features of a male bird including the larger comb and the presence of a wattle (c).

including the larger comb and the presence of a wattle (c). The combs and wattles should be homogeneous and pink, whereas the eyes,

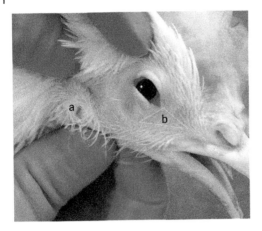

Figure 25.4 The opening of the ear is located caudal and ventral to the eye and can be exposed by spreading the feathers away from the area (a). The infraorbital sinus is located deep to the skin, between the nares and eye (b).

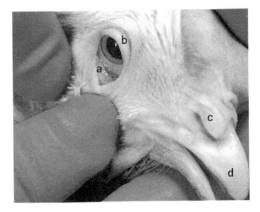

Figure 25.5 The inner conjunctiva is well vascularized and moist but not overly red (a). The eyelids (b) are rims of skin with small sparse feathers (b). The external covering of the nares and the cere (c) are smooth, homogenous structures and the outer coverings of the beak (rhamphotheca, d), are normally smooth, and free of fissures and cracks.

nares, and mouth should be free of exudate and debris.

Ears

The opening of the ear (Figure 25.4) is located caudal and ventral to the eye and can be exposed by spreading the feathers away from the area (a). The infraorbital sinus is located deep to the skin, between the nares and eye (b). Exudates in this area may cause swelling of this area of the face. Pressing on this area can cause exudates to exude from the nares and can be an indication of viral or bacterial respiratory disease.

Eyes

The eyes and conjunctivae should be clear and smooth. The inner conjunctiva is well vascularized and moist but not overly red (Figure 25.5a). The eyelids (b) are rims of skin with small sparse feathers (b). The external covering of the nares and the cere (c) are smooth, homogeneous structures, and the outer coverings of the beak (rhamphotheca, d), are normally smooth and free of fissures and cracks. In some cases, the beak may be trimmed and blunt. Overgrowth of the beak can indicate systemic disease and over exuberant beak trimming may cause infection or interfere with feeding.

Oral Cavity

Open the mouth and examine the choanal slit (Figure 25.6a), oral cavity and tongue (b). The choanal slit is the connection between the oral and nasopharynx and is surrounded by rows of papillae. The tongue is stiff compared to a

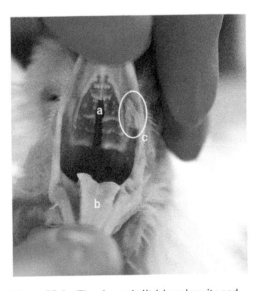

Figure 25.6 The choanal slit (a), oral cavity and tongue (b) are shown. Note the yellow plaques at the commissure of the beak (c), these are lesions consistent with exposure to mycotoxins and are relatively common in adult laying hens.

mammal's as it is supported by bone and cartilage. The tracheal opening is located at the base of the tongue. Note the yellow plaques at the commissure of the beak (c); these are lesions consistent with exposure to mycotoxins and are relatively common in adult laying hens.

Feet

Examination of the feet included assessment of the leg scales and metatarsal and digital pads. (Figure 25.7) Roosters and some hens may have a spur (a), which is similar in composition to the claws. The metatarsal pad (b) is the large pad from which the digital pads extend. It should be smooth, bulge slightly and be free of ulcers, erosions, or scabs. This is a common site of infection (bumble foot) in birds on improper or contaminated substrate.

Wing

The ventral aspect of the wing has a feather-free tract from removal of small feathers for better visualization of veins (Figure 25.8). The ulnar vein and its branches can be visualized beneath the thin skin (a).

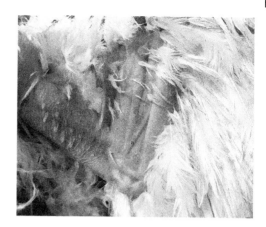

Figure 25.8 The ventral aspect of the wing has a feather free tract from removal of small feathers for better visualization of veins. The ulnar vein and its branches can be visualized beneath the thin skin (a).

Initial Incision and Skin Removal

Once the external examination is completed, the bird should be dunked in a solution of water and disinfectant (Figure 25.9). The bird's head should not be submerged as disinfectant may enter the upper respiratory or gastrointestinal tracts and interfere with potential laboratory testing. The bird should be wet enough to keep the feathers out of the dissection field and prevent feather dust from being released during the post mortem. After the bird has been

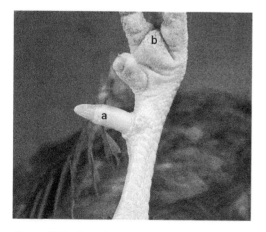

Figure 25.7 Examination of the feet included assessment of the leg scales, and metatarsal and digital pads. Roosters and some hens may have a spur (a) which is similar in composition to the claws. The metatarsal pad (b) is the large pad from which the digital pads extend.

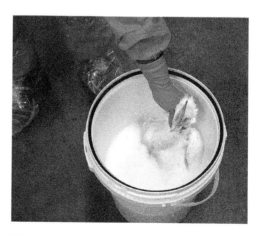

Figure 25.9 Once the external examination is completed, the bird should be dipped in a solution of water and disinfectant.

wet down, place it in dorsal recumbency and begin the internal examination (Figure 25.10). First, open the skin from the cloaca to the base of the mandible. The initial incision can be made at the caudal point of the sternum and extended cranially and caudally, either by incision or by blunt dissection. The skin is very thin. The skin should be peeled laterally to expose the pectoral muscles and the coxofemoral joints. Remove the skin on the ventral thigh to expose the muscle and connective tissue in this area (Figure 25.11). In order to facilitate

exposure of the internal organs, and cause the bird to lay flat, grasp the femurs and pull them dorsally to disarticulate the coxofemoral joint (Figure 25.12). This also allows examination of the articular cartilage of the femoral head, a common site of degenerative joint disease. Normal cartilage should be smooth, coated by a thin layer of synovial fluid that is light blue. As the bird becomes autolyzed, this cartilage may slough off the femoral head with manipulation.

Removal of the skin (Figure 25.13) reveals the ventral edge of the keel (a), pectoral muscles, and the thigh muscles (b). The pectoral muscles should form a semicircular silhouette with the ventral edge of the keel. As the bird loses condition, this silhouette will become more concave, while overconditioned or heavily muscled birds will have a convex silhouette, due to either muscle development or an overlay of adipose tissue. Note the difference in color of the pectoral and thigh muscles. This is normal, as chickens are largely terrestrial so

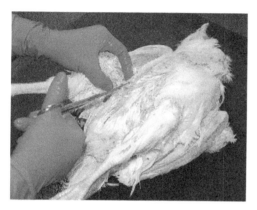

Figure 25.10 After the bird has been wet down, place it in dorsal recumbency and begin the internal examination.

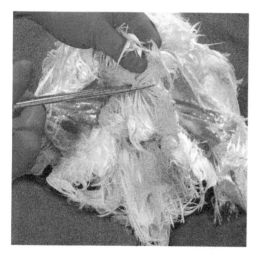

Figure 25.11 Remove the skin on the ventral thigh to expose the muscle and connective tissue in this area.

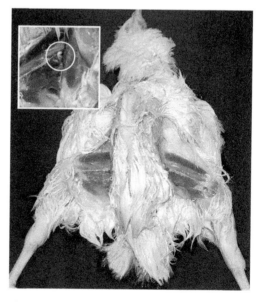

Figure 25.12 In order to facilitate exposure of the internal organs, and cause the bird to lay flat, grasp the femurs and pull them dorsally to disarticulate the coxofemoral joint.

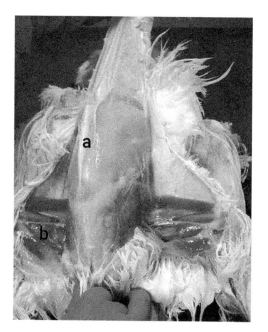

Figure 25.13 Removal of the skin reveals the ventral edge of the keel (a), pectoral muscles and the thigh muscles (b).

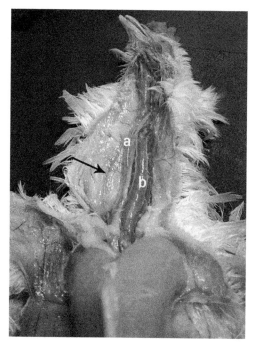

Figure 25.14 The structures of the neck lie just beneath the skin and can be exposed with minimal fascial dissection. The trachea (a) and esophagus lie in close approximation and track ventral and slightly to the right of the cervical spine and musculature (b). The arrow points to the vagus nerve running parallel to the tubular cervical structures.

they have more myoglobin in their leg muscle than in the flight muscles.

Structures of the Neck

The structures of the neck lie just beneath the skin and can be exposed with minimal fascial dissection (Figure 25.14). The trachea (a) and esophagus lie in close approximation and track ventral and slightly to the right of the cervical spine and musculature (b). The arrow points to the vagus nerve running parallel to the tubular cervical structures. Additional structures of the neck are variably prominent (Figure 25.15). The right jugular vein (a) is larger than the left and runs parallel to the esophagus. The thymus (b) in young birds lies in this jugular furrow and consists of seven lobes of soft, nodular glandular tissue that extend the length of the neck. This organ regresses with age. The crop (c) is a diverticulum of the cervical esophagus that lies at the thoracic inlet and acts as a storage sac for food prior to passage into the deeper gastrointestinal tract. It is tightly adhered to the underlying skin and its size varies with the amount of content.

The thymus (Figure 25.16) regresses as the bird ages and is grossly absent by the time the bird is sexually mature. As the thymus regresses, remnants of thymic tissue can often be found in the fascia of the neck (circle) and can vary in size and range from pink to red depending on the age of the bird.

Figure 25.17 is a closeup view of the thoracic inlet. This closer view of the crop (a) shows it slightly distended by content and its relationship with the thoracic inlet. The V-shaped inlet (b) is formed by the intersection of the right and left coracoid and furcular (wishbone) bones.

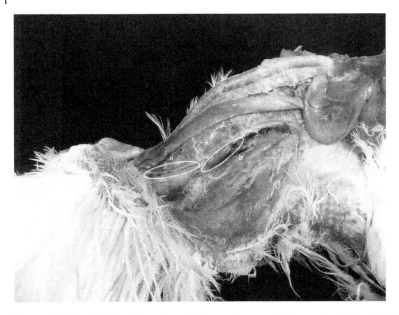

Figure 25.15 Additional structures of the neck are variably prominent. The right jugular vein (a) is larger than the left and runs parallel to the esophagus. The thymus (b) in young birds, lies in this jugular furrow and consists of 7 lobes of soft, nodular glandular tissue that extend the length of the neck. The crop (c) is a diverticulum of the cervical esophagus that lies at the thoracic inlet and acts as a storage sac for food prior to passage into the deeper gastrointestinal tract.

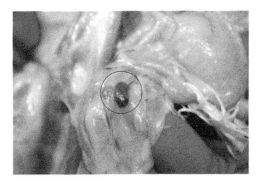

Figure 25.16 The thymus (Figure 25.16) regresses as the bird ages and is grossly absent by the time the bird is sexually mature.

Entering the Body Cavity

In order to enter the coelomic cavity, dissect the muscle and fascias overlying the abdomen, caudal to the keel (Figure 25.18). This will expose the caudal coelomic cavity. Well-fed or overfed birds will have a large fat pad over the organs contained in a mesenteric reflection

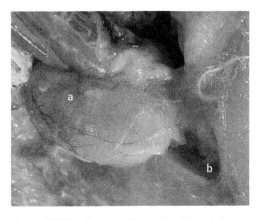

Figure 25.17 Close up view of the thoracic inlet. This closer view of the crop (a) shows it slightly distended by content and its relationship with the thoracic inlet. The V shaped inlet (b) is formed by the intersection of the right and left coracoid and furcular (wishbone) bones.

called the post hepatic septum. To remove the sternum, ribs, and keel, grasp the caudal point of the keel and sternum and reflect cranially (Figure 25.19). Using the poultry shears, incise

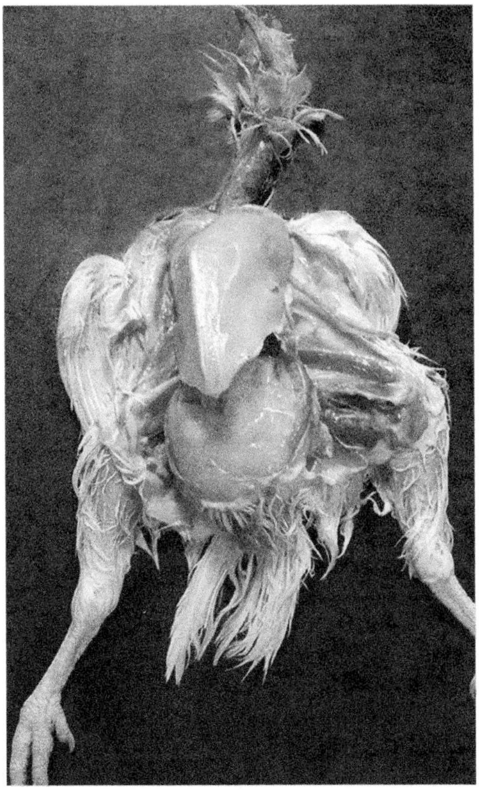

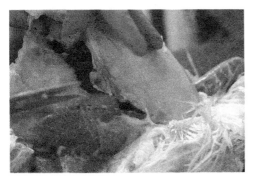

Figure 25.18 In order to enter the coelomic cavity, dissect the muscle and fascias overlying the abdomen, caudal to the keel. This will expose the caudal ceolomic cavity.

the pectoral muscles, and ribs at the level of the costochondral junction, aiming the cuts toward the thoracic inlet.

As the ribs are cut, and the sternum freed, continue to reflect it forward (Figure 25.20). This will provide you with your first view of the viscera and the first view of the air sacs. The thin, clear to slightly opaque membranes evident as you reflect the keel are the walls of the abdominal air sac (a). If fluid, fibrin, or other exudates are present in the air sacs, they will be visible at this time. Infections affecting the air sacs cause thickening and increased opacity. Given that manipulation of these structures has been minimal, any cultures necessary may be taken at this time. Sections of air sac can also be collected for histopathology. As the air sac is very thin, and will contract once incised, sections of air sac to be submitted for histopathology should be placed in a plastic tissue cassette prior to fixation so they are not lost in the formalin. You will also notice that the pericardium is partially adhered to the ventral sternum. This is normal.

Continue cutting the ribs (Figure 25.21). As you approach the thoracic inlet, aim the cuts slightly medially. At the thoracic inlet, you will encounter two bones that make up what

Figure 25.19 To remove the sternum, ribs and keel, grasp the caudal point of the keel and sternum and reflect cranially. Using the poultry shears, incise the pectoral muscles, and ribs at the level of the costochondral junction, aiming the cuts toward the thoracic inlet.

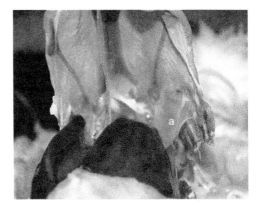

Figure 25.20 As the ribs are cut, and the sternum freed, continue to reflect it forward. This will provide you with your first view of the viscera and the first view of the air sacs (a).

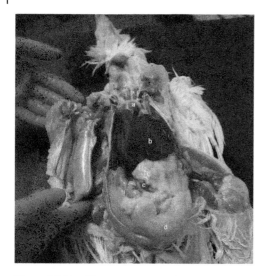

Figure 25.21 The two most prominent organs are the heart (a) and the liver (b). Since birds have no diaphragm, the two organs are only separated by thin membranes and lie in close approximation. The ventriculus (c) is partially visible beneath the fat pad (d).

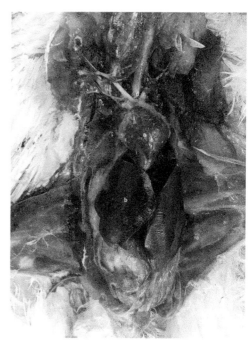

Figure 25.22 Remove the fat pad and the ventriculus (c) can be seen along with the heart (a) and liver (b). Observe the trachea (d) extending from the cervical region and tracking behind the heart.

would be the thoracic girdle. The largest of these is the coracoid, the smaller is the furcula (also known as the wishbone). Being thicker than the ribs, it can take some effort to cut these bones, particularly the coracoid. If the poultry shears are inadequate, rongeurs can be used. Remove the keel, pectoral muscles and sternum as a whole and examine the viscera in situ. The two most prominent organs are the heart (a) and the liver (b). Since birds have no diaphragm, the two organs are only separated by thin membranes and lie in close approximation. The ventriculus (c) is partially visible beneath the fat pad (d). Remove the fat pad (Figure 25.22), and the ventriculus (c) can be seen along with the heart (a) and liver. Observe the trachea (d) extending from the cervical region and tracking behind the heart. The avian trachea has complete rings that are generally cartilaginous but can ossify, particularly in older animals.

Heart and Syrinx

By pushing the heart caudally (Figure 25.23), additional features of the respiratory system

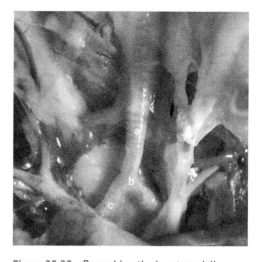

Figure 25.23 By pushing the heart caudally, additional features of the respiratory system are evident. The trachea (a) terminates in a segment that abruptly decreases in diameter and is slightly flattened. This is the syrinx (b), the "voice box" of the bird.

are evident. The trachea (a) terminates in a segment that abruptly decreases in diameter and is slightly flattened. This is the syrinx (b), the "voice box" of the bird. Given the acute decrease in diameter in this area, foreign bodies, parasites, and exudates can lodge in this area and cause acute death. Examination of the syrinx will be an important part of the dissection of the respiratory system that will be discussed later. The primary bronchi bifurcate just caudal to the syrinx.

Thyroid and Parathyroid

The avian thyroid and parathyroid gland are also located at the thoracic inlet, lateral to the trachea and in the fascia near the brachiocephalic trunk (Figure 25.24a). The location of the thyroids is not symmetrical, with one of them sometimes slightly cranial to the other. The parathyroid glands are small and, as in the pictured bird, not visible due to fat. They will be located either directly adjacent to the caudal pole of the thyroid gland or slightly distal to it. Collection of the thyroid and parathyroid

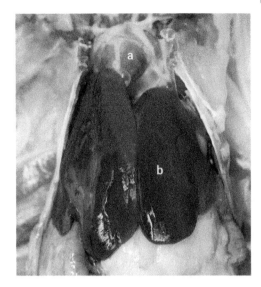

Figure 25.25 The liver (b) is located directly caudal to the heart (a).

glands for histopathology should be done at this time, and because of their small size, they should be placed in a tissue cassette prior to being placed in the formalin container.

Liver

The liver (Figure 25.25), (b) is located directly caudal to the heart (a). The avian liver has two lobes and, unlike in a mammal, the normal liver may extend past the last rib. The right lobe is often larger than the left lobe. The liver should be homogenous, deep brown-red, with a smooth glistening capsule and fill the entire width of the coelomic cavity. The edges of the liver lobes should be thin and sharp. The edges of the lobes in enlarged livers are thickened and blunt. A small liver that does not fill the width of the cavity may be seen in emaciated birds.

Gallbladder

Expose the gallbladder (Figure 25.26), (a) by gently separating the liver lobes (b). The size of the gall bladder varies with the nutritional state of the bird and postprandial period. Enlarged gallbladders are evidence of anorexia. Discoloration of the liver tissue adjacent

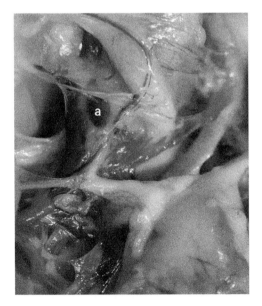

Figure 25.24 The avian thyroid (a) and parathyroid gland are also located at the thoracic inlet, lateral to the trachea and in the fascia near the brachiocephalic trunk.

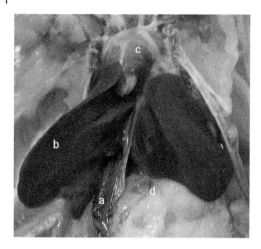

Figure 25.26 Expose the gall bladder (a) by gently separating the liver lobes (b).

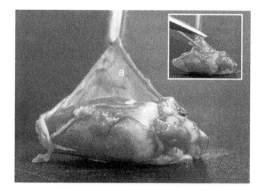

Figure 25.27 Cut through the brachiocephalic trunks and surrounding facia to remove the heart. The pericardium should be opened by tenting the tissue and incising. This can be done while the heart is in situ or after removal.

to the gallbladder is a normal post mortem artifact (bile imbibition) and is of no significance. Similar staining may be seen on the surface of the ventriculus (d) adjacent to the gallbladder. Note the proximity of the heart (c) to the liver.

Organ Removal and Examination: Stage 1

Heart

Cut through the brachiocephalic trunks and surrounding fascia to remove the heart (Figure 25.27). The pericardium should be opened by tenting the tissue and incising. This can be done while the heart is in situ or after removal. Only a small amount of clear fluid should be present in the pericardial space and the outer membrane should not be adhered to the epicardium.

The myocardial surface (Figure 25.28), (a) should be smooth and slightly glistening. Color will depend on the amount of fat and post mortem interval as well as the amount of blood in the auricles. Blood pooling in and enlarging of the right auricle is a common incidental finding. In general, the myocardium should be light red. Fat may be present at the base of the heart and small amounts of fat may surround the coronary vessels.

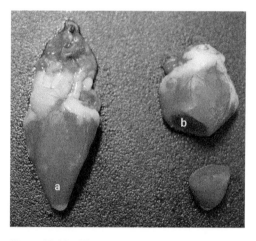

Figure 25.28 The myocardial surface (a) should be smooth and slightly glistening. Make a transverse cut through the heart, approximately one-third the distance proximal to the apex. Examine the cross section (b).

Make a transverse cut through the heart, approximately one-third the distance proximal to the apex. Examine the cross section (b). The left ventricular free wall and septum should be approximately equal in thickness with a small ventricular space. The right ventricular wall is very thin, and the ventricular cavity only a small slit between the free wall and the septum.

Insert the scissors into the ventricular lumina and cut through the free walls in order to open the ventricles and atria (Figure 25.29). The mural side of the right atrioventricular

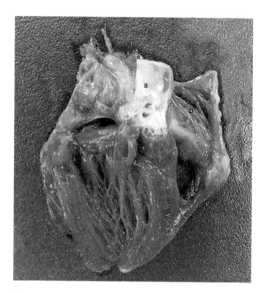

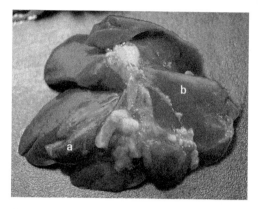

Figure 25.30 Being careful not to rupture the gall bladder (a), gently dissect the attachments of the liver (b) and remove it and the gall bladder in whole.

Figure 25.29 Insert the scissors into the ventricular lumina and cut through the free walls in order to open the ventricles and atria. The intimal surfaces of the great vessels (a) are smooth, and pale yellow to white. Moderator bands are evident on the endocardial surfaces of the atria (b) and ventricles (c).

valve is muscular while the rest of the valve is membranous. The left atrioventricular valve is completely membranous. Semilunar valves are present at the base of the pulmonary artery and aorta. The intimal surfaces of the great vessels (a) are smooth and pale yellow to white. As the post mortem interval increases, the intima may become stained with hemoglobin (hemoglobin imbibition) imparting a red tinge to the tissue. Moderator bands are evident on the endocardial surfaces of the atria (b) and ventricles (c). For small birds, the entire heart can be placed in formalin for histopathology. If the heart is too large, sections through the valves, ventricles, and atria can be taken and fixed for histologic examination.

Liver and Gallbladder

Being careful not to rupture the gallbladder (Figure 25.30a); gently dissect the attachments of the liver (b) and remove it and the gallbladder in whole. Make parallel cuts through the

hepatic parenchyma and examine the cut surfaces looking for lesions such as areas of necrosis, hemorrhage, inflammation, or fibrosis. Submit any lesions for histopathology and/or laboratory testing. If no lesions are present, submit a representative section from each lobe for histopathology.

Spleen, Proventriculus, Ventriculus, and Oviduct

Now that the heart and liver are removed, and deeper organs become visible (Figure 25.31). The spleen (a) is a small, round, red organ located to the left and slightly dorsal to the proventriculus (b), near the junction with the ventriculus (c). The proventriculus is the glandular stomach and can be recognized by its pale tan color and slightly cobblestone appearance. The ventriculus is the grinding stomach and portions are coated in a thick, white fascia while other areas are a darker red muscle. In mature birds, particularly those who are in lay, the oviduct (d) may become apparent. This long, tortuous tubular organ has a prominent vasculature and is pale tan, distinguishing it from the smaller diameter loops of intestine (e), the color of which varies with the color of the content.

Remove the spleen (Figure 25.32). In chickens the spleen is round, slightly turgid and has

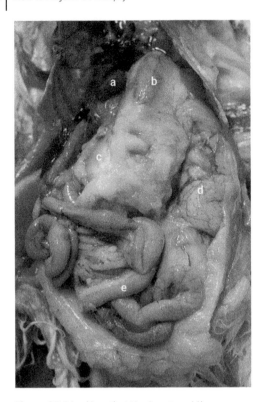

Figure 25.31 Now that the heart and liver are removed, deeper organs become visible. The spleen (a) is a small, round, red organ located to the left and slightly dorsal to the proventriculus (b), near the junction with the ventriculus (c). In mature birds, particularly those who are in lay, the oviduct (d) may become apparent. This long, tortuous tubular organ has a prominent vasculature, and is pale tan, distinguishing it from the smaller diameter loops of intestine (e), the color of which varies with the color of the content.

a slightly marbled surface depending on the prominence of the lymphoid tissue. The avian spleen does not store blood in the same way as the mammalian spleen, and thus the texture tends to be slightly firmer. The spleen should be approximately one-third the size of the proventriculus. Enlarged soft spleens can be evidence of systemic bacterial infection, while some viral infections result in a smaller spleen. Increased amounts of lymphoid tissue may cause the spleen to be more marbled and softer. If the spleen cannot be located, check the ventral surface of the liver as it is sometimes inadvertently removed with this larger organ.

Organ Removal and Examination: Stage 2

Examination of the gastrointestinal tract begins with opening the esophagus (Figure 25.33). Insert your scissors in the right commissure of the beak and into the cranial esophagus. Cut through the commissure, freeing the right side of the mandible and extend the cut caudally into the esophageal lumen (c). This also allows for further examination of the oral structures including the choanal slit (a) with papillae and the oral mucosa (b). Note the jugular vein running parallel to the esophagus (d).

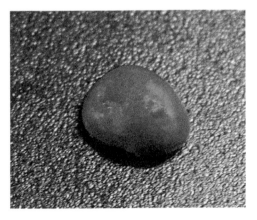

Figure 25.32 Remove the spleen.

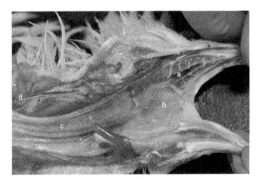

Figure 25.33 Insert your scissors in the right commissure of the beak and into the cranial esophagus.

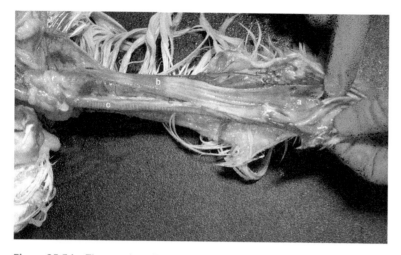

Figure 25.34 The opening of the esophagus lies at the back of the throat (oropharynx), dorsal to the tongue (a). The esophageal mucosa (b) is white but may become pink with livor mortis (hypostasis).

Esophagus

The opening of the esophagus (Figure 25.34) lies at the back of the throat (oropharynx), dorsal to the tongue (a). The esophageal mucosa (b) is white but may become pink with livor mortis (hypostasis). The mucosal surface is faintly stippled by numerous, small glands, giving it a slightly cobblestone texture. Variable amounts of clear, to slightly opaque mucus coats the mucosa as well as ingesta. Ingesta can sometimes be mistaken for an exudate, but in contrast to ingesta, which will rinse easily away from the tissue, exudates such as fibrin will adhere. A section of the esophagus should be removed and submitted for histopathology.

Proventriculus, Ventriculus, and Intestinal Tract

Incise the esophagus just cranial to the entry into the proventriculus and reflect the proventriculus caudally (Figure 25.35). Use the proventriculus to apply traction to the mesenteric attachments. Cut these attachments as you remove the entire digestive tract, including the cloaca. Linearize the intestine with the exception of the duodenum and lay them out on the dissection table for examination. The lower digestive tract lies dorsal to the liver (a)

and from cranial to caudal includes the proventriculus (b), ventriculus (c), jejunum (e), ileum (g), paired ceca (f), descending colon (h), and cloaca (i). The gastrointestinal, urinary, and

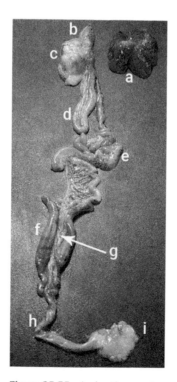

Figure 25.35 Incise the esophagus just cranial to the entry into the proventriculus and reflect the proventriculus caudally.

reproductive tracts all empty into the cloaca, but it is most easily removed with the descending colon. In young birds, the bursa of Fabricius, a round, soft lymphoid organ, will be located on the dorsal surface of the junction of the descending colon and cloaca (see anatomy chapter).

The proventriculus (Figure 25.36a) and ventriculus (b) are the glandular and grinding gastric compartments respectively. These two compartments are separated by a short isthmus. The ventriculus empties into the duodenum (c). Separate the ventriculus and proventriculus from the duodenum and use the scissors to open the gastric compartments (Figure 25.37). The proventricular glands and their luminal openings are clearly evident on the proventricular mucosa (a). As chickens are granivorous birds, the proventricular muscles (b) are extremely thick and firm, and significant effort may be required to cut through the muscle and the fascia on the adventitial surface. The ventricular content consists of feed material (c) in varying stages of breakdown.

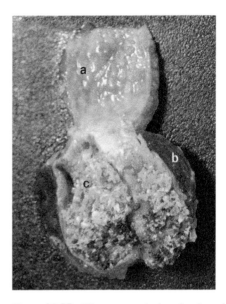

Figure 25.37 The proventricular glands and their luminal openings are clearly evident on the proventricular mucosa (a). As chickens are granivorous birds, the proventricular muscles (b) are extremely thick, and firm and significant effort may be required to cut through the muscle and the fascia on the adventitial surface. The ventricular content consists of feed material (c) in varying stages of breakdown.

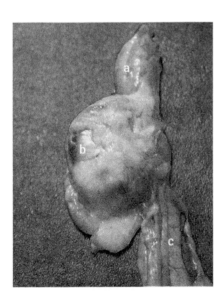

Figure 25.36 The proventriculus (a) and ventriculus (b) are the glandular and grinding gastric compartments respectively. These two compartments are separated by a short isthmus. The ventriculus empties into the duodenum (c).

Small pebbles or even rocks may be ingested by the bird to help with the grinding process.

Rinse the content out of the ventriculus and proventriculus (Figure 25.38). This will reveal the contrast in the mucosal appearance of the glandular proventriculus (a), the smoother isthmus (b) and the ventricular mucosa, which is coated by a thick protein called koilin (c). The color of the koilin will vary depending on the color of feed but is generally a shade of yellow or green. Using the forceps, peel off the koilin to reveal the mucosal surface. The mucosa should be smooth, pale white to red and the koilin should not adhere strongly to any area. Adherence may indicate inflammation or neoplasia. When submitting tissues for histopathology, it is important to include full thickness sections through the proventriculus, isthmus, and ventriculus. Inclusion of the isthmus is important as this is the area is which the acid pH of the proventriculus transitions to the

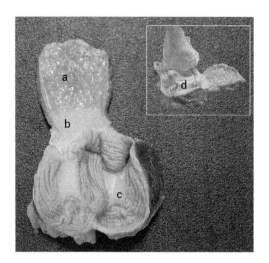

Figure 25.38 Rinse the content out of the ventriculus and proventriculus. This will reveal the contrast in the mucosal appearance of the glandular proventriculus (a), the smoother isthmus (b) and the ventricular mucosa which is coated by a thick protein called koilin (c).

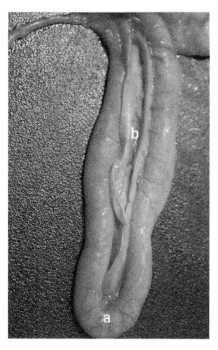

Figure 25.39 The loops of the duodenum (a) surround the pancreas (b).

more neutral pH of the ventriculus, giving pathogens a variety of microenvironments in which to propagate.

The loops of the duodenum (Figure 25.39a) surround the pancreas (b). The color of the tissue varies with content and post mortem interval, but the pancreas generally retains its pink color. The duodenum should be opened on the antimesenteric side and the mucosa and content examined. When examining any portion of the intestine, special attention should be paid to any ulcers, erosions, or areas of mural thickening. The color of the intestinal loops can change markedly after death and thus is not a good metric by which to evaluate the tissue. Intestinal content is an important feature to evaluate as abnormal content indicates intestinal dysfunction, regardless of the gross appearance of the tissue. Samples of duodenum and pancreas should be submitted for histology, maintaining the pancreatic attachment to the duodenum, as this allows the pathologist to easily identify this section of tissue.

The duodenum empties into the jejunum, which leads to a short ileum (Figure 25.40).

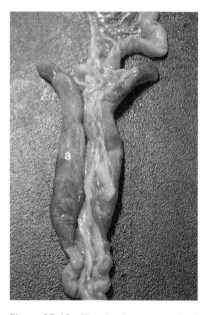

Figure 25.40 The duodenum empties into the jejunum, which leads to a short ileum. The ileum ends at the ileo-ceco-colic junction. The chicken has two, large, ceca (a) extending cranially from this junction.

The ileum and jejunum are separated by Meckel's diverticulum, a small flap of tissue on the antimesenteric side of the intestine that is the remnant of the yolk sac attachment in the neonatal bird (see anatomy chapter). The ileum ends at the ileo-ceco-colic junction. The chicken has two, large, ceca (a) extending cranially from this junction. The content of the ceca is thicker and darker than the content of the other sections of the intestine. Sections of the intestine should be opened and examined as described for the duodenum. Samples of each, including the ceca, attached to the ileum, should be submitted for histopathology. Care should be taken not to manipulate the mucosa of the samples for histopathology; this can damage the mucosa, preventing adequate histologic evaluation.

The ileo-ceco-colic junction is characterized by a slight swelling at the base of the ceca (Figure 25.41). This swelling is the cecal tonsil, an important lymphoid organ of the bird. The cecal tonsils are the largest lymphoid aggregates of avian gut-associated lymphoid tissue. The inset shows the open, mucosal surface of the tonsil. Note the slightly roughened area, this corresponds to the lymphoid aggregates in the submucosa. A cross section through the junction, including the cecal tonsil should be submitted for histopathology. The unfixed cecal tonsil can also be submitted for laboratory evaluation for certain viral infections. Viruses such as infectious bronchitis virus survive for long periods in the cecal tonsils and can be isolated during virus isolation testing.

Organ Removal and Examination: Stage 3

With the intestines removed, the deepest organs become visible (Figure 25.42). These include the lungs and the reproductive system. The inset shows the oviduct in situ with the intestinal structures. The large picture is of this same bird with the intestine removed, revealing the ovaries, and the oviduct, just caudal to the lungs. The large yellow spherical structures are the mature ova. These are covered in a thin vascular membrane. By gently reflecting these structures caudally, traction can be placed in the attachments of the ovary and the oviduct, facilitating incision of these attachments and removal of the reproductive tract. Unlike mammals, female birds only have a left ovary and oviduct. Remnants of embryonic, right-sided oviduct may be maintained in

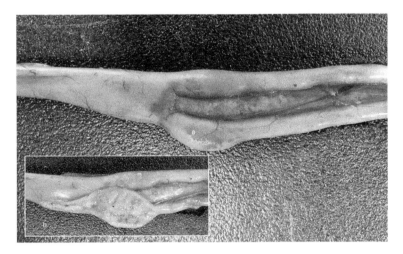

Figure 25.41 The ileo-ceco-colic junction is characterized by a slight swelling at the base of the ceca. This swelling is the cecal tonsil, an important lymphoid organ of the bird.

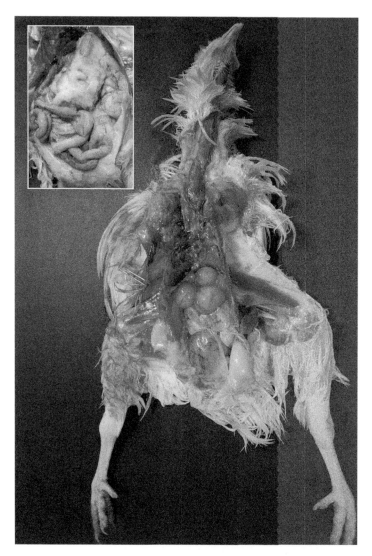

Figure 25.42 With the intestines removed, the deepest organs become visible. These include the lungs and the reproductive system. The inset shows the oviduct in situ with the intestinal structures. The large picture is of this same bird with the intestine removed, revealing the ovaries, and the oviduct, just caudal to the lungs. The large yellow spherical structures are the mature ova.

the adult bird (Figure 25.43). These appear as cystic structures located laterally and to the right of the most caudal portion of the fully developed oviduct. In this photograph, the cyst (b) is adjacent to the shell gland (uterus) (a). The shell gland is quite enlarged due to the presence of an egg in the tract. Cystic oviducts are thin-walled and translucent and often filled with a small amount of clear, watery to slightly viscous fluid.

Testes

In the male bird, the testicles are located at the cranial pole of the kidneys, just caudal to the lungs (Figure 25.44). The size of the testes varies with age and reproductive status. They are round to elongate structures and generally pale but may be pigmented in dark-colored chickens such as Silkies. Because this bird is in breeding condition, the testes are quite large

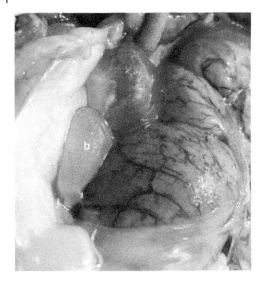

Figure 25.43 Remnants of embryonic, right-sided oviduct may be maintained in the adult bird. These appear as cystic structures located laterally and to the right of the most caudal portion of the fully developed oviduct. In this photograph, the cyst (b) is adjacent to the shell gland (uterus) (a). The shell gland is quite enlarged due to the presence of an egg in the tract.

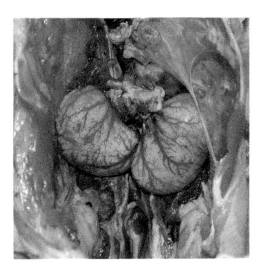

Figure 25.44 In the male bird, the testicles are located at the cranial pole of the kidneys, just caudal to the lungs. The size of the testes varies with age and reproductive status. Because this bird is in breeding condition, the testes are quite large, and vascular.

They are small, slightly yellow and, unlike in mammals, do not have a clearly defined cortex and medulla.

Ovary and Oviduct

The complete reproductive tract of the female bird includes the ovary (Figure 25.45a) and oviduct (b). The oviduct terminates in the cloaca (c), which is discussed with the gastrointestinal tract. The ovary contains ova in various stages of development (Figure 25.46a). The

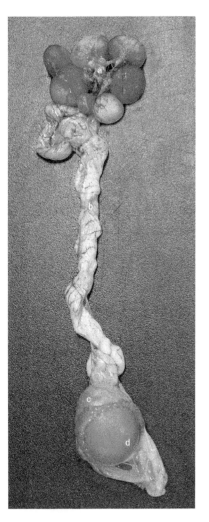

Figure 25.45 The complete reproductive tract of the female bird includes the ovary (Figure 25.45, a), and oviduct (b). The oviduct terminates in the cloaca (c). This photograph shows an egg at the cloaca.

and vascular. The adrenal glands, not evident in the photographs, are located dorsal to the gonads in both the male and female birds.

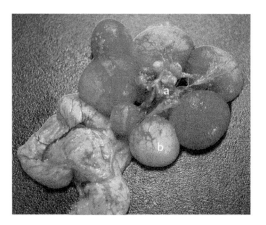

Figure 25.46 The ovary contains ova in various stages of development (a). The mature ova (b) are large, yellow and covered in a thin vascular membrane. There is a thin avascular band in this membrane called the stigma.

mature ova (b) are large and yellow and covered in a thin vascular membrane. There is a thin avascular band in this membrane called the stigma. This is the location in which the membrane will rupture, releasing the ova into the oviduct.

The oviduct, which is about 50 cm long, has multiple segments including the infundibulum, which catches the ovulated ova; the largest section, the magnum (b), secretes the albumen, the isthmus adds the shell membrane, and the shell gland or uterus (c) encases the egg (d) in a hard shell. The fully formed egg passes through the last part of the oviduct called the vagina before oviposition. A protective cuticle (bloom) forms on the egg while it passes through the vagina. Sperm host glands that can store sperm for as long as a couple of weeks can be found at the junction of the uterus and the vagina. The finding of an egg in the oviduct is normal and does not, in and of itself indicate impaction (Figure 25.47). Impacted eggs will be surrounded by inflamed tissue and may be adhered to the oviduct wall. Normal eggs are easily removed. Note that during a post mortem, a shelled egg may be found in segments of the oviduct cranial to the shell gland. This is due to post mortem movement of the egg and is not a lesion.

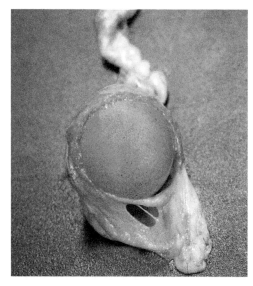

Figure 25.47 The finding of an egg in the oviduct is normal and does not, in and of itself indicate impaction.

Lungs and Respiratory Tract

The avian lungs (Figure 25.48a) are tightly adhered to the ribs (b). They can be removed by bluntly dissecting them away from the costal attachments, beginning at the base of the lungs where the attachment is less tight. Normal avian lungs are bright pink but will

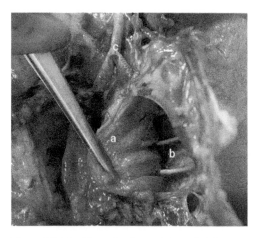

Figure 25.48 The avian lungs (a) are tightly adhered to the ribs (b). As the lungs are retracted cranially, they can be removed with the upper respiratory structures including the syrinx (c), trachea, and primary bronchi.

darken as the post mortem interval increases. Rib impressions on the dorsal aspect of the lungs are normal. A small amount of fluid may exude from the lungs with manipulation. As the lungs are retracted cranially, they can be removed with the upper respiratory structures including the syrinx (c), trachea, and primary bronchi. Figure 25.49 shows the fully removed respiratory tract, including the trachea (a) and lungs (b). The inset is a closer view of the syrinx in situ. Note the abrupt decrease in the diameter of the airway at the level of the syrinx. The lungs should be sectioned to examine the tissue for lesions and the tubular structures

opened in order to examine the mucosa. Representative sections of trachea, syrinx, and lungs should be submitted for histopathology. Scissors should be used to open the trachea (Figure 25.50) and examine the mucosa, taking care to limit disruption of the mucosa in order to preserve it for microscopic evaluation. As previously noted, the avian trachea has complete tracheal rings, so it will not fully open with the ease we see in mammalian trachea. The normal distal trachea may contain a small amount of fluid or froth due to agonal breathing and ingesta may be present in the lumen due to terminal aspiration. This latter change should not be interpreted as significant unless it is accompanied by tissue reaction, indicating a pre-mortem aspiration. The tracheal rings range from cartilaginous to ossified. In the larger photograph, a segment of esophagus is still present along the right side of the trachea.

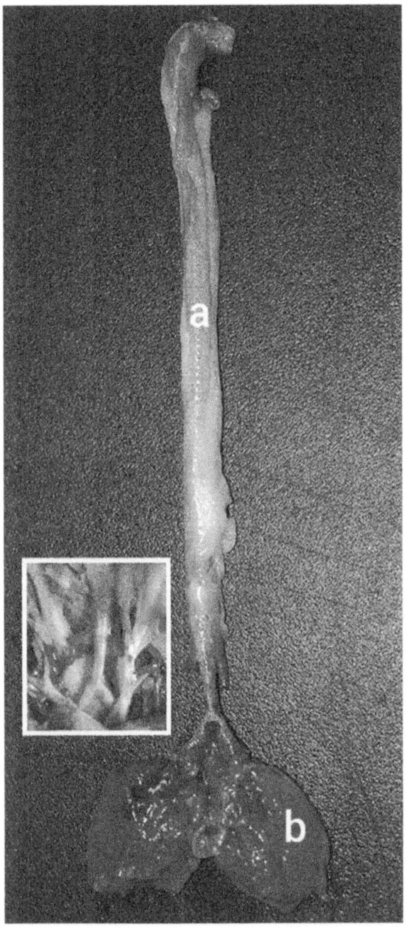

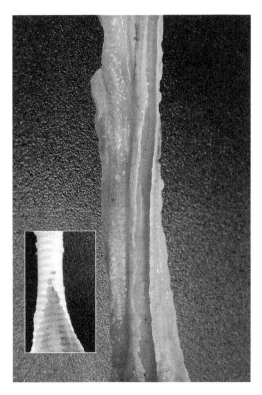

Figure 25.49 A fully removed respiratory tract, including the trachea (a) and lungs (b). The inset is a closer view of the syrinx in situ. Note the abrupt decrease in the diameter of the airway at the level of the syrinx.

Figure 25.50 Scissors should be used to open the trachea and examine the mucosa, taking care to limit disruption of the mucosa in order to preserve it for microscopic evaluation.

Kidneys

Removal of the reproductive organs exposes the kidneys (Figure 25.51). Each kidney has three divisions: cranial (a), middle (b), and caudal (c). These are embedded in the renal fossa of the synsacrum and can be bluntly dissected away from the bone in a similar manner to the lungs. The cranial division is less deeply embedded in the fossa and is a good place to begin removal of the organ. The tortuous, white tubules running medial to the kidneys are the vas deferens (d) remaining after removal of the testes. The kidneys should be sectioned, examined for lesions and appropriate samples submitted for histopathology. The thin, straight tubules located caudal to the kidneys (Figure 25.52, circled) and entering the cloaca are the ureters. In a normal bird, these structures are relatively inapparent, but if the bird is dehydrated or is retaining urates for any reason, they may become more prominent.

Sciatic Nerve

Post mortem examination of any chicken must include detailed examination of the sciatic (ischiadic) nerves and plexus (Figure 25.53). The sciatic nerve runs parallel to the femur and can be exposed by reflecting or removing the adductor muscle (a). The arrow delineates the sciatic nerve after removal of the superficial

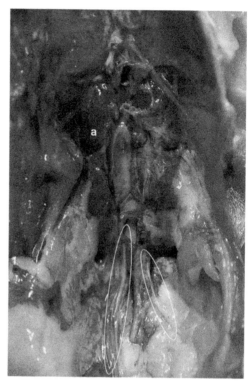

Figure 25.52 The thin, straight tubules (circled) located caudal to the kidneys and entering the cloaca are the ureters.

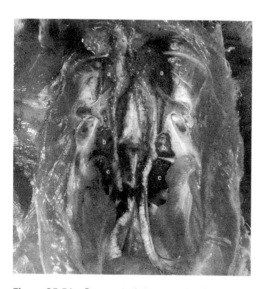

Figure 25.51 Removal of the reproductive organs exposes the kidneys. Each kidney has three divisions, cranial (a), middle (b) and caudal (c).

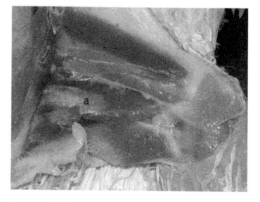

Figure 25.53 Post mortem examination of any chicken must include detailed examination of the sciatic (ischiadic) nerves and plexus. The sciatic nerve, runs parallel to the femur and can be exposed by reflecting or removing the adductor muscle (a).

muscle (Figure 25.54). Note the cross striations along the length of the nerve and the smooth, even contour to the nerve. Irregularity along the length of the nerve or loss of cross striation can be indicative of cellular infiltrates, the most common of which would be due to Marek's disease. After removal of the kidney (remnants labeled Figure 25.55a,b), the sciatic plexus is evident. In the photo, the plexus (circle) can be seen traversing the body wall (c) and emerging as the sciatic nerve (d). It is

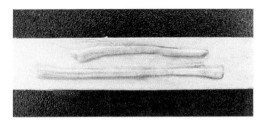

Figure 25.56 The longest sections of sciatic nerve possible should be collected.

important to examine both the right and left sciatic plexi and both sciatic nerves, as Marek's disease lesions may be segmental. Full evaluation of the sciatic nerves to look for evidence of Marek's disease includes histopathology. Both nerves should be submitted. The longest sections of nerve possible should be collected (Figure 25.56). In order to prevent fixation artifact due to submersion in formalin, the nerves should be laid out on a tongue depressor and allowed to adhere to the surface. Once they are adhered, the tongue depressor can be placed in fixative with the nerves.

Nasal Passages and Sinuses

Examination of the nasal passages and the infraorbital sinus can be accomplished by using the shears to remove the beak at the level of the

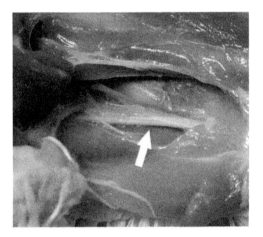

Figure 25.54 The arrow delineates the sciatic nerve after removal of the superficial muscle. Note the cross striations along the length of the nerve and the smooth, even contour to the nerve.

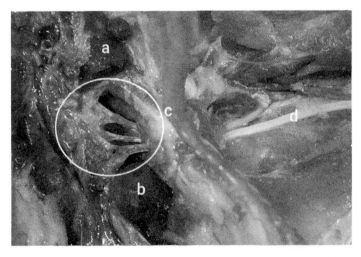

Figure 25.55 After removal of the kidney (remnants labeled a and b), the sciatic plexus is evident. In the photo, the plexus (circle) can be seen traversing the body wall (c) and emerging as the sciatic nerve (d).

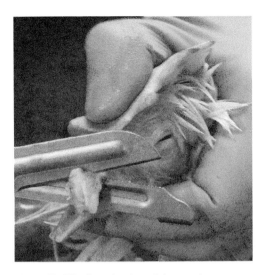

Figure 25.57 Examination of the nasal passages and the infraorbital sinus can be accomplished by using the shears to remove the beak at the level of the mid nares.

mid nares (Figure 25.57). The presence of mucus or caseous exudates in the sinuses is associated with a wide range of respiratory viral and bacterial diseases. The nasal passages and sinuses should be clear of exudate and only contain a small amount of mucus (Figure 25.58).

The turbinates should be smooth and symmetrical. The color may range from tan to red depending on degree of autolysis and livor mortis. In larger birds, where cutting the beak may not be possible, the infraorbital sinus can be examined by inserting the point of the scissors in the medial canthus of the eye and cutting through the tissues between the eye and the nares. The area to excise is illustrated in Figure 25.4.

Once the sinuses are examined, the head can be removed and skinned to reveal the skull (Figure 25.59). The skull should be examined for fractures or protuberances. The red coloring to the bone should not be interpreted as hemorrhage as blood does pool in the calvarial bones post mortem and hematopoiesis may occur in the tissue.

Brain

Brain removal can be challenging and can be done with rongeurs in smaller birds, but a hand saw may be needed in larger or older birds (Figure 25.60). A transverse cut can be

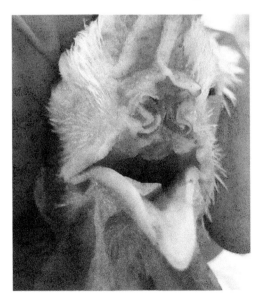

Figure 25.58 The nasal passages and sinuses should be clear of exudate and only contain a small amount of mucus. The turbinates should be smooth and symmetrical.

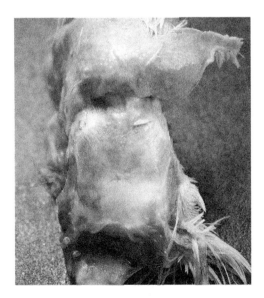

Figure 25.59 Once the sinuses are examined, the head can be removed and skinned to reveal the skull. The skull should be examined for fractures or protuberances.

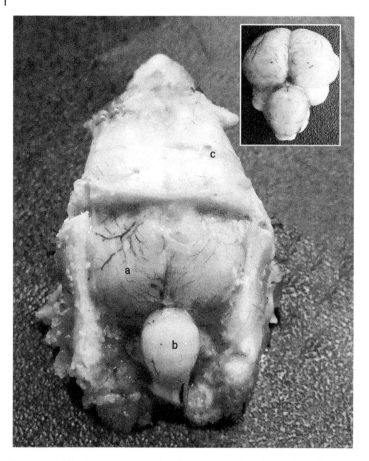

Figure 25.60 A transverse cut can be made in the mid portion of the calvarium (c) and connected to two more lateral cuts extending to the foramen magnum. Once this wedge of skull has been cut, it can be pulled off to expose the brain. The cerebral hemispheres (a) are devoid of gyri and sulci, and the cerebellum (b), with prominent folia is located caudal and slightly ventral to the cerebrum.

made in the mid portion of the calvarium (c) and connected to two more lateral cuts extending to the foramen magnum. Once this wedge of skull has been cut, it can be pulled off to expose the brain. The cerebral hemispheres (a) are devoid of gyri and sulci, and the cerebellum (b), with prominent folia, is located caudal and slightly ventral to the cerebrum. In order to remove the brain, the caudal skull can be tapped gently on the table to loosen the brain attachments and the skull held upside down so as to use gravity, along with gentle dissection to remove the organ (inset).

Joints

The last step of the necropsy is to open a sampling of joints (Figure 25.61). The skin of the joint should be removed, and the joint capsule incised in order to facilitate disarticulation. As described with the coxofemoral joint, the articular cartilages should be light colored, smooth and glistening, and covered in a small amount of clear, viscous synovial fluid. The surrounding capsule and connective tissue should not be swollen, red or gelatinous. Note: The defects on the condylar cartilages in the photographs are knife artifacts introduced during dissection.

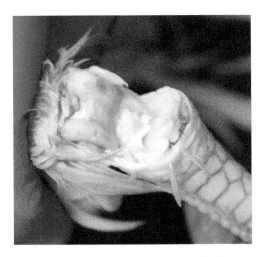

Figure 25.61 The skin of the joint should be removed, and the joint capsule incised in order to facilitate disarticulation. Note: The defects on the condylar cartilages in the photographs are knife artifacts introduced during dissection.

References

1 www.heritageacresmarket.com A list of poultry laboratories by state. (accessed 7 June 2019).

2 United States Department of Agriculture. Animal Plant Health Inspection Service. status of reportable diseases in the United States. http://www.aphis.usda.gov (accessed 7 June 2019).

3 Gregory, N.G. and Robins, J.K. (1998). A body condition scoring system for layer hens. *New Zeal. J. Agr. Res.* 41 (4): 555–559. Also available on line at www.tandfonline.com.

26

Diagnostic Laboratory Sampling

Rocio Crespo[1] and H.L. Shivaprasad[2]

[1] *Department of Population Health and Pathobiology, North Carolina State University, Raleigh, NC, USA*
[2] *California Animal Health and Food Safety Laboratory System, Tulare, CA, USA*

Introduction

Veterinarians are educated and trained to diagnose and treat animal diseases. Many practicing veterinarians do not specialize in poultry medicine/diagnostics. However, for veterinarians with an interest in treating backyard poultry, the advantages of incorporating these patients into the practice are numerous. With only minimal equipment additions and continuing education in the field of poultry, the practitioner can increase patient diversity and practice volume and gain an introduction to the challenge of poultry diagnostics and therapeutics.

Diseases that affect poultry have a wide range of overlapping clinical signs and visible lesions. Most veterinarians should be able to perform a basic physical exam, quickly diagnose most common avian problems, and send appropriate tissue samples to the diagnostic laboratory for further testing if necessary. This is especially important when a foreign or notifiable disease, such as avian influenza, Newcastle disease, or infectious laryngotracheitis, is suspected. In this chapter, where and how to obtain appropriate diagnostic samples is discussed. Additionally, guidelines on how to best collect and preserve samples and considerations for sending samples to an outside laboratory are provided.

History

Clinical examination is a key part of diagnosis of diseases in birds. Even before a bird is handled for examination, there are important prerequisites. The first of these is to ensure one has as complete a history as possible. Good background information increases the chances of an accurate and rapid diagnosis. At the clinic, veterinarians are normally confronted with the individual bird, but a visit to inspect the premises where a flock is kept may be helpful and is sometimes necessary.

The collection of clinical history is very similar to the gathering of information in general veterinary practice. However, clinical signs in mammals are more obvious to owners than those of birds. Therefore, careful, methodical, and logical questioning is essential when dealing with birds. History should include information not only about the bird(s) itself but also about the environment in which the bird lives and the management to which the flock is subjected.

First, it is important to collect basic information regarding the owner and the patient, such as owner's name, address, and contact information, patient's name or other identification (e.g. leg band), species, breed, gender, age, source, and duration of ownership. It is also pertinent to ask the reason for the visit. The patient may be submitted for routine health assessment, inspection of the flock (e.g. for export purposes), or a medical condition.*

Start gathering clinical information with general questions, proceeding to more specific ones. A thorough history frequently provides clues that may identify risk factors that are important in diagnosing and resolving a patient's problems. Important aspects to consider during the gathering of the clinical history include general clinical details, housing, and feeding, vaccinations, and medications if any (Table 26.1).

Table 26.1 Important aspects to consider during clinical history collection.

History of the problem

Where possible list dates of onset and/or duration.

- General abnormalities – sudden death, morbidity (the number of clinically sick birds), droopiness, depression, lack of appetite, ruffled or missing feathers, abnormal color of wattles and combs, dehydration, loss of feathers, etc.
- Respiratory system – sound of fluid mucus in the airways (rales), gasping, coughing, swelling of areas around eyes, inflamed sinuses, watery eyes, nasal exudates, etc.
- Digestive system – loose droppings, diarrhea, abnormal color of feces, big belly, etc.
- Nervous system – head shaking, neck twisting, abnormal extension of legs, circling, etc.
- Skin and musculoskeletal system – scratches, abnormal discoloration, lumps, lameness, scaly legs, twisted legs, abnormal back curvature, etc.
- Reproductive system – drop in egg production, poor egg quality: Thin shell, abnormal shape, color, and size, etc.

Table 26.1 (Continued)

Flock description and history

- Size of the flock/Number of birds at risk.
- Number (or %) sick.
- Number (or %) dead (distinguish natural deaths vs. culls), in the last week and last 3 mo.
- New bird arrivals? Where did they come from; their medication/vaccination history?
- Are there other species on the farm? How much contact is there with these other species and the birds?
- Have the birds been to a show or race recently?
- Have they been moved from one barn/loft to another recently?
- Have they had normal molting and brooding behavior?

Management practices – feed and water

- What type of feed – any recent changes in feed or feed supplier?
- Are there any feed additives? Do you give treats (i.e. scratch, garden vegetables, kitchen scraps)?
- What is the source of water (city, well, surface, cistern, etc.) and any recent changes in the source?
- What watering system is used (i.e. trough, bell, nipple, etc.)? Any changes in the watering system (i.e. from troughs to nipple drinkers)?
- Is the drinking water treated or has the treatment changed? (i.e. filtered, chlorinated, etc.).
- Any water additives used (i.e. apple cider vinegar, vitamin packs, antibiotics, etc.)?

Management practices – housing

- Access to outside.
- Access to open water.
- Access to wildlife (mainly wild bird populations).

History of the problem

- Cage or housing system.
- Litter/bedding materials, (type of bedding, changes, source).
- Other: Ventilation problems, weather or temperature changes, abnormal noise, electrical surges, blackout, recent use of insecticides and/or herbicides, etc.

Source: Adapted from Hunter et al. [5].

Sample Collection

A variety of samples may be collected, including blood, swabs, and tissues samples. Collected samples may be used for a variety of analyses. The tests to be carried out may dictate how the sample is taken, preserved, transported, and processed (Table 26.2). It is therefore important to plan carefully and to make sure that appropriate materials are available when taking samples.

The following rules apply generally to samples for clinical investigation:

1) As a general rule, be prepared to take blood, swabs, and other samples from every case. Have tubes, syringes, bottles, slides, and so on ready before clinical examination starts
2) Use the best-quality equipment, as poor samples can yield erroneous results. Swabs and reagent should be stored properly and used before the expiration date
3) Follow standard techniques when sampling poultry and ensure that this is performed efficiently and humanely
4) Ensure that all samples taken are properly labeled and recorded
5) Monitor the bird carefully following sampling. This is not just good practice, but it may provide further information on the condition of the bird
6) Be aware of the possible risks to human health when taking samples and follow appropriate guidelines. Do not expose staff or owners to hazards unnecessarily.

Collection of Blood Samples

The total blood volume of a bird is approximately 10% of its body weight, and ideally, for phlebotomy purposes, no more than 10% of the blood volume (or 1% of the body weight) should be removed from healthy adult chickens. If the bird is unhealthy, young, or elderly then even less should be removed. For example, the blood volume of a 2 kg bird (2×0.1) is 200 ml, and if it is healthy then a maximum of ($200\,ml \times 0.1$) 20 ml can be removed. Rarely is that large amount needed for diagnostic purposes as it is possible to run a full hematology profile on 0.3 ml of blood. On the other hand, 0.5–1 ml of whole blood is needed for each immunologic test (on average 0.3 ml of serum or plasma is required per test). Blood collection tubes should only be 1/2–3/4 full.

Blood or serum samples can yield a surprising amount of valuable information. Techniques that can be carried out on blood include hematology, biochemistry, and immunology. Immunology or serology can test for antibodies to various viruses and bacteria, and are very important tests as they can be quick and economical. Blood can also be used to perform microbiology, parasitology, toxicology, and molecular studies.

The site for collection may depend on the age of the bird, species, and competency of the blood collector. The jugular vein is commonly used on day-old or very young birds (Figure 26.1a) but can be used in birds of any age. The wing or brachial vein is the most commonly used to draw blood in poultry (Figure 26.1b). It is also used for collecting blood from small poultry breeds, such as quail, pigeons, or bantam (dwarf) chickens. The metatarsal vein is the vein of choice when collecting blood from waterfowl (Figure 26.1c). Blood can also be collected from occipital venous sinus and heart with the bird under anesthesia, but these techniques should be reserved for birds that are used in research, commercial poultry facilities, or prior to euthanasia. These sites may cause severe injuries or even kill the bird if performed improperly. Vacuum tubes apply too much pressure on the vein, causing collapse, and are not recommended.

Blood samples for hematologic or biochemistry analyses are collected in tubes containing anticoagulant. Ethylenediaminetetraacetic acid (EDTA) and heparin are most common. Because anticoagulants may cause artifacts on the blood cells, it is recommended to prepare a blood film and to submit this along with the

Table 26.2 Guidelines for sample collection and transportation.

Sample type	Test type	Suspected condition	Medium	Transportation
Blood	Hematology		Blood collection tube with anticoagulant (i.e. EDTA, heparin)	Chill
	Biochemistry		Blood collection tube with anticoagulant (i.e. EDTA, heparin)	Chill
	Serology	AI, NDV, IBV, Mycoplasma (MG, MS, MM), Salmonella Pullorum and S. gallinarum, etc.	Blood collection tube with or without anticoagulant	Chill
	Microbiologic evaluation[a]	Septic bacteria (i.e. Pasteurella)	Swab in Aimes or Stuart medium	Chill
	PCR	Marek's disease	FTA card[b]	Room temp.
	Toxicology	Heavy metal exposure	Blood collection tube with non-EDTA anticoagulant	Chill
		Trace minerals	Plasma or serum (without RBC)	Chill
Oropharyngeal, sinus, and trachea	Microbiologic evaluation	Mycoplasma sp., coryza	Swab in Aimes or Stuart medium	Chill
	PCR	AI, NDV, IBV, ILT, Mycoplasma	Polyester swab in BHI	Chill
			FTA card	Room temp.
	Virus isolation	AI, NDV, IBV, ILT, pox	Swab in BHI or VTM	Freeze
Fecal	Microbiologic evaluation	Salmonella	Fresh feces in sterile container or swab in Aimes or Stuart medium	Chill
	Parasite	Oocysts and eggs	Fresh feces in sterile container	Room temp.

(Continued)

Table 26.2 (Continued)

Sample type	Test type	Suspected condition	Medium	Transportation
Tissue/carcass	Gross evaluation[c]		*Slide smear* (heat or acetone fixed)	Room temp.
			Sealed container	Chill
	Histologic evaluation[c]	Infectious and non-infectious conditions	Formalin fixed	Room temp.
			Slide smear (heat or acetone fixed)[d]	Room temp.
	Microbiologic evaluation	Aerobic and anaerobic microorganisms	Fresh tissue in sterile container or swab in Aimes or Stuart medium	Chill
	PCR	Various viruses and bacteria	Sterile container	Chill
			FTA card	Room temp.
	Virus isolation	Various viruses	BHI or VTM	Freeze
	Toxicology	Various	Consult with lab	Consult with lab

[a] Microbiologic evaluation includes bacteria and fungus isolation.

[b] FTA cards are used for identification only. Samples submitted on FTA cards cannot be used for isolation of pathogens.

[c] Gross and histologic evaluation may be used for the identification of infectious diseases, as well as nutritional, toxic, and neoplastic problems.

[d] Special stains such as gram, acid fast, or Giemsa.

(a) (b) (c)

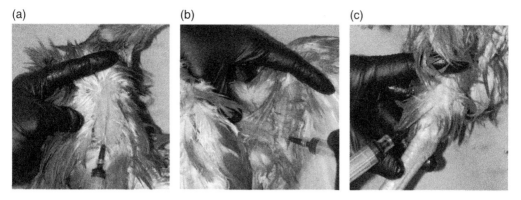

Figure 26.1 Demonstration of phlebotomy sites used in chickens. a Blood can be drawn from the jugular vein of chickens of any age and is especially good for small poultry breeds such as quail. b Blood being drawn from the wing or brachial vein (also known as the basilic or cutaneous ulnar vein). c Blood being drawn from the medial metatarsal vein.

blood sample. The standard two-slide wedge technique works well with avian blood (Figure 26.2).

Blood samples for immunologic tests are collected aseptically in sterile blood collection tubes without anticoagulants, separator tubes, or other non-EDTA/heparin tubes. For maximum serum yield, do not fill the tubes to more than two-thirds of their capacity, and lay the

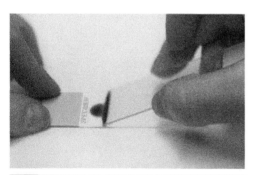

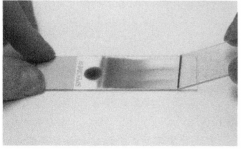

Figure 26.2 Preparing a blood film using avian blood. The standard wedge technique can be used.

tubes containing freshly drawn blood on their sides. Once the blood has clotted, the serum can be processed from the clot and sent to the laboratory, or the tubes containing clotted blood can be sent to the laboratory. Submit a minimum of 0.3 ml (300 μl) of serum per test, or 1–3 ml of clotted blood, depending on the number of tests requested. Refrigerate the serum or clotted blood until shipment. Whole blood that is kept refrigerated may be used for immunologic testing within five days of collection. If testing cannot be performed in that time, separate the serum/plasma and freeze it. Do not freeze whole clotted blood.

Live Bird Sampling

Any sample collection from a live bird should be performed after the bird has been fully evaluated. Swabs, aspirates, skin scrapings, and biopsy samples can yield valuable information that may assist in diagnosis. Examples of sites in birds from which swabs can be taken include the oropharynx and cloaca. Aspirates can be taken from joints (synovial fluid) and purulent exudates or transudates in the body cavity. Individual ectoparasites and feathers that contain eggs can be collected in a sealed container and submitted for identification. Many external parasites have preference to certain parts of the body, for instance the region around the cloaca is the best place to examine the bird for Northern fowl mites. For identification, these parasites should be fixed and stored in 70% alcohol.

Swabs from the oropharynx and cloaca often provide good samples for detection of respiratory viruses (such as avian influenza, Newcastle, or infectious bronchitis), and bacteria including *Mycoplasma* spp. Label containers holding the samples with the animal ID, date of collection, and body region from which the samples are taken.

There are a variety of swabs and media available. In general, avoid using calcium alginate swabs, cotton tips swabs, and swabs mounted on a wooden shaft. Chemicals on these swabs can interfere with some tests. It is also important to select the appropriate transport media for the test. Transport tubes containing Aimes and Stuart media are good not only for bacteria and *Mycoplasma* isolation but also for virus isolation. Media that contain antibiotics may be good for virus isolation, but they are not suitable for bacteria culture. For anaerobic isolation, Cary-Blair medium is recommended.

Oropharyngeal Swabs

The bird should be held securely to prevent stress and injury. It may be tucked under the arm with the ventral side facing up. Use one hand to open the beak (a finger may be inserted in the side to hold the beak open). Use the other hand for sample collection by swabbing the mucosa around the oropharynx and the choanal cleft (Figure 26.3). The goal of swabbing is to collect as much mucus as possible. Avoid blood in the swab, as this interferes with some tests.

Cloaca Swabs

The bird should be held securely to prevent stress and injury. Gently lift the tail feathers of the bird with one hand and then insert the swab in the cloaca. Shake off excess fecal material to prevent bacterial contamination.

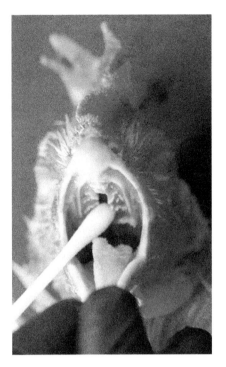

Figure 26.3 Demonstration of swabbing the choanal cleft of a chicken.

Postmortem Sampling

Practitioners may choose to perform their own necropsy evaluation and then submit tissue samples to the lab. Before necropsy starts, soak the bird's feathers with soapy water to prevent aerosol buildup. If the necropsy is performed on the premises in which the birds are housed, the examination should be performed away from the pen to reduce the risk of spreading infection. The selected location should also have easy access to water for cleaning and disinfection after the necropsy is completed. Figure 26.4 provides a list of items that are recommended for inclusion in a necropsy field kit.

In sick flocks, it is important to select birds with typical clinical signs. If the main problem is increased mortality without any other sign, choose birds that have died recently for the necropsy examination. It is important to examine *all* organs, with or without gross lesions. In most cases, gross examination does not provide

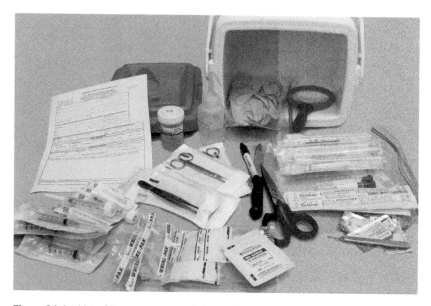

Figure 26.4 List of items recommended to be included in a necropsy field kit: Cooler/container, disposable gloves, pen (waterproof), submission forms, gauze, 70% alcohol, syringes (1, 3, and 6 ml), needles (25, 22, and 21 g), blood collection tubes, dry swabs, tubes with transport media, swabs with media, disposable cotton applicators, sterile scissors, sterile forceps, sterile scalpel blades (and handle), disinfected knife, disinfected shears (or large scissors), 10% formalin, clear sealable plastic bags, magnifying lens, camera/video.

full diagnosis and additional samples need to be tested to confirm a diagnosis and rule out other possible problems. Bird samples that can be submitted to the lab include blood, tissues, and swabs. Environmental samples can be also submitted. If a nutritional problem is suspected, also submit feed and water samples for analysis.

Tissue swab or tissue samples that are submitted for microbiologic evaluation must be collected and transported in a sterile container. Depending on the sample size, media may be needed to keep the sample moist. As indicated above (see section "Live bird sampling"), Aimes and Stuart media are good not only for bacteria and *Mycoplasma* isolation but also for virus isolation. Broth that contains antibiotics may be used to preserve samples in which virus isolation is desired but cannot be used for bacterial isolation.

If samples are submitted for molecular testing, several poultry labs accept not only tissue samples, preserved in standard transport media, but also tissue impressions, scrapings,

or swab samples made on FTA™ cards (Fisher Scientific, US, 1-800-766-7000) (Figure 26.5). The FTA card allows for easier shipment because there is no required transport media or special preservation (i.e. chill or frozen) of the sample. Additionally, because the pathogen is inactivated on the card, it eliminates the transportation of potentially harmful pathogens or hazardous materials (i.e. phenol). Nucleotide sequencing of PCR products allows for the characterization of the bacteria or viruses detected. On the other hand, if isolation of a specific pathogen is desired (for instance for antibiotic sensitivity testing) submission of a fresh sample or swab in the appropriate transport media is required.

When tissues are submitted for histologic evaluation, the selected tissue sample needs to be converted from a three-dimensional tissue into a stained section, approximately 4 mm thick, adhered to a glass slide that can be examined under the microscope. As with any other sample, it is important to collect a representative tissue sample and use appropriate fixation.

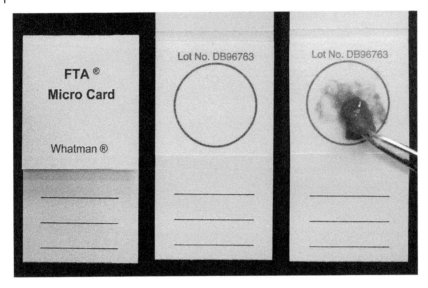

Figure 26.5 If samples are submitted for molecular testing, tissue impressions, scrapings, or swab samples can be made on FTA cards (Fisher Scientific, US, 1-800-766-7000) as shown without the need for transport media or special preservation of the sample.

The aim of fixation is to maintain fresh tissue in a state that stabilizes its architecture and chemical components in a form that enables it to be processed for histological staining and long-term preservation. Buffered 4–10% formaldehyde solutions are best. Because formaldehyde penetrates tissue at a rate of about 5 mm per 24 hours, it is important to avoid submitting samples that are too big. In general, the volume of fixative should be at least 10 times the volume of the piece of tissue. It is best to add the tissue to the fixative to avoid one surface of the sample adhering to the wall of the container. For larger samples, or multiple tissues following postmortem examination, the volume of fixative required may be too great to send through the mail. The excess fixative should be poured off before submission and the tissues should be sent to the laboratory moist with a small amount of fixative in a sealed container.

If whole birds are submitted to a diagnostic laboratory for evaluation, live and freshly deceased birds should be submitted. In most cases, live birds would have to be hand delivered, as most commercial couriers only accept carcasses. In order to slow down decomposition of dead birds, wet all the feathers on the body with cool soapy water. Place the carcass in a sealed bag and refrigerate as soon as possible. Do not freeze the carcasses unless they are going to be delivered more than five days after death. Freezing produces some artifacts, but a decomposed carcass is worse.

Submitting Samples

While it is frequently convenient for results of a test to be available during the patient's visit, the results have to be accurate and reliable, as well as cost-effective. The decision regarding which tests to perform in-house and which to send to other laboratories depends on several factors: Speed of desired results; effect of results on therapeutics decisions; staff ability to perform tests accurately and proficiently; equipment sensitivity and suitability for sample volume; consultation; and trouble shooting. Considerations for choosing an outside laboratory include experience in poultry diagnostics; types of services and tests available;

sensitivity and specificity of the tests offered; policies regarding lab supplies and transport media; mailers, billing, and invoice policies; turnaround time; and method of reporting (telephone, fax, computer, or mail).

When submitting samples, select specimens and/or freshly dead carcasses that are representative of the problem. Whenever possible, make sure that they have not been treated with antibiotics. Call ahead so that the veterinarian or laboratory knows that you will be submitting samples and to determine the information that is required, so that your submission can be analyzed as quickly as possible.

Obtaining useful/accurate results from the diagnostic laboratory requires good samples and a complete history. It is important to become familiar with laboratory submission and shipment protocol and methods of reporting results. Submitted samples should always be clearly identified and accompanied by a completed submission form that indicates the tests requested, a brief history of clinical signs, differential or tentative diagnoses, and medications being used. A summary of management practices and vaccinations are also helpful. Most diagnostic laboratory submission forms require standard information such as the species, breed, age, sex, weight of the bird(s), flock statistics, and relevant bird/flock history. It is advisable to keep appropriate transport media and shipping containers in the hospital.

Packing and Shipping Samples

When shipping samples it is important to maintain the integrity of the specimen, prevent leaking, and avoid cross contamination or misidentification of samples. The following tips will hopefully help limit any damage to samples during transportation to the lab.

If delivering carcasses, prepare the body as described above in the section on postmortem sampling. When ready to ship, place the bagged bird and a few ice packs (e.g. blue ice) within a second plastic bag and seal. Place the bundle in an inexpensive, leak-proof Styrofoam cooler, such as those found at a grocery store, and then place in a cardboard box or a cardboard box with additional loosely wadded paper for extra insulation.

If delivering tissues or other samples, place each individual sample in a bag or container that is leak-proof and secure properly. It is good practice to use a double-sealed container or bag within a sturdy cardboard box or padded envelope for shipping. If the sample needs to be refrigerated or frozen, include the appropriate frozen freezer packs to preserve sample integrity during transport.

Remember to complete the lab submission form and include it in the box (Figure 26.6). It is a good idea to place the paperwork in a Ziploc bag to prevent the paper from getting wet and becoming contaminated. Seal the box appropriately and mail or ship the package overnight. If the samples are shipped using a commercial carrier, it is necessary to pack samples in compliance with local postal regulations. Furthermore, if the samples need to be transported refrigerated or frozen, unless you have made previous arrangement with the lab, avoid shipping on Friday, Saturday, or immediately before a holiday to ensure prompt delivery before the coolant is exhausted.

Conclusions

1) Provide a complete and detailed history of the problem.
2) When birds are sick be sure to carefully select representative samples for testing.
3) Preserve samples in the appropriate medium for the requested test.
4) Identify samples properly and avoid cross contamination.
5) Follow local postal regulations for packing when shipping samples using a commercial carrier.

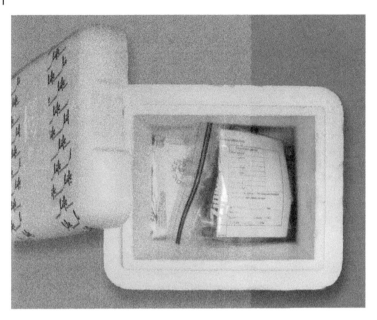

Figure 26.6 The laboratory submission form is included in the box with the sample, but it is a good idea to place the paperwork in a sealable plastic bag to prevent the paper from getting wet and becoming contaminated.

References

1 Barger, K. (2011). Taking proper samples and submitting them to the laboratory. In: A Practical Guide for Managing Risk in Poultry Production (ed. R.L. Owen), 199–211. Jacksonville, FL: American Association of Avian Pathologists, Inc.

2 Bermudez, A.J. (2008). Principles of disease prevention: diagnosis and control, chap. 1. In: Diseases of Poultry (eds. Y.M. Saif, A.M. Fadly, J.R. Glisson, et al.), 3–46. Ames, IA: Blackwell Publishing.

3 Buckles, E., Morich, J., Ruiz, J. et al. (2008). Avian diagnostic sample collection. In: Poultry Examination and Diagnostics. Ithaca, NY: College of Veterinary Medicine Partners in Animal Health, Cornell University www.partnersah.vet.cornell.edu.

4 Doufour-Zavala, L., Swayne, D.E., Pearson, J.E. et al. (eds.) (2008). Isolation, Identification, and Characterization of Avian Pathogens, 5e. Athens, GA: The American Association of Avian Pathologists.

5 Hunter, B., Whiteman, A., Sanei, B. et al. (2011). Responding to disease. In: Small Flock Poultry Health (ed. W. Cox), 81–84. Abbotsford, British Colombia: Animal Health Centre, BC Ministry of Agriculture www.agf.gov.bc.ca/ahc/poultry/small_flock_manual.pdf.

6 Johnson-Delaney, C. (1994). Practice dynamics, chap. 7. In: Avian Medicine: Principles and Applications (eds. B.W. Ritchie, G.J. Harrison and L.R. Harrison), 131–143. Lake Worth, FL: Wingers Publishing, Inc.

7 Samour, J. (2006). Diagnostic value of hematology. In: Clinical Avian Medicine (eds. G.J. Harrison and T.L. Lightfoot), 587–609. Palm Beach, FL: Spix Publishing.

8 Samour, J. (2008). Clinical and diagnostic procedures. In: Avian Medicine (ed. J. Samour). Edinburgh: Mosby Elsevier.

27

Interpretation of Laboratory Results and Values
Rocio Crespo[1] and H.L. Shivaprasad[2]

[1] *Department of Population Health and Pathobiology, North Carolina State University, Raleigh, NC, USA*
[2] *California Animal Health and Food Safety Laboratory System, Tulare, CA, USA*

Introduction

Accurate diagnosis of disease in birds, including poultry, depends upon a series of carefully carried out investigations. Meticulous evaluation of the clinical history and examination of the bird should aid the collection of appropriate samples to carry out a variety of analyses. In the previous chapter, collection and handling of samples were reviewed. In this chapter, an overview of the diagnostic testing (serology, microbiology, histopathology, and molecular biology) that is available and information gained from testing, including normal hematologic and biochemical parameters are discussed.

Hematology

Hematology is the discipline of medical science that studies the blood and blood-forming tissues. Hematology assays seldom provide etiologic diagnosis, but they remain an important tool to evaluate the health in individuals, to monitor the response and progress of therapeutic regimens, and to offer prognosis. Serology is still the predominant method of disease monitoring in commercial poultry, and

examination of blood smears and blood chemistry is rarely performed.

Although chickens have been used as research animal models for establishing normal parameters for other avian species, little information has been published on hematology of domestic poultry in clinical settings. Backyard poultry has become more popular in recent years and visits to veterinarians are increasing. Most of the current information about routine hematologic parameters is extracted from clinical values that have been established for psittacines. Serology is still the predominant method of disease monitoring in commercial poultry, and examination of blood smears and blood chemistry is rarely performed.

Hematocrit or Packed Cell Volume

The packed cell volume (PCV) is a quick assay that serves to evaluate the hemoglobin concentration and cell count. The PCV is obtained by centrifuging a microhematocrit tube full of blood at 12,000G for five minutes. Many standard textbooks on avian medicine, such as those edited by Samour (2006), Campbell (2005), and Ritchie et al. (1994), provide PCV values for specific poultry species, including chickens,

Backyard Poultry Medicine and Surgery: A Guide for Veterinary Practitioners, Second Edition.
Edited by Cheryl B. Greenacre and Teresa Y. Morishita.
Companion website: www.wiley.com/go/greenacre/medicine

quail, pheasants, and ducks. A recent study in healthy adult backyard chickens demonstrated the PCV value ranges between 24 and 36%, with an average value around 30% [3].

Blood Smears

Blood smears can provide information about cell morphology, differential white cell count, and blood parasites. A variety of stains can be used to evaluate the air-dried blood or methanol-fixed films. Slides can be stained with Wright's and Giemsa stains or Diff-Quick kit. Avian white cells are more difficult to find than the corresponding mammalian cells. One reason is that avian red cells and thrombocytes are nucleated. In addition, the avian leucocytes are scattered throughout the slide and are not aggregated in the margins of the slide as in mammals. Blood smears are not recommended for manual counting of cells because they are often inaccurate. However, blood smears can be used if no other systems are available.

Hematogram

Evaluation of the hematogram involves counting the various blood cells as well as cytological evaluation of the cells. Normal blood values of chickens and turkeys are presented in Table 27.1. The processing of avian hematology samples can be performed using automatic analytical systems. However, these systems are useful to differentiate between heterophils and lymphocytes but are not so useful for segregating all cell types. Otherwise, most laboratories use a manual method, such as the Natt and Herrick method or the eosinophilic pipette method, to differentiate white blood cells.

Erythrocytes are elliptic and large (Figure 27.1). They also have an elongated nucleus. The erythrocyte life span is 20–35 days. The total red blood cell count is not only an important value in hematology, but is also essential for the estimation of the mean corpuscular volume (MCV) and the mean corpuscular hemoglobin (MCH). Many labs today use

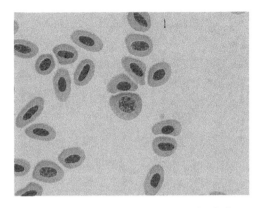

Figure 27.1 Wright's stain of red blood cells from a 2-year-old female white leghorn chicken with egg-related peritonitis. Note that the cell in the center is a polychromatophil (young RBC) with bluer cytoplasm and plumper, less dense, nucleus than the mature RBCs. It is acceptable to see up to 8% polychromasia in a normal sample. (Thank you to Dr. Jennifer Scruggs for assistance in producing this picture.)

automatic systems, rather than manual methods. As with PCV, younger birds have lower total erythrocyte count and MCH than adult birds. There are also variations between males and females. As with other bird species, MCV lies between 121 and 200 fL. Anemia causes changes in these values. Causes of anemia in poultry are summarized in Table 27.2. Acute blood loss (hemorrhagic and hemolytic anemia) is usually characterized by normal cell morphology, but the PCV and Hb are reduced if the blood sample is taken immediately after the acute event. However, if the sample is taken even a few hours after the loss of blood has occurred the MCV will be increased. In regenerative anemia, where the hemopoietic tissue is trying to replace the depleted erythrocytes, the morphology is characterized by polychromasia of erythrocytes. Polychromatic cells are precursors of mature red blood cells. Sometimes in regenerative anemia, an increase and/or variation of red blood size is also observed. In chronic nonregenerative anemia, the cell morphology may be normocytic or microcytic (MCV value may be normal or depressed) and the reticulocytes are depressed or absent. In most birds, up to 8% polychromasia is

Table 27.1 Hematologic values for the domestic chicken (*Gallus gallus domesticus*), turkey (*Meleagris gallopavo*), quail (*Coturnix spp.*), and ring-necked pheasant (*Phasianus colchicus*).

Analyte (abbreviation)	Units, SI [conventional]	Chicken	Turkey	Quail	Ring-necked pheasant
White blood cell count (WBC)	$\times 10^9$/l = [$\times 10^3$/μl]	9–32[8] 12–30[19]	16–25.5[8] 10.3–46.5[19]	12.5–24.6[19]	18–39[19]
Heterophils absolute	$\times 10^9$/l = [$\times 10^3$/μl]	3–6[19]	4–27.6[19]		
Heterophils	Proportion of 1.0[%]	0.15–0.5 [15–50][8]	0.29–0.52 [29–52][8]	0.25–0.50 [25–50][8]	0.12–0.30 [12–30][8]
Lymphocytes absolute	$\times 10^9$/l = [$\times 10^3$/μl]	7–17.5[19]	4.2–34.3[19]		
Lymphocytes	Proportion of 1.0 [%]	0.29–0.84 [29–84][8]	0.35–0.48 [35–48][8]	0.50–0.70 [50–70][8]	0.63–0.83 [63–83][8]
Monocytes absolute	$\times 10^9$/l = [$\times 10^3$/μl]	0.15–2[19]	0–3.9[19]		
Monocytes	Proportion of 1.0 [%]	0.001–0.07 [0.1–7][8]	0.03–0.1 [3–10][8]	0.005–0.038 [0.5–3.8][8]	0.02–0.09 [2–9][8]
Eosinophils absolute	$\times 10^9$/L = [$\times 10^3$/μl]	0–1[19]	0–1[19]		
Eosinophils	Proportion of 1.0 [%]	0–0.16 [0–16][8]	0–0.05 [0–5][8]	0–0.15 [0–15][8]	0[4]
Basophils absolute	$\times 10^9$/l = [$\times 10^3$/μl]	Rare[19]	0–2[19]		
Basophils	Proportion of 1.0 [%]	0–0.08 [0–8][8]	0.01–0.09 [1–9][8]	0–0.0015 [0–0.15][8]	0–0.03 [0–3][8]
Hematocrit (packed cell volume = PCV)	Proportion of 1.0 [%]	22–55[8] 22–35[19] 24–36[3]	30.4–45.6[8] 31–42[19]	30–45.1[8]	–
Hemoglobin	g/l [g/dl]	70–186[8] [7–18.6][8] 70–130[19] [7–13][19]	88–134[8] [8.8–13.4][8] 103–152[19] [10.3–15.2][19]	107–143[8] [10.7–14.3][8]	80–112[8] [8.0–11.2][8]
Red Blood Cell (RBC) Count, (Erythrocytes)	$\times 10^{12}$/l = [$\times 10^6$/μl]	1.3–4.4[8] 2.5–3.5[19]	1.74–3.7[8] 2.3–3.8[19]	4–5.2[8]	1.2–3.5[8]
Reticulocytes	Proportion of 1.0 [%]	0–0.6[19]	–	–	–
Mean Corpuscular Volume (MCV)	μm^3 = fL	100–139[8] 90–140[19]	112–168[8] 129[19]	60–100[8]	–
Mean Corpuscular Hemoglobin (MCH)	pg/cell	25–48[8] 33–47[19]	32–49.3[8] 42.9[19]	23–35[8]	–
Mean corpuscular hemoglobin concentration (MCHC)	g/dl	20–34[8] 26–35[19]	23.2–35.3[8] 29.6[19]	28–38.5[8]	–

Sources: Board et al. [3], Hawkins et al. [8], and Wakenell [19].

Table 27.2   Causes of anemia in poultry.

Type of anemia	Causes
Hemorrhagic	Hemorrhage: Trauma, cannibalism, aortic rupture, fatty liver hemorrhagic syndrome
	Parasitic: Ticks, mites, helmiths, coccidiosis
Hemolytic	Parasites: Hemoprotozoa
	Bacterial infections: Salmonellosis, spirochetosis
	Toxic: Aflatoxin, lead (acute), copper, dimethyl disulfide, phenylhydrazine
Nutritional	Minerals: Iron deficiency (ochratoxin-induced), copper deficiency
	Vitamins: Pyridoxine, folic acid
Anaplastic/ pancytopenia	Viral infections: Chicken anemia virus, infectious bursal disease, adenovirus, retrovirus, Marek's disease virus
	Toxic: Sulfonamides, lead (chronic), trichothecene mycotoxin, penicillum citrium, irradiation
Inherited Undetermined	

acceptable because of the relatively short erythrocyte lifespan and high turnover. An increase in PCV usually represents hemoconcentration or polycythemia (many cells) and it can be caused by dehydration.

The leucocyte numerical value is variable, even in birds of the same species. Therefore it is more helpful to compare leucocyte counts over time. In general, white blood cell counts vary from 10 to $45 \times 10^3/\mu l$. *Leucopenia* is an overall decrease in the number of all types of circulating white blood cells. It usually occurs with an overwhelming bacterial infection or immuno-suppressive diseases. Leucocytosis is an overall increase in the number of white blood cells. This could be a result of infection (bacteria, fungi, or parasite), trauma (resulting in massive tissue necrosis), or neoplasia (with extensive tissue necrosis or because of lymphoid leucosis complex).

Heterophils are the counterpart of the neutrophils that are found in mammalian species. They have a segmented nucleus and cytoplasmic granules that are elongated (fusiform shaped) and highly eosinophilic in chickens and turkeys (Figure 27.2). Heterophils from

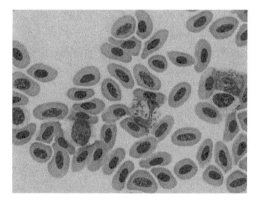

Figure 27.2   Wright's stain of two heterophils from a 2-year-old female white leghorn chicken with egg-related peritonitis. Note the rod-shaped pink (eosinophilic) granules. (Thank you to Dr. Jennifer Scruggs for assistance in producing this picture.)

poultry show increased phagocytic activity and killing activity compared to macrophages. A relative increase of heterophils is suggestive of an acute infection (bacteria or fungal), acute tissue damage, myeloid leukemia, and so on. Coccidiosis and *Escherichia coli* septicemia are examples of infectious diseases in poultry that are associated with an increase of heterophils. A decrease of heterophils may be caused by bone marrow damage, viremia, and aleukemic leukemia.

Lymphocytes are the predominant leukocyte in the peripheral blood of chickens and turkeys. Lymphocytes may be small or medium. Small lymphocytes are round with a round nucleus, high nuclear: cytoplasmic ratio, and a small amount of basophilic cytoplasm (Figure 27.3). Medium lymphocytes are more abundant, may be difficult to differentiate from monocytes, and may be increased in some infectious and metabolic diseases, as well as in lymphoid leucosis; while they are decreased in cases of stress, uremia, and immunosup-pressive conditions such as Marek's disease, chicken infectious anemia, and infectious bursal disease.

Thrombocytes are also nucleated (Figure 27.4). They may be confused with small lymphocytes. Thrombocytes participate in hemostasis and also have phagocytic properties. Thrombocytosis or increase of thrombocytes is observed in response to bacterial infection and as a result of excessive hemorrhage.

Monocytes are the largest of the leucocytes and are macrophages. As mentioned above, they need to be differentiated from lymphocytes. Monocytes are round cells, and usually have indented nuclei and abundant pale

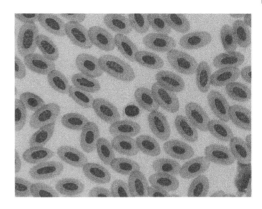

Figure 27.4 Wright's stain of thrombocyte from a 2-year-old female white leghorn chicken with egg-related peritonitis. Note the scant clear cytoplasm and small size of the cell compared to the RBCs. (Thank you to Dr. Jennifer Scruggs for assistance in producing this picture.)

cytoplasm, which contain fine azurophilic granules (Figure 27.5). An increase of these cells or monocytosis usually indicates a chronic bacterial infection or tissue necrosis. It is seen in cases of Chlamydiosis and Mycobacteriosis.

Eosinophils have irregular shape and their granules are round. The function of *eosinophils* in birds is unclear; therefore an increase of eosinophils may not necessarily be an indication of a parasitic infection. In raptors, eosinophils

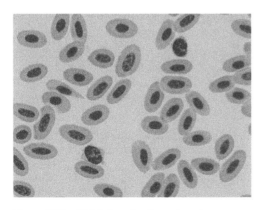

Figure 27.3 Wright's stain of two lymphocytes from a 2-year-old female white leghorn chicken with egg-related peritonitis. Note the scant cytoplasm and pseudopodia. (Thank you to Dr. Jennifer Scruggs for assistance in producing this picture.)

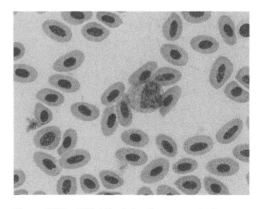

Figure 27.5 Wright's stain of a monocyte from a 2-year-old female white leghorn chicken with egg-related peritonitis. Note the relatively large size of this cell and the abundant light blue foamy cytoplasm, and a nucleus that is less dense than that of a lymphocyte. (Thank you to Dr. Jennifer Scruggs for assistance in producing this picture.)

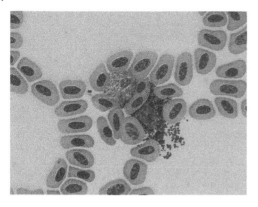

Figure 27.6 Wright's stain of a basophil and a heterophil from a 2-year-old female white leghorn chicken with egg-related peritonitis. Note that the basophil has dark purple cytoplasmic granules. (Thank you to Dr. Jennifer Scruggs for assistance in producing this picture.)

can increase in response to trauma. It is believed that basophils have the same function in birds as in mammals, and they are involved in early acute inflammatory reaction and in reaction to neoplasms with significant tissue necrosis.

Basophils are round cells with deeply basophilic granules in the cytoplasm (Figure 27.6). Basophils are one of the first leucocytes to enter tissue as part of an early inflammatory response.

Blood Chemistry

In many species, blood clinical chemistries are essential for medical assessment and diagnosis. For some diseases, they are essential for the diagnosis and treatment of affected birds. On the other hand, the results of the biochemical analysis in poultry should be taken as a rough guide to a final diagnosis. Blood clinical chemistries have rarely been used to assess diseases in poultry. There is only limited information regarding chemistry in poultry, as these species have been traditionally considered food animals and diagnosis has been attained through other means, such as microbiology investigation and necropsy. Other factors that contribute to the lack of established standard values

for poultry is the variability among breeds or strains of birds, wide variation in the physiological conditions (i.e. age, gender, egg laying, molting), and environmental differences (i.e. husbandry, nutrition).

Another reason for lack of standardized blood chemical values in poultry is that rarely poultry is taken to a clinic where analysis can be done promptly. Sample handling and transportation can alter blood gasses, potassium, or ionized calcium concentrations. Fortunately progress has been made in the knowledge of standard blood chemical values in poultry thanks to the use of handheld and small analyzers such as i-STAT® or VetScan2 (Table 19.3) that allow blood analysis directly in the field. Published reference values for poultry can be found in the *Exotic Animal Formulary* (Carpenter and Marion 2013) and *Schalm's Veterinary Hematology* (Weiss and Wardrop 2010). Unfortunately, the origin of most of these interval values cannot not be traced or validated. Blood biochemistry intervals in backyard hens have been recently validated using a VetScan2 [3].

Blood plasma proteins participate in the maintenance of colloid osmotic pressure, gluconeogenesis, transport of minerals and hormones, and production of enzymes and immunoglobins. Because plasma/serum proteins have numerous roles in the physiology of birds, they are a significant indicator of the condition of animals' health. Total plasma protein is probably the most used. As with most other avian species, the total value is 3–5 g/dl and concentration of proteins is significantly lower in young animals than in adults. Serum protein increases with prior egg laying and with age. As the liver produces most of the serum proteins, a reduction in total serum protein may be one indicator of liver disease. Other possible causes of reduced serum protein are anemia, malnutrition, malabsorption (secondary to gastrointestinal disease), intestinal parasitism, glomerulonephritis, severe trauma, prolonged stress, and heavy metal poisoning. On the other hand, hyperproteinemia

Table 27.3 Blood biochemical and gas values for the domestic chicken (*Gallus gallus domesticus*), turkey (*Meleagris gallopavo*), quail (*Coturnix* spp.), and ring-necked pheasant (*Phasianus colchicus*).

Analyte (abbreviation)	Units, SI [conventional]	Chicken	Turkey	Quail	Ring-necked pheasant
Calcium	mmol/l	3.3–5.9[8]	2.9–9.7[8]	–	–
	[mg/dl]	[13.2–23.7][8]	[11.7–38.7][8]		
		[≥10.9] [3]			
Ionized calcium	mmol/l	1.20–1.73[19]			
	[mg/dl]	[4.8–6.9][19]			–
Phosphorus Sodium	mmol/l	2–2.5[8]	1.7–2.3[8]	–	
	[mg/dl]	1.6–7.2 [3]	[5.4–7.1][8]		
		[6.2–7.9][8]			
		[4.1–5.7][19]			
	mmol/l = mEq/l	133–151 [3]	149–155[8]	180[8]	–
		141.6–152.6[19]			
Potassium	mmol/l = mEq/l	3–7.3[8]	6–6.4[8]	1.4[8]	–
Bicarbonate	mmol/l	3.2–6.1 [3]			
	mmol/l =	18.9–30.3[19]			
pH		7.28–7.57[19]	–		–
Carbon dioxide partial pressure	mmHg	25.9–49.5[19]			
Oxygen partial pressure	mmHg	32.0–60.5[19]			
Carbon dioxide	mmol/l =	19.9–31.5[19]			
	[mEq/l]				
Base excess	mmol/l	6.8–7.2[19]			
Oxygen saturation	%	70.6–93.3[19]			

(*Continued*)

Table 27.3 (Continued)

Analyte (abbreviation)	Units, SI [conventional]	Chicken	Turkey	Quail	Ring-necked pheasant
Creatinine	µmol/l	80–160[8]	71–80[8]	4.4[8]	–
	[mg/dl]	[0.9–1.8][8]	[0.8–0.9][8]	[0.05][8]	
	U/l	107–1780[3]			
Uric acid	µmol/l	149–483[8]	203–310[8]	322–328[8]	334–357[8]
	[mg/dl]	0.9–8.9 [3]	[3.4–5.2][8]	[5.4–5.5][8]	[5.6–6][8]
Glucose	mmol/l	12.63–16.69[8]	15.30–23.65[8]	14.41–17.36[8]	–
	[mg/dl]	[227–300][8]	[275–425][8]	[259–312][8]	
		11.53–14.51[19]			
		[207.2–260.7][19]			
Cholesterol	mmol/l	2.3–5.5[8]	2.1–3.8[8]	–	–
	[mg/dl]	[86–211][8]	[81–129][8]		
ALT	U/l = [IU/l]	–	–	6.5–9.6[8]	–
AST	U/l = [IU/l]	118–298[3]	–	402–422[8]	–
BA	(umol/l)	≤45 [3]			
GGT	U/l = [IU/l]			1.7–1.9[8]	
Total protein	g/l	33–55[8]	49–76[8]	34–36[8]	45–51[8]
	[g/dl]	[3.9–7] [3]	[4.9–7.6][8]	[3.4–3.6][8]	[4.5–5.1][8]
Globulin	g/l	15–41[8]	17–19[8]	–	19–21[8]
	[g/dl]	[1.6–4.3] [3]	[1.7–1.9][8]		[1.9–2.1][8]
Albumin	g/l	13–28[8]	30–59[8]	13–15[8]	26–27[17]
	[g/dl]	[1.2–3.7] [3]	[3–5.9][8]	[1.3–1.5][8]	[2.6–2.7][8]

Source: Board et al. [3], Hawkins et al. [8], and Wakenell [19].

is encountered in cases of dehydration (PCV is also elevated), shock, or acute infection.

To evaluate the health status of birds, in addition to the total concentration of total plasma proteins, it is important to determine the concentration of individual fractions. Albumins serve as a source of amino acids during insufficient intake of food, and participate in transporting fatty acids, minerals, vitamins, and thyroid hormones. Inflammatory processes induce an increase of globulins and a decrease of albumin.

Serologic Investigation

The laboratory examination of serum sample can be a valuable aid for assessing if a bird has been exposed to a specific pathogen. Serology is most powerful and accurate when used in association with other sources of information (i.e. clinical signs, production data, vaccination, necropsy findings, etc.) When poultry are moved between states or out of the country, serologic testing may be required to demonstrate that birds have not been exposed to certain diseases. There are a variety of serological tests available, such as enzyme-linked immunosorbent assay (ELISA), agar gel immune diffusion (AGID), agglutination test, hemagglutination inhibition (HI), and complement fixation (Table 27.4).

It is essential to know the uses and limitations of this procedure to ensure that maximum benefit is realized. Most serological tests have the following limitations:

1) Most tests only evaluate circulating antibodies, and take no account of mucosal antibody or cell mediated immunity. Serology testing has little value for diseases in which protection depends on cellular immunity (such as Marek's disease, infectious laryngotracheitis or pox virus infection), rather than antibody production
2) Lack of antibodies against a particular pathogen may be interpreted as the lack of exposure to such a pathogen. However, in acute infections, antibodies may not be measurable at the time of testing. Birds remain negative for at least 4 days after infection. For clinical diagnostic situations, paired serum testing is critical. Paired serum involves testing of serum samples collected two weeks apart, during the acute and convalescent periods of a disease. By using a paired serum sample the bird can be shown to be actively responding to the infection immunologically by a rising titer. On the other hand, if titers plateau or decrease it is generally an indication that no recent exposure has occurred. The antibodies persist in the circulating blood of the bird for months, even after the pathogen is no longer present
3) Antibodies to antigenically related agents might cause confusion as a result of cross-reactions
4) Serologic assays cannot "type" the immune responses against specific variants, such as differentiation between of avian influenza or the strain of infectious bronchitis
5) There is an inherent risk of false positive and false negative reactions.

An agglutination test (Figure 27.7) is probably the simplest of the serologic tests. It is a qualitative method and cannot be automated. This assay is inexpensive. It is commonly used for the detection of antibodies of *Salmonella* Pullorum (pullorum disease), *S.* Gallinarum (fowl typhoid), *Mycoplasma gallisepticum* (MG), and *M. synoviae* (MS). However, because false positive reactions may occur, it is only used as a screening tool. Positive results need to be confirmed with other serologic tests.

The HI test is considered the gold standard for serology assays. It is a quantitative assay, because HI is highly specific and consequently requires specific reagents for each antigen or antiserum tested. There are only a few false positive reactions. It requires homologous red blood cells for the test at hand. It is used for determination of the avian influenza subtype (Hemagglutinin and Neuraminidase groups), infectious bronchitis serotype (i.e. Arkansas,

Table 27.4 Selected serologic immunoassays available for poultry.

Disease	Serologic test	Comments
Avian Influenza	ELISA	Chickens and turkeys. Only a few labs offer a multispecies ELISA (includes waterfowl and game fowl).
		If positive, confirm with AGID.
	AGID	All species.
		If positive perform HI.
	HI	H and N groups determination
Newcastle disease	ELISA	Chickens and turkeys only
	HI	All species
Infectious bronchitis	ELISA	Chickens only
Mycoplasma	ELISA (MG, MS)	Chickens and turkeys only
		If positive confirm with HI
	Agglutination (MG, MS)	All species. If positive confirm with
		HI
	HI (MG, MS, MM)	All species
Salmonella Pullorum/ thyphoid	Agglutination	If positive confirm with microtiter
Reovirus (viral arthritis)	Microtiter ELISA	Chickens only
Infectious bursal disease	ELISA	Chickens only
Avian encephalomyelitis	ELISA	Chickens only

The AGID test (Figure 27.9) is based on the passive diffusion of soluble antigens and/or antibodies toward each other, leading to their precipitation in a gel matrix. It is commonly used for the detection of avian influenza antibodies. It is a semi-quantitative method and cannot be automated. In addition, it is difficult to interpret; this is especially true of weak positive sera.

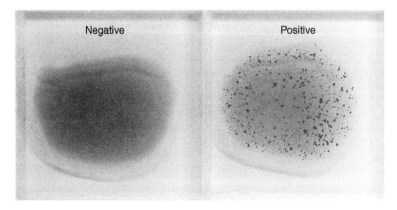

Figure 27.7 Agglutination test. The interaction of particulate antigens with antibodies leads to agglutination reactions. In a positive agglutination reaction (right) sufficient antibodies are present in the serum to link the antigens together, forming clumps of antigen-antibody complexes.

Connecticut, Delaware, and Massachusetts), and confirmation of MG and MS. In general, titers >1:8 are suggestive of previous exposure.

ELISA is a qualitative method that is easily automated and is more sensitive than other assays. For poultry serum samples, ELISA measures IgY (equivalent to the IgG antibodies in mammals) (Table 27.5). ELISA (Figure 27.8) is currently the preferred serologic testing method in commercial poultry. Because it can be automated, large numbers of samples can be processed in a single day to detect and measure antibodies against a variety of poultry pathogens. It is known to lead to false positive reactions occasionally; consequently, positive results may need confirmation by different methods. Finally, ELISA is species specific and most of the assays have been validated for chickens and turkeys. ELISA cannot be performed to measure antibodies in pigeons, waterfowl, and game fowl. Other types of assays can also be sensitive, specific, and possibly less costly, but they often require more complex procedures and intensive labor.

Histology

Samples that are taken for histopathology can provide diagnostic results that are timely and relatively inexpensive for the clinicians when performed properly. Histologic examination allows differentiation between infectious and non-infectious conditions. It can also narrow down whether an infectious problem is caused by bacteria, virus, fungus, or parasite, as well as if a non-infectious condition may be caused by a neoplasia, nutritional deficiency, or toxicity. Histology is an invaluable tool for diagnosing such common diseases in backyard chickens as Marek's disease and ovarian carcinoma. Special stains performed on the sections, such as Gram, Giemsa, PAS, GMS, Acid Fast, Tri-chrome, Warthin Starry, Von Kossa, Brown and Hopps, and Perl's Iron, can further identify or narrow down the possible causes of the disease. Specific pathogens, such as Avian paramyxovirus, Avian Influenza, Infectious bronchitis, and *Mycoplasma gallisepticum*, can be identified in the tissues by using immunohistochemistry. But these tests are not available in most laboratories. Formalin-fixed and

Table 27.5 Guidelines for interpretation of ELISA titers in poultry. In general, titer group 0 is interpreted as negative (not exposed to pathogen) and titer groups >1 are positive (exposed or vaccinated).

Doubling dilutions	Log titers	Interpretation	
1	0	Negative or no exposure	Negative or no exposure
2	1	No immunity	Maternal Immunity (*up to 4 wk of age*)
4	2		Live Prime Vaccine
8	3	Poor immunity	
16	4		
32	5		2nd Live Prime Vaccine
64	6	Protection Against mortality	
128	7		
256	8		
512	9		Prime Plus Killed Vaccine
1024	10	Field Challenge	
2048	11		

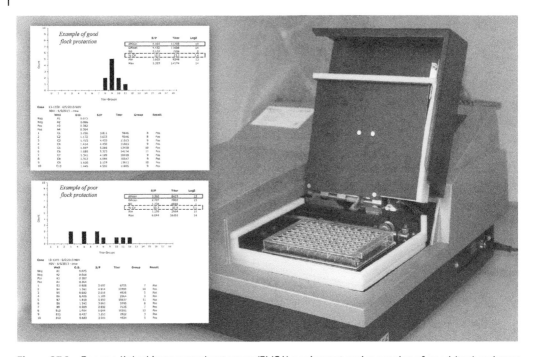

Figure 27.8 Enzyme-linked immunosorbent assay (ELISA) equipment and examples of good (top) and poor (bottom) results in a poultry flock. The mean titer of the tested birds within a flock indicates the strength of the antibody response of a flock. It basically provides a measure of the immune response of the flock. The coefficient of variation, or CV%, provides an indication of mean titer response variability of a flock. The lower the %CV, the more uniform the distribution of titers and the better the vaccination. For most diseases, the %CV after a correctly applied vaccination should be less than 40%. A CV% greater than 60% indicates uneven immune status of the flock or poor vaccination.

paraffin-embedded samples can also be cut into sections for molecular testing, from cases where fresh samples are not sent, cannot be shipped, or are not available, to identify potential pathogens.

Microbiological Investigations

Poultry become infected with multiple microorganisms from contact with wild birds, rodents, humans, and the environment. Birds that are newly introduced in the aviary can bring a disease such as infectious laryngotracheitis or mycoplasma. The primary goal of microbiologic testing is the detection of bacteria, viruses, and fungi that are possibly involved in a disease process.

The harvesting of the microorganism from a particular site is easier than determining whether the finding is significant. In reality, microbiologic testing can be misused as an indication of avian health. It is very easy to make a quick decision and conclude that a particular microorganism is the sole or primary cause of the disease process. The best way to interpret microbiology findings is to closely examine the patient, even before attempting to identify a possible pathogen. Then the clinician should establish if the bacteria, viruses, or fungi are actually involved in the clinical condition. Additionally, the clinician needs to determine whether the microorganisms that are detected are the primary cause of the disease or are secondary to another condition (i.e. malnutrition, contamination of the water source, immunodepression).

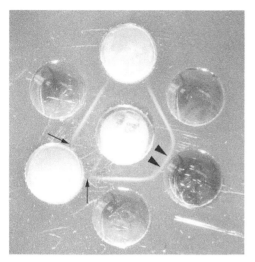

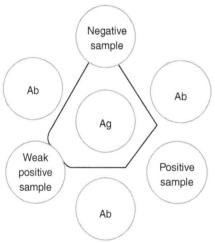

Figure 27.9 Agar gel immune-diffusion (AGID) is the passive diffusion of soluble antigens and/or antibodies toward each other leading to their precipitation in a gel matrix. There is slight bending of the lines associated with the weak positive sample (arrows), while in strong positives the precipitation line is clearly formed between the antigen and positive sample wells (arrowheads). Ab, antibody; Ag, antigen.

Bacteria Culture

The harvesting of bacteria from a particular site and their subsequent identification and testing for antibiotic susceptibility is a relatively easy process; more difficult is determining the significance of the findings. In reality, bacterial culture/sensitivity testing may be misused as an indicator of avian health. The best way to interpret bacterial findings is to closely examine the patient, even before attempting to identify a possible pathogen. The first question to be addressed is whether or not there are any visible clinical signs of infection.

A bacterial culture from a perfectly normal oropharynx may be irrelevant, regardless of the bacteria that might be isolated. It should be noted that a wide variety of bacteria are normal commensals of the gut of birds. Apparently undesirable bacteria may actually be harmless, or they may be present secondary to another condition (i.e. malnutrition, contamination of the water source). For instance, *Escherichia coli* is a normal inhabitant of the gut in poultry and *Salmonella* sp. may not cause enteritis in mature poultry. However, these bacteria may be pathogenic if the bird is stressed. Furthermore, when taking samples from postmortem specimens, one should take into account that cultures obtained from specimens that have been dead for more than 24 hours may not be representative. Some organisms, such as *Proteus* sp., present in the gut, may rapidly invade other organs after death, and may overgrow other pathogens on a culture plate. Only when a direct specific disease condition can be directly linked to a possible pathogen should a culture be considered significant. Rarely should a patient be treated with antibiotics merely because of the presence of suspect bacteria.

The laboratory may not be able to recover certain bacteria, even if present, or if the patient has been treated with antibiotics. Antibiotics in the sample may inhibit the growth of bacteria. Furthermore, bacteria may not be isolated if the specimen is not cultured in the proper media and under optimal environmental conditions. Bacterial cultures are routinely set on standard aerobic media, such as streaking of the sample onto Blood and McConkey agars and incubating at 37 °C for 24 hours. However, some bacteria may require special conditions to grow in the laboratory. Failure to use the appropriate culture medium or environment may result in no recovery of the desired microorganism. A few important bacterial groups that may be found in poultry samples, do not grow in standard media and/or conditions, and require special handling to be isolated include Avibacterium, Campylobacter, Clostridium, and Mycoplasma. When submitting to a laboratory for bacteria isolation, the submission form should include a list of suspected conditions or pathogens to avoid lack of isolation.

Sensitivity to a particular antibiotic can be done by disk diffusion (Kirby-Bauer) or minimum inhibitory concentration (MIC) method. The latter is preferred nowadays, as this assay provides the precise concentration of antibiotic required to inhibit growth of a bacterium. Because poultry is classified as a food animal, there are very few approved antibiotics. A list of currently approved antibiotics for poultry and their withdrawal time is available online at http://www.farad.org/members/index.html. Practitioners for back yard poultry flocks must be cautious when prescribing antibiotics to these birds. Many people who keep poultry in their backyard consume their eggs. Some of these drugs may pass through the egg, and may cause the development of antibiotic-resistant bacteria, or induce allergic reactions, if the eggs containing antibiotics are consumed. Please refer to the chapter on appropriate drug use in this book.

Parasite Examination

Parasites that affect poultry range from single-celled protozoans to multicellular helminths and arthropods. Parasitic life cycles may be direct or indirect. Parasites also may invade various organs. It is important to stress that identifying a parasite (or parasite egg) does not always mean clinical disease. Many parasites coexist with their hosts without causing pathologic changes. For instance, poultry older than four months of age have usually built up immunity to coccidia; therefore detection of a few coccidial oocysts in their feces may not be relevant. Poultry may become infected with

these parasites from multiple sources, that is, contaminated equipment, humans, or the feces of other animals. Parasitic infections may be diagnosed through examining samples from living animals or through necropsy of affected individuals or representatives of the flock.

In living animals, the most common diagnostic samples are feces, blood, and skin/feathers for the detection of parasites, eggs, or intermediate life forms. From dead birds, investigation can be performed from gross and histopathologic observations. It is a good idea to consult with a specialist who can help to classify the parasite. Fecal samples should be collected and examined on a routine basis. Standard flotation and centrifugation concentrating techniques are usually performed from fecal samples to look for protozoan (*Cryptosporidium, Coccidia,* and *Giardia* spp.) and nematode eggs

Table 27.6 Fecal flotation protocol.

Preparation of flotation medium
Heat 355 ml (1.5 cups) tap water and add 454 g (1 lb) sugar while stirring.
Continue stirring the solution on low heat until sugar is dissolved.
The solution will last about 3 wk.
Sample preparation
Transfer approximately one gram of feces into a vacutainer tube.
Note: If needed, filter sample out coarse material using a funnel covered with the gauze.
Fill tube half way with the sugar solution and vortex. Continue filling the tube until a slight positive meniscus is formed.
Let rest for 20 min.
Then float a cover slip over the tube, making contact with the sample.
Examine microscopically for ova, cysts, and oocytes.
Interpretation
Positive: Presence of ova, cysts, and/or oocytes and identified to genus. *For coccidia it can be qualified as high: >50, moderate: 20–50, low: <20 oocytes per field at a 100x.*
Negative: No ova, cyst or oocysts observed.

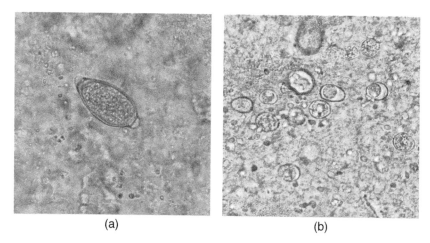

(a) (b)

Figure 27.10 Example of parasite eggs found in fecal samples of poultry: (a) *Capillaria* sp. form a pigeon fecal sample. *Note* the bi-polar poles. (b) Coccidia (*Eimeria* sp.) from a chicken fecal sample. *Note* that a couple of stages (oocyst and schizoonts) are present.

(Table 27.6). Identification of ova or oocytes can be performed by flotation by examining fresh feces (Figure 27.10). Please refer to the Parasitology chapter for further detail.

A direct smear is best for detecting motile protozoa (i.e. *Coclosoma, Giardia, Trichomonas*). Samples are not diagnostic if they are more than 15 minutes old. Feces or oral scrapings are mixed with lactate Ringer's solution or physiologic saline solution, rather than tap water. Examine the sample under the microscope and look for flagellar movement. To confirm the morphology of the parasites, a slide with the sample can be fixed in polyvinyl alcohol and stained with trichrome.

Blood films are used to detect hematozoa. Some examples of the parasites found in poultry are Plasmodium (mostly in pigeons) and Leucozytozoon (occasionally seen in turkeys). Giemsa or Wright's stains provide excellent results. It is also possible to use the Diff-Quick kit to stain the blood film.

Fungal Culture

The primary fungi of concern in poultry are *Candida albicans* and *Aspergillus fumigatus*. When isolated, their significance must be interpreted in light of clinical signs, hematology data, and so on. As it occurs with other microorganisms, their presence alone does not confirm disease.

Viral Culture

Viruses can be cultured from a variety of tissues in chick embryos and living cells. Embryos from specific-pathogen-free dams should be used for virus isolation. Samples may be from ante- and post-mortem cases. Virus isolation is currently offered in a few laboratories. The test is time consuming, it may take weeks to get results back, and it is expensive. It may require inoculation of embryos at different ages or routes and the use of multiple cell cultures. However, virus isolation is still considered the golden standard for identification of viruses. If a suspected foreign animal disease or a disease that would be costly to the poultry industry is suspected, such as vND (velogenic Newcastle's disease), AI (avian influenza), or ILT (infectious laryngotracheitis), please contact your state veterinarian and state laboratory regarding testing, which is often available at no or minimal cost. Please refer to the AI chapter for further detail on this important pathogen.

Molecular Testing

Diagnostic microbiology has been transformed with the use of molecular technology. Molecular techniques have become a crucial tool for identifying microorganisms that are important in animal production and health. Molecular techniques can complement the work of immunologists, microbiologists, and veterinarians. The incorporation of molecular techniques has been of great importance in the identification and characterization of many viruses, including avian influenza and velogenic Newcastle.

Essentially, molecular techniques are based on a polymerase chain reaction (PCR), a method for detection of specific DNA or RNA (Figure 27.11). There are many modifications of the PCR method, that is, conventional PCR, multiplex PCR (simultaneous amplification of several DNA sequences), nested PCR, semi-quantitative PCR, reverse transciptase PCR or RT-PCR (for the amplification of RNA), and real time PCR (aka quantitative PCR).

As these techniques develop, the number of tests available for the identification of pathogens, including viruses, bacteria, parasites, and fungi in any samples (i.e. blood, feces, exudates, tissues) increases. PCR is sensitive, specific, and can provide quick results. PCR has advantages as a diagnostic tool in conventional microbiology, particularly in the detection of

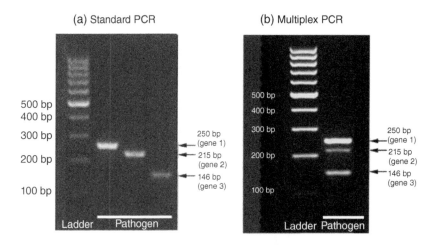

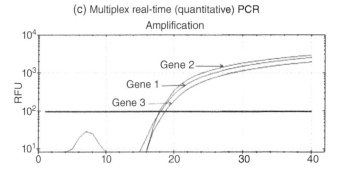

Figure 27.11 Different outputs for a given pathogen using different PCR methods. (a) For standard PCR a single genetic marker is tested per reaction. It needs three reactions (lanes) to identify the three markers. (b) For multiplex PCR multiple, the three genetic markers are tested in a single reaction (lane). (c) In a multiplex real time PCR, the presence of the three genetic markers is also tested in a single reaction, in addition the concentration of the pathogen can be calculated. In (a) and (b) only positive (presence) or negative (absence) results are provided.

slow-growing or difficult to cultivate microorganisms, or under special situations in which conventional methods are expensive or hazardous. As a result of the stability of DNA, nucleic-acid based detection methods can be also used when inhibitory substances, such as antibiotics or formalin, are present. Newer molecular assays, such as next generation or high-throughput sequencing can sequence multiple pathogens directly to avoid biases, they can even conduct genomic analysis directly on the cell. However, sequencing is still too expensive to be used as a routine diagnostic method. It also requires careful analysis of data, as the sequences may be of poor quality causing sequencing errors.

Finally, it is important to point out that molecular techniques, although they are powerful diagnostic tools, they should be used as another tool for diagnosis and the results from these tests should be interpreted in the context of the other findings, that is, clinical signs, serology, and pathology. Molecular assays only indicate the presence of DNA or RNA of a potentially infective microorganism; they do not give any indication of the activity of the infection.

Conclusions

1) An accurate diagnosis in poultry is usually obtained after a series of evaluations of multiple analyses. No one test is more important than another
2) Although chickens have been extensively used in research settings, there is limited published information on hematology of domestic poultry in clinical settings. However, because of technical advances and the interest in backyard poultry as pets the situation is changing
3) Traditionally, serology has been the preferred method of monitoring health and disease in poultry species
4) Histologic examination allows morphologic examination of the tissues and allows for the differentiation of infectious from non-infectious disorders
5) Microbiologic testing is used for the detection of bacteria, viruses, and fungi. The role a microorganism plays on a particular condition should be evaluated in the context of other diagnostic findings, that is, clinical signs, serology, and pathology.

References

1 Bermudez, A.J. (2008). Principles of disease prevention: diagnosis and control, Chapter 1,. In: Diseases of Poultry (eds. Y.M. Saif, A.M. Fadly, J.R. Glisson, et al.), 3–46. Ames, IA: Blackwell Publishing.
2 Bounous, D.I., Wyatt, R.D., Gibbs, P.S. et al. (2000). Normal hematologic and serum biochemical reference intervals for juvenile wild turkeys. *J. Wild. Dis.* 32 (2): 393–396.
3 Board, M.M., Crespo, R., Shah, D.H., and Faux, C.M. (2018). Blood chemistry reference intervals for backyard hens. *J. Avian Med. Surg.*, in Press.
4 Carpenter, J.W. and Marion, C.J. (eds.) (2013). Exotic Animal Formulary. MO, Elsevier: St. Louis.
5 Doufour-Zavala, L., Swayne, D.E., Pearson, J.E. et al. (eds.) (2008). Isolation, identification, and characterization of avian pathogens. In: The American Association of Avian Pathologists, 5e. GA: Athens.
6 Griminer, P. and Scanes, C.G. (1986). Protein metabolism. In: Avian Physiology (ed. P.D. Sturkie), 326–345. New York: Springer Verlag.
7 Harr, K.E. (2006). Diagnostic value of biochemistry. In: Clinical Avian Medicine (eds. G.J. Harrison and T.L. Lightfoot), 611–629. Palm Beach, FL: Spix Publishing.
8 Hawkins, M.G., Barron, H.W., Speer, B.L. et al. (2013). Exotic Animal Formulary, 4e, vol. 2013

(eds. J.W. Carpenter and C.J. Marion), 184–438. Elsevier.

9 Hernández-Rodríguez, P. and Gomez Ramirez, A. (2012). Polymerase chain reaction: types, utilities and limitations, Chapter 8. In: Polymerase Chain Reaction (ed. P. Hernández-Rodríguez), 157–172. InTech.

10 Kaneko, J.J. (1997). Serum proteins and the dysproteinemias. In: Clinical Biochemistry of Domestic Animals (eds. J.J. Kaneko, J.W. Harvey and M.L. Bruss), 117–138. San Diego, CA: Academic Press Available from: http://www.intechopen.com/books/polymerase-chain-reaction/polymerase-chain-reaction-types-utilities-and-limitations.

11 Krautwald-Junghanns, M. (2007). Aids to diagnosis, Chapter 4. In: Essentials of Avian Medicine and Surgery (ed. B. Coles), 56–102. Oxford, UK: Wiley-Blackwell.

12 Lilliehook, I., Wall, H., Tauson, R., and Tvedten, H. (2004). Differential leukocyte counts determined in chicken blood using the cell-dyn 3500. *Vet. Clin. Path.* 33 (3): 133–138.

13 Lumeij, J.T. and MacLean, B. (1996). Total protein determination in pigeon plasma and serum: comparison of refractory methods with the biuret method. *J. Avian Med. Surg.* 10 (3): 150–152.

14 Martin, M.P., Wineland, M., and Barnes, H.J. (2010). Selected blood chemistry and gas reference ranges for broiler breeders using the i-stat handheld clinical analyzer. *Avian Dis.* 54 (3): 1016–1020.

15 McNabb, F.M. and Hughes, T.E. (1983). The role of serum binding proteins in determining free thyroid hormone concentrations during development in quail. *Endocrinology* 113: 957–963.

16 dos Santos, M., Schmidt, E., Paulillo, A.C. et al. (2009). Hematology of the bronze Turkey (meleagris gallopavo): variations with age and gender. *Int. J. Poult. Sci.* 8 (8): 752–754.

17 Samour, J. (2006). Diagnostic value of hematology. In: Clinical Avian Medicine (eds. G.J. Harrison and T.L. Lightfoot), 587–609. Palm Beach, FL: Spix Publishing.

18 Sharma, J.M. (2008). Host factors for disease resistance, Chapter 2. In: Diseases of Poultry (eds. Y.M. Saif, A.M. Fadly, J.R. Glisson, et al.), 47–58. Ames, IA: Wiley-Blackwell.

19 Wakenell, P.S. (2010). Normal avian hematology: chicken and Turkey, Chapter 122,. In: Schalm's Veterinary Hematology (eds. D.J. Weiss and K.J. Wardrop), 958–967. Baltimore, MD: Lippincott Williams & Wilkins.

Section 6

Treatment and Prevention of Disease

28

Regulatory Considerations for Medication Use in Poultry

Lisa Tell[1], Tara Marmulak[2] and Krysta Martin[1]

[1] *Food Animal Residue Avoidance and Depletion Program and Department of Medicine and Epidemiology, School of Veterinary Medicine, University of California, Davis, CA, USA*
[2] *Veterinary Teaching Hospital, College of Veterinary Medicine and Biomedical Sciences, Colorado State University, Fort Collins, CO, USA*

Introduction/Overview

Medicating poultry is a worldwide practice regardless of whether it applies to an individual bird or a large commercial flock. However, medication use in poultry has both rewards and challenges. It prevents or treats illness, thus producing healthier animals. In addition, flocks with multiple birds have the advantage of increased production. However, consumers, regulators, and legislators are increasingly concerned about direct and indirect hazards of drug use and potential impacts on public health. For example, when medications are administered to poultry, drug residues can be present within edible products if an insufficient drug withdrawal time (WDT) is not observed. In order to help minimize drug residues in poultry food products, it is important that all veterinarians, whether they treat individual birds or advise large-scale operations, are educated and inform their clients about how to minimize drug residues in the human food chain.

Veterinarians who treat individual or small numbers of poultry patients face several challenges. Many of the approved products for poultry are formulated for large-scale commercial operations, because only a few poultry products are approved for laying hens, and pet owners are often willing to treat individual birds with complex treatment regimens that lack approved WDTs for poultry. This chapter is designed to provide veterinarians with information that will help them navigate the legal and logistical hoops of medication use in poultry, provide resources for finding WDTs for drugs approved for poultry, provide guidance for estimating withdrawal intervals (WDIs) when drugs are used in an extra-label manner, and highlight guidance recommendations regarding prudent use of antibiotics. The information presented in this chapter is the authors' interpretation of the legislation, guidelines, and literature; however, the regulatory agencies have the ultimate authority and should be contacted with any questions. For most of the chapter, the resources and legislative/legal information are focused on the United States, but information relative to other worldwide geographic areas is briefly highlighted.

Definition of Poultry

In the United States, the Food, Drug, and Cosmetics Act defines the term "poultry" to include birds that are deemed to be major animal species (chickens and turkeys). The US Center of Veterinary Medicine (CVM), a branch of the Food and Drug Administration (FDA), has a list of definitions (Table 28.1) for poultry species and classes of chickens and turkeys [1]. In a broader sense, the term "poultry" also encompasses avian species that are "minor" animal species. The Code of Federal Regulations (CFR) defines "minor" animal species by exclusion, meaning that the "major" animal species have been identified and all others are deemed "minor." Major animal species are dogs, cats, horses, cattle, swine, chickens, and turkeys. Therefore, examples of "minor" poultry would include ducks, geese, game birds, pigeons, and so on. For the purposes of this chapter, "poultry" is deemed to refer to any avian species that has the potential for its meat, eggs, offal (entrails and internal organs of an animal used as food), by-products (i.e. feathers), or manure to directly or indirectly enter or influence any portion of the human food chain.

Drug Administration, On-Label and Extra-Label Drug Use in Poultry

In poultry medicine, medications can be administered to an individual bird or an entire flock depending on numbers of birds needing treatment, disease, and/or overall management practices. The types of medications commonly administered to poultry include antibiotics, anticoccidials, and antiparasitics. Similar to any other animal species that are in need of medications, administration routes can be oral or parenteral. Because they require lower labor efforts, oral routes of drug administration for birds commonly include medicated water or feed regardless of whether or not the flock is small or large. Parenteral administration routes for medications are typically reserved for individual patients that might have a severe illness and have a high likelihood of not entering the human food chain because parenteral administration routes have a higher likelihood of resulting in drug residues. When medicating poultry, practitioners should consider their unique gastrointestinal anatomy, physiology, and drug elimination processes that differ from mammals [2]. Practitioners treating poultry in the United States can use FDA-approved veterinary products according to the label or in an extra-label manner. Use of medications according to the label directions is termed "on-label drug use," meaning that all of the drug label specifications (animal species and class, administration route, dose, dosing frequency/interval, indication, limitations, and WDT) are fulfilled and the FDA-approved WDT is observed. The FDA-approved WDT is the amount of time that must be observed after the last dose is administered and before the meat, eggs, or offal that is intended for human consumption can enter the food chain.

In contrast to on-label drug use, medications for poultry in the United States can also be prescribed by a veterinarian for "extra-label drug use." Extra-label drug use (ELDU) occurs when the animal species/class, administration route, dose, dosing frequency/interval, or indication differs from the FDA-approved label. In the United States, ELDU was legalized with the passage of the Animal Medicinal Drug Use Clarification Act (AMDUCA) of 1994. When veterinary products are used in an extra-label manner, a withdrawal "interval" must be estimated based on scientific evidence and must be extended beyond the FDA-approved WDT regardless of the dose, route, or indication. It should be mentioned that legal ELDU does not include the use of prohibited drugs (such as fluoroquinolones in chickens). More details on the prohibition of certain drugs and drug classes in food-producing species will be discussed later in this chapter.

Table 28.1 United States of America Food and Drug Administration's definitions of species and classes of chickens and turkeys.

Species	Class	Definition
Chickens	Egg	From in ovo until hatching.
	Laying hens (or layers)	Hens that produce eggs for human consumption.
	Chicks	Chickens from day of hatch until they are able to survive in ambient temperature (no longer brooded).
	Broiler chickens (or fryers or frying chickens)	Meat-type chickens normally grown to a market age of 35–49 d and market weights between approximately 4 and 7 lb (1.80 and 3.2 kg).
	Roasters (or roasting chickens)	Meat-type chickens grown to market weights between approximately 6 and 9 lb (2.7 and 4.1 kg).
	Replacement chickens	Chickens intended to become laying hens or breeding chickens. Sexually mature male and female
	Breeding chickens	chickens of any type intended for the production of fertile eggs; the eggs are not intended for human consumption.
Turkeys	Egg	From in ovo until hatching.
	Laying hens (or layers)	Hens that produce eggs for human consumption.
	Poults	Turkeys from day of hatch until they are able to survive in ambient temperature (no longer brooded).
	Growing turkeys	Turkeys grown for meat purposes to a market age of approximately 17 (female) or 22 (male) weeks; may be further divided into heavy or light turkey strains.
	Finishing turkeys	Turkeys intended for meat production during the last two to four weeks of growth.
	Replacement turkeys	Turkeys intended to become laying hens or breeding turkeys.
	Breeding turkeys	Sexually mature male or female turkeys intended to produce fertile eggs; their eggs are not intended for human food use.

Source: US Food and Drug Administration: Animal & Veterinary [1].

Definition of Residues

The word "residue" is defined in many ways by the literature and worldwide regulatory agencies. For the purposes of this chapter, a residue is deemed to be either the parent compound or metabolite of a parent compound that may accumulate, deposit, or otherwise be stored within the cells, tissues, organs, or edible products (e.g. milk, eggs) of an animal following its use to prevent, control, or treat animal disease or to enhance production [3]. According to the FDA, a residue is any compound that is present in edible tissues of the target animal that results from the use of the sponsored compound, including the sponsored compound, its metabolites, and any other substances formed in or on food because of the sponsored compound's use (21 CFR 500.82). The focus of this chapter is on drug residues; however, residues can also originate from pesticides [4], biotoxins, heavy metals, radionuclides, and so on. In general, residues that accumulate in food products can be problematic from a human health standpoint and should be considered when estimating how long to withhold poultry meat, eggs, and/or offal before they enter the human food chain.

Human Health Hazards of Drug Residues

The human health hazards of drug residues can be classified as direct or indirect impacts [5]. Direct impacts are those that result more immediately and include toxic reactions that impact consumers directly, such as the clenbuterol exposure of 135 residents of Spain in 1990; and similarly, 15 residents of Italy in 1997 that consumed contaminated beef [6, 7]. Other examples of direct impacts include allergic/hypersensitivity reactions or bone marrow toxicity. Indirect impacts usually have negative effects over a longer time period and include carcinogenicity, mutagenicity, reproductive disorders, immunopathological effects, and transfer of antibiotic-resistant bacteria to the human population. The US FDA-CVM assesses the risks of veterinary drugs on public health prior to granting approval [8–11]. However, when drugs are used in an extra-label manner, these risk assessments have not been performed by a regulatory agency. A review of how risk assessment principles can be applied to evaluate the human health risks posed by different classes of drugs used in extra-label manner has been published [9].

Regulatory Monitoring of Drug Residues in Animal Products

Monitoring of drug residues in food-producing animals has been previously described [12]. In addition, regulatory systems for Europe, Australia, Canada, and Japan have also been reviewed [13].

In the United States, the primary mission of the National Residue Program (NRP) is to verify control of animal drug residues, pesticides, environmental contaminants, and any other chemical hazards in or on meat, poultry, or egg products. The principal agencies that work together to achieve the mission of the NRP include the Food Safety and Inspection Service (FSIS), the Environmental Protection Agency (EPA) and the FDA. Through the Federal Food, Drug and Cosmetic Act, the FDA is given the authority to establish drug tolerances (maximum permissible concentrations) that are published in Title 21 of the CFR. Title 21 also contains tolerances set by the FDA for heavy metals, industrial chemicals, and pesticides that are no longer approved for use. The EPA is provided a similar responsibility for pesticide tolerances under the Federal Insecticide, Fungicide and Rodenticide Act (FIFRA). The tolerances for pesticides are published in Title 40 of the CFR.

The United States Department of Agriculture (USDA) oversees FSIS, an agency that is responsible for the analytical testing program for residues in domestic and imported meat, poultry, and egg products. In particular, the NRP Sampling Plan, known as the Blue Book, is developed yearly and made publicly available, whereas the Red Book contains NRP drug residue testing results from previous years. Both the Blue and Red Books are available online by linking to their URLs, which are listed in Table 28.2.

Through the NRP, poultry and egg products are tested in federally inspected establishments according to the sampling plan that is listed in the Blue Book. An inspector may also sample products that, according to his/her professional judgment, warrant testing and include analysis for approved and unapproved drugs, pesticides, hormones, and environmental contaminants. Overall, the number of violative

Table 28.2   World-wide web URL links for on-line resources that provide veterinary drug and/or poultry specific information.

Website	Description	URL website address
Drugs @ FDA	FDA's searchable database of approved human drugs	https://www.accessdata.fda.gov/scripts/cder/daf
Animal Drugs @ FDA	FDA's searchable database of approved animal drugs and tolerances	https://animaldrugsatfda.fda.gov/adafda/views/#/search
Vetgram	FARAD's searchable drug database for food animal drugs and tolerances	http://www.farad.org/vetgram
Bayer Animal Health	Searchable US compendium of veterinary products database; use charts tab for summarized label and WDT information	https://bayerall.cvpservice.com
Canadian Compendium of Veterinary Products presented by Bio Agri Mix Total Solutions	Searchable Canadian compendium of veterinary products database; use charts tab for summarized label and WDT information	http://www.bioagrimix.com/compendium
Drugs.com	Searchable database of veterinary drugs; can search by animal groups; also lists Canadian veterinary drugs	http://www.drugs.com/vet
Centre for Agriculture and Bioscience International (CABI)'s Animal Health and Production Compendium	List of international animal drug databases	https://www.cabi.org/ahpc/more-resources/drug-databases
Australian Pesticides and Veterinary Medicines Authority	Pubcris is a searchable database of registered pesticides and veterinary drugs.	https://portal.apvma.gov.au/pubcris
National Office of Animal Health	UK site with searchable drug compendium of approved drugs	www.noahcompendium.co.uk/Compendium/Overview
Health Products Regulatory Authority	Searchable compendium of approved drugs in Ireland	http://www.hpra.ie

(Continued)

Table 28.2 (Continued)

Website	Description	URL website address
European Medicines Agency Database	Public database providing on-line access to information about human and veterinary medicines available to European Union (EU) citizens	http://www.eudrapharm.eu/eudrapharm
USDA Foreign Agricultural Service	Veterinary drug and pesticide tolerance and MRL searchable database	https://www.fas.usda.gov/maximum-residue-limits-mrl-database
FAO/WHO Food Standards Codex alimentarius	Definitions of terms used in discussing veterinary drug residues in food animals	http://www.fao.org/fao-who-codexalimentarius/codex-texts/dbs/vetdrugs/glossary/en
Joint FAO/WHO Expert Committee on Food Additives (JECFA)	Description of JECFA and links to publications	http://www.fao.org/food/food-safety-quality scientific-advice/jecfa/en/
JECFA "Residues of some veterinary drugs in foods and animals"	Searchable database of maximum residue levels for veterinary drugs as recommended by JECFA that includes pharmacokinetic data summaries	http://www.fao.org/food/food-safety-quality scientific-advice/jecfa/jecfa-vetdrugs/en/
Codex alimentarius international food standards	Homepage for codex alimentarius	http://www.fao.org/fao-who-codexalimentarius/about-codex/en
European Medicines Agency European Public MRL Assessment Report	Summary report on the established MRL and the data supporting the MRL	http://www.ema.europa.eu/ema/index.jsp?curl=pages/medicines/landing/vet_mrl_search.jsp&mid=WC0b01ac058008d7ad
USDA/FSIS science chemistry page	Includes FSIS sampling plan (Blue Book) and results (Red Book)	https://www.fsis.usda.gov/wps/portal/fsis/topics/data-collection-and-reports/chemistry/residue-chemistry
USDA Food Safety and Inspection Service (FSIS)	Homepage with contact information and links to resources	http://www.fsis.usda.gov
FDA Center for Veterinary Medicine	Homepage with contact information and links to resources	http://www.fda.gov/AnimalVeterinary/default.htm 240-276-9300 AskCVM@fda.hhs.gov
FDA-CVM Compliance Policy Guide	AMDUCA	http://www.fda.gov/AnimalVeterinary/Guidance ComplianceEnforcement/ActsRules Regulations/ucm085377.htm
AVMA: Animal Medicinal Drug Use Clarification Act (AMDUCA)	Reviews components of AMDUCA and includes list of prohibited drugs	https://www.avma.org/KB/Resources/Reference/Pages/AMDUCA.aspx
AVMA: VCPR Reference Guide	AVMA's definition of a valid VCPR	https://www.avma.org/KB/Resources/Reference/Pages/VCPR.aspx
FDA-CVM Compliance Policy Guide	Extra-label use of medicated feeds for minor species	http://www.fda.gov/ICECI/ComplianceManuals Compliance PolicyGuidanceManual/UCM074659

Table 28.2 (Continued)

Website	Description	URL website address
FARAD	Restricted and prohibited drugs in food animals	http://www.farad.org/prohibited-and-restricted-drugs.html
FARAD regulatory information	Details of the published law on compounding and AMDUCA	http://www.farad.org/amduca-law.html
FARAD species and topics pages	FARAD website pages that cover species related information and topics related to drug use in food animals.	http://www.usfarad.org
AVMA Compounding	AVMA brochure on veterinary compounding	https://ebusiness.avma.org/ProductCatalog/Product.aspx?ID=155
Society of Veterinary Hospital Pharmacists statement on compounding	Position statement on the compounding of drugs for use in animals	http://svhp.org/position-statements
FARAD	Site where ELDU withdrawal requests may be made online and other resources for food animal veterinarians	http://farad.org
Canadian gFARAD	Canadian program providing withdrawal recommendations following extra-label drug use.	https://cgfarad.usask.ca/index.php
National Pesticide Information Center	NPIC provides objective, science-based information about pesticides and pesticide-related topics	http://npic.orst.edu
US Environmental Protection Agency (EPA)	Home page for EPA; pesticide information	http://www.epa.gov
Center for Disease Control and Prevention (CDC)	CDC's Food Safety Program	https://www.cdc.gov/vitalsigns/food-safety.html
Minor Use Animal Drug Program (MUADP)	Searchable database for drugs approved in minor food animal species. MUADP project requests can be submitted via this web site.	http://www.nrsp7.org
American Association of Veterinary Laboratory Diagnosticians (AAVLD)	Listing of AAVLD labs in USA by state	https://aavld.memberclicks.net/accredited-laboratories
US Food and Drug Administration: Animal & Veterinary. *CVM Guidance For Industry #152*	Appendix A identifies antibiotics deemed medically important by FDA and affected by Guidance #213	https://www.fda.gov/downloads/AnimalVeterinary/GuidanceComplianceEnforcement/GuidanceforIndustry/UCM052519.pdf
Australian Pesticides and Veterinary Medicines Authority Food safety studies for veterinary drugs used in food-producing animals	Guideline describing the food safety study design to determine maximum residue limits and withholding periods; contains sections specific to poultry.	https://apvma.gov.au/node/746

(Continued)

Table 28.3 (Continued)

Website	Description	URL website address
Alabama Cooperative Extension	Downloadable publication on pest management in poultry	http://www.aces.edu/pubs/docs/A/ANR-0483/ANR-0483.pdf
Poultry Science Association	Resources for poultry veterinarians	http://www.poultryscience.org/index.asp
Chicken Farmers of Canada	Organization representing the chicken industry in Canada	http://chicken.ca
Poultry Med	International website that provides information pertinent to poultry veterinarians including drug and residue information	http://www.poultrymed.com/Poultry/index.asp
National Chicken Council	A national, non-profit trade association representing the US chicken industry	http://www.nationalchickencouncil.org
FARAD Digests	FARAD digests are publications providing guidance specific to drug use in food-producing animals. A digest on drug use in game birds is available through this URL.	http://www.farad.org/publications/digests.asp

residues found in poultry and poultry products from large commercial operations are relatively low [14, 15].

In July 2012, FSIS announced that it was restructuring the way in which the NRP sampling plan will be scheduled [16]. In particular, the number of overall samples per production class will be reduced with the adoption of new analytical methods that allow samples to be analyzed for more chemical compounds than was previously possible.

In contrast to federally inspected large-scale commercial operations are the mid-size, smaller scale, and individual producers that are involved with local, farmers', or flea market sales. To the knowledge of the authors of this chapter, for these operations there is minimal regulatory oversight; therefore, it is critical that the advising veterinarians take responsibility and educate their clients regarding best practices for avoiding drug residues.

Legislation, Regulations, and Programs Related to Drug Use and Drug Residues in Poultry Species

Minor Use/Minor Species (MUMS) Animal Health Act

The MUMS Animal Health Act was passed in 2004. This legislation added new options for approving limited-use drugs and provided a new mechanism to legally market some unapproved products. The intention of this legislation was to increase the number of FDA approvals for minor food animal species (i.e. game birds such as ducks or quail) and to provide sponsors with incentives to seek label claims for veterinary products that would have "minor uses" in major species of animals (for poultry, these would include chickens and turkeys). "Minor use" is determined by frequency of use and geography. More specifically, minor use means that a drug can be used in a major species for an indication that occurs infrequently and in a small number of animals, or in a limited geographical area and in only a small number of animals annually.

The MUMS Animal Health Act modifies the Federal Food, Drug and Cosmetic Act to include conditional approval, designation, and indexing for veterinary drugs used in minor animal species [17]. Conditional approval and designation provide incentives to drug sponsors with the ultimate goal of drug approval. Drugs that are conditionally approved have shown a reasonable expectation of effectiveness, but the sponsor is granted up to five years to provide all the necessary data proving effectiveness. Conditionally approved drugs cannot be used in an extra-label manner. Designation provides incentives for approvals, including grants to support the studies required for approval, and up to seven years exclusive marketing rights by the sponsor. MUMS legislation also allows for medications to be categorized as "indexed" drugs. Indexed drugs have not undergone a formal drug approval process but the designation allows drug companies to market and sell these medications for selected populations. Indexing is intended for drug treatment of diagnosed conditions in minor non-food producing animal species, specifically targeting laboratory animals and zoological collection specimens. The purpose of indexing is to make products available that cannot meet requirements of the drug approval process as a result of a limited animal population and a wide variety of species. Indexed drugs may not be legally used in an extra-label manner in food-producing animals. More details regarding MUMS legislation have been previously described [18].

Minor Use Animal Drug Program (MUADP)

The Minor Use Animal Drug Program (MUADP) (formerly known as National Research Support Project-7; NRSP-7) is a multi-institutional collaborative research program. The mission of MUADP is to identify animal drug needs for minor species and minor uses in major species, to generate and disseminate data for safe and effective therapeutic applications in minor species, and to facilitate FDA/CVM approvals for drugs that are identified as a priority for a minor species or minor use in a major species. To accomplish these goals, NRSP-7 functions through the coordination of efforts among animal producers, pharmaceutical manufacturers, FDA/CVM, USDA/Cooperative State Research, Education, and Extension Service, universities, State Agricultural Experiment Stations, and veterinary medical colleges throughout the country. The MUADP home web page (Table 28.2) lists FDA-approved veterinary products that have been approved for minor food-producing animal species including various poultry. Historically, via the MUADP web site, individuals could fill out a request form asking for programmatic consideration to seek FDA approval for a drug that is intended for use in a minor species or for a drug that would have a minor use in a major species. The process for selecting drugs that the MUADP would pursue for FDA approval is represented in a schematic on the web site. For a number of reasons, including manufacturer interest, known side effects of the drug, importance of the disease being treated, and the targeted animal species for treatment, some proposals have higher priority than others. Funds are limited, so the program must select projects carefully.

It should be noted that the MUADP is currently applying to establish a formal structure for the program since the sunsetting of NRSP-7. It is also important to highlight that this program was a cooperative research program and was different from the MUMS congressional act. However, the MUMS legislation benefitted MUADP by including a provision for competitive grants to help support studies that are necessary to seek label claims for minor species and minor uses in a major animal species.

The Animal Medicinal Drug Use Clarification Act (AMDUCA) of 1994

The AMDUCA of 1994 made ELDU of FDA-approved medications by veterinarians in the United States legal. "Extra-label use" is defined in the CFR as: "Actual use or intended use of a drug in an animal in a manner that is not in accordance with the approved labeling. This includes, but is not limited to, use in species not listed in the labeling, use for indications (disease and other conditions) not listed in the labeling, use at dosage levels, frequencies, or routes of administration other than those stated in the labeling, and deviation from labeled WDT based on these different uses" [21CFR530.3 (a)].

The requirements of AMDUCA are listed in Table 28.3. Key points within AMDUCA include (i) ELDU can only occur on the order of a veterinarian within the context of a veterinarian-client-patient relationship (VCPR); (ii) ELDU must be limited to a therapeutic purpose to treat a sick or dying animal; (iii) ELDU in food-producing animals requires that no violative residues occur; (iv) Certain compounds are prohibited from ELDU. The

Table 28.3 Requirements of the Animal Medicinal Drug Use Clarification Act (AMDUCA) of 1994.

Requirement	Explanation
Therapeutic purpose	Extra-label drug use can only occur for therapeutic purposes when an animal's health is suffering or threatened. Extra-label drug use for reproductive purposes, growth promotion and efficiency is not allowable under AMDUCA.
No effective labeled drugs	ELDU should not occur unless FDA approved drugs as labeled are clinically ineffective for their intended use.
VCPR	A valid veterinarian-client-patient relationship (VCPR) must exist. Table 28.2 includes the website address to AVMA's definition of a valid VCPR.
Veterinarian's supervision	ELDU is permitted only under the supervision of a veterinarian. This includes the extra-label use of over-the-counter (OTC) medications. Also, any over-the-counter product that is compounded in veterinary medicine is deemed a prescription drug and may only be used under veterinarian supervision.
FDA approved drugs	ELDU is permitted using only FDA-approved animal and human drugs. When using medications extra-label, medications approved for other food animal species should be used before medications approved only for non-food animal species which should be used preferentially over drugs approved for humans only. Using bulk chemical or active pharmaceutical ingredient (API) is not allowed as they are not FDA-approved.
Not in feed	Extra-label use of an approved animal drug or human drug or feed additive in or on an animal feed is prohibited. Also, using combinations of medicated feed or feed additives not approved to be used together is not considered AMDUCA compliant. Extra-label drug use in water is permitted.
No residues	ELDU must not result in violative residues.
Additional food animal requirements	Make a careful diagnosis and evaluation of the conditions for which the drug is to be used. Establish a substantially extended withdrawal period supported by scientific information. Institute procedures to assure that the identity of the treated animal or animals is carefully maintained. If the individual animal cannot be identified for the extended withdrawal interval, then the extended withdrawal interval must be applied to the entire group. Take appropriate measures to assure that assigned timeframes for withdrawal are met and no illegal drug residues occur in any food-producing animal subjected to extra-label treatment.

Source: [21 CFR530.3 (a)].

American Veterinary Medical Association (AVMA) has defined what constitutes a legal VCPR and the website address for this definition is included in Table 28.2. AMDUCA stipulates that ELDU only applies to FDA-approved human and veterinary medications. It does not legalize the extra-label use of EPA regulated pesticides or USDA regulated biologics. For example, fipronil cannot be administered to a chicken for diminishing ectoparasitism, because this product is deemed an insecticide and is regulated by EPA and not FDA. As all FDA-approved veterinary products are assigned either a new animal drug application (NADA) or an abbreviated new animal drug applications (ANADA) number, if a veterinary product does not have an NADA or ANADA number its use is most likely not AMDUCA-compliant in an extra-label manner. In addition, drugs that are approved for humans have new drug application (NDA) numbers for pioneer drugs or abbreviated new drug application (ANDA) numbers for generic medications. Approval status of both animal and human drugs can be found on the FDA-CVM and FDA websites, respectively. The web site URLs are included in Table 28.2.

Compliance Policy Guide (CPG) 615.115 Extra-Label Use of Medicated Feeds for Minor Species

Extra-label use of medicated feed or drugs used extra-label in or on feed is prohibited by AMDUCA. However, for some minor food-producing species, especially poultry, medicating via the feed might be essential. In many circumstances, medicating poultry may not be practical via water or other drug administration routes. Therefore, the CPG 615.115 was created. This Compliance Policy Guide (CPG) allows veterinarians to prescribe FDA-approved medicated feeds to be fed to minor food-producing animals in an extra-label manner. As the FDA considers chickens and turkeys to be major animal species, the CPG does not apply to them. However, for the "minor"

poultry species, such as ducks, geese, pheasants, and quail, medicated feeds that are approved for major species (turkeys or chickens) can be used for the minor poultry species under the supervision of a veterinarian. In other words, the CPG does not make it legal to use medicated feed for these minor poultry species. However, the CPG does give field investigators "regulatory discretion," and if all of the CPG requirements are followed correctly, field investigators do not have to take any action against the producer or veterinarian.

When medicated feeds are being used under the auspices of the CPG, the other requirements of AMDUCA should be met. Additional stipulations for the ELDU of medicated feed in minor species include:

1) A written recommendation that includes the medical rationale and dated within three months prior to use is required. The producer and veterinarian must keep copies of the written recommendation that would be available in the case of an FDA inspection.
2) A medicated feed to be used in a minor food-producing species must be approved in a similar food-producing species. Only medicated feeds approved for use in avian species can be used extra label in a minor poultry species.
3) No changes in the formulation of the FDA-approved medicated feed may be made. For example, the percentage of protein in a medicated feed that is approved for chickens cannot be changed to meet the nutritional requirements of pheasants. The medicated feed that is approved for chickens must keep the original chicken label and the feed must be used "as is" for the minor species.

Prohibited Drugs/Prohibited Drug Use in Poultry

In the United States, the FDA has established a list of drugs or drug classes that are either completely prohibited or prohibited from ELDU in food-producing animals. Other countries have their own lists of drugs of high regulatory concern. Table 28.4 lists the veterinary products that the FDA-CVM prohibits from use in poultry or drug classes that the FDA-CVM prohibits from extra-label use in poultry in the United States. A complete listing of the FDA-CVM prohibited drugs for all animal species can also be found at web site links referenced in Table 28.2. It is advised that the FDA prohibited drug list be checked on a regular basis for updates as it is subject to change. If any of these prohibited drugs are mistakenly used in poultry, then the affected animal and its by-products (i.e. eggs or poultry litter used as feed for other food-producing animals) should never be allowed to enter the human food chain, and ideally the animal should be isolated from other birds that are used as food producers for humans.

In the United States, any animal that has the potential to enter the human food chain or directly or indirectly impact public health should not be administered a prohibited drug. More specifically, in poultry medicine, regardless of whether a bird is in a social (i.e. a companion or "pet chicken") or production (i.e. small flock of backyard laying chickens) setting, it should not be administered FDA-prohibited medication. The FDA has established this prohibited drug list as a measure to protect public health. Examples highlighting how poultry might directly or indirectly impact public health include eggs from backyard chickens that are given to neighbors and/or sold at local farmer's markets; the feces of a companion chicken that might be co-mingled with excrement from other birds being used to produce eggs for human consumption; or chicken feces that might be fed to cattle intended for human consumption [20]. In all

Table 28.4 United States of America Food and Drug Administration-Center of Veterinary Medicine prohibited drugs that have relevance to poultry and reported adverse reaction(s) in humans.

Prohibited drug	Adverse reaction(s) reported in humans
Chloramphenicol	Idiosyncratic, non-dose dependent, irreversible, aplastic anemia
Clenbuterol	B-adrenergic toxicities
Diethylstilbestrol (DES)	Reproductive tract abnormalities and tumors in female offspring, Infertility
Nitroimidazoles such as metronidazole	Potential for carcinogenesis
Nitrofurans-including topical applications	Potential for carcinogenesis
Fluoroquinolones such as enrofloxacin can be used on label only	Potential to cause development of resistant human pathogens
Glycopeptides such as vancomycin	Potential to cause development of resistant human pathogens
Gentian violet – prohibited from use in feed	Human food safety has not been assessed
Antivirals (adamantine and neuramidase inhibitors) in poultry	Potential to cause development of resistant human pathogens
Cephalosporins, not including cephapirin, must be used on label in cattle, swine, chickens, and turkeys. They may be used extra-label only in the above species to treat a disease indication not labeled.	Potential to cause development of resistant human pathogens

Source: Davis, J.L., Smith, G.W., Baynes, R.E., et al. [19].

these cases, there are potential direct or indirect impacts on public health. Therefore, even if an owner thinks that a companion pet chicken would never be used for human consumption, it should not be administered an FDA-prohibited drug as there is no guarantee that the chicken would remain in a companion status and/or there are other ways that bird could indirectly impact human health.

There are three prohibitions proclaimed by the FDA that impact poultry: The prohibition of extra-label use of cephalosporins, the prohibition of fluoroquinolones, and the prohibition of antiviral medications.

Prohibition of Extra-Label Drug Use of Cephalosporins in Major Food-Producing Animals

On 5 April 2012, a prohibition of the extra-label use of cephalosporins in major food-producing animal species, including chickens and turkeys, took effect. The FDA enacted this prohibition because of concerns for increasing bacterial resistance to cephalosporins, many of which are used for treating humans. At the time that this chapter was authored, there was only one cephalosporin that was approved for poultry, ceftiofur sodium. Ceftiofur sodium is labeled for use in day-old chicks and turkey poults for control of early mortality associated with *Escherichia coli* infections. From a legal standpoint, ceftiofur sodium can only be used in an extra-label manner in the aforementioned species/class for a different indication. In other words, the label dose, administration route, treatment duration, and species (in this case, day old chicks and turkey poults) must all be on-label. *In ovo* administration would be deemed prohibited. At the time that this chapter was authored, the minor food-producing poultry species (ducks, geese, etc.), were excluded from this ban; thus cephalosporins may continue to be used responsibly in an extra-label manner.

Prohibition of Fluoroquinolones

In the early 1990s, there was a rapid increase in fluoroquinolone-resistant *Campylobacter* spp., a known contributor to foodborne illness in humans, that was associated with increased use of fluoroquinolones in poultry [21]. As a result, the extra-label use of fluoroquinolones was banned in the United States in 1997. At that time, sarafloxacin and enrofloxacin were approved for use in poultry. Even with this prohibition, increased fluoroquinolone-resistant *Campylobacter* spp. in poultry were linked with resistant infections in humans, leading to the voluntary withdrawal of sarafloxacin products in 2001. In 2005, the FDA approval for enrofloxacin was withdrawn [22]. At the time that this chapter was written, the use of any fluoroquinolones in US poultry is prohibited.

Prohibition of Specific Antiviral Medications

In 1999, avian influenza entered the limelight in the United States as a deadly zoonotic disease on a global scale. Given the serious nature of avian influenza infection, the antivirals rimantadine, amantadine, oseltamivir, and zanamivir were prohibited from use in poultry in the United States in order to preserve their effectiveness for treatment of human beings. It has been reported that countries that have previously allowed the use of these medications in poultry have observed development of drug resistance [23, 24].

Compounding of Medications for Poultry

Compounding is the term used for combining, mixing, or altering ingredients to create a medication that is tailored to the needs of an individual patient. It involves making a new drug for which safety and efficacy have not been demonstrated with the kind of data that FDA requires for new drug approval. In virtually all cases, FDA regards compounded drugs as unapproved new drugs [25].

According to the CFR, a veterinarian may consider using a compounded product in poultry "when there is no approved new animal or approved new human drug that, when used as labeled or in conformity with criteria established in this part, will, in the available dosage form and concentration, appropriately treat the condition diagnosed" [21CFR530.13].

Given that poultry are deemed food-producing animals, there are specific requirements for legal use of a compounded product in poultry (and any other food-producing animal) [21CFR530.13]. These requirements are listed in Table 28.5.

Using compounded medications is deemed to be ELDU of an approved animal or human drug. As compounding falls under AMDUCA, the requirements for ELDU and compounded medications under AMDUCA are listed in Table 28.3.

Often, bulk chemicals or active pharmaceutical ingredients (APIs) are used in commercial compounding. This is not deemed legal under AMDUCA for food animal species because this chemical is not an FDA-approved drug. Defined in 21 CFR 207.3, "bulk drug

substance means any substance that is represented for use in a drug and that, when used in the manufacturing, processing, or packaging of a drug, becomes an active ingredient or a finished dosage form of the drug, but the term does not include intermediates used in the synthesis of such substances." In other words, by bulk chemical, we mean the drug in powdered chemical form, which is often used for research purposes and may not be of pharmaceutical grade. Compounding with bulk chemicals can be less expensive than using an FDA-approved medication. However, according to AMDUCA, ELDU (in this case compounding) is legal for therapeutic purposes only; therefore, cost is not an acceptable reason for compounding.

In order to be AMDUCA compliant, when compounded products or medications are used in poultry in an extra-label manner, the information listed in Tables 28.6 and 28.7 needs to be documented in the patient's medical records and on the prescription label respectively. These records must be kept for two years and be accessible to FDA inspectors, so that they can estimate the risk to public health.

There can be some liability associated with the use of compounded medications, as they generally do not undergo the same quality assurance testing as commercially manufactured

Table 28.5 Requirements for legal use of compounded products in food-producing animals.

All requirements for ELDU under AMDUCA are met
An approved animal drug should be used for compounding before a human drug
Compounding is performed by the veterinarian or pharmacist within their scope of practice
Adequate procedures are followed to ensure the safety and effectiveness of the compounded product
Scale of compounding is in line with the need for the product and is for a particular patient. Compounding in anticipation of receiving prescriptions, except in limited quantities, is illegal. The compounding of large quantities can fall under "manufacturing" and thus the compounded product would be deemed a drug in need of FDA approval. Also, compounding for third parties to resell or selling it at wholesale to another individual or entity for resale is illegal. So, it would not be legal for a compounding pharmacy to make a product for a veterinarian to keep on his truck to sell to dairies.
All state laws relating to compounding are followed

Table 28.6 Required Information to be included in the patient's medical record with extra-label drug use or compounded medication use.

Identity of the animals, either as individuals or a group
Animal species
Number of animals treated
Condition being treated
Established name of the drug and active ingredient
Dosage prescribed or used
Duration of treatment
Specified withdrawal, withholding, or discard time(s), if applicable, for meat, eggs, or animal-derived food

Table 28.7 Required information to be included on the prescription label with extra-label drug use or compounded medication use.

Name and address of the prescribing veterinarian

Established name of the drug or each ingredient

Any specified directions for use including the class/species or identification of the animal or herd, flock, pen, lot, or other group; dose, frequency, and route of administration; and the duration of therapy

Any cautionary statements

The veterinarian's specified withdrawal, withholding, or discard time for meat, eggs, or any other food that might be derived from the treated animal or animals

---

medications. In addition, AMDUCA requires that there be sufficient scientific data to estimate a WDI. In general, scientific pharmacokinetic data for compounded medication use in food-producing animals is limited, so estimating a WDI can be difficult. Recommending a WDI to the client is the legal responsibility of the veterinarian. It is particularly important that the veterinarian be aware of this, especially if a pharmacy is performing the drug compounding, as the pharmacy may not be aware of all the legal ramifications. If there is insufficient data to estimate a WDI, then the veterinarian must assure that the animal and its products never enter the human food chain.

It is also important to remember that medications can only be compounded for an individual patient with whom the veterinarian has a valid VCPR.

Overall, the compounding of medications for poultry and other food-producing animals should be rarely used. When treating an animal whose tissues or products have the potential to enter the human food chain, it is important to remember that food safety and public health come first. Additional resources regarding compounding and a link to AVMA's brochure on veterinary compounding and choosing a compounding pharmacy are listed in Table 28.2.

FDA-CVM Guidance Documents Impacting Poultry

In April 2012, the FDA-CVM released the final version of Guidance for Industry (GFI) #209, "The judicious use of medically important antimicrobial (MIA) drugs in food-producing animals" [26]. This document summarizes the agency's findings that have suggested that food-producing animals that have been treated with antimicrobials affect the bacterial populations of humans who consume them. Based on the interpretations of these findings, the FDA has determined that use of antimicrobials that are important for therapeutic use in humans in food-producing animals should be limited to therapies necessary to maintain animal health only. In addition, the FDA has determined that there should be veterinary oversight for any use of MIAs in food-producing animals to ensure the judicious use of these important medications. MIA drugs as identified by the FDA are listed in Appendix A of FDA-CVM's GFI #152. The web URL for GFI #152 can be found in Table 28.2 of this chapter.

GFI #213, "New animal drugs and new animal drug combination products, administered in or on medicated feed or drinking water of food-producing animals: recommendations for drug sponsors for voluntarily aligning product use conditions with GFI #209" goes further [27]. As of January 2017, GFI #213 has been fully implemented.

This document outlines changes that involved the withdrawal of marketed feed or water antibiotics, deemed medically important in the treatment of humans, that were labeled for production purposes, including weight gain and feed efficiency. Any remaining over-the-counter medicated feed or water treatments that contain MIAs with therapeutic indications, including treatment, control, and prevention of specific diseases were reclassified as prescription drugs or veterinary feed directive (VFD). The guidance outlines the steps involved for manufacturers of the previously over-the-counter medicated feeds or drinking water products to seek approvals for therapeutic claims, making them VFDs or prescription drugs. A VFD is a written statement issued by a veterinarian with a valid VCPR for the use of a VFD drug or VFD combination drug in or on animal feed. A list of sponsor applications that are being impacted by the FDA rulings can be found at https://www.fda.gov/AnimalVeterinary/SafetyHealth/AntimicrobialResistance/JudiciousUseofAntimicrobials/ucm390429.htm. A list of drugs and approved VFD drug combinations can be found on the Food Animal Residue Avoidance and Depletion Program (FARAD) website (http://www.farad.org/vfd-drug-combinations.html). In order for a veterinarian to write for a VFD drug, the veterinarian must be licensed to practice in the state the animals reside in, have a valid VCPR, and issue the VFD in compliance with the drugs approved labeling and conditions. Extra-label use of VFD drugs is prohibited.

In the state of California, Senate Bill 27 (SB 27) became effective on January 1, 2018. SB 27 was created to address antimicrobial resistance. It is similar to the federal regulations on judicious use of MIA; however, it extends veterinary oversite of MIA further. For animals being treated in California, all forms of MIA, including oral, injectable, topical, intramammary now require a prescription from a veterinarian. This means that MIA formulations that are designated as OTC at the federal level will be designated as Rx in the state of California. This prescription status for medications impacted by this ruling can be found on VetGram on the FARAD website.

Proposed legislation that will have an impact on medication use in veterinary medicine if passed into law includes the Preservation of Antibiotics for Medical Treatment Act (PAMTA). This legislation proposes to preserve the effectiveness of antimicrobials for use in treating human diseases by phasing out what the bill calls "non-therapeutic uses" in food-producing animals. If passed, this legislation will ban any use of MIAs as a feed or water additive for an animal in the absence of any

clinical sign of disease for the purposes of growth promotion, feed efficiency, weight gain, routine disease prevention, or other routine purpose.

The bill would also require the withdrawal of antibiotics that are used for "non-therapeutic" reasons in food-producing animals unless it could be proven that they pose no harm to human health, a difficult task to prove.

Considerations for Avoiding Residues in Poultry Products Intended for Human Consumption

General Recommendations

Some general recommendations to help avoid residues include the following:

- All waterers should be thoroughly rinsed and cleaned once the course of medication is complete
- All equipment used for mixing and storing medicated feed and feeders should be cleaned once treatment is complete
- If the label WDT requires it, all birds should be switched to a non-medicated feed to allow residues to deplete prior to slaughter. Medicated feeds are a common source of drug residues if the proper WDT is not observed
- Calculations of dosages for medicated water and feeds should be carefully performed and even double checked by a second party in cases where large numbers of birds are to be treated. A list of conversions commonly used in poultry production has been previously published [28]
- Bedding litter should be changed after completing treatment as any remaining litter may serve as a source of drug exposure to both birds and humans from feces or dropped feed [29]. This could contribute to antimicrobial resistance and possible residues. Nicarbazin has been shown to be

stable in litter for prolonged periods and cause persistent residues in the feces and eggs of hens that are kept on unchanged litter after treatment [30]

- If the units for the WDTs are days, a full 24-hour period per day, beginning from the last treatment/dose, must be observed. For example, if the WDT is two days, 48 hours must pass after the last treatment/dose before an animal can be slaughtered
- Proper records and identification of treated animals must be maintained. Inadequate treatment records or failure to identify treated animals lead to insufficient WDTs and violative residues
- When using rodenticides, bait stations that are inaccessible to birds should be used and dead rodents should be promptly disposed of
- Label instructions and WDTs should be followed when using pesticides and insecticides. Consult the EPA web site for guidance (Table 28.2).

When using medicated water to treat poultry there are some factors that may affect treatment efficacy. For example, serum concentrations of medications can vary considerably because of differences in water uptake by individual birds. Factors affecting water intake include environmental temperature, feed quality and amount of feed ingested, species, age, health, and circadian rhythm and accessibility [2]. Table 28.8 lists some factors known to affect water consumption in poultry. Tables 28.9 and 28.10 list estimated water and feed consumption rates that may be used as a guide when determining treatment regimens for poultry [31].

Characteristics of the water itself, including hardness and pH, should be evaluated when administering medications in water. Tetracyclines form less soluble complexes if the water is hard, reducing bioavailability in the treated birds. Additionally, many drugs have only a certain pH range at which they are stable for any length of time. Therefore, the pH of the water is also an important consideration when determining a drug regimen.

Table 28.8 Factors increasing and decreasing water uptake in poultry.

Factors increasing water consumption	Factors decreasing water consumption
Soybean meal diet	High energy diets
High fiber diet	Nighttime
High environmental temperature	Sickness
Dawn and dusk	Poor palatability
Age	Decreased feed intake
Electrolytes	
Increased feed intake	

Source: Vermeulen, B., De Backer, P. and, Remon, J.P. [2].

Table 28.9 Estimated water consumptions for chickens.

Hens-nonlaying	5.0 gal/100 birds	19 l/100 birds
Hens-laying	5–7.5 gal/100 birds	19–28 l/100 birds
Chickens 4 wk	2.0 gal/100 birds	7.6 l/100 birds
Chickens 8 wk	4.1 gal/100 birds	15.5 l/100 birds
Chickens 12 wk	5.5 gal/100 birds	21 l/100 birds

Source: Buck, B.B. [31].

Table 28.10 Estimated feed consumption rates for chickens.

Chicken body weight (lb)	Chicken body weight (kg)	Weight of food eaten per day expressed as percentage body weight
0.5	0.23	14
1.0	0.45	11.4
1.5	0.68	9.7
3.5	1.59	6.7
5.5	2.5	5.0

Source: Buck, B.B. [31].

In order to increase the likelihood of achieving therapeutic dosages, a fresh solution of drug should be prepared daily. The solution should be mixed thoroughly and checked to ensure that the drug goes into and remains in solution.

On-Label Drug Use: The Gold Standard for Minimizing Drug Residues

The ideal scenario for minimizing drug residues in poultry products is to use an approved product according to the label directions and comply with the label WDT as established by the regulatory agency. Tables with summarized WDTs for poultry drugs approved in the United States and Canada can be found on the Compendium of Veterinary Products Web Site (Table 28.2). In the United States, a variety of web sites also provide the ability to search for approved poultry products (Table 28.2); however, it is the veterinarian's ultimate responsibility to consult the product information contained on the product label or package insert. Lists of US veterinary products that are approved for game birds have been published [32], but the information should be compared to the FDA-approved veterinary drug web site because the approvals might have changed since the publication date.

In the United States, the Office of New Animal Drug Evaluation (ONADE) within the FDA-CVM is responsible for reviewing and approving NDAs. For a drug to be approved, the drug sponsor must demonstrate that the drug is safe in the intended species and is effective for the indication or disease condition that is being treated using the labeled dose and administration route. The sponsor must also demonstrate that the drug is safe for the person administering it, that use of the drug will not harm the environment, and that the drug can be consistently manufactured to standards of strength and purity. If the drug is to be labeled for food-producing animals, human food safety is also a major component of the approval process. In other words, for the product to gain approval there must be reasonable certainty of no harm occurring to human health from the ingestion of foodstuffs from food-producing animals that are treated with the drug.

Part of the approval process is to estimate a safe time for which the meat, organs, by-products, or eggs must be withheld before entering the human food chain. This WDT is dependent on the maximum concentration of the drug or its metabolite allowed in the edible tissue that has the longest elimination. In the United States, this is known as tolerance, whereas in Europe and other parts of the world this concentration is known as the maximum residue limit (MRL). Calculations of tolerances or MRLs have been previously described [33, 34].

When WDTs are established by the FDA, they are calculated so that 99% of the animals are below the tolerance when the drug is used according to label directions. This is based on data provided by the sponsor (i.e. a pharmaceutical company or any other entity applying for drug approval in healthy animals). Keep in mind that animals that are systemically compromised, suffering from liver or renal dysfunction, or a septic illness, may take longer to eliminate the drug and require an extended WDT even when label directions are followed.

Other countries have their own approval processes that are not detailed in this chapter; however, for reference purposes a summary of approved poultry medications and their WDTs for the United Kingdom and Australia, respectively, can be found on this book's accompanying website. It is important to remember that this information is dynamic, thus veterinarians should always consult the product label or package insert to ensure accuracy (Table 28.2).

Extra-Label Drug Use: Strategies for Minimizing Drug Residues

In the United States, AMDUCA stipulates that it is the legal responsibility of the prescribing veterinarian to make a withdrawal recommendation based on scientific evidence when drugs are used in an extra-label manner. In addition, ELDU must be assigned a substantially "extended" WDT. This "extended" WDT(s) is/are referred to as withdrawal interval(s) or WDI(s) in this chapter. The WDI must be longer than the FDA-approved WDT, regardless of the dose, duration/frequency of treatment, or dosing frequency, even if any of these dosing factors are less than those listed on the FDA-approved label. For example, if a hypothetical drug label dosage is 10 mg/kg, the corresponding FDA-approved WDT is five days, and the drug is administered in an extra-label manner at 5 mg/kg, then the WDI must be longer than five days.

A US program that provides advice regarding on-label and ELDU and provides WDIs based on scientific data is the FARAD. FARAD was previously known as the Food Animal Residue Avoidance Databank, but because the program serves many more functions besides data banking, the program's name was changed in 2011. A similar program exists in Canada (Canadian gFARAD), but they are a separate entity from the US program. Any comments in this chapter regarding FARAD are specific to the US program.

US FARAD is a national, congressionally-funded, USDA-administered, cooperative program, with a primary mission to prevent or mitigate illegal residues of drugs, pesticides, and other chemicals in foods of animal origin. FARAD collects, analyzes, and evaluates scientific data to provide WDIs when drugs are used in an extra-label manner. FARAD also advises on pesticide exposure and accidental contaminations (biotoxins, heavy metals, radionuclides, mistaken feeding of a batch of higher than label dose-medicated feed to a flock of chickens where there was an error in the dose calculation, etc.)

When veterinarians prescribe drugs according to the label or in an extra-label manner, they can contact FARAD for WDTs or WDI recommendations, respectively, via the telephone hotline (1-888-873-2723) or submit withdrawal requests online at www.farad.org. Withdrawal recommendations are provided to the prescribing veterinarian on a case-by-case basis.

FARAD does not recommend generation of WDI "lists," as these lists can become outdated as a result of new information in the literature changing a WDI, tolerances being changed, or FDA-approved WDTs being modified.

Strategies and techniques for estimating WDIs when drugs are used in an extra-label manner in livestock have been previously published [35, 36]. Additionally, factors or information that FARAD takes into consideration for estimating a WDI for poultry and other food-producing animals when they are treated with veterinary products in an extra-label manner have been previously published [37] and include those listed in the following sub-sections.

General Factors Impacting Pharmacokinetic Parameters and Drug Residues

When recommending a WDI after ELDU or a contamination incident, FARAD takes into account conditions that might impact drug absorption and elimination. Some treatment conditions include dose, duration of treatment, and administration route.

Egg withdrawal recommendations can be difficult to estimate, as the variables involved in residue deposition in eggs have not been fully elucidated. Systemic administration of medications generally results in exposure of the ovary, follicle, and oviduct potentially leading to egg residues. It has been reported that with some medications, egg white concentrations mirror plasma concentrations, with higher doses resulting in higher residue concentrations [38]. Imaging studies have found that during yolk formation, drugs are incorporated into the yolk through daily layering of yolk material. Consequently, drug exposure in early stages of yolk development results in drug residues in the inner rings of yolk, while exposure in the later stages of development results in residues in the outer portion of the yolk [39, 40]. This means that even drugs with short elimination times may still cause detectable egg residues for prolonged periods as a result of exposure of early stage egg yolks [39, 41]. Physical-chemical properties of the drug itself, including lipophilicity, hydrophilicity, protein binding, pKa, drug dose, and treatment length influences the extent of drug transfer to the yolk or albumin [38, 42]. Two excellent review articles addressing the issues of modeling drug residues in edible poultry tissues and eggs have been published [43, 44] and a literature review of scientific studies with egg residue data is also available [45].

Physiological Factors/Compromised Health Conditions Impacting Pharmacokinetic Parameters and Drug Elimination

Drug clearance can be affected by the clinical condition of the patient receiving the treatment. Dehydration might impact how the drug is absorbed, especially if the drug is administered subcutaneously. If the drug has an extended absorption time, then this could lengthen the elimination time. Another important factor to consider when estimating a WDI is the overall function of the slowest organ to eliminate the drug. Most antibiotics are excreted via the kidney. Any clinical condition affecting the kidney could also impact drug elimination. For example, renal failure could result in prolonged drug elimination of most antibiotics including beta-lactams. Liver failure affects drugs that require hepatic activation, undergo biotransformation, or are affected by hypoproteinemia (i.e. highly protein bound drugs). As a result, avian-unique characteristics in drug metabolism and clearance should always be considered [2]. Similar to mammals, gastrointestinal diseases in birds may limit drug absorption because of altered intestinal absorption [2].

Pharmacokinetic Parameters: Drug Residue Serum, Tissue or Egg Data from Published Studies

FARAD commonly uses published data (especially time versus concentration data) to calculate pharmacokinetic parameters that are

subsequently used for recommending WDIs following ELDU. The principal pharmacokinetic parameters of a veterinary drug that are useful for predicting the concentrations of residues after a drug has been administered have been described [46]. In order for FARAD to deem published data to be useful, the time versus concentration data must derive from live animal studies, all of the dosing information must be provided, and the matrix, that is, serum, plasma, tissue, egg, and so on, that is analyzed must be clearly identified. Tissue or egg concentration data are more helpful than serum or plasma data as they represent the edible products that would be consumed by humans. In addition, plasma or serum data may or may not reflect residue concentrations in the tissues or eggs [39, 41, 47, 48]. In some published studies, authors report that residues were still detectable on the last sampling day, thus FARAD is conservative when estimating a withdrawal recommendation, especially if no tolerance exists. Even if residues were not detected on a sampling day post-treatment, FARAD would compare the assay's limit of detection with the tolerance for the drug, poultry species, and matrix (i.e. tissue type, egg component, serum, or plasma, etc.). If the assay's limit of detection is higher than the tolerance, then violative residues could still be present in the edible poultry products. According to AMDUCA, following ELDU in the United States, if there is no approved tolerance, no residues (i.e. the tolerance would be deemed to be 0) should be detected in products intended for human consumption. Therefore, if the analytical method is extremely sensitive, an extended WDI is necessary.

Established Tolerance or MRL

Another factor that FARAD takes into account when recommending a WDI, is whether a tolerance has been established for the marker residue and matrix of interest for the bird species that was treated. A marker residue is the residue the concentration of which maintains a known relationship to the concentration of total residue in an edible tissue [49]. When the concentration of the marker residue is below the tolerance in the target tissue, the total residues in all the edible tissues are less than their respective safe concentrations [33].

In certain countries, MRLs are the focus. The USDA Foreign Agricultural Service MRL database, is a searchable international database for pesticide and veterinary drug MRLs for various commodities and markets. Worldwide web site URLs for on-line resources listing tolerances or MRLs can be found in Table 28.2. The Food and Agriculture Organization (FAO) and World Health Organization (WHO) have a joint program known as Codex Alimentarius Commission that publishes a collection of international food standards and guidance documents. The Codex Committee on Residues of Veterinary Drugs in Foods (CCRVDF) is responsible for establishing MRLs for veterinary drugs in foods and related details. Efforts related to international harmonization of MRLs are of interest to countries participating in trade of food animal products and to pharmaceutical companies that wish to market their products in multiple countries [50].

If a drug is not approved in a species, then a tolerance probably does not exist. If no tolerance exists, any detectable residue would be deemed violative following ELDU. Therefore, the WDI needs to be long enough to allow for residue depletion below the limit of detection for analytical methods used by regulatory authorities. This concept can result in a significantly extended WDI recommendation by FARAD in some cases.

Analytical Testing Method and Limits of Detection

Limits of detection for analytical methods that are used to measure residues are an important consideration when FARAD estimates WDIs, especially when there is no established tolerance. As mentioned previously, the WDI may need to be extended to achieve residue concentrations below the detection capability of the

analytical method. FSIS publishes the results of the NRP on a yearly basis known as the Red Book, which describes the analytical methods used by FSIS and their limits of detection (Table 28.2).

Foreign Drug Approval Data

In some cases, a drug might lack US FDA approval, but be approved in another country. In these circumstances, FARAD may use foreign WDTs as a guide for recommending a WDI after ELDU. However, one should be mindful that the WDT or withdrawal period for the drug with an approved foreign label would be based on an MRL that was established by that country, while there would be no FDA-approved tolerance for the drug in the United States. Therefore, when foreign labels are used to estimate WDI recommendations following ELDU in the United States, the WDI must always be conservatively longer to allow the drug residues to deplete below the FSIS analytical methods' limit of detection. Table 28.2 includes a listing of international drug databases that have foreign-approved drug label information, including dose and WDTs.

Testing for Drug Residues

The analytical methods for detecting drug residues have a wide spectrum of needs when it comes to equipment, personnel expertise, reagents, and so on. Some analytical methods are cost-efficient, do not require highly skilled personnel, have simple equipment needs, and offer advantages of rapid testing. The opposite end of the spectrum includes sophisticated expensive techniques that are labor- and equipment-intensive. Sample preparation and drug residue analysis in poultry products have been previously described [51].

If a practitioner or producer/owner wants to confirm that poultry products (i.e. meat or eggs) are at or below the tolerance, they can consider submitting a limited number of flock-representative birds for drug residue testing.

Age range, disease status, and gender representation are just a few things to consider when choosing birds to be representative of the flock. Samples or carcasses can be submitted to a commercial laboratory for residue testing. Another option for sample submission would be a state veterinary diagnostic laboratory. The web site URL for state veterinary laboratories in the United States is listed under AAVLD in Table 28.2.

Commercial rapid tests for drug residue testing in poultry are very limited in availability compared to those available for other food-producing animals. The commercial rapid tests for drug residue screening are typically either FDA or Association of Official Analytical Chemists (AOAC) approved. These rapid tests are evaluated for their ability to detect the targeted analyte in a matrix from the animal species from which the samples originated. An example of a manufacturer of rapid "commercial" chicken-side tests is Charm Sciences (http://charmsciences.com). Similar to recommendations made previously for other analytical tests, the limit of detection for the rapid tests should be at or below the tolerances in order to ensure that the poultry product can enter the human food chain.

Pharmacovigilence: Guidelines for Prudent Antibiotic Drug Use when Medicating Poultry

It is of upmost importance for veterinarians to use careful consideration when selecting antimicrobial therapy for poultry because of ongoing concerns regarding antimicrobial use in food-producing animals, the potential for microbial resistance, and growing concerns for protecting human public health. In some cases, especially with extremely resistant organisms, a veterinarian might have to advise as to whether or not treatment is appropriate or if euthanasia should be considered. This is especially important in households with immunocompromised individuals. In general, prolonged use of antimicrobials in a poultry population should be avoided to prevent the formation of antimicrobial-resistant reservoirs within the birds' normal bacterial flora.

When choosing an antibiotic, one with a narrow spectrum should be selected over a broad-spectrum agent when possible. Use of a broad-spectrum antibiotic can put selective pressure on non-target bacteria, thus increasing the likelihood of the development of resistance.

Guidelines for prudent antimicrobial use when treating poultry include

1) All antimicrobials (including over-the-counter medications) should be used under the supervision of a veterinarian
2) Good husbandry practices, including good hygiene, preventative strategies such as vaccination, probiotics, nutrition [52], and routine health monitoring, should be used to reduce the need for antimicrobials
3) Extra-label use of antimicrobials should be the exception (not the rule) and should only be performed under the supervision of a veterinarian and in compliance with stipulations set forth by AMDUCA
4) Antimicrobial therapy should be administered over as short a treatment period as possible at therapeutic doses to ill or at risk birds only
5) Culture and sensitivity results should be used when possible to guide antimicrobial selection
6) Records should be kept of all antimicrobial administration and may be used to evaluate efficacy and treatment protocols
7) Immunocompetent statuses of humans in direct or indirect contact with the medicated avian patient should be taken into account, especially when targeting highly resistant organisms. In some cases, if there are immunocompromised humans that will be in contact with the bird, a decision as to whether or not to treat the bird may be

necessary. In some cases, euthanasia of the bird might need to be discussed.

Antimicrobials that are deemed less important for treating serious infections in humans should be used before more important antimicrobials are used. Canada Health has classified antimicrobials based on their importance for use in humans and the necessity of preserving their effectiveness [53]. These rankings are listed in Table 28.11.

Conclusion

Veterinarians treating individual birds or poultry flocks have the challenging responsibility of protecting human public health while simultaneously ensuring avian health. It was the intent of the authors of this chapter to provide a comprehensive review of medication use in poultry and approaches for judicious and responsible drug use, because veterinari-

Table 28.11 Health Canada's categorization of antimicrobial drugs based on importance in human medicine.

Category I: very high importance

These antimicrobials are deemed to be of very high importance in human medicine as they meet the criteria of being essential for the treatment of serious bacterial infections and limited or no availability of alternative antimicrobials for effective treatment in case of emergence of resistance to these agents. Examples include:

Carbapenems
Cephalosporins- 3rd and 4th generation
Fluoroquinolones
Glycopeptides
Glycylcyclines
Ketolides
Lipopeptides
Monobactams
Nitroimidazoles (metronidazole)
Oxazolidinones
Penicillin-β-lactamase inhibitor combinations
Polymyxins (colistin)
Therapeutic agents for tuberculosis (e.g. ethambutol, isoniazid, pyrazinamide, and rifampin)

Category II: high importance

Antimicrobials in this category consist of those that can be used to treat a variety of infections including serious infections and for which alternatives are generally available. Bacteria that are resistant to drugs of this category are generally susceptible to Category I drugs, which could be used as alternatives. Examples include:

Aminoglycosides (except topical agents)
Cephalosporins- 1st and 2nd generations (including cephamycins)
Fusidic acid
Lincosamides
Macrolides
Penicillins
Quinolones (except fluoroquinolones)
Streptogramins
Trimethoprim/sulfamethoxazole

(Continued)

Table 28.11 (Continued)

Category III: medium importance

Antimicrobials in this category are used for treatment of bacterial infections for which alternatives are generally available. Infections caused by bacteria that are resistant to these drugs can, in general, be treated by Category II or I antimicrobials. Examples include:

Aminocyclitols

Aminoglycosides (topical agents)

Bacitracins

Fosfomycin

Nitrofurans

Phenicols

Sulphonamides

Tetracyclines

Trimethoprim

Category IV: low importance

Antimicrobials in this category are currently not used in human medicine. Examples include:

Flavophospholipols

Ionophores

Source: Health Canada. [53].

ans are professionals who are well-suited to the task of educating owners and producers. To aid in this endeavor, readers were provided with information regarding US legislation affecting medication use in poultry, guidance recommendations regarding legal and prudent on-label and ELDU in poultry, and approaches for establishing WDIs when drugs are used in an extra-label manner. In addition, resources listing WDTs for approved poultry drugs in the United States and other countries were provided. After reading this chapter, veterinarians will hopefully be more informed about how to better serve their clients and patients while still helping to protect the human food chain.

Acknowledgments

The authors gratefully acknowledge the editorial comments and advice provided by Dr. Aliki Dragona of the UC Davis University Writing Program. In addition, the assistance provided by Ms. Valerie Goetting, Ms. Roan Chiong, and Mr. Ruben Pacheco were greatly appreciated.

References

1 US Food and Drug Administration: Animal & Veterinary. (2012). Appendix III, species and classes of major food animals. *CVM's Guidance for Industry (GFI) #191: Changes to Approved NADAs – New NADAs vs. Category II Supplemental NADAs.* https://www.fda.gov/downloads/AnimalVeterinary/ GuidanceComplianceEnforcement/ GuidanceforIndustry/ucm052460.pdf (accessed 20 August 2018).

2 Vermeulen, B., De Backer, P., and Remon, J.P. (2002). Drug administration to poultry. *Adv. Drug Delivery Rev.* 54: 795–803.

3 Riviere, J.E. and Sundlof, S.F. (2009). Chemical residues in tissues of food animals. In: Veterinary Pharmacology & Therapeutics, 9e (eds. J.E. Riviere and M.G. Papich), 1453–1462. Oxford: Blackwell Publishing.

4 Landy, R.B. (1999). Regulatory approaches for controlling pesticide residues in food animals. *Vet. Clin. North Am. Food Anim. Pract.* 3: 89–107.

5 Paige, J.C. (1999). Health implications of residues of veterinary drugs and chemicals in animal tissues. *Vet. Clin. North Am. Food Anim. Pract.* 15: 31–43.

6 Martínez-Navarro, J.F. (1990). Food poisoning related to consumption of illicit β-agonist in liver. *Lancet* 336: 1311.

7 Brambilla, G., Loizzo, A., Fontana, L. et al. (1997). Food poisoning following consumption of clenbuterol-treated veal in Italy. *J. Am. Med. Assoc.* 278: 635–635.

8 Greenlees, K.J., Friedlander, L.G., and Boxall, A. (2011). Antibiotic residues in food and drinking water, and food safety regulations. In: Chemical Analysis of Antibiotic Residues in Food (eds. J. Wang, J.D. MacNeil and J.F. Kay), 111–123. Hoboken: Wiley.

9 Greenlees, K.J. (2003). Animal drug human food safety toxicology and antimicrobial resistance-the square peg. *Int. J. Toxicol.* 22: 131–134.

10 Cerniglia, C.E. and Kotarski, S. (2005). Approaches in the safety evaluations of veterinary antimicrobial agents in food to determine the effects on the human intestinal microflora. *J. Vet. Pharmacol. Ther.* 28: 3–20.

11 Cerniglia, C.E. and Kotarski, S. (1999). Evaluation of veterinary drug residues in food for their potential to affect human intestinal microflora. *Regul. Toxicol. Pharm.* 29: 238–261.

12 National Research Council (1999). Drug residues and microbial contamination in food. In: The Use of Drugs in Food Animals: Benefits and Risks, 110–144. Washington, DC: The National Academies Press.

13 Fletouris, D.J. (2000). Drug Residues in Foods: Pharmacology: Food Safety, and Analysis. ProQuest Ebook Central. https://ebookcentral.proquest.com/lib/ucdavis/detail.action?docID=216467.

14 United States Department of Agriculture Food Safety and Inspection Service. (2014). *U.S. National Residue Program Data ("Red Book")*. https://www.fsis.usda.gov/wps/wcm/connect/93ae550c-6fac-42cf-8c11-006748a4d817/2017-Red-Book.pdf?MOD=AJPERES (accessed 10 September 2018).

15 Donoghue, D.J. (2003). Antibiotic residues in poultry tissues and eggs: human health concerns? *Poult. Sci.* 82: 618–621.

16 Federal Register notice announcing changes to FSIS testing methodology (Docket No. FSIS-2012-0012). (2012). http://www.fsis.usda.gov/OPPDE/rdad/FRPubs/2012-0012.pdf (accessed 20 August 2018).

17 United States Government Printing Office (2012). *Public Law 108–282 - An act to amend the Federal Food, Drug, and Cosmetic Act with regard to new animal drugs, and for other purposes.* https://www.gpo.gov/fdsys/pkg/PLAW-108publ282/content-detail.html (accessed 20 August 2018).

18 Tell, L.A., Oeller, M., and Craigmill, A.L. (2009). Considerations for treating minor food-producing animals with veterinary pharmaceuticals. In: Veterinary Pharmacology & Therapeutics, 9e (eds. J.E. Riviere and M.G. Papich), 1331–1342. Oxford: Blackwell Publishing.

19 Davis, J.L., Smith, G.W., Baynes, R.E. et al. (2009). Update on drugs prohibited from extralabel use in food animals. *J. Am. Vet. Med. Assoc.* 235: 528–534.

20 Love, D.C., Halden, R.U., Davis, M.F. et al. (2012). Feather meal: a previously unrecognized route for reentry into the food supply of multiple pharmaceuticals and personal care products (PPCPs). *Environ. Sci. Technol.* 46: 3795–3802.

21 Lathers, C.M. (2001). Role of veterinary medicine in public health: antibiotic use in food animals and humans and the effect on evolution of antibacterial resistance. *J. Clin. Pharmacol.* 41: 595–599.

22 Nelson, J.M., Chiller, T.M., Powers, J.H. et al. (2007). Fluoroquinolone-resistant *Campylobacter* species and the withdrawal of fluoroquinolones from use in poultry: a public health success story. *Clin. Infect. Dis.* 44: 977–980.

23 Parry, J. (2005). Use of antiviral drug in poultry is blamed for drug resistant strains of avian flu. *Br. Med. J.* 331: 10.

24 He, G., Qiao, J., Dong, C. et al. (2008). Amantadine-resistance among H5N1 avian influenza viruses isolated in Northern China. *Antiviral Res.* 77: 72–76.

25 US Food and Drug Administration (2006). *Limited FDA survey of compounded drug products.* https://www.fda.gov/drugs/guidan cecomplianceregulatoryinformation/ pharmacycompounding/ucm155725.htm (accessed 20 August 2018).

26 US Food and Drug Administration: Animal & Veterinary (2012). *CVM guidance for industry #209 - the judicious use of medically important antimicrobial drugs in food-producing animals.* https://www.fda.gov/ downloads/AnimalVeterinary/ GuidanceComplianceEnforcement/ GuidanceforIndustry/UCM216936.pdf (accessed 20 August 2018).

27 US Food and Drug Administration: Animal & Veterinary (2012). *CVM guidance for industry #213 – new animal drugs and new animal drug combination products administered in or on medicated feed or drinking water of food-producing animals: recommendations for drug sponsors for voluntarily aligning product use conditions with GFI #209.* https://www.fda.gov/ downloads/AnimalVeterinary/ GuidanceComplianceEnforcement/ GuidanceforIndustry/UCM299624.pdf (accessed 20 August 2018).

28 Walleghem, D.V. Appendix 2: common conversions. In: The Responsible Use of Health Management Products for Poultry Production: A Home Study Course for Alberta Producers (eds. R. Chernos, T. Inglis, and J. Martin),

29 SafeFood (2014). *A review of coccidiostat residues in poultry.* https://www.safefood.eu/ Publications/Research-reports/A-Review- of-Coccidiostat-Residues-in-Poultry.aspx (accessed 20 August 2018).

30 Kan, K. (2005). Chemical residues in poultry and eggs produced in free-range or organic systems. In: Proceedings of the XVII European Symposium on the Quality of Poultry Meat and XI European Symposium on the Quality of Eggs and Egg Products, 28–36. Doorwerth, Netherlands, 23–26 May 2005: Golden Tulip Parkhotel Doorwerth.

31 Buck, B.B. (1985). Calculations in toxicology. In: Clinical and Diagnostic Veterinary Toxicology, 3e (ed. G.A. Van Gelder), 9–16. Dubuque: Kendall/Hunt Publishing Company.

32 Needham, M.L., Webb, A.I., Baynes, R.E. et al. (2007). Current update on drugs for game bird species. *J. Am. Vet. Med. Assoc.* 231: 1506–1508.

33 Martinez, M., Berson, M., Dunham, B. et al. (2009). Drug approval process. In: Veterinary Pharmacology & Therapeutics, 9e (eds. J.E. Riviere and M.G. Papich), 1365–1406. Oxford: Blackwell Publishing.

34 Food and Agriculture Organization of the United Nations; World Health Organization (2009). Maximum residue limits for pesticides and veterinary drugs. In: Principles and Methods for the Risk Assessment of Chemicals in Food; Environmental Health Criteria 240, 1–53. Geneva, Chapter 8: FAO/WHO.

35 Baynes, R.E., Martin-Jimenez, T., Craigmill, A.L. et al. (1999). Estimating provisional acceptable residues for extralabel drug use in livestock. *Regul. Toxicol. Pharm.* 29: 287–299.

36 Martin-Jimenez, T., Bayens, R.E., Craigmill, A. et al. (2002). Extrapolated withdrawal-interval estimator (EWE) algorithm: a quantitative approach to establishing extralabel withdrawal times. *Regul. Toxicol. Pharm.* 36: 131–137.

37 Riviere, J.E., Webb, A.I., and Craigmill, A.L. (1998). Primer on estimating withdrawal times after extralabel drug use. *J. Am. Vet. Med. Assoc.* 213: 966–968.

38 Kan, C.A. and Petz, M. (2001). Detecting residues of veterinary drugs in eggs. *World Poult.* 17: 16–17.

39 Donoghue, D.J. (2001). Mechanisms regulating drug and pesticide residue uptake by egg yolks: development of predictive models. *World's Poult. Sci. J.* 57: 373–380.

40 Donoghue, D.J. and Myers, K. (2000). Imaging residue transfer into egg yolks. *J. Agric. Food. Chem.* 48: 6428–6430.

41 Donoghue, D.J., Hairston, H., Henderson, M. et al. (1997). Modeling drug residue uptake by eggs: yolks contain ampicillin residues even after drug withdrawal and nondetectability in the plasma. *Poult. Sci.* 76: 458–462.

42 Kan, C.A. and Petz, M. (2000). Residues of veterinary drugs in eggs and their distribution between yolk and white. *J. Agric. Food. Chem.* 48: 6397–6403.

43 Donoghue, D.J. (2005). Modelling risks from antibiotic and other residues in poultry and eggs. In: Food Safety Control in the Poultry Industry (ed. G.C. Mead), 83–100. Cambridge: Woodhead Publishing.

44 Hekman, P. and Schefferlie, G.J. (2011). Kinetic modeling and residue depletion of drugs in eggs. *Br. Poult. Sci.* 52: 376–380.

45 Goetting, V., Lee, K.A., and Tell, L.A. (2011). Pharmacokinetics of veterinary drugs in laying hens and residues in eggs: a review of the literature. *J. Vet. Pharmacol. Ther.* 34: 521–556.

46 Ludwig, B. (1989). Use of pharmacokinetics when dealing with the drug residue problem of food-producing animals. *Dtsch. Tierarztl. Wochenschr.* 96: 243–248.

47 Afifi, N.A. and Abo El-Sooud, K. (1997). Tissue concentrations and pharmacokinetics of florfenicol in broiler chickens. *Br. Poult. Sci.* 38: 425–428.

48 Reyes-Herrera, I., Schneider, M.J., Blore, P.J., and Donoghue, D.J. (2011). The relationship between blood and muscle samples to monitor for residues of the antibiotic enrofloxacin in chickens. *Poult. Sci.* 90: 481–485.

49 US Food and Drug Administration: Animal & Veterinary (2012) *CVM guidance for industry* #207 (VICH GL48) studies to evaluate the metabolism and residue kinetics of veterinary drugs in food-producing animals: marker residue depletion studies to establish product withdrawal periods. https://www.fda.gov/downloads/AnimalVeterinary/GuidanceComplianceEnforcement/GuidanceforIndustry/UCM207941.pdf (accessed 20 August 2018).

50 Thompson, S.R. (1999). International harmonization issues. *Vet. Clin. North Am. Food Anim. Pract.* 15: 181–195.

51 Hagren, V., Peippo, P., and Lovgren, T. (2005). Detecting and controlling veterinary drug residues in poultry. In: Food Safety Control in the Poultry Industry, 1e (ed. G.C. Mead), 44–82. Boca Raton: CRC Press.

52 Abbas, R.Z., Colwell, D.D., and Gilleard, J. (2012). Botanicals: an alternative approach for the control of avian coccidiosis. *World's Poult. Sci. J.* 68: 203–215.

53 Health Canada (2014). *Categorization of antimicrobial drugs based on importance in human medicine.* https://www.canada.ca/en/health-canada/services/drugs-health-products/veterinary-drugs/antimicrobial-resistance/categorization-antimicrobial-drugs-based-importance-human-medicine.html (accessed 20 August 2018).

29

Commonly Used Medications

Cheryl B. Greenacre

Department of Small Animal Clinical Sciences, College of Veterinary Medicine, University of Tennessee, Knoxville, Knoxville, TN, USA

Introduction

Backyard poultry are commonly being presented to veterinary practices for individualized and small flock care. Veterinarians should realize that even if an individual chicken or turkey is never used for food, it is still regulated as a food animal *species* by the United States Food and Drug Administration (FDA). The FDA prohibits the use of certain drugs, with no allowable extra-label drug use (ELDU), in any food-producing animal species and their regulations must be followed. There are very few FDA-approved labeled medications that can be administered to a chicken that lays eggs for human consumption. For laying hens, the FDA-approved withdrawal time is 0 days, thus there are a limited number of FDA-approved medications available for egg-laying chickens.

The goal of this chapter is to provide practical information on what is commonly used and available to treat backyard poultry within the current laws and regulations.

Scope and Disclaimer

This chapter is not intended to provide an exhaustive list of all medications used in poultry as it would be beyond the scope and size of this book. Also, there are entire books and websites available on this subject, which are outlined later under "Sources of Information Available." Nor will this chapter detail the laws and regulations as this information is well described in the previous chapter (Chapter 28, Regulatory Considerations for Medication Use in Poultry), where it states that the chapter "is designed to provide veterinarians with information that will help them navigate the legal and logistical hoops of medication use in poultry, provide resources for finding withdrawal times for drugs approved for poultry, provide guidance for estimating withdrawal intervals when drugs are used in an extra-label manner, and highlight guidance recommendations regarding prudent use of antibiotics."

The author attempted to verify all references, dosages, and other information contained within this chapter. However, despite this diligence, errors in the original sources or in the preparation of this chapter may have occurred. Therefore, users of this chapter should empirically evaluate all dosages to determine that they are reasonable prior to use. The author does not necessarily endorse specific products, procedures, or dosages reported in this chapter. The listing of a drug or commercial product in this chapter does not indicate approval by the FDA or the manufacturer for use in poultry. Also, laws and regulations change

Backyard Poultry Medicine and Surgery: A Guide for Veterinary Practitioners, Second Edition.
Edited by Cheryl B. Greenacre and Teresa Y. Morishita.
© 2021 John Wiley & Sons, Inc. Published 2021 by John Wiley & Sons, Inc.
Companion website: www.wiley.com/go/greenacre/medicine

constantly; therefore, information in this chapter may become outdated, and the reader is encouraged to refer to the regulatory websites listed here and in the previous chapter before use of medications.

Sources of Information Available

Food Animal Residue Avoidance Databank (FARAD) and the Veterinarian's Guide to Residue Avoidance Management (VetGRAM)

The Food Animal Residue Avoidance Databank (FARAD) website (under Veterinarian's Guide to Residue Avoidance Management [VetGRAM]) lists more than 200 approved medications for poultry (chickens, turkeys, and ducks) [1, 2]. Each of these listed medications has specific guidelines on its use in an approved manner, including such specifics as the type, size, and age of the bird, dose, formulation, duration, and indications for use. VetGRAM is a user-friendly resource that has sorting capabilities and withdrawal time tables for FDA-approved veterinary food animal drugs/products, including Abbreviated New or New Animal Drug Application (A/NADA) numbers and can be found on the FARAD website at http://wwww. http://farad.org [1].

The FARAD website also provides an online request system by clicking the "Request Advice" icon to ask withdrawal time for ELDU medications, with a response time of less than 72 hours [3]. There is no fee for this service, and their response can be documented in the patient's record. There is also a request area for Canadian veterinarians [4].

Exotic Animal Formulary

A detailed source of doses for various medications for poultry and other birds, including extensive references to research published in the literature, is available in both the Backyard Poultry chapter and the Avian chapter of the *Exotic Animal Formulary, 5th edition*, by James W. Carpenter. It includes doses for individuals as well as flocks, with references to research

and anecdotal information, for more than 100 medications for ring-necked pheasants, chickens, waterfowl, poultry, Galliformes, quail, and peafowl [5, 6].

US FDA Center for Veterinary Medicine

The US FDA also has a searchable database called "Animal Drugs @ FDA" where you can search for drugs by trade name or A/NADA number; the database can be found at https://animaldrugsatfda.fda.gov/adafda/views/#/search [7].

Minor Use Animal Drug Program

The Minor Use Animal Drug Program has a database on their web site (http://www.nrsp7.org/mumsrx/Species) to search for approved drugs, either by active ingredient or trade name, and has an avian-specific section for minor species such as ducks, pheasants, partridges, and quail [8].

Drugs.com

A list of veterinary drugs, label directions, and A/NADA numbers can also be found at https://www.drugs.com/vet [9].

Legalities

Prohibited Drugs

The FDA prohibits the use of certain drugs with no allowable ELDU in any food-producing animal *species* such as chickens and turkeys [1]. Please refer to Tables 29.1 and 29.2 for a complete list of medications the FDA currently considers prohibited in food animal species. These regulations are in place because edible tissues containing veterinary drug residues can be a risk to human health via direct toxic effects, allergic reactions, or increased bacterial resistance to common antibiotics [10, 11].

Note that one class of drugs prohibited by the FDA in food-producing animals since 1997 are the fluoroquinolones, including enrofloxacin. Never use fluoroquinolones in poultry, as these drugs are prohibited by the US FDA. As stated by the FDA, "Currently, no fluoroquinolones

Table 29.1 FDA Prohibited Drugs - Group 1. The FDA considers these as drugs with no allowable extra-label uses in any food producing animal species. The US Food and Drug Administration (FDA) considers chickens and turkeys food animal species. For more information go to www.farad.org [1].

Prohibited drugs – Group 1	• Chloramphenicol • Clenbuterol • Diethylstilbesterol (DES) • Fluoroquinolone–class antibiotics • Glycopeptides – all agents, including vancomycin • Medicated feeds • Nitroimidazoles – all agents, including dimetridazole, ipronidazole, metronidazole, and others • Nitrofurans – all agents, including furazolidine, nitrofurazone, and others

Table 29.2 FDA Prohibited Drugs - Group 2. The FDA considers these as drugs with restricted extra-label uses in food producing animal species. For more information go to www.farad.org [1].

Prohibited drugs – Group 2	• Adamantane and neuraminidase inhibitors – (Like amantadine/rimantidine known as Flumadine or oseltamivir known as Tamiflu) extra-label use (ELDU) of these drugs is *prohibited* in poultry including chickens, turkeys, and ducks in the United States. Although these drugs are *not approved for use in animals in the United States,* some of these drugs are used in other countries for the treatment or prevention of avian influenza in chickens, turkeys, and ducks. • **Cephalosporins** – ELDU of all cephalosporin antibiotics, except cephapirin is *restricted* in the United States. – ELDU restrictions differ for Major vs. Minor Food Animal Species as noted below: • **Major Food Animal Species** (cattle, pigs, chickens, and turkeys): ELDU is permissible *only for therapeutic indications* that are not included on the product label. However, ELDU of cephalosporin antibiotics is *prohibited* in all of the following situations: – the intended use of the product deviates from the approved dose, treatment duration, frequency, or administration route on the product label, – the intended use of a product in an unapproved major species or animal production class, – the intended use of the product for the purpose of disease prevention. • **Minor Food Animal Species** (all species that are not major species): ELDU of cephalosporin antimicrobial agents is permitted in these species. • **Gentian violet** – use is *prohibited* in food or feed of all food-producing animal species • **Indexed drugs** – ELDU of these drugs is *prohibited* in all food producing animals, with some exceptions for minor-use animal species that are not used as food for humans or other animals. • **Phenylbutazone** – all uses of this drug is *prohibited* in female dairy cattle greater than 20 mo of age. • **Sulfonamide–class antibiotics** – ELDU of all sulfonamides and potentiated sulfonamides is prohibited in adult lactating dairy cattle or dairy cattle greater than 20 mo of age. – only labeled uses of approved sulfonamides are allowed. – ELDU of sulfonamides in milking sheep and goats is discouraged but not prohibited.

are approved for use in poultry in the U.S. Due to the extralabel use prohibition in place for fluoroquinolones, use in poultry is currently illegal in the U.S." [12]. Prohibited drugs cannot be given in an extra-label manner, even if the patient is a rooster that will never lay an egg, even if it is written in the record to never eat the bird or its eggs, even if the owner signs a document saying they will never eat the eggs or bird, and even if the owner would never think of eating the bird. In the case of fluoroquinolones, one serious concern is that chickens can amplify the creation of antibiotic resistant *Campylobacter* spp. which would create a situation in which a human could get a severe, even life-threatening, diarrhea from these organisms and physicians would have very limited to no treatment options.

Cephalosporins are also prohibited for use in food-producing animal species such as poultry since 2012, but there are two exceptions: (i) use of ceftiofur in one-day-old chicks as per label or, as an allowable exception, for a different indication (disease) than on the label but still only allows use in one-day-old chicks. (ii) Use in an extra-label manner in ducks, a food-producing minor species [13].

Extra-Label Drug Use (ELDU)

The FDA defines ELDU as: "Actual use or intended use of a drug in an animal in a manner that is not in accordance with the approved labeling. This includes, but is not limited to, use in species not listed in the labeling, use for indications (disease and other conditions) not listed in the labeling, use at dosage levels, frequencies, or routes of administration other than those stated in the labeling, and deviation from labeled withdrawal time based on these different uses" [14]. Many of the drugs used in individually owned poultry fall under the FDA rules of ELDU since very few studies have been performed evaluating and commercializing individual dosing in poultry. Use the VetGRAM program at www.farad.org for specific information and instructions on ELDU in poultry.

Labeled Drugs

A labeled drug must be used *exactly* as is written on the label to be considered as labeled drug use. If the labeled drug is an antibiotic that is to be given in the food, then a Veterinary Feed Directive (VFD) or prescription is needed. Labeled drugs will have an A/NADA (Abbreviated/New Animal Drug Application) number and current information can be easily accessed by looking up a labeled drug by this number. A NADA (New Animal Drug Application) is used to seek approval of a new animal drug. An ANADA (Abbreviated New Animal Drug Application) is used to seek approval of a generic new animal drug, which is a copy of an approved new animal drug for which patents or other periods of exclusivity are near expiration [15]. At the time of writing, there were only 21 drugs labeled for use in laying hens, and most were feed additives with the exception of formulations of amprolium (NADA #033-165, 200-463, 200-488, 200-496, 013-149, 200-630, 013-663) and fenbendazole (NADA #141-449) for drinking water and topical proparacaine (NADA #009-035) [2].

Veterinary Feed Directive (VFD)

A VFD is used for any labeled feed additive given to a food animal and must be written *exactly* as is written on the medication label. All labeled drugs have an A/NADA number that can be used to access labeling information. Manufacturers of specific labeled drugs can provide a prefilled VFD with their product's information already typed into the form, or if you are a member of the American Veterinary Medical Association (AVMA), there is blank form available on their website www.avma.org [16]. A valid veterinary client–patient relationship (VCPR) must exist. See Table 29.3 detailing what must be on a VFD or consult the FDA website. [17](Table 29.3).

Table 29.3 A veterinary feed directive (VFD) must be written *exactly* as written on the drug label and include the following written directions on the order.

- Veterinarian's information with signature
- Client information
- Where animals are located
- Type and number of animals
- Date issued
- Expiration date
- Indication for use, dose, withdrawal time
- And this specific verbiage "Use of feed containing this VFD drug in a manner other than as directed on the labeling (extralabel use), is not permitted"

Routes of Administration

The pros and cons of the various routes of administration of medications in poultry are listed in Table 29.4.

Technique for Crop Gavage (Tube Feeding)

Birds have a high basal metabolic rate with very little in reserves; therefore, if a bird is not maintaining or gaining weight in the hospital, then it needs crop gavage (tube feeding). While hospitalized the bird should be weighed on a gram scale daily in the morning. Generally, birds are tube fed 1–4 times/day at a rate of 30–60 ml/kg body weight per feeding.

Before crop gavage, be sure the patient is hydrated. The first gavage should be a small amount and thin; then gradually increase amount and thickness. Use omnivore-specific critical care formulas that are available for best results. These are high in calories and easy to digest. See Table 29.5 for detailed technique on how to gavage a chicken (Table 29.5).

Dehydration and Fluid Therapy

Most sick birds are 5–10% dehydrated. Clinical signs of dehydration include depression, reduced skin elasticity over digits, sunken eyes, cool digits, stringy mucus in oral cavity, and decreased refill time of the basilic (a.k.a. cutaneous ulnar, wing) vein. Maintenance fluids are 50 ml/kg/day. The most commonly used fluids are LRS or Normosol-R since they most closely resemble the fluid lost. Warm (about 90–100 °F) fluids are imperative since the normal average body temperature of a chicken is about 105 °F. Subcutaneous fluids are generally administered into the inguinal area in birds where there is the most loose skin. It is easier on the chicken to administer these while they are in a standing position. Severe dehydration or shock requires rapid circulatory expansion with IV or IO (intraosseous) fluids. Although peripheral indwelling (IV) catheters have been avoided in parrots due to small fragile veins, hematoma formation, highly mobile dermis, refractory temperaments, and a powerful beak, chickens seems to tolerate IV catheters well. The medial metatarsal vein seems best since it can be secured very well, although other veins could be used (basilic or jugular vein). Intraosseous catheters are most commonly placed in the distal ulna but can also be placed in the proximal tibiotarsus. The IO catheters should not be placed in a pneumatic bone as this will drown the bird when fluids are administered, since pneumatic bones communicate directly with the respiratory system. Likewise, intracoelomic fluids are generally avoided as these can easily go into an air sac and drown the bird. See Table 29.6 for detailed technique on how to place an IO catheter (Table 29.6).

Topical

In birds, avoid greasy topical compounds that reduce the insulation capacity of feathers. If ointments must be used in birds, then use sparingly.

Table 29.4 Routes of medication administration used in birds.

Route	Advantages	Disadvantages
Water additive	• Easy to administer • Bird self-medicates • Reduce specific water borne disease	• Inexact dose • Poor palatability reduces water and drug intake • Some medications unstable in water • Underdosing increases organism resistance • Poorly or slowly absorbed • Overdosing in hot weather or if polydipsic
Food additive	• Easy to administer • Food consumption fairly consistent	• Inexact dose • Poor palatability reduces food and drug intake • Some medications unstable in food • Underdosing increases organism resistance • Poorly or slowly absorbed • Realize sick birds are often anorectic
Direct Oral	• Precise dose (unless they spit the drug out or do not swallow) • Pediatric suspensions available • Tube/gavage feed at same time	• Stress of capture and restraint • Aspiration of drug • Drug may be poorly or slowly absorbed • Malabsorption (if for example the bird is in shock or has a GI disorder)
IM	• Exact dose • Quick and easy to administer • Quickly absorbed	• Not all drugs available as IM • Pain and necrosis • Muscle may be damaged
IV	• Exact dose • Rapid therapeutic levels	• Stress of prolonged restraint • Fragile veins • Maintaining catheter
IO (distal ulna)	• Exact dose • Can be left in place up to 5 d	• Painful to place (need anesthesia) • Maintaining catheter
SC	• Exact dose • Quick and easy to administer • Less stressful if given with the bird standing in a normal position	• Some drugs are irritating SQ • Severely debilitated birds may not absorb SQ fluids or drugs

It is better to use water-soluble creams such as silver sulfadiazine or, even better, medical-grade Manuka honey for wounds. Remember to consult FARAD for withdrawal times even with topical medications.

Nebulization

Nebulization is used to deliver medications for respiratory infections. Nebulization is the atomization of a liquid into small droplets that

Table 29.5 Detailed technique for gavage (tube feeding) poultry.

- On a table restrain the bird with a towel wrapped around the body secured at the base of the neck like a cape; have the bird in a normal upright position so as to avoid regurgitation and aspiration.
- Have a 60 cc syringe and a 12 or 16 French red-rubber catheter pre-filled with warm formula; using the non-dominant hand gently pinch the commissures of the mouth and place thumb in the mouth to keep it open.
- Aim the catheter from the bird's left commissure to the crop area; avoid the opening to the large trachea (the glottis) and avoid excessive force so as not to puncture the esophagus.
- Be absolutely sure of placement by palpating the trachea and the feeding tube at the same time (you should feel two tubes – one being the trachea and the other being the red rubber catheter) or look down the open mouth to see that the red rubber catheter is not going into the glottis.
- Close the mouth over the catheter and hold the head and catheter as one so the bird cannot sling its head and move the catheter.
- Gently extend the neck or place thumb over proximal esophagus to help prevent food coming up the esophagus; push plunger of syringe to give food quickly but not forcefully (stop if you feel pressure).
- If the bird regurgitates, or becomes overly stressed then release it immediately.
- Kink the tube to prevent spillage and aspiration as you gently pull the tube out; do not push on the full crop during further restraint. This should be your last procedure to minimize handling after gavage.

Table 29.6 How to place an intraosseous (IO) catheter.

- Preferably anesthetize the bird (since going through the periosteum is painful), pluck and aseptically prepare the dorsal carpus
- Instill up to 2 mg/kg lidocaine SC at distal ulna.
- Position needle (20 gauge) in center of distal ulna and push and twist needle until it pops through the periosteum into the medullary area of the ulna.
- Affix a catheter cap or line to the catheter and flush with 1–3 ml saline and visualize the fluid going through basilic vein for confirmation of proper placement.
- Anchor catheter to soft tissue of carpus with suture or tape, and apply a Figure-of-8 bandage for added security.

can be inhaled. Since birds have small air capillaries (about 3 μm) compared to the smallest mammalian alveoli (about 10 μm), be sure to use a nebulizer that forms the smaller droplets. Usually nebulization is performed for 10–30 minutes by forcing oxygen or air through a solution (containing antibiotics or antifungals, etc.). The Bird chapter for Carpenter's *Exotic Animal Formulary* is an excellent source of information regarding doses for nebulizing

birds [6]. Remember to consult FARAD for withdrawal times.

Therapy Overview

Most infections in birds are due to Gram-negative organisms. Pharmacokinetic and pharmacodynamic studies on various medications used in poultry are available in the literature, but the doses studied may not be applicable to individual bird care due to studying one-time doses, studying healthy young animals or a single species of bird, given to a flock via food or drinking water, or a dose or medication that is prohibited, deemed ELDU, or does not pertain to the patient at hand for some other reason.

Some drug dosages are arrived at empirically or anecdotally if no pharmacodynamic and pharmacokinetic studies have been performed on chickens or other poultry species. Realize that there is no generic bird and that even different chicken *breeds* have been shown to respond differently to different drugs. For example, white Leghorn hens were found to metabolize a single oral dose of meloxicam significantly faster than Wyandotte hens [18].

Table 29.7 Comparison of the average weight of a Rhode Island red pullet (a layer breed), a Rhode Island red cockerel, and a Cornish Cross broiler (a fast growing meat breed) as they grow their first 6 wk.

Age	Rhode Island red pullet Grams (oz)	Rhode Island red cockerel Grams (oz)	Cornish Cross broiler Grams (oz)
3 d	35 (1.23)	36 (1.27)	43 (1.53)
1 wk	49 (1.73)	51 (1.80)	77 (2.70)
2 wk	103 (3.63)	104 (3.67)	240 (8.45)
3 wk	192 (6.77)	187 (6.60)	638 (22.50)
4 wk	284 (10.03)	292 (10.30)	941 (33.20)
5 wk	377 (13.30)	422 (14.90)	1379 (48.65)
6 wk	459 (16.20)	608 (21.45)	2024 (77.75)

For accurate dosing calculations, always weigh individual birds prior to medicating, but if the remainder of a flock needs to be treated this chart of average weights can be used as a rough estimate. Please refer to the Common Breeds of Backyard Poultry Chapter (Chapter 2) for average weights of adult birds [19].

The goal of therapy is to achieve antimicrobial tissue levels at the site of infection that are greater than the minimum inhibitory concentration (MIC), but realize tissue penetrations vary. Also realize that drug excretion is rapid in birds compared to mammals. Antibiotics can cause immunosuppression and change normal flora producing a secondary fungal infection, therefore only use antibiotics when indicated so as not to upset the delicate balance of normal flora in birds. Whenever possible, choose bacteriocidal instead of bacteriostatic antimicrobials. An accurate weight of the patient is needed for accurate dosing calculations, but an average weight for the age of the bird is provided in cases of calculating needed in flock situations (Table 29.7) [19].

Water and Feed Consumption Rates

For many medications, a mg/kg dose for individual dosing is sometimes difficult to find. Many labels describe dosing 1000 birds at a time in water or feed. Realize the disadvantages of treating in water include that a sick bird may not drink enough medicated water to reach treatment levels, and that water consumption also changes with breed, strain, environmental temperature and humidity, gender, age, size, and quality of water. Note that chickens can drink 30–50% more water when the environmental temperature is hot (>75° F). Birds do not sweat, so when hot they pant, which causes them to lose large amounts of moisture.

As a generalization, 100 turkeys will drink 1 gallon of water per day for each week of age; chickens will consume one-half this amount [20]. Please see Tables 29.8 and 29.9 for published average water consumption rates of chickens and turkeys shown in L/1000 birds/day (Tables 29.8 and 29.9) [21, 22]. Also see Tables 28.8 and 28.9 from the previous chapter regarding factors that affect water consumption rates, and water consumption rates shown in gallons or L/100 birds/day. For calculating feed additives, the feed consumption rates of various sized birds is included in Table 28.10 in the previous chapter [5]

Adverse Event Reporting

If there is an adverse event associated with an animal vaccine, then contact USDA APHIS Center

Table 29.8 Average drinking water (DW) consumption rate in liters DW/1000 birds/day of various types and ages of birds at various environmental temperatures [21, 22].

Type of bird (Production stage/age)	20C [21]	21C [21]	32C [22]	10–21C [22]	27–35C [22]
Broiler (1 wk)	50–65		50		
Broiler (2 wk)	120				
Broiler (3 wk)	180				
Broiler (4 wk)	245–260		415		
Broiler (5 wk)	290–345		550		
Broiler (6 wk)	330				
Broiler (7 wk)	355				
Broiler (8 wk)	370–470		770		
Layer pullet (4 wk)		100			
Layer pullet (12 wk)		160			
Layer pullet (18 wk)		200			
Laying hens (50% production)		220			
Laying hens (90% production)		270			
Turkey poult (1–7 wk)				38–327	38–448
Turkey poult (8–14 wk)				403–737	508–1063
Turkey poult (15–21 wk)				747–795	1077–1139

Table 29.9 Drinking water (DW) consumption rate in liters DW/1000 birds/day of various types and weights of birds. Range (average over a year) [21].

Type of bird	Weight range	Liters DW/1000 birds/day; range (average over a year)
Pullets	0.05–1.5 kg	30–180 (105)
Laying hens	1.6–1.9 kg	180–320 (250)
Broiler breeders	3.0–3.5 kg	180–320 (250)

for Veterinary Biologics at https://cvbpv.aphis.usda.gov/PVXClient/index.html#pageStart . [23]

If there is an adverse event associated with an FDA-approved drug, then the company can be called (the phone number is on the package or on the company website) and ask to speak to the "technical services veterinarian." They are required to forward a report to the FDA's Center for Veterinary Medicine (CVM).

If there is an adverse event associated with any animal drug, either approved or not, you can report it directly yourself to the FDA (Department of Health and Human Services, FDA, CVM) by submitting FORM FDA 1932a, also known as the "Veterinary Adverse Experience, Lack of Effectiveness or Product Defect Report" by going to https://www.fda.gov/animal-veterinary/report-problem/how-report-animal-drug-side-effects-and-product-problems [24].

Commonly Used Medications

Examples of medications commonly used in backyard individual poultry are listed in tables below. Drug labels, dosages, and withdrawal times for all classes of labeled medications can be found at https://animaldrugsatfda.fda.gov/adafda/views/#/search and http://www.fda.gov/AnimalVeterinary/Products/default.htm [7, 25]. For ELDU consult http://farad.org and click on icon to ask for recommended withdrawal times [1]. Information on dosages and other information can also be found at https://www.drugs.com/vet/chickens-a.html [9].

Antiparasiticides and Anticoccidial Medications

Coccidiosis is very common, especially in young poultry. Chicks from hatch to six to eight weeks of age should be on a medicated starter feed, usually medicated with amprolium to help control coccidia until the chick develops immunity. The exception would be if the chicks have been vaccinated against coccidia since vaccine immunity develops by reinfection with the non-virulent strain. Anticoccidial drugs are not allowed for use in organic poultry production, therefore vaccines are popular with this group [26]. Chickens with clinical disease due to coccidia include young not on mediated feed, exposure in naïve individuals, having a particular strain of coccidia such as *Eimeria tenella* or one that has developed resistance to amprolium, or being immunosuppressed or stressed in some way [27]. Adult chickens with a low number of coccidia and no clinical signs typically do not need treatment due to protective immunity from past exposure. For more information on cocciciosis, see Chapter 11, the Parasitology chapter.

Generally, the treatment for coccidiosis starts with improving hygiene and administering amprolium or a sulfa drug, such as sulfamethazine, sulfadimethoxine, sulfaquinoxaline, sulfadimethoxine/ometoprim, sulfadimethoxine,

sulfadiazine/trimethoprim, or trimethoprim/sulfamethoxazole. There are numerous other anticoccidial medications available that can be divided into two categories: the polyether ionphores or the enzymatic compounds. The polyether ionophores include lasolocid, salinomycin, maduromycin, monensin, narasin, lonomycin, and semduramicin. Ionophores have a narrow therapeutic margin with the therapeutic dose close to the toxic dose. Sulfonamides potentiate monensin, and erythromycin potentiates monensin, narasin, and salinomycin, therefore they should not be given together. Narasin and salinomycin are toxic to turkeys, ducks, and guinea fowl, and should not be given to them. Please refer to Chapter 20 on Toxicology for further information. The enzymatic compounds include amprolium, clopidol, diclazuril, decoquinate, reobenidine, roxarsone, sulfonamides, salinomycin, and zoalene.

Please see Tables 29.10 and 29.11 for an example of antiparasiticides used in commercial, backyard and individual poultry (Tables 29.10 and 29.11) [5, 6, 9, 28–30].

Antimicrobials

Examples of labeled antibiotics for use in drinking water of poultry are in Table 29.12 with ANADA numbers for ease of searching on-line at https://animaldrugsatfda.fda.gov. Meat and egg withdrawal times listed are for when the drug is used exactly as written on the label (Table 29.12) [2, 9, 20].

The list of antimicrobial and other drugs in Table 29.13 and Table 29.14 refers to drugs commonly used in an extra-label manner in individual birds. Consult http://FARAD.org regarding recommended meat and egg withdrawal times prior to use in an extra-label manner in chickens or turkeys (Table 29.13) [5, 6, 18, 31–40] and Table 29.14 [5, 6, 18, 29, 32, 41].

Table 29.10 Examples of labeled anticoccidial medications and antiparasiticides used in the drinking water of poultry. Labeled drugs are accompanied by their A/NADA number for easy information access on-line. DW, drinking water [9].

Medication	Dose	Comment
Amprolium 20% soluble powder, (NADA #33–165, Amprol 128, Huvepharma); (NADA #200–488, AmproMed-P for Poultry, Bimeda); each packet will make 128 gal DW at 0.012%; 4 oz. = 16 Tbs will make 50 gal at 0.012%	0.012–0.024% in DW × 3–5 d, then 0.006% × 1–2 wk	Growing chickens, turkeys, laying hens: For the treatment of coccidiosis.
Amprolium 9.6% solution (NADA # 200–496, CocciCure®-P for Poultry, Aspen; AmproMed-P, Bimeda); (ANADA #200–630, CocciAid* Amprolium 9.6% Oral Solution Cocidiostat, Aurora Pharmaceutical); 8 fl. oz. makes 50 gal DW at 0.012%	0.012–0.024% in DW × 3–5 d, then 0.006% × 1–2 wk	Growing chickens, turkeys, laying hens: For treatment of coccidiosis.
Fenbendazole, 200 mg/ml, (NADA 141–449, Safe-Guard Aqua-Sol for Chickens, or Safe-Guard Aquasol for Chickens and Swine, Intervet)	1 mg/kg BW/d × 5 d in DW (25 ml in DW will treat 5000 kg BW of chickens/d)	Broiler and Replacement Chickens: For the treatment and control of adult *Ascaridia galli.* No withdrawal period. Breeding Chickens and Laying Hens: For the treatment and control of adult *A. galli* and *Heterakis gallinarum.* No withdrawal period.
Piperazine sulfate, (NADA #10–005, Wazine-17*, Fleming Laboratories); each 100 ml contains 17 g of piperazine		For the removal of large roundworms (*Ascaridia spp.*) from turkeys and chickens.
	For each 100 birds, use 1 fl. oz. = 30 ml per gal (3.8 l) DW. Can repeat every 30 d.	Chickens 4–6 wk of age. Meat withdrawal 21 d.
	For each 100 birds, use 2 fl. oz. = 60 ml per 2 gal (7.6 l) DW. Can repeat every 30 d.	Chickens over 6 wk of age. Meat withdrawal 21 d.
	For each 100 birds, use 2 fl. oz. = 60 ml per 2 gal (7.6 l) DW. Can repeat every 30 d.	Turkeys Under 12 wk of age.
	For each 100 birds, use 4 fl. oz. = 120 ml per 4 gal (15 l) DW. Can repeat every 30 d.	Turkeys over 12 wk of age.

DW = drinking water; BW = body weight.

Table 29.11 Examples of anticoccidial medications and antiparasiticides commonly used in an extra-label manner in individual poultry. Please consult www.farad.org prior to use for recommended meat and egg withdrawal times. DW = drinking water. [5, 6, 9, 28–30].

Agent	Dose	Comment
Albendazole	10 mg/kg PO once;	Poultry/PK [5, 28];
	47 mg/kg PO once, repeat in 4 wk	Chickens: Heterakis [5]
Amprolium	13–26 mg/kg PO	Chickens [5]
Fenbendazole	–	Antihelmenthic active against cestodes, nematodes, trematodes, *Giardia*, acanthocephalans [5]
	20 mg/kg PO; repeat in 10–14 d;	Waterfowl [5, 29];
	10–50 mg/kg PO, repeat in 10–14 d;	Chickens: Ascarids [5];
	10–50 mg/kg q24h PO × 5 d	Chickens: *Capillaria* [5, 30]
Ivermectin injectable (1% = 10 mg/ml = 10 000 µg/ml)	0.2 mg/kg SQ, PO repeat in 10–14 d	Poultry: Nematodes, leeches, mites [5, 29]
Permethrin, Y-Tex GardStar 40% EC Livestock and Premise Insecticide*	Dilute 1–4 fl. oz. (30–118 ml) to 3.75 gals and use as course spray (1 gal of diluted course spray will treat 100 birds);	Poultry: Northern fowl mites, lice. Follow label precautions for human and honey bee safety while applying. [9]
	Dilute 4 fl. oz. (118 ml) in 10 gals water to treat environment. For severe infestation it is permissible to use 4 fl. oz. to 4 gals. Spray crevices of roost poles, cracks in walls and cracks in nest and nest boxes.	Environment: Bed bugs and Chicken mites, lice, ticks, and fleas. Follow label precautions for human and honey bee safety while applying. [9]
Permethrin (0.25%), Y-Tex GardStar Garden & Poultry Dust*	Apply directly to birds at a rate of 1 lb. per 100 birds. Ensure thorough treatment of vent area.	Poultry: To control Northern Fowl Mites and Lice [9]
	Use at a rate of 1 lb. per 40 sq. ft. to treat environment. Apply to floors, roosts and interior surfaces. Do not apply directly to eggs or nest litter. Do not contaminate feed or drinking water.	Environment: To control Northern Fowl Mite, Poultry Mite and Lice in poultry houses [9]
Piperazine	45–200 mg/kg once PO;	Waterfowl: *Tetrameres, Capillaria* [5];
	50–100 mg/kg once PO;	Chickens [5];
	100–500 mg/kg once PO, repeat in 10–14 d	Game birds [5]
Praziquantel	10 mg/kg PO,SC, repeat in 10–14 d	Waterfowl, chickens: Trematodes, cestodes [5]
Sulfamethazine	125–185 mg/kg PO q24h × d, then 64–94 mg/kg × d	Chickens [5]

Table 29.12 Examples of labeled antibiotics for use in drinking water of poultry with ANADA numbers for ease of searching on-line at https:// animaldrugsatfda.fda.gov. Meat and egg withdrawal times listed are for when the drug is used exactly as written on the label, but check the FARAD website prior to use as these can change. If a drinking water medication is listed as "X" mg/kg BW/day, then in a 24 hr period the bird must drink a certain amount of drinking water to obtain that many mg based on calculations of average water consumption (see Tables 28.8, 28.9, 29.7, and 29.8 for water consumption rates of various types of poultry). (DW = drinking water; BW = body weight) [2, 9, 20].

Drug	Dose	Comments
Bacitracin methylenedisalicylate soluble powder (NADA #065-470, BMD Soluble, Zoetis)	100 mg/gal DW (prevention);	Broiler and replacement chickens: Necrotic enteritis caused by *Clostridium perfringens*;
	200–400 mg/gal (control);	Growing turkeys: Transmissible enteritis (blue comb, mud fever) complicated by organisms susceptible to bacitracin.
	400 mg/gal DW (control) OR 400 mg/gal DW (prevention)	Growing quail: Ulcerative enteritis due to *Clostridium colinum*.
Ceftiofur sodium (NADA 140-338, Naxcel®, Zoetis);(ANADA #200-420, Ceftiflex®, Aspen; Ceftiflex Powder®, Vet One)	0.08–0.20 mg ceftiofur/chick SC in neck region	Day-old chicks: For the control of early mortality, associated with *E. coli* organisms susceptible to ceftiofur.
	0.17–0.5 mg ceftiofur/poult SC in the neck region	Day-old turkey poults: For the control of early mortality, associated with *E. coli* organisms susceptible to ceftiofur.
Chlortetracycline (CTC) hydrochloride, (NADA 65-440, Chloronex Soluble Powder, Huvepharma); (ANADA #200-441, Aureomycin® Soluble Powder Concentrate, Huvepharma) (each lb. contains 64 g of CTC)	200–400 mg/gal DW × 7–14 d	Chickens: For control of infectious synovitis caused by *Mycoplasma synoviae* sensitive to tetracycline hydrochloride;
	400–800 mg/gal DW × 7–14 d	Chickens: For control of chronic respiratory disease and air sac disease caused by *Mycoplasma gallisepticum* and *Escherichia coli*;
(each 25.6 oz. packet contains 102.4 g of CTC)	1000 mg/gal DW × 7–14 d	
	400 mg/gal DW × 7–14 d	Chickens: Control of mortality due to fowl cholera caused by *Pasteurella multocida*.
	25 mg/lb. BW/day × 7–14 d	Growing turkeys: Control of infectious synovitis caused by *Mycoplasma synoviae*.
	25 mg/lb. body weight/day × 7–14 d	Growing turkeys: Control of complicating bacterial organisms associated with bluecomb (transmissible enteritis, coronaviral enteritis) susceptible to chlortetracycline.

Drug (NADA/Product)	Dosage	Indication
Erythromycin phosphate* (NADA #035-157, Gallimycin PFC Water Soluble®, Bimeda)	500 mg/gal DW × 5d (provides 5.0–17.8 mg/lbBW/d)	Broilers and Replacement Chickens: As an aid in the control of Chronic Respiratory Disease due to *Mycoplasma gallisepticum* susceptible to erythromycin. Withdraw 1 d before slaughter.
	500 mg/gal DW × 7 d (provides 5.0–17.8 mg/lbBW/d)	Replacement Chickens (<16wk of age) and Chicken Breeders: As an aid in the control of Infectious Coryza due to *Haemophilus gallinarum* susceptible to erythromycin. Withdraw 1 d before slaughter.
	500 mg/gal DW × 7 d (provides 3.1 to 34.2 mg/lbBW/d)	Growing Turkeys: As an aid in the control Bluecomb (Non-specific Infectious Enteritis) caused by organisms susceptible to erythromycin. Withdraw 1 d before slaughter.
Gentamycin sulfate, (NADA #101–862, Garasol® Injection 100 mg/ml, Intervet); (ANADA #200–468, Genta-Med-P for Poultry Injection, Bimeda)	0.2 mg/chick SC in neck (usual volume is made to 0.2 ml)	1-d-old chicks: For the prevention of early mortality associated with *Escherichia coli*, *Salmonella typhimurium*, and *Pseudomonas aeruginosa*. Must not be slaughtered for food for at least 5 wk following treatment.
	1 mg/poult SC in neck (usual volume is made to 0.2 ml)	1–3-d-old poults: To aid in the prevention of early mortality associated with *Arizona paracolon* infections. Must not be slaughtered for food for at least 9 wk following treatment.
Lincomycin HCl soluble powder* (NADA #111-636, Lincomix Soluble Powder, Zoetis); (ANADA #200-189, Lincomycin Soluble Powder, Huvepharma);(ANADA #200-377, Linx-Med-SP, Bimeda)	64 mg/gal DW × 7 d	Broiler Chickens: Indicated for the control of necrotic enteritis caused by *Clostridium perfringens* susceptible to lincomycin.
Lincomycin HCl and Spectinomycin sulfate tetrahydrate, (NADA#46–109, LS-50 Water Soluble Powder, Zoetis)	50–65 mg/lb. BW (1 bottle/25 gal DW)	Chickens up to 7d of age: For air sacculitis caused by either *Mycoplasma synoviae* or *Mycoplasma gallisepticum*, or Complicated Chronic Respiratory Disease caused by *Escherichia coli* and *M. gallisepticum*.

(Continued)

Table 29.12 (Continued)

Drug	Dose	Comments
Oxytetracycline HCl soluble powder*, varying concentrations (NADA#130-435, Oxytet, Huvepharma), (ANADA #200–146, Tetroxy 25 Soluble Powder with 10 g oxytetracycline per packet, Bimeda); (ANADA #200–247, Tetroxy 343 Soluble Powder with 102.4 g of oxytetracycline/packet, Bimeda)	200–400 mg/gal DW no more than 14 d	Chickens: Control of infectious synovitis caused by *Mycoplasma synoviae*, susceptible to oxytetracycline. Turkeys: Control of hexamitiasis caused by *Hexamita meleagridis*, susceptible to oxytetracycline.
	400–800 mg/gal DW no more than 14 d	Chickens: Control of chronic respiratory disease (CRD) and air sac infections caused by *Mycoplasma gallisepticum* and *Escherichia coli*, susceptible to oxytetracycline. Control of fowl cholera caused by *Pasteurella multocida*, susceptible to oxytetracycline.
	400–800 mg/gal DW no more than 14 d	Turkeys: Control of infectious synovitis caused by *Mycoplasma synoviae*, susceptible to oxytetracycline.
	25 mg/lb. BW no more than 14 d	Growing Turkeys: Control of complicating bacterial organisms associated with bluecomb (transmissible enteritis, coronaviral enteritis), susceptible to oxytetracycline.
Spectinomycin, (NADA 038-661, SpectoGard Water Soluble Powder, Bimeda)(Each 1000 g of product contains 500 g of spectinomycin)	2 g/gal DW × first 3 d of life and 1 d following each vaccination;	Chickens, Broilers: As an aid in the prevention or control of losses due to CRD associated with *M. gallisepticum*. Do not give within 5 d of slaughter. Do not administer to laying chickens.
	1 g/gal DW × first 3–5 d of life	Chickens, Broiler: As an aid in controlling infectious synovitis due to *Mycoplasma synoviae*. Do not give within 5 d of slaughter. Do not administer to laying chickens. Note: Rarely, humans can develop serious reactions after handling.
Sulfadimethoxine (ANADA #200-238, Sulfadimethoxine 107 g powder, Vet One); (Sulfadived soluble powder, VedCo Inc.; Sulfasol, Med Pharmex); (ANADA #200–376, Sulfa Med G Soluble Powder, Bimeda)	0.05% (1 packet per 50 gal DW)× 6 d	Broiler, Replacement Chickens: for the treatment of disease outbreaks of coccidiosis, fowl cholera, and infectious coryza. Meat >5d. Do not administer to chickens over 16 wk (112 d) of age.
	0.025% (1 packet per 100 gal DW) × 6 d	Meat-producing Turkeys: for the treatment of disease outbreaks of coccidiosis and fowl cholera. Meat >5d. Do not administer to turkeys over 24 wk (168 d) of age.

Drug	Dosage	Indications
Sulfadimethoxine Concentrated Solution 12.5% (ANADA #200–251, Aspen Veterinary Resources; Sulfadived 12.5% solution, VedCo Inc.; Sulforal, Med Pharmex)	0.05% (Add 1 fl oz. to 2 gal of drinking water, OR 25 fl oz. to 50 gal DW)× 6 d	Broiler, Replacement Chickens: for the treatment of disease outbreaks of coccidiosis, fowl cholera, and infectious coryza. Meat >5d. Do not administer to chickens over 16 wk (112d) of age.
	0.025% DW(Add 1 fl oz. to 4 gal of drinking water or 25 fl oz. to 100 gal DW) × 6 d	Meat-producing Turkeys: for the treatment of disease outbreaks of coccidiosis and fowl cholera. Meat >5d. Do not administer to turkeys over 24 wk (168d) of age.
Sulfamerazine, sulfamethazine and sulfaquinoxaline combination soluble powder, (NADA #100-094, PoultrySulfa® by Huvepharma, each packet contains: 78g Sodium Sulfamerazine Activity, 78g Sodium Sulfamethazine Activity, 39g Sodium Sulfaquinoxaline Activity, each packet makes 128 gal of 0.04% OR 206 gal of 0.025% DW solution)	0.04% DW × 2–3 d, can be repeated	Chickens and turkeys: For acute fowl cholera caused by Pasteurella multocida. Meat withdrawal 14d.
	0.04% DW × 2–3 d, then plain water × 3d, then 0.025% DW × 2d. If needed, repeat at 0.025% level ×2d. DO NOT CHANGE LITTER.	Chickens: For coccidiosis caused by Eimeria tenella and E. necatrix. Meat withdrawal 14d.
	0.025% DW × 2d, then plain water × 3d, repeated 3 times. DO NOT CHANGE LITTER.	Turkeys: For coccidiosis caused by Eimeria meleagrimitis and E. adenoeides. Meat withdrawal 14 d (Note: Do not mix or administer in galvanized containers.)
Sulfamethazine (sodium sulfamethazine, 1 lb. pouch), (NADA #122–272, Sulmet® Soluble Powder = Huvepharma) (ANADA #200–434, SMZ-Med454®, Bimeda)	58–85 mg/lb. BW/d (128–187 mg/kgBW/d) (Add 1 lb. pouch to 128 gal DW OR make a 12% stock solution of 1 lb. pouch to 1 gal water and then add 2 Tbs = 1 fluid ounce = 30 ml of this stock solution to each gal of DW)	Chickens: For Infectious Coryza (Avibacterium paragallinarum) treat 2d, coccidiosis (Eimeria tenella, Eimeria necatrix) treat 2d then half dose for additional 4d, acute Fowl Cholera (Pasteurella multocida) treat 6d, Pullorum Disease (Salmonella Pullorum) treat 6d. Edible flesh withdrawal 10d.
	50–124 mg/lbBW/d (110–273 mg/kg BW/d) (Add 1 lb. pouch to 128 gal DW OR make a 12% stock solution of 1 lb. pouch to 1 gal water and then add 2 Tbs = 1 fluid ounce = 30 ml of this stock solution to each gal of DW)	Turkeys: For Coccidiosis (Eimeria meleagrimitis, Eimeria adenoeides) treat 2 d then half dose for an additional 4 d. Edible flesh withdrawal 10d.
Sulfamethazine sodium 12.5% solution (ANADA 006–084, Sulmet Drinking Water Solution, Huvepharma)	61–89 mg/lbBW/d (Add 2 Tbs = 1 fl oz. = 30 ml to each gallon of DW)	Chicken, excluding layers: For Infectious Coryza (Avibacterium paragallinarum treat 2 d), Coccidiosis (Eimeria tenella, Eimeria necatrix) treat 2 d then half dose for additional 4 d. Acute Fowl Cholera (Pasteurella multocida) treat 6d, Pullorum Disease (Salmonella Pullorum) treat 6d; Edible flesh withdrawal 10d.
	53–130 mg/lbBW/d	Turkey, excluding layers: For Coccidiosis (Eimeria meleagrimitis, Eimeria adenoeides) treat 2 d then half dose for an additional 4 d. Edible flesh withdrawal 10d.

(Continued)

Table 29.12 (Continued)

Drug	Dose	Comments
Tetracycline HCl Soluble Powder 324, each lb. contains 324 g of tetracycline (ANADA #200–234, Vedco Inc.; Tetrasol® Soluble powder, Vet Pharmex); (ANADA #200–374, Aspen Veterinary Resources; Tetra-Med® 324 HCA Soluble Powder, Bimeda); (Duramycin®, Vet Tek)	400–800 mg/gal DW × 7–14 d	Poultry: Do not slaughter birds for food within 4 d of treatment.
		Chickens: For chronic respiratory disease and air sac disease caused by *Mycoplasma gallisepticum* and *Escherichia coli*
	200–400 mg/gal DW × 7–14 d	Chickens: For infectious synovitis caused by *Mycoplasma synoviae* sensitive to tetracycline hydrochloride.
	400 mg/gal DW × 7–14 d (to make stock solution add 5 oz. packet to 2 gal water then add 30 ml = 1 oz = 2 Tbs to each gal DW)	Turkeys: For infectious synovitis caused by a *Mycoplasma synoviae*
	25 mg/lbBW/d in divided doses × 7–14 d	Bluecomb (transmissible enteritis, coronaviral enteritis) complicated by organisms sensitive to tetracycline hydrochloride.
Tylosin tartarate soluble (100 g packet makes 70–117 gal of 851–1419 mg/gal OR makes 50 gal of 2000 mg/gal),(NADA 13–076, Elanco)	851–1419 mg/gal (225–375 ppm) in DW × 5 d; to consume ~50 mg/lb./d	Broiler chickens: (for necrotic enteritis associated with *Clostridium perfringens*); Meat >1 d
Tylosin (tartarate) soluble powder (100 g packet makes 50 gal of 2000 mg/gal (NADA 13–076, Tylan®, Elanco);(ANADA 200–455, Tylosin Tartarate soluble Powder, Aspen Veterinary Resources; Tylosin Soluble Powder, Vet One); BiloVet® Soluble Powder, Bimeda), (ANADA 200–473, Tylovet® Soluble, Huvepharma)	2000 mg/gal (528 ppm) in DW × 3–5 d; to consume ~50 mg/lb./d	Broiler and replacement chickens: (for chronic respiratory disease associated with *Mycoplasma gallisepticum* or *Mycoplasma synoviae*); Meat >1 d
	2000 mg/gal (528 ppm) in DW × 3–5 d; to consume ~60 mg/lb./d	Turkeys: For infectious sinusitis associated with *Mycoplasma gallisepticum*; Meat >5 d

Table 29.13 Antimicrobial drugs. Below is a list of antimicrobial drugs that have anecdotally been administered parenterally to individual poultry, often used in an extra-label manner, but with no study to reference. Always consult http://farad.org before use for recommended meat and egg withdrawal times and appropriateness of use [5, 6, 18, 31–40].

Drug	Dose	Comments/Use
Amikacin	5.3 mg/kg IV-RLP (once for 15 min)	Chickens with pododermatitis: Regional limb perfusion (RLP) into medial metatarsal vein with tourniquet proximal to hock joint [5, 31]
Amoxicillin sodium (injectable 250 mg/ml)	100 mg/kg q4–8 hr IM, IV; 50–250 mg/kg IM q12–24 hr	Extrapolated from other avian species. Can decrease blood potassium levels [6]
Amoxicillin trihydrate (50 mg/ml oral suspension, or 50, 100, 200, or 400 mg tablets)	15–20 mg/kg q24hr PO; 100–200 mg/kg q4–8 hr PO	The low dose is extrapolated from drinking water dose. The higher dose is extrapolated from other species. Can decrease blood potassium levels [6]
Amoxycillin with clavulanate, (62.5 mg/ml oral suspension, or various sized tablets and chewables)	125–250 mg/kg q8hr PO	Poultry, other avian species: Recent study showed therapeutic levels (0.5ug/ml) were never reached at the 125 mg/kg dose in White Leghorn hens with tablet form of drug [5, 18]
Ampicillin trihydrate	55–110 mg/kg q8–12 IM	Poultry: Clostridiosis [5]
Ampicillin sodium and sulbactam sodium	200–300 mg/kg IM, IV q8h	Chickens/PK, Turkeys/PK [32–34]
Clindamycin	100 mg/kg q24hr PO × 3–5 d	Quail: Clostridiosis [5, 29]
Doxycycline 10 mg/ml oral suspension	25–50 mg/kg q12hr PO; 20 mg/kg q24hr PO	Waterfowl/PK: Chlamydiosis; [5, 29] Chickens/PK Chlamydiosis [5, 35, 36]
Doxycycline monohydrate (Vibramycin, Zoetis)	20–50 mg/kg/d PO × 3–7 d	Poultry [5]
Erythromycin	55–110 mg/kg q12hr PO	Poultry: Mycoplasmosis, Infectious Coryza (chickens) [5]
Itraconazole	10 mg/kg q24hr PO × 7–10d; 10 mg/kg q24hr × 4–6 wk	Waterfowl (Aspergillosis prophylaxis) [29]; Waterfowl (Aspergillosis treatment) [29]
Nystatin	300 000 U/kg q12hr PO × 7d	Waterfowl: Candidiasis [29]
Oxytetracycline		IM route causes muscle necrosis
	5 mg/kg q12–24 hr SC, IM	Chicks/PD [5]
	23 mg/kg q6–8 hr IV	Pheasants/PK [37]
	43 mg/kg q24 hr IM	Pheasants/PD [37]
Oxytetracycline HCl injectable, 100 mg/ml [38]	Chickens and turkeys: 1 d–2 wk of age give 6.25 mg SC/bird diluted 1 part drug to 3 parts sterile water × 1–4 d 2–4 wk of age give 12.5 mg SC/bird diluted 1 part drug to 3 parts sterile water × 1–4 d	Chickens (broilers, breeders) and turkeys: Used for the treatment of air sacculitis (air sac disease, chronic respiratory disease) caused by *Mycoplasma gallisepticum* and *Escherichia coli;* fowl cholera caused by *Pasteurella multocida;* infectious sinusitis caused by *Mycoplasma gallisepticum;* and infectious synovitis caused by *Mycoplasma synoviae*

(Continued)

Table 29.13 (Continued)

Drug	Dose	Comments/Use
	Chickens: 4–8 wk of age give 25 mg/bird undiluted.	
	8 wk of age give 50 mg SC undiluted.	
	Adults give 100 mg/bird SC undiluted × 1–4 d	
	Turkeys: 4–6 wk of age give 50 mg/bird SC undiluted	Turkeys: If light turkey breed then no more than 25 mg/lb BW SC
	9–12 wk of age give 150 mg/bird SC undiluted	For infectious sinusitis in turkeys can give 0.25–0.5 ml injection directly into each swollen sinus depending on age of bird and severity of the condition while simultaneously giving the SC dose. Can be repeated in 5–7 d
	>12 wk of age give 200 mg/bird SC undiluted	
	5 mg/kg SC, IM q12–24 hr	Poultry [5]: If given IM can cause muscle necrosis at injection site
Penicillin	50 000 IU/kg IM	Waterfowl: *Erysipelas* [29]
Penicillin benzathine/ procaine	200 mg/kg q24 hr IM	Extrapolated from other avian species. Birds <1 kg may have toxic effects [32]
Trimethoprim/ Sulfamethoxazole		Antibacterial/ anticoccidial
	50 mg/kg q12 hr PO	Chickens [5]
	20–50 mg/kg q12 hr PO	Ducks [5]
		(Most species of birds the dose is 100 mg/kg q12 hr PO) [6]
Tylosin	10–40 mg/kg q6–8 hr IM	Poultry: Mycoplasmosis
	20–30 mg/kg q8 hr × 3–7 d	Waterfowl: Mycoplasmosis [5, 29]
	25 mg/kg q6 hr IM	Quail/PK: Necrotic enteritis [5]
Voraconazole		Aspergillosis
	10 mg/kg q12 hr PO, IV	Chickens/PK [5, 39]
	20 mg/kg q8–12 hr PO, IV	Ducks/PD [32]
	40 mg/kg q24 hr PO	Quail/PD [5, 40]

BW=body weight

Table 29.14 Miscellaneous Drugs. Below is a list of miscellaneous drugs that have anecdotally been administered parenterally to individual poultry, often used in an extra-label manner, but with no study to reference. Always consult http://farad.org before use for recommended meat and egg withdrawal times and appropriateness of use [5, 6, 18, 29, 32, 41].

Agent	Dose	Comments
Bupivacaine HCl	2 mg/kg infused SC	Mallard ducks/PD: High plasma levels at 6 and 12 post-administration so delayed toxicity possible [5]
	2–8 mg/kg perineurally	Mallard ducks: Variable effectiveness for brachial plexus nerve blocks [5]
Butorphanol	0.5–2 mg/kg IM	Ducks: Isoflurane sparing effects shown [5]
	2 mg/kg IM	Chickens [5]
Calcium EDTA (edetate calcium disodium)	10–40 mg/kg IM q12 hr × 5–10 d	Waterfowl: Chelates +2 cations such as lead and zinc [29]
Dimercaptosuccinic acid (DMSA)	25–35 mg/kg q12–24 hr PO 5 d/wk × 3–5 wk	Waterfowl: Chelates +2 cations such as lead and zinc. Crosses blood-brain barrier [29]
Iron dextran	10 mg/kg IM, repeat in 1 wk	Waterfowl: Iron deficiency [29]
Ketoprofen	5–10 mg/kg IM	Waterfowl: Analgesia [5, 29, 32]
Meloxicam	1 mg/kg q12–24 hr PO, IM	Chickens/PK [5]: White Leghorns metabolized the oral drug faster than Wyandotte chickens [18]
Midazolam	2 mg/kg IM	Canada geese: Sedation for 15–20 min [5]
Tramadol	7.5 mg/kg PO	Peafowl/PK: Only 2/6 birds reached human tramadol analgesic concentrations, while 5/6 reached human O-tramadol metabolite analgesic concentrations for 10–12 hr and 3/6 for 24 hr [41]
Thiamine (vitamin B$_1$)	1–3 mg/kg IM	Avian: Thiamine deficiency [6, 32]

References

1 www.farad.org (accessed 30 October 2019).
2 http://www.farad.org/vetgram/search.asp (accessed 30 October 2019).
3 http://cafarad.ucdavis.edu/FARMWeb (accessed 30 October 2019).
4 http://www.cgfarad.usask.ca (accessed 30 October 2019).
5 Greenacre, C.B., Luna, G.L., and Morishita, T.M. (2018). Backyard poultry and waterfowl. In: *Exotic Animal Formulary*, 5e (ed. J.W. Carpenter), 377–432. St. Louis, Missouri: Elsevier.
6 Hawkins, M.G., Sanchez-Migallon Guzman, D., Beaufrere, H. et al. (2018). Birds. In: *Exotic Animal Formulary*, 5e (ed. J.W. Carpenter), 168–376. St. Louis, Missouri: Elsevier.
7 https://animaldrugsatfda.fda.gov/adafda/views/#/search (accessed 30 October 2019).
8 http://www.nrsp7.org/mumsrx/Species (accessed 30 October 2019).

9 https://www.drugs.com/vet (accessed 30 October 2019).

10 Goetting, V., Lee, K.A., and Tell, L.A. (2011). Pharmacokinetics of veterinary drugs in laying hens and residues in eggs: a review of the literature. *J. Vet. Pharmacol. Ther.* 34: 521–556.

11 Marmulak, T., Tell, L.A., Gehring, R. et al. (2015). Egg residue considerations during the treatment of backyard poultry. *J. Amer. Vet. Med. Assoc.* 247: 1388–1395.

12 https://www.fda.gov/animal-veterinary/antimicrobial-resistance/extralabel-use-and-antimicrobials (accessed 30 October 2019).

13 https://www.fda.gov/animal-veterinary/antimicrobial-resistance/cephalosporin-order-prohibition-questions-and-answers (accessed 30 October 2019).

14 https://www.fda.gov/animal-veterinary/acts-rules-regulations/animal-medicinal-drug-use-clarification-act-1994-amduca (accessed 30 October 2019).

15 https://www.fda.gov/animal-veterinary/development-approval-process/new-animal-drug-applications (accessed 30 October 2019).

16 www.avma.org Must be an AVMA member to access the blank VFD form. (accessed 30 October 2019).

17 https://www.fda.gov/animal-veterinary/development-approval-process/veterinary-feed-directive-vfd (accessed 30 October 2019).

18 Souza, M.J., Gerhardt, L., Shannon, L. et al. Breed Differences in the pharamcokinetics after oral administration of meloxicam in domestic chickens (Gallus domesticus). *J. Am. Vet. Med. Assoc.* In press.

19 Damerow, G. (2013). *Hatching and Brooding your Own Chicks*, 74–91. North Adams, MA, What to expect as they grow.: Storey Publishing.

20 https://dailymed.nlm.nih.gov/dailymed/drugInfo.cfm?setid=9ae5dab7-d2a5-4631-a51b-1aa93bba88fa (accessed 30 October 2019).

21 http://www.poultryhub.org/nutrition/nutrient-requirements/water-consumption-rates-for-chickens (accessed 30 October 2019).

22 Daniel Ward - Engineer, Poultry and Other Livestock - Housing and Equipment/OMAFRA; Kevin McKague - Engineer, Water Quality/OMAFRA Ontario Ministry of Agriculture, Food, and Rural Affairs, www.omafra.gov.on.ca/english/engineer/facts/07-023.htm (accessed 30 October 2019).

23 https://cvbpv.aphis.usda.gov/PVXClient/index.html#pageStart (accessed 30 October 2019).

24 https://www.fda.gov/animal-veterinary/report-problem/how-report-animal-drug-side-effects-and-product-problems (accessed 30 October 2019).

25 http://www.fda.gov/AnimalVeterinary/Products/default.htm (accessed 30 October 2019).

26 Jacob J. Use of Anticoccidial Medications and Vaccines in Poultry Production. https://articles.extension.org/pages/66917/use-of-anticoccidial-medications-and-vaccines-in-poultry-production, (accessed 30 November 2019).

27 Gerhold RW. Overview of Coccidiosis in Poultry. Merck Veterinary Manual, https://www.merckvetmanual.com/poultry/coccidiosis/overview-of-coccidiosis-in-poultry, (accessed 30 November 2019).

28 Csikó, G.Y., Banhidi, G.Y., Semjén, G. et al. (1996). Metabolism and pharmacokinetics of albendazole after oral administration to chickens. *J. Vet. Pharmacol. Therap.* 19: 322–325.

29 Carpenter, N.A. (2000). Anseriform and Galliform therapeutics. *Vet. Clin. No. Amer.* 3 (1): 1–17.

30 Macklin KS. Overview of helminthiasis in poultry. Merck Veterinary Manual. http://www.merckvetmanual.com/poultry/helminthiasis/overview-of-helminthiasis-in-poultry (accessed 30 October 2019).

31 Ratliff, C.M. and Zafarano, B.A. (2017). Therapeutic use of regional limb perfusion in a chicken. *J. Avian. Med. Surg.* 31: 29–32.

32 Carpenter, J.W., Hawkins, M.G., and Barron, H. (2016). Table of common drugs and approximate doses. In: *Current Therapy in Avian Medicine and Surgery* (ed. B.L. Speer), 795–824. St. Louis, MO: Elsevier.

33 Fernandez-Varón, E., Carceles, C., Espuny, A. et al. (2004). Pharmacokinetics of a combination preparation of ampicillin and sulbactam in turkeys. *Am. J. Vet. Res.* 65: 1658–1663.

34 Fernandez-Varón, E., Carceles, C., Espuny, A. et al. (2006). Pharmacokinetics of an ampicillin:sulbactam (2,1) combination after intravenous and intramuscular administration to chickens. *Vet. Res. Commun.* 30: 285–291.

35 Yang, F., Si, H.B., Wang, Y.Q. et al. (2016). Pharmacokinetics of doxycycline in laying hens after intravenous and oral administration. *Br. Poult. Sci.* 57 (4): 576–580.

36 Yang, F., Yang, F., Wang, G., and Kong, T. (2018). Pharmacokinetics of doxycycline after oral administration of single and multiple dose in broiler chickens. *J. Vet.*

Pharmacol. Ther. 41 (6): 919–923. https://doi.org/10.1111/jvp.12699.Epub.

37 Teare, J.A., Schwark, W.S., Shin, S.J. et al. (1985). Pharmacokinetics of a long-acting oxytetracycline preparation in ring-necked pheasants, great horned owls and Amazon parrots. *Am. J. Vet. Res.* 46: 2639–2643.

38 https://www.law.cornell.edu/cfr/text/21/522.1662a Legal Information Institute. (accessed 30 October 2019).

39 Burhenne, J., Haefeli, W.E., Hess, M. et al. (2008). Pharmacokinetics, tissue concentrations, and safety of the antifungal agent voriconazole in chickens. *J. Avian. Med. Surg.* 22: 199–120.

40 Tell, L.A., Clemons, K.V., Kline, Y. et al. (2010). Efficacy of voriconazole in Japanese quail (*Coturnix japonica*) experimentally infected with *Aspergillus fumigatus*. *Med. Mycol.* 48: 234–244.

41 Black, P.A., Cox, S.K., Macek, M. et al. (2010). Pharmacokinetics of tramadol hydrochloride and its metabolite O-desmethyltramadol in peafowl (*Pavo cristatus*). *J. Zoo. Wild. Med.* 41: 671–676.

30

Vaccination of Poultry
Robert Porter

Veterinary Diagnostic Laboratory, St. Paul, MN, USA

Vaccines that are available for commercial poultry are rarely used in backyard poultry; nonetheless, a description of the available vaccines is presented here for reference and understanding. Chicks for backyard use should be purchased previously vaccinated for Marek's disease in ovo (in the egg) or injected at one day of age [1, 2]. Vaccination for other agents might be considered if a small flock incurs an abnormally severe or yearly challenge with an infectious agent such as infectious laryngotracheitis virus or fowl pox [3]. Live vaccines should applied judiciously in small flocks, especially if the flock will not remain closed, and these vaccines should be used under the guidance of a licensed veterinarian who is trained to handle and apply biological materials. Transporting vaccinated birds to poultry exhibitions is a breach of biosecurity and can allow for transmission of live vaccine agent to nonvaccinated birds (e.g. Newcastle disease virus, infectious laryngotracheitis virus, *Mycoplasma gallisepticum*). For this reason, application of live vaccines to birds that intermittently leave the flock for exhibition purposes is discouraged. An example of a vaccination program for a small flock is proposed in this chapter.

Poultry vaccines are used to immunize birds against three groups of agents: viruses, bacteria, and parasites. Vaccines are applied in several forms: inactivated (killed), live, or live recombinant vaccines [4, 5]. Routes of administration of vaccines varies and includes injection, in ovo (in the egg) injection, drinking water, spray, wing web, and eye drop. The choice of the route of administration depends on various factors such as the type of animal (broilers vs. turkeys vs. commercial layers), age of animal (one-day-old vs. eight weeks), disease for the vaccination (Marek's disease or Newcastle disease), type of vaccine (Infectious laryngotracheitis – tissue culture vs. chick embryo origin, or genetically engineered/recombinant) and the labor involved in administering the vaccine (availability and cost of labor).

Inactivated (Killed) Vaccines

Inactivated (killed) vaccines usually apply to either viruses or bacteria. Killed vaccines usually result in high, long lasting, and uniform immunity. Killed antigen (the water phase) is encapsulated in oil or aluminum hydroxide and is therefore called a "water in oil emulsion." Inactivated vaccines are given by either intramuscular (IM) or subcutaneous (SQ) injection [6].

Backyard Poultry Medicine and Surgery: A Guide for Veterinary Practitioners, Second Edition.
Edited by Cheryl B. Greenacre and Teresa Y. Morishita.
© 2021 John Wiley & Sons, Inc. Published 2021 by John Wiley & Sons, Inc.
Companion website: www.wiley.com/go/greenacre/medicine

Advantages of Inactivated (Killed) Vaccines

Killed vaccines should have fewer systemic reactions than other forms of vaccine since there is no live agent. Fewer revaccinations are needed with the use of inactivated vaccines (more direct hits). There is no risk of the antigen spreading to other birds. A longer-term immune response is generated compared to live vaccines; therefore, it is usually used in breeders. Inactivated vaccines reduce the risk of interference when using multiple antigen combinations when compared to live vaccines. There are a number of ways to properly give an injection with a killed vaccine, as long as a full dose of the vaccine gets under the skin (not on the feathers) or in the muscle (not in the abdominal cavity or in blood vessels or in bones), it should be effective [7, 8].

Disadvantages of an Inactivated (Killed) Vaccine

Disadvantages of an inactivated vaccine include the need to handle the birds (labor cost increased), and adjuvant in the vaccine can adulterate tissue or leave residual oil, contaminated needles can transmit bacterial infection, and the vaccine can cause an exaggerated tissue reaction (usually caused by the adjuvant) [6, 9].

Routes of Administration of Inactivated (Killed) Vaccines

Intramuscular Injection

Intramuscular injections of inactivated vaccines are usually given in the leg, breast, or possibly wing in turkey breeders. The leg is usually only recommended for commercial layers and is given by injecting toward the head of the bird on the outside of the leg [9–11]. This should help to avoid nerves and major blood vessels. The breast (pectoral muscle) injection is injected in the thickest portion

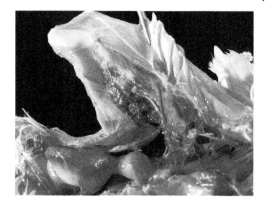

Figure 30.1 Layer pullet. Killed vaccine adjuvant and associated inflammatory reaction around the liver resulted from vaccination needle penetrating both the breast muscle and thorax, depositing vaccine directly into coelomic cavity.

of the breast, angled injection toward the head is recommended. The breast should be the easiest target area to hit with very few misses; however, the breast should be injected at an angle to the skin surface to prevent direct injection into the thoracic cavity (Figure 30.1). Spent hen processors do not like to find residual oil in the white breast muscle. This residual oil from the vaccine can show up as dark spots in the white meat after cooking. The wing injection, which can be done in turkey breeders, is done on the ventral side of the wing [9, 12].

Subcutaneous Injection

SQ injections are used for both viral and bacterial killed vaccines and is the most common route for administration of Marek's disease vaccine. The preferred route for SQ injections is the neck in case there are tissue reactions [10, 13]. Injection should be done in the lower third of the neck where there is room for skin to expand. Avoid the esophagus or crop. If injection is placed too rostral on the neck there might be adverse swelling of the neck and head [6, 9, 14]. Both SQ and intramuscular injections of killed vaccines over the breast muscle should be avoided in meat-type birds to prevent adulteration of meat that is to be consumed (Figure 30.2).

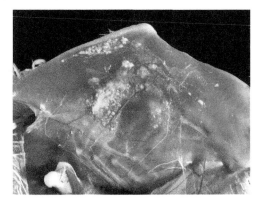

Figure 30.2 Killed vaccine injected into breast muscle or adjacent subcutis can result in adulterated tissue that is unfit for consumption.

Directions for Injection

Always warm the inactivated vaccine to at least room temperature or preferably to 90 °F prior to use. Cold vaccine can irritate the birds (make them uncomfortable) and does not flow well (low viscosity) through the needle. This creates more effort to inject and can increase wear on the syringe. Usually ¼- to ½-in. needle length is used. Needle guards can be used to protect vaccinator, but this may require a longer needle. Change needles at least every 1000 birds in commercial settings [6, 14].

Live Vaccines

Most vaccines, particularly viruses, are administered as live agents because of the advantages, but procedures for administration must be closely followed to ensure that birds are adequately exposed and the live agent is not inactivated during administration.

Advantages of Live Vaccines

Live vaccines are usually easier to apply compared to killed vaccines, there is often a faster application time, they are superior in inducing mucosal immunity compared to inactivated vaccines, they can be stored for longer periods (freeze dried) than killed emulsion vaccines, and there are no skin or muscle reactions [15, 16].

Disadvantages of Live Vaccines

Live vaccines can induce adverse reactions in the respiratory tract, they require rapid application (careful attention to time is required), they have a limited half-life for microorganisms in suspension, and induce a shorter humoral immune response compared to killed vaccines [6, 15, 17].

Routes of Administration for Live Vaccines

Injection

Injection into the cervical or pipping muscle is used for Marek's disease vaccination in one-day-old chicks as well as recombinant Newcastle disease vaccines in one-day-old turkeys [18–20]. This practice for Marek's disease vaccination has largely been replaced in large chicken hatcheries by in ovo injection but is still used in small hatcheries. Bacterial contamination of the injection needle can cause localized infection and death in young birds.

In Ovo

In ovo vaccines are used for vaccinating with Marek's disease and possibly IBD, coccidiosis and some recombinant vaccines in embryos before hatch at transfer time from the incubator to the hatcher. For optimal performance, in ovo inoculation must be done between 18 and 19 days of incubation either via the amniotic or the intraembryonic route. This greatly reduces labor costs in the hatchery but must be closely monitored to avoid contamination [2].

Eye Drop and Nasal

Eye drop and nasal vaccines can be used for infectious laryngotracheitis virus and *Mycoplasma gallisepticum* (ts-11) vaccination. A blue dye mixed with the vaccine greatly aids in checking vaccination procedures. A single drop should be placed into the open eye,

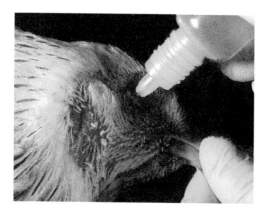

Figure 30.3 Respiratory virus vaccines, such as infectious laryngotracheitis, can be applied by eye drop. Place the edge of dropper close to the palpebral fissure so that the drop enters the conjunctival sac, but do not touch adjacent skin or cornea with the dropper.

getting the end of the dropper close to the eye for accuracy, but not touching the eyelids to avoid contamination between birds (Figure 30.3). The back of the bird's tongue will be stained blue for a short time after vaccination, so check for the staining within 10 minutes of vaccination. If vial cannot be used in one hour, discard the remaining vaccine and mix a fresh bottle. Better yet, mix a 1000-dose bottle and split between two people on vaccination crew to ensure fresh vaccine is being used at all times [7, 21, 22]

Wing Web Vaccine

The wing web (patagium) vaccine is used for fowl pox, Avian encephalomyelitis virus, *Pasteurella multocida* (fowl cholera), and chicken anemia virus (CAV). In small flocks the technique is most often used for avipoxvirus vaccination. A dye is used to monitor application as the birds are being vaccinated. Two different colors should be used if there are two separate wing web vaccinations, e.g., fowl pox and *P. multocida*. The applicator is a double-pronged needle that picks up fluid when immersed in the vaccine diluent (Figure 30.4) and is then immediately inserted through the skin (Figure 30.5). Take care not to wipe off the vaccine on the feathers prior to piercing the

wing web. Immediately after applying vaccine the wing web should show dye between the layers of the skin (Figure 30.6). The needle placement should be in the center of the wing web (patagium). Successful application of pox or cholera to the skin results in localized skin inflammation ("reactions" or "takes") [14, 23]. These should be checked 7–10 days after vaccination, and appear as a scab or thickening of the wing web (Figure 30.7). Less than 90% takes may require revaccination of the flock. Keep an accurate and detailed record of who was applying the vaccine in case trouble shooting is necessary [8, 14].

Drinking Water

Drinking water vaccines are used for Newcastle disease virus, infectious bronchitis virus, Infectious bursal disease virus, infectious laryngotracheitis virus, avian encephalomyelitis virus, and others [24]. Water vaccination appears easy – mix up the vaccine and run it

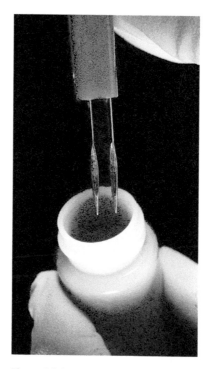

Figure 30.4 Vaccine viruses such as fowl pox virus are often colored and are applied by double prong needle that is dipped into the diluent.

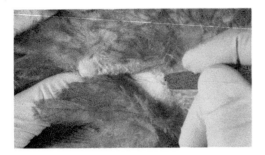

Figure 30.5 Fowl pox virus is applied as a wing web stick, piercing the entire skin layer in the center of the wing web (patagium).

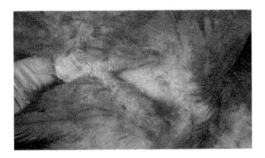

Figure 30.6 Following inoculation of fowl pox virus with the inoculation needle, the dye in the diluent should be observed in the entire thickness of the skin with a minimal amount on the feathers.

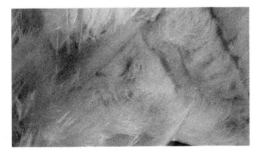

Figure 30.7 Vaccine "take": Nodules or scabs in the wing web skin, indicative of successful reaction to vaccine, should be observed at 7–10 days after inoculation with fowl pox virus.

through the proportioner – and might be less labor intensive than spray or injection, but there are challenges to proper administration. Consider the following points: What is the capacity of the water lines? What is the daily water consumption of the flock? Do all the birds drink when you are vaccinating? Is the water being treated with sanitizers or antibiotics? Have you applied a stabilizer to protect the vaccine in the drinking water? The following are recommended procedures for drinking water vaccination: (i) Clean the water lines before vaccination. (ii) Birds should be water deprived ("water starve") for about two hours prior to vaccinating and the lights should be turned off [25]. (iii) Fill the water lines with vaccine, approved dye and vaccine stabilizer either while the lines are raised above the birds or before the lights are turned on. (iv) Make sure all water lines contain vaccine by observing the dye at the end of the water lines; consider allowing at least an extra 15 seconds of vaccine water to flow through to make sure there is adequate vaccine in the entire line. (iv) Lower the water lines to bird level or turn on the lights. (vi) The remaining vaccine stock solution should last for at least 30 minutes. After the birds begin to drink, if the vaccine was successfully applied one should observe vaccine dye on the tongues of most birds during the procedure (Figure 30.8). (vii) Running automatic feeders during vaccination can increase water consumption [7, 25, 26].

Spray Vaccination

Spray vaccination includes coarse spray, fine spray, and very fine spray or aerosol and can also be used for most of the drinking water

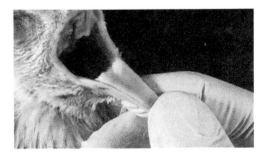

Figure 30.8 Vaccines that are administered as an eye drop or in drinking water often contain a dye that results in staining of the tongue if applied effectively, as demonstrated by blue stain on tongue of pullet.

vaccines. A coarse spray is defined as 100 µm or larger. A medium spray is 50–100 µm, and a fine spray is less than 50 µm. Important factors to consider are the size droplet should be used for each vaccine. Finer droplets will penetrate deeper into the respiratory tract to increase the chance of vaccine reaction. You should be familiar with the type sprayer that you plan to use and clean it thoroughly after each use. There are many models of commercial sprayers with a variety of features from which to choose. Other factors to consider include the volume of water to spray on the birds and how long these droplets are to remain suspended in the air. Automated ventilation (fans and blowers) should remain off during spray vaccination to prevent drawing vaccine to the outside of the house but should be immediately turned back on after administration to prevent overheating of the flock [16, 26].

Spray vaccination is an excellent method for mass administration of vaccine. Distilled water is recommended to avoid contaminants or additives that could inactivate live vaccine. A strong local immunity can elicited if the spray reaches the mucous membranes, but respiratory tissues can react in exaggerated fashion (conjunctivitis, respiratory distress) if birds receive a high dose of vaccine or spray droplets travel too deep into the respiratory tract [13, 27]. The depth of penetration of the spray depends upon the size of the droplets. Evaporation can change a coarse spray into a fine spray. Low spray pressure usually produces a coarse spray and high pressure produces a fine spray. The use of water-sensitive paper can show the droplet size and where the spray is actually going inside the house [16, 28]. It is best to spray during the cooler portion of the day because house fans will be turned off while the spray is applied to the birds. Birds that are overheated will pant and can inhale a coarse droplet even deeper into the respiratory tract to cause a harsh reaction. Dim or shut off the lights to calm the birds when spraying.

Coarse spray (100–200 µm and larger) is used for initial vaccinations and when low reaction is desired. This spray falls out of the air very quickly, having the appearance of a "wet fog" [16]. Birds shake their heads to indicate that the spray is getting into the eyes; therefore, you can directly observe if the birds are being vaccinated. The spray should be directed at or slightly above the head of the birds. Some vaccines like IBD and Salmonella should only be given by coarse spray when sprayed. One hundred-micron droplets fall 10 ft in 11 seconds [28].

Medium spray (about 50–100 µm) is used for revaccination of Newcastle and bronchitis. Direct the spray slightly above the head of the birds to allow them to breathe in the spray. Fifty-micron droplets fall 10 ft in 40 seconds and have the appearance of "misty rain" [11, 16, 28].

Fine spray (20–50 µm or smaller) can also be used for revaccination of Newcastle and bronchitis, but a greater vaccine reaction might occur. It can be used for initial vaccination of *Mycoplasma gallisepticum* (Mycovac-L). With this very small droplet size the person applying the vaccine should slow the walking pace to allow the vaccine to reach all birds [6, 26]. Ten-micron droplets fall 10 ft in 1020 seconds (17 minutes) [28]. Use of medium to fine spray vaccine in susceptible birds can promote excessive vaccine reactions as a result of virus extending deeper into the respiratory tract (Figure 30.9).

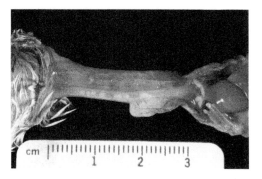

Figure 30.9 Bantam chick received a fine droplet aerosol of LaSota strain of Newcastle disease, resulting in exaggerated inflammatory response ("vaccine reaction") observed as white bubbles within the tracheal lumen.

Vaccination Program for Backyard Chickens

Both live and inactivated vaccines should be applied through the guidance of a veterinarian who is versed on the proper preparation, application, and disposal of biological agents. The vaccine program listed in Table 30.3 serves as a guideline for the veterinarian who can establish a protocol based on the potential disease risks and the uses of a particular flock. The vaccines are based on the author's experience of what diseases occur most often in small flocks. A flock owner might consider the costs of vaccination to be cost-prohibitive, but a veterinarian's involvement in vaccination will encourage a veterinary-client relationship and allow the professional to provide advice on biosecurity and management. Owners of small chicken flocks used as breeders for production marketing of specialty breeds would be excellent candidates for vaccination. Vaccination programs are best applied to small flocks with closed management in which birds remain on the premise at all times and new birds are quarantined before adding to the preexisting flock. Birds that have received live vaccines should not leave the premise for at least 30 days, which would minimize potential shedding of virus to other naive birds. The most important is Marek's disease virus, a cell-associated virus that is best applied at one day of age at the hatchery. It is strongly recommended that flock owners purchase chicks from hatcheries that can apply MD vaccine at hatch [3]. Additional vaccines to be applied to the birds

Table 30.1 Vaccination program for layers.

Vaccine	Age	Comment	Administration
Marek's disease	1 d	HVT, SB-1, Rispens	SC injection
Infectious Bronchitis	1 d	Mass-Conn,	Coarse spray (100 μm)
Newcastle disease	1 d	B1-B1	Coarse spray (100 μm)
Infectious bursal Dz	14 d	Intermediate strain	Water or coarse spray
Infectious Bronchitis	14 d	Mass-Conn,	Coarse spray (100 μm)
Newcastle disease	14 d	B1-B1	Coarse spray (100 μm)
Infectious bursal Dz	28 d	Intermediate strain	Water or coarse spray
Infectious Bronchitis	28 d	Mass-Conn,	Coarse spray (100 μm)
Newcastle disease	28 d	B1-B1	Coarse spray (100 μm)
Infectious Bronchitis	6 wk	Mass-Conn,	Medium spray (50 μm)
Newcastle disease	6 wk	Lasota	Medium spray (50 μm)
Infectious laryngo.	7–8 wk	Eye drop/drinking water tracheitis	
Mycoplasma gallisepticum	10 wk	F strain or 6/85	Fine spray (20 μm)
Infectious Bronchitis	12 wk	Holland	Fine spray (20 μm)
Newcastle disease	12 wk	Lasota	Fine spray (20 μm)
Avipoxvirus	12 wk	Fowl/quail pox combo	Wing web stick
Avian Encephalomyelitis	12 wk	Combined with pox	Wing web stick
Infectious coryza	12 wk	In problem flocks	Subcutaneous injection
Infectious Bronchitis	Every 8 wk	Mass-Conn	Medium spray
Newcastle disease	Every 8 wk	B1-B1	Medium spray

on farm can be administered as eye drop or wing web stick. Live attenuated vaccines that can be applied to a flock through eye drop include infectious laryngotracheitis, Newcastle disease virus, infectious bronchitis, and *M. gallisepticum*. State regulations should always be consulted before purchasing and administering these vaccines. Additionally, the use of tissue culture origin vaccine products rather than chicken embryo origin vaccines is recommended to reduce both vaccine reactions and bird-to-bird spread

of vaccine. Vaccines to apply as wing web stick include avian encephalomyelitis virus – to be given to breeder chickens to prevent transmission to hatchlings – and fowl pox virus [29]. Antibody titers to these agents can abate over time so yearly vaccination may be required, particularly in flocks used for breeder purposes.

For examples of vaccination programs for chickens see Table 30.1 for Layers, Table 30.2 for Broilers and Table 30.3 for Backyard/Small chicken flocks.

Table 30.2 Vaccination program for broilers.

Vaccine	Age	Comment	Administration
Marek's disease	−3 to 1 d	HVT, SB-1, Rispens	SC injection or in ovo
Infectious bursal Dz	−3 to 1 d	Variant strain	SC injection or in ovo
Infectious Bronchitis	1 d	Mild Mass-Conn,	Coarse spray (100 μm)
Newcastle disease	1 d	B1-B1	Coarse spray (100 μm)
Infectious Bursal Dz	7 d	Classic/Variant strain	Water or coarse spray
Infectious Bronchitis	14 d	Mass-Conn,	Coarse spray (100 μm)
Newcastle disease	14 d	B1-B1	Coarse spray (100 μm)

Table 30.3 Vaccination program for backyard chickens/small flocks.

Vaccine	Age	Comment	Administration
Marek's disease	1 d	HVT, SB-1, Rispens	SC injection
Infectious bronchitis	10 d	Mild Mass-Conn	Eyedrop
Newcastle disease	10 d	B1-B1	Eye drop
Infectious Laryngotracheitis	6 wk	Tissue culture strain	Eye drop
Avipoxvirus	6–10 wk	Fowl pox	Wing web
Avian Encephalomyelitis	6–10 wk	For breeder chickens	Wing web
Mycoplasma gallisepticum	10 wk	Tissue culture strain	Eye drop
Infectious bronchitis	35 d	Mass-Conn	Eye drop
Newcastle disease	35 d	B1-B1	Eye drop

References

1 Purchase, H.G., Okazaki, W., and Burmester, B.R. (1972). Long term field trials with the herpesvirus of turkeys vaccine against Marek's disease. *Avian Dis.* 16: 57–71.

2 Sharma, J.M. and Burmeister, B.R. (1982). Resistance to Marek's disease at hatching in chickens vaccinated as embryos with the Turkey herpesvirus. *Avian Dis.* 26: 134–149.

3 Sato, Y. and Wakenell, P.S. Vaccination of backyard poultry, in Backyard Poultry, MSD Online Veterinary Manual, www. merckvetmanual.com, 2018.

4 Boursnell, M.E.G., Green, P.F., Campbell, J.I.A. et al. (1990). Insertion of the fusion gene from Newcastle disease virus into a non-essential region in the terminal repeats of fowlpox virus and demonstration of protective immunity by the recombinant. *J. Gen. Virol.* 71: 621–628.

5 Danforth, H.D., McCandliss, R., Libel, M. et al. (1985). Development of an avian coccidial antigen by recombinant DNA technology. *Poultry Sci.* 64: 85–92.

6 Stone, H. Oil emulsion vaccines. Vineland Update, No. 63 January 1999, Vineland Laboratories, Vineland, NJ.

7 Baxendale, W. Current methods of delivery of poultry vaccines. In: *Poultry Immunology* (eds. T.F. Davison, T.R. Morris and L.N. Payne), 375–387. Abingdon: Carfax.

8 McCarty, J. F. Understanding the basics of your breeder vaccination program. Vineland Update, No. 54 April 1996. Vineland Laboratories, Vineland, NJ.

9 Lovell, E. J. Farm vaccination-injection method for oil emulsion vaccines. Proceedings, Poultry Vaccination Techniques and Evaluation Workshop. St. Paul, MN, Sept. 16, 1995. American College of Poultry Veterinarians. pp. 55–57.

10 Gingerich, E. Common errors in vaccinating pullet flocks, Part II. DeKalb Management Newsletter, Sept 30, 1996, DeKalb Poultry Research, DeKalb, IL.

11 Sander, J. Principles of vaccination programs for poultry health. Poultry Digest, March 1991, p. 14–24, Watt Publishing Co., Mount Morris, IL.

12 Hildebrand, D.G., Page, D.E., and Berg, J.R. (1983). Mycoplasma gallisepticum (MG) – laboratory and field studies evaluating the safety and efficacy of an inactivated MG bacterin. *Avian Dis.* 27: 792–802.

13 Sander, J. Vaccination reactions. Vineland Update, No. 55 July 1995, Vineland Laboratories, Vineland, NJ.

14 Howell, L.M. Farm vaccination- wing web method. Proceedings, Poultry Vaccination Techniques and Evaluation Workshop. St. Paul, MN, Sept. 16, 1995. American College of Poultry Veterinarians., pp. 40–45.

15 Klopp, S. (1986). *Effects of vaccine handling on immunization. Poultry Digest*, 124–126. Mount Morris, IL: Watt Publishing Co.

16 Stewart-Brown, B. Applying poultry vaccines via the aerosol route on the farm: technique and critique. Proceedings, Poultry Vaccination Techniques and Evaluation Workshop. St. Paul, MN, Sept. 16, 1995. American College of Poultry Veterinarians, pp. 30–39.

17 Bancroft, B.J. and Spradrow, P.B. (1977). The spread of V4 strain of Newcastle disease virus between chickens vaccinated by drinking water administration. *Aus. Vet. J.* 1977 (54): 500–501.

18 Gilbert, R. Marek's vaccine mixing and handling procedure. Proceedings, Poultry Vaccination Techniques and Evaluation Workshop. St. Paul, MN, Sept. 16, 1995. American College of Poultry Veterinarians., pp. 10–15.

19 Okazaki, W., Purchase, H.G., and Burmester, B.R. (1970). Protection against Marek's disease by vaccination with a herpesvirus of turkeys. *Avian Dis.* 14: 413–429.

20 Powell, P.C. (1985). Immunity. In: *Marek's Disease* (ed. L.N. Payne), 177–201. Boston: Martinus Nijhoff.

21 Davelaar, F.G. and Kouwenhoven, B. (1981). Study on the local effect of eye-drop vaccination against infectious bronchitis in 1-day-old chicks with maternal antibodies. *Avian Pathol.* 10: 83–90.

22 Jordan, F.T.W. (1981). Immunity-to infectious laryngotracheitis. In: *Avian Immunology* (eds. M.E. Ross, L.N. Payne and B.M. Freeman), 245–254. Edinburgh: British Poultry Science Ltd.

23 Baxendale, W. Immunity to Fowl Pox. *Avian Immunology,* Poultry Science Symposium No. 16 (Eds. Rose, M.E., Payne, L.N., and Freeman, B.M.) British Poultry Science, Edinburgh 1984, pp. 255–262.

24 Cervantes, H. (1995). Farm evaluation-water method. In: *Proceedings, Poultry Vaccination Techniques and Evaluation Workshop*, 16–24. St. Paul, MN: American College of Poultry Veterinarians.

25 Grieve, D. (1995). Factors affecting the delivery of live vaccines through the drinking water. In: *Proceedings, Poultry Vaccination Techniques and Evaluation Workshop*, 30–39. St. Paul, MN: American College of Poultry Veterinarians.

26 Takeshita, K. Your vaccination program. In Vineland Update, No. 58 March 1997, Vineland Laboratories, Vineland, NJ.

27 Parry, S.H. and Aitken, I.D. (1977). Local immunity in the respiratory tract of the chicken. II. The secretory immune response to Newcastle disease virus and the role of IgA. *Vet. Microbiol.* 2: 143–165.

28 Steinberger, E. Trouble-shooting vaccine administration in layers. Proceedings, Poultry Health Management School, Madison, WI., May 21, 2004. pp. 34–42.

29 Ebako, G.M., and Scheideler, S. Preventative medicine for backyard poultry flocks. Document G1453. Neb Guide-University of Nebraska-Lincoln Extension, Institute of Agricultural and Natural Resources. July 2002

Index

a

"abdominal" (coelom/coelomic)
133, 135, 138
  air sac 147, 180–182, 360,
    390, 397, 404, 416, 424,
    485
  aorta 154, 327
  cavity 125, 303, 312, 468, 585
  detail 326
  distension 324
  fat 81, 85, 304, 321
  oblique muscle 138
  sepsis 403
  viscera 150
  wall 145, 150
abnormal
  activities 91
  behavior(s) 53, 91, 102, 434,
    444, 448, 452
  body parts 473
  cartilage 249
  cholesterol accumulations
    272
  comb 162, 163, 231, 244,
    246, 270, 272, 273, 290,
    291, 295, 297, 299, 303,
    304, 308, 317, 325, 384,
    444, 505
  contents 493
  egg(s) 286, 475, 505
  feather 133
  feet/foot 234

  filling 165
  finding 133, 159
  fluid retention 174
  forces 254
  hatches 475
  humerus 179
  imprinting 91
  joint 57, 249, 253
  lead levels 370
  ovary 189
  palpation 166
  position 256, 505
  radiographic findings 505
  respiratory effort 165
  shell 224
  skin 166, 167, 505
  smell 160, 168
  sounds 165, 505
  stance 161, 167, 250, 251
  stool 362
  testes 425, 426
  tissue(s) 190, 349, 385, 393,
    404, 410, 420, 427
  troponin T 324
abnormality 388
  cardiac 126, 317, 318,
    322–326, 328–330,
    333–335, 347
  identification 177, 187, 328,
    359, 470
  leg 235
abnormally shaped eggs 186

acaricides 262
access, outdoor 32, 46, 50, 54,
  56, 79, 93, 102, 357
accessory
  arteries
    ovarian 419
    testicular 423
  gland 150
  parathyroid 154
  spleen 155
accommodation, corneal 156
accreditation, veterinary 13, 14
accumulation
  brain DHA 84
  cartilage 249
  cholesterol, abnormal 272
  colloid 153, 154
  exudate 222, 277, 385
  fat 80, 88
  fecal 89, 265, 425
  fluid 211, 277, 280, 385, 423
  lipid 80
  moisture 47, 259, 471
acid(s)
  amino 80–82, 87, 117, 122,
    125–128, 281, 282, 285,
    302, 304, 523
  arachidonic 83, 84
  bile 87, 318, 402
  delta-aminolevulinic 369
  dimercaptosuccinic (DMSA)
    370–372, 375, 581

Backyard Poultry Medicine and Surgery: A Guide for Veterinary Practitioners, Second Edition.
Edited by Cheryl B. Greenacre and Teresa Y. Morishita.
© 2021 John Wiley & Sons, Inc. Published 2021 by John Wiley & Sons, Inc.
Companion website: www.wiley.com/go/greenacre/medicine

erucic   334, 379
ethylenediaminetetraacetic
    (EDTA)   370–372, 375,
    376, 506, 507, 509, 581
fatty   82–85, 117, 126, 127,
    326, 335, 379, 424, 523
folic   120, 518
fusidic   557
linoleic   83, 85
linolenic   83
nicotinic (niacin)   86, 120
nucleic   531
oleic   85
organic   127
oxalic   379
pantothenic   86, 120
pH   492
phytic   119, 379
polyglycolic   392
propionic   127
prussic   378
ribonucleic (RNA)   124, 229,
    232, 297, 302, 308, 530, 531
salicylic   356
Schiff, periodic   405
uric   289, 310, 406, 469, 522
acid-base   351
acid-fast   201, 292, 300, 508, 525
acidic environment   375
acidosis   329
acoustic
    meatus, external   133, 136,
        156, 163
    window   322, 323
Act
    Egg Products Inspection Act
        16, 17
    Federal Food, Drug and
        Cosmetic   538, 543
    Minor Use/Minor Species
        Animal Health (MUMS)
        542, 543
    Poultry Products Inspection
        (PPIA)   15
    Preservation of Antibiotics
        for Medical Treatment
        (PAMTA)   550

activity(ies)
    abnormal   91
    electrical   319, 334, 344
    level   77
additives   589
    enzyme   87
    feed   77, 87, 88, 124, 127,
        128, 505, 540, 544, 550,
        565, 567, 569
    intravenous fluid   351
    water   550, 567
adipose tissue   146, 400, 482
administration
    colloid   351, 352, 520
    medication routes   536, 544,
        545, 547, 549, 552, 553,
        564–567, 579
adrenal
    cortex   154, 496
    gland(s)   153, 154, 247, 256,
        406, 421, 424, 425, 496
    veins   423
    weight   154
aerosol
    build-up   510
    dust   310
    transmission   220–224, 226,
        231, 232, 303, 304
    vaccine administration   588,
        589
aerosolization   200, 310, 478,
    589
African goose/geese (breed)
    60, 63, 66, 67, 72, 74, 391
aflatoxin   88, 124, 376, 518
agar
    blood   470, 471, 527
        sheep   471
    gel immunodiffusion   203,
        231, 305, 523, 527
    MacConkey's media   471
age, market   537
agent identification   220–222,
    231, 269, 303, 527, 529,
    530
agglutination   523, 524
    crop   295

modified (MAT) test   214
    Mycoplasma   524
    plate   220, 295
    Salmonella   524
    serum plate   220
    tube   295
    whole blood   202, 295
aggression behavior   51, 53, 59,
    61, 62, 80, 90, 91, 94,
    166, 167, 265, 266, 268,
    391, 424, 434, 437–439,
    444, 448, 450
AGID (agar gel
    immunodiffusion)   203,
    231, 523, 524, 527
agonist, gonadotropin releasing
    hormone (GnRH)   99,
    102, 409
Aimes transport media   507,
    508, 510, 511
air
    capillaries (terminal
        bronchus/i)   147, 568
    cell   466, 471
    chamber   464
    circulation   47, 378, 461,
        568
    dry   471, 516
    exposure   241, 378
    fuzzy growth   227
    gasping   108, 211, 212
    humidification   359
    incubator
        forced   461
        still   461
    leakage   390
    lucency   179
    moisture   219
    movement   46, 360, 390
    quality   283
    shipment carriers   13
    storage   147
    subcutaneous   361
    temperature   47, 219
air sac   146, 147, 150, 155,
    179–182, 220, 381, 390,
    391, 397, 485

air sac (*cont'd*)
abdominal 147, 150,
180–182, 360, 390, 397,
404, 416, 424, 485
auscultation 166
cannula 344, 349, 359, 360,
387
cervical 147, 180, 182
clavicular 175, 180–182, 388
compression 361
endoscopy 349, 360
evaluation 348, 349
fluid avoidance 350, 402,
566
fuzzy growth 227
healing 361
intubation 360
penetration 399, 416, 424
thoracic 154, 180, 181, 183,
226, 360, 397, 424
trauma 361, 458
volume 182
air sacculitis 182, 220, 221,
226, 304, 309, 474, 475
airway disease, lower 361
albumen 426, 463–465, 497
sac 469
thick 463–465, 474
thin 463–466, 474
algae, green 56
alginate swab, calcium 510
Alimentarius Commission,
Codex (FAO/WHO Food
Standards) 540, 555
allantois 469, 470
alpha
cell 146
islets 146
toxins 299
alular
muscle 136
patagium 133, 135
aluminosilicate, calcium 124
alveoli 147, 568
AMDUCA 536, 540, 541, 544,
545, 548, 549, 552, 554,
556
Ameraucana (breed) 24, 27

American 10
Association of Avian
Pathologists (AAAP) 4
Association of Veterinary
Laboratory
Diagnosticians
(AAVLD) 541
Bantam Association (ABA) 63
Board of Veterinary
Practitioners (ABVP) 4
Buff (breed) 63, 66
city(ies) 5
Class(es)(Standard of
Perfection breeds) 24,
25, 31, 37, 63
College of Poultry
Veterinarians (ACPV) 3
Game Bantam (breed) 30,
36, 38, 40
migratory waterfowl, North
102, 108, 229, 230
Poultry Association
(APA) 62, 63
Standard of Perfection
23, 24, 63
Veterinary Medical
Association (AVMA)
457, 545, 565
widgeon (breed) 70, 97
amino acid(s) 80–82, 87, 117,
122, 125–128, 281, 282,
285, 302, 304, 523
ammonia 47, 88, 110, 218,
219, 361, 406
excess 47
amnion 469
amputation
phallus 363, 427
toe 243, 267
analgesia 265, 267, 346, 355,
363, 381
butorphanol 267, 355, 358,
458
carprofen 355, 356
local 267, 355, 360, 363
NSAIDs (non-steroidal anti-
inflammatory drugs)
355

opioids 355
pain 235, 268, 355, 381, 382
salicylic acid 356
tramadol 356, 581
waterfowl 581
analog
gonadotropin releasing
hormone (GnRH) 407
methyl hydroxyl
(methionine) 126
Analytical Chemists,
Association of
(AOAC) 556
anastomosis, resection
and 388, 389, 394, 397
anatomy
egg 464, 466
eye 34, 155, 156, 290, 332,
357, 387, 473, 480, 501
radiograph(s) 177, 179, 187
androgen hormone(s) 139
anemia 120, 121, 215, 216,
263, 264, 271, 308, 352,
369, 371, 376, 516, 518,
520, 546
chicken (disease) 114, 271,
519
virus, chicken (CAV;
infectious chicken
anemia) 260, 271, 518,
587
hemorrhagic 516, 518
infectious chicken (CAV;
chicken anemia virus)
260, 271, 518, 587
anesthetic monitoring 240
aneurysm(s) 320, 327, 329,
335
aortic 329
dissecting 327
angel wing 72, 82, 256
animal
companion 4, 14, 23, 100,
323, 324, 438, 448, 546,
547
control 5, 6, 9, 12, 54
Drug Evaluation, Office of
New (ONADE) 552

Health Act, Minor Use/
Minor Species (MUMS)
542, 543
Health Laboratory (AHL)
317, 330
Network, National
(NAHLN) 231, 232
Medicinal Drug Use
Clarification Act of, 1994
(AMDUCA) 536, 540,
541, 544, 545, 548, 549,
552, 554, 556
Plant Health Inspection
Service (APHIS) 5,
13–15, 19, 107, 108,
569, 570
Residue Avoidance and
Depletion Program,
Food (FARAD) 261,
323, 528, 539, 541, 542,
550, 553–555, 563–565,
567, 568, 571, 573, 574,
579, 581
Welfare Act (AWA) 14, 15
animation, suspended 467
Anseriformes management
56–106
anterior chamber 161, 357
antibiotic(s) 127, 128, 183,
198, 199, 219–223, 235,
236, 240, 245, 265, 268,
271, 276, 279, 281, 291,
292, 298, 300, 302, 303,
305, 310, 353, 356, 358,
361, 363, 364, 385, 389,
391, 392, 396, 399, 401,
412, 413, 416, 422, 426,
427, 505, 510, 511, 513,
527, 528, 531, 535, 536,
538, 541, 549, 550, 554,
556, 562–565, 568, 569,
571, 574, 588
Medical Treatment Act,
Preservation of (PAMTA)
550
antibody 200, 220, 257, 271,
308, 523, 524, 526, 527,
591

anticoccidial medications/drugs
208, 209, 297, 376, 473,
571–573, 580
antimicrobial(s) 127, 271, 323,
333, 334, 363, 381, 382,
412, 416, 426, 549, 550,
556–558, 564, 569, 571, 579
resistance 550
antiparasitic medications/drugs
536, 571–573
antiviral medications/drugs
202, 353, 546, 547
prohibited 547
aorta 318, 327, 335, 410, 419,
423, 489
abdominal 154, 327
aortic
aneurism 329
rupture 327, 335, 518
APMV-1(avian paramyxovirus
serotype 1) 232
aponeurotic region 143
coccygeal 153
apparatus, hyoid 136, 141, 391
approval, drug 539, 543, 544,
548, 555, 563, 570
apterylae 137
arachidonic acid 83, 84
Araucana (breed) 27, 464
arch, nasal 133, 134
area
brooding 49–51
floor 45, 46, 438, 451
nesting 45, 46, 54, 71, 96,
100, 281, 284, 295, 306,
438, 444–446, 451, 468,
471, 573
opaca 468
pellucida 468
thermoneutral 47
arginine 80–82, 125, 326
dietary arginine 81
arrest
cardiac 343, 345, 358, 381
cardiopulmonary 343
vagal 345
artery(ies)
accessory

ovarian 419
testicular 423
celiac 155
carotid 153
femoral 138
iliac 147–149, 327, 410,
419–421
ischiadic (ischiatic;
sciatic) 138, 410
metatarsal 347
ovarian 419, 421
oviductal 410, 416
pudendal 410
radial 240, 347
renal 410, 419, 423
stalk 419
testicular 423
arthritis 57, 60, 73, 91, 93
septic 186, 187, 295
viral 524
articular gout 310
artificial insemination 466
ascariasis 298, 299
Ascaridia 293, 572
dissimilis 215
galli 287, 298, 572
ascending duodenum 397
ascites 84, 166, 249, 278, 317,
318, 320, 324–326, 329,
332, 334, 346, 361, 377,
390, 401, 410–412, 422
syndrome 317, 318, 326,
330, 333, 334
Asian
geese (breed) 67, 70
strain (avian influenza
H5N1) 230
Asiatic Class (Standard of
Perfection) 24, 25, 31, 37
aspergillosis 114, 183,
211–213, 226, 290, 292,
301, 329, 360
medication 579, 580
Aspergillus
flavus 376
fumigatus 226, 529
parasiticus 376
spp. 331

aspirate(s) 235, 278, 349, 363, 398, 412, 415, 417, 420, 422, 426, 509

aspiration
coelomic 361, 420, 422
crop 256, 292, 362
drug 567
duodenal 398
fine needle 361
ovarian 420, 422
oviductal 412, 416
pneumonia 292, 350, 361, 375, 568
pre-mortem 498
sinus 385
terminal 498
testicular 426

assay, enzyme-linked immunosorbent (ELISA) 200, 203, 220, 224, 231, 248, 257, 308, 523–526

association(s) 458
Avian Pathologists (AAAP), American 4
Avian Veterinarians (AAV) 4
Bantam (ABA), American 63
homeowners 4, 5
neighborhood 4, 5
Official Analytical Chemists (AOAC) 556
Poultry (APA), American 23, 24, 62, 63
APA Standard of Perfection 23, 24, 63
Poultry Science (PSA) 542, 545
State Public Health Veterinarians, National 199
Veterinary Laboratory Diagnosticians, American (AAVLD) 541
Veterinary Medical, American (AVMA) 457, 545, 565

asymptomatic (disease)
carriers 18, 110, 198, 200, 220, 222, 246, 257, 271, 294, 296, 298, 301, 306, 308
atheroma (lipid core) 335
atheromatous build-up 335
atherosclerosis 326, 327, 330, 335

atrial
repolarization 320
rupture 327
attack, dog 54, 55, 252, 265, 356
auditory 266, 436
tube (Eustachian) 142
auscultation
air sac 166
cardiac (heart) 162, 164, 165, 172, 318, 343, 470
lung (pulmo) 165, 166, 172
Australorp (breed) 24–26
avian
chlamydiosis 195, 199–201, 301, 330, 332, 334
cholera 111
encephalomyelitis (epidemic tremor) 113, 257, 331, 524, 587, 590, 591
vaccine 113, 587, 590, 591
influenza 10–14, 18, 19, 108, 111, 202, 203, 223, 224, 229, 230, 233, 281, 283, 288, 301, 304, 331, 332, 361, 504, 510, 523–525, 529, 530, 547, 564
high pathogenicity (HPAI) 19, 229–231, 304, 305
low pathogenicity (LPAI) 19, 230, 231, 304, 305
leucosis (leukosis) 246, 248–250, 307, 308, 331, 384, 388, 518, 519
virus 246, 249, 250, 331
malaria 214
mycobacteriosis 201, 202, 300, 301, 306, 519

paramyxovirusserotype 1(APMV-1; Newcastle disease) 203, 232, 279, 287, 302, 331, 525
Pathologists (AAAP), American Association of 4
pox 113, 114, 171, 211–213, 223–226, 270, 271, 290–292, 384, 391, 507, 523, 567, 584, 588, 590, 591
retroviruses 248, 330
tuberculosis (mycobacteriosis) 111, 114, 201, 300, 557
Veterinarians, Association of (AAV) 4
Avibacterium paragallinarum 221, 528, 577
Avipoxvirus 290, 587, 590, 591
avocado 334, 378
avoidance 438, 444
fluid 350
predator 73, 435, 437, 442
residue 261, 323, 350, 550, 563
avulsion
brachial plexus(es) 255, 256
tracheal 389
AWA (Animal Welfare Act) 14, 15

b
backbone (spine; vertebral column) 142, 177, 234, 483
bacteria 16, 52, 107, 110, 119, 127, 187, 197–199, 201, 222, 234, 235, 239, 245, 256, 263, 271, 276, 279, 290, 294, 295, 300, 309, 310, 323, 330, 363, 377, 412, 415, 470–472, 506–508, 510, 511, 518, 525–528, 530, 531, 538, 556–558, 584
intracellular (obligate) 301

bacterial
  contamination 309, 426,
    471–473, 510, 586
  culture(s) 198, 199, 201,
    220–222, 235, 239, 240,
    245, 265, 269, 271, 281,
    294–296, 299–301, 310,
    318, 333, 349, 356, 362,
    364, 385, 398, 401, 402,
    412, 413, 416–418, 422,
    426, 466, 471, 472, 477–479,
    485, 510, 527, 556
  diarrhea 239, 294, 296,
    300–302, 308
  egg culture 466, 470, 471
  media 471, 472
  overgrowth 398, 478, 527
bacterin (vaccine), fowl
    cholera 113, 587
ball, bandage 354, 364
band
  identification 98, 99, 201,
    478, 505
  leg 98, 201
  wing 478, 505
bandage 354
  ball 354, 364
  figure-of-8 (eight) 82, 255,
    350, 568
  leg 240, 242, 250, 251
  Robert-Jones 254, 354
  tie-over 268
  wing 72, 82, 255, 444
bandaging 235, 251, 252, 353,
    357, 364
bantam 23, 24, 29–31, 36–38,
    40, 44, 63, 64, 163, 168,
    278, 506, 589
Bantam
  American Game (breed) 30,
    36, 38, 40
  Association (ABA),
    American 63
  Class (Standard of Perfection
    breed) 23–25, 30, 31,
    37, 63, 64, 506
Barred Plymouth Rock (breed)
    24, 25, 28, 161, 163, 169,
    224, 244, 273, 307

Barren, Cape (breed) 61, 69
barrier, moisture 236
basophil 517, 520
bathing, dust 373, 437, 440,
    444, 446, 451
Baylisascaris 214
beak 59, 96, 99, 134, 140, 141,
    161, 162, 168, 172, 234,
    290, 345, 385, 391, 436,
    437, 441, 446, 447, 450,
    468, 470, 480, 490, 500,
    501, 510, 566
  deformities 257
  injury 356, 437
  lesion(s) 91, 118, 120, 125,
    172, 257, 270, 273, 356,
    385, 392, 437, 473, 480,
    481
  midline (culmen) 140
  modification 53, 54, 59, 91,
    141, 275, 281, 282, 306,
    480
  overgrowth 480
  surgery 391
  trephination 385
  trimming 53, 54, 59, 91,
    141, 275, 281, 282, 306,
    480
beam, cross 173
beard(s/ed) 23, 27, 30, 36, 38,
    40, 42, 44
bearing, weight 170, 364
bedbug(s) 263, 264
bedding 47, 49, 51, 110, 113,
    259, 451, 505, 550
behavior(s) 55, 60, 102, 112,
    159, 434, 452, 458
  abnormal 53, 91, 102, 434,
    444, 448, 452
  aggression 51, 53, 62, 391,
    438, 450
  broodiness 54, 70, 284,
    444–446, 505
  cannibalism 53, 91, 139,
    141, 222, 270, 271,
    275–277, 281, 291, 305,
    357, 415, 450, 518
  comfort 91, 440, 441
  defensive 446

developmental 437
  disorder 53
  drinking 94, 118, 160, 447,
    570
  egg eating 54, 451
  enrichment 451
  fear 91, 447, 452
  foraging 54, 76, 122, 437, 446
  grooming 440, 441
  guarding 437
  herding 73
  imprinting 60, 61
  inactivity 91
  mating 91, 99, 100, 424,
    444, 450
  modification 100, 391, 401,
    424, 438
  pecking 450
  predator avoidance 442
  receptive 99, 444
  reproductive 100, 102, 408,
    435, 443
  sensory perception 436
  social/group behaviors 442,
    447
  social order (pecking
    order) 39, 62, 438, 467
  vent pecking 450
bent ribs 284, 363
beta(β)
  aminopropionitrile (peas'
    toxin) 327
  cell(s) 146
  islets 146
  lactams 554
  toxin(s) 299
biceps brachii muscles 136–138
bile 146, 215, 308
  acid(s) 87, 318, 402
  duct 143, 146, 215, 402, 403
  imbibition 488
bill 58, 67, 70, 437
  Senate (SB27; Senate Bill)
    550
binding (bound), egg 184, 250,
    277, 412
biochemistry 289, 333, 348,
    362, 363, 365, 506, 507,
    515, 520, 540

biopsy 200, 269, 270, 272, 290, 384, 391, 401–406, 416, 422, 423, 426, 509
  cup 402, 404, 405
  forcep 400, 402
  hepatic 402
  needle 402
biosafety level 200
biosecurity 13, 19, 46, 107–109, 113, 195, 197, 198, 221, 224, 280, 287, 298, 303, 305, 478, 584, 590
biotin 120, 240
  deficiency 120, 240
  treatment 240, 312, 362
biphenyls, chlorinated 334
bird(s)
  deceased 512
  flu 229
  market, live 18, 304
  meat 46, 48, 201, 221
  sampling, live 509, 511
bird breeder's lung (hypersensitivity pneumonitis) 204
birnavirus 271, 296
Black Star (crossbreed) 24, 245
blackhead 209, 210, 215, 305, 311
bladder
  gall 146, 403, 487–489
  pod 378
blastoderm 464–466, 468, 470
blastodisc 464, 465, 470
blister, breast 164, 272
blocker, calcium channel 324
blood
  agar 470, 471, 527
    sheep 471
  agglutination, whole 202, 295
  brain barrier 581
  calcium 154, 277, 283, 363, 365, 395, 520, 521
  capillaries 143, 148, 149, 154, 216, 318

cell, red (RBC; erythrocyte) 215, 216, 369, 371, 507, 516–518, 523
chemistry (biochemistry) 289, 333, 348, 362, 363, 365, 506, 507, 515, 520, 540
cholesterol 83, 85, 335, 522
clot 120, 401, 509
feather 99, 261
film 506, 509, 529
loss 294, 297, 346, 352, 516
pressure 318, 326, 329, 347, 351, 355, 358, 382, 445
ring, static 470
smear(s) 318, 333, 508, 515, 516, 529
spots (egg) 285, 286, 462, 473, 474
stained eggs 275
transfusion 271, 347, 352, 370
vessel(s)
  branching (embryo) 470
  refill 347
  usage, whole 202, 285, 506, 509
blood-strained
  egg(s) 275
  feather(s) 223, 298, 450
bloody droppings 297, 298
blue
  Book 539, 540
  color vision 436
  wing disease 271
Board of Veterinary Practitioners (ABVP), American 4
body
  checks 287
  condition score 77–79, 123, 172, 328, 478, 479
  fat 77, 85
    decreased 298, 300
    excess 80, 362
  louse (*Menacanthus stramineus*) 259–261

regions 133, 135, 510
glycogen 153
temperature (core) 147, 166, 347, 348, 358, 448, 566
vitreous 156
weight 17, 25, 31, 37, 46, 50, 63, 76–81, 84, 86, 93, 94, 101, 102, 117, 123, 125, 147, 168, 177, 201, 206, 209, 211, 212, 226, 234, 235, 237, 240, 245, 246, 251, 256, 259, 262, 270, 275–277, 293, 296, 298, 299, 301, 312, 322, 345, 348, 352, 369, 402, 407, 424, 426, 478, 506, 513, 549–551, 566, 569–572, 574, 580
body parts, abnormal 473
bone(s)
  breast (sternum) 69, 135, 136, 155, 166, 321, 344, 349, 390, 391, 402, 482, 484–486
  calvarium 501, 502
  catheter (intraosseous) 265, 345, 350, 351, 458, 566, 568
  clavicle(s) 136, 137, 175, 177, 178
  color 30, 35, 185, 187, 501
  comparison (to mammals) 251
  concentration, lead 369–371, 374
  coracoid 137, 175, 177, 483, 484, 486
  cortex 251
  curved keel 122, 284
  deformities 86, 249, 251, 284, 308, 363
  disorders 118, 121, 464
  femur 118, 177, 178, 187, 251, 255, 350, 360, 458, 499
  formation 84, 283
  fracture(s) 122, 167, 184, 186–188, 251–253, 255, 328, 345, 348, 354, 356, 357, 362, 364, 391, 407, 501

furcula (wishbone) 483, 484, 486
growth 251
healing 251–255, 356
health 83
humerus 118
hyoid apparatus 136, 391, 481
infections 300, 308, 385
keel 112, 136, 272, 289, 306, 321, 478, 585
leg 172, 442
marrow 125, 185, 187, 300, 519, 538
  nodules 300
meal, eat and 119, 126, 373
melanoma 273
metacarpal 177
mineralization 84, 93, 119, 122, 464
pectoral girdle 136, 175
pneumatic 179, 187, 251, 350, 458, 566
pubic 99
quadrate 134
quality 84
remodeling 122
resorption 84, 121, 122, 127, 464
scleral ring 136
skull 136
soft (pliable) 118, 121, 283
spur 186
sternum 69, 135, 136, 155, 166, 321, 344, 349, 390, 391, 402, 482, 484–486
synsacrum 499
tarsometatarsal 177, 187, 188, 244
thoracic girdle 137, 485, 486
tibia 118
true rib 135
wing 82, 172, 255
Book
  Blue 539, 540
  Red 539, 555
botulism (limberneck) 76, 113, 114, 214, 233, 256, 284, 368, 377

bound (binding), egg 184, 250, 277, 362, 411, 412, 415, 418
box(es)
  dust 262
  nest (nestbox) 45, 46, 53, 54, 100, 159, 275, 281, 282, 443–446, 450, 451, 573
brachial
  nerve 237, 255, 256, 307, 581
  plexus(es) 255, 256, 581
    avulsion 255, 256
  vein (wing vein) 506, 509, 566
Brahma (breed) 29–33, 166
brain 67, 84, 152, 153, 199, 216, 257, 302, 303, 332, 348, 372, 437, 444, 473, 501, 502
  barrier, blood 581
  stem 152, 153
brain-heart infusion broth 471, 472
branching
  blood vessels (embryo) 470
  cords (islets) 146
  ducts (kidney) 148
breakout, egg 472, 473
breast 67, 70, 71, 73, 78, 79, 81, 83, 85, 164, 165, 289, 298, 300, 478
  blister 164, 272
  bone (sternum) 69, 135, 136, 155, 166, 321, 344, 349, 390, 391, 402, 482, 484–486
  cellulitis 309
  feather loss 70, 71, 282, 283
  injection 585, 586
  skin 269, 271
breed 25, 26, 29, 31, 32, 36–39, 62, 63, 67, 69, 77, 80, 140, 154, 159, 448, 450, 464, 477, 478, 505, 513, 569
  African 60, 63, 66, 67, 72, 74, 391

Ameraucana 24, 27
American Buff 63, 66
American Game
  Bantam 30, 36, 38, 40
Araucana 27, 464
Australorp (breed) 24–26
Barred Plymouth Rock 24, 25, 28, 161, 163, 169, 224, 244, 273, 307
Black Star (crossbreed) 24, 245
Brahma 29–33, 166
Buff Orpington 29–34
Buttercup (Sicilian) 30, 37, 39, 43, 44
Cape Barren 61, 69
Chinese 57, 63, 66, 67, 70, 186, 384
Classes
  chicken(s) 23, 24, 536, 537, 569
  duck(s) 63, 64
  goose/geese 63, 66
Cochin 30, 36, 38, 40, 41
congenital deformities 169, 234, 272, 318, 325, 326, 410
Cornish 29–33, 164
Delaware 24, 29, 31–33, 525
dual purpose 23, 24, 26, 29, 32, 38, 469
egg (laying breeds) 23–26, 29, 141, 298, 412, 446, 464, 569
Embden 63, 66, 67, 86
Hamburg 24–28
Hawaiian goose/geese 69
Jersey Giant 29–32
Lakenvelder 24, 26
Leghorn 23–26, 28, 29, 84, 161, 164, 237, 238, 246, 298, 319, 322, 327, 446, 448, 459, 516, 518–520, 568, 579, 581
Mallard 57–60, 63, 64, 67, 69–71, 73, 74, 76, 87–90, 94, 99, 182, 184, 389, 581
Maran 24–29

breed (*cont'd*)
  meat   23, 29, 31, 32, 272, 469, 569
  mixed   61, 72, 73, 101, 408, 414
  Muscovy   57, 58, 60, 62–64, 67, 68, 71, 80, 81, 83, 91, 331, 426, 467
  New Hampshire   24, 29, 31, 32
  Orloff   30, 36, 39, 42, 236
  ornamental   23, 26, 30, 36, 38
  Orpington   29–32, 170, 247
  Pekin   57, 63, 64, 77, 79–81, 87, 93, 99, 102, 171, 199, 235, 238, 239, 252, 266, 318–320, 370, 382, 403, 404, 413, 417, 419, 423
  Plymouth Rock   23–26, 224, 298, 317
  Polish   23, 29, 30, 36, 39, 42, 43
  Red Star (crossbreed)   24
  Roman   63, 67
  Rouen   63, 68
  Rhode Island Red   24–26, 164, 410, 569
  Sebastopol   57, 66
  selection   12, 23, 47, 53, 317, 323, 325, 329
  show(s)   223
  Silkie   30, 35, 37, 39, 44, 167, 168, 187, 272, 273, 278, 352, 358, 446, 495
  Sussex   29, 31, 32, 34, 160, 170, 235
    Speckled Sussex   34, 160, 170, 235
  Toulouse   63, 67, 70, 405
  Welsummer   24–26, 28, 29, 225, 241
  widgeon, American   70, 97
  Wyandotte   24, 29–32, 34, 35, 364, 568, 581
breeder's lung (hypersensitivity pneumonitis)   204
  bird   204
  pigeon   204

broiler (chicken)   86, 117, 123, 124, 128, 129, 161, 162, 208, 219, 220, 249, 259, 271, 280, 299, 300, 309, 322, 326–328, 333, 407, 452, 537, 569, 570, 572, 574–578
bronchitis, infectious   113, 114, 123, 161, 166, 204, 220, 221, 223, 224, 279–284, 286, 287, 305, 309, 310, 359, 383, 406, 463, 474, 494, 510, 523–525
  vaccine   233, 304, 587, 589–591
bronch(us/i)   359
  primary   69, 147, 487, 497, 498
  secondary   147
  terminal (air capillaries)   147, 568
  tertiary (parabronchi)   147
brooder pneumonia   226
brooding   45, 49–51, 55, 226, 227, 448
broodiness (behavior)   29, 54, 70, 284, 444–446, 468, 505
broody hen   29, 54
broth
  brain-heart infusion broth   471, 472
  enrichment   472
  virus isolation   511
brown egg(s)   25–27, 29, 32, 37–39, 286, 287, 448, 464, 474
Buff Orpington (breed)   29–34
build-up
  aerosol   510
  atheromatous   335
  organic debris   111
bulb
  heat (lamp)   49, 50, 361, 377, 378, 448, 450
  light   50
  olfactory   152
bulk chemical(s)   544, 548

bulla(ae), syringeal
  osseous   69, 182, 184, 388, 389
  radiograph   67, 69, 389
bumble foot (pododermatitis)   57, 60, 93, 171, 186, 187, 234–239, 241, 251, 252, 266, 330, 348, 354, 364, 579
  radiograph   186
bursal disease, infectious (IBD)   114, 260, 271, 296, 300, 518, 519, 524, 590
  vaccine   586, 587, 589, 591
bursa
  cloacal (of Fabricius)   155, 156, 271, 296, 297, 307, 308, 400, 492
  hemorrhagic   296
  proctodeum diverticulum (bursa)   155
  sternal   245, 272
butorphanol, analgesia   267, 355, 358, 458
Buttercup
  cup comb   44, 161
  Sicillian (breed)   30, 37, 39, 43, 44
by-product(s), feather   536, 546, 552

C
C cell(s) (parafollicular cell)   153, 154
cage
  layer fatigue (osteomalacia)   283, 363, 464
  mate   59, 110, 260
calamus   140
calcite crystals   466
calcium
  alginate swab   510
  carbonate, crystallized   277, 464
  channel blocker   324
  deficiency   121, 122, 283, 412
  depletion   283, 284

dietary   77, 89, 119, 121–124, 126–128, 277, 281, 283, 284, 310, 362, 363, 369–373, 395, 406, 464, 581
intracellular   328
low blood   154, 277, 283, 363, 365, 395, 520, 521
metabolism   154, 283, 284, 287, 335, 369, 372, 375, 376, 412, 444, 445, 464, 581
tetany   121, 277, 283
uroliths   406
calcite crystal(s)   466
calcium   154, 277, 283, 284, 287, 328, 335, 363, 365, 369, 395, 406, 445, 464, 520, 521
alginate   510
alumino silicate   124
blood   277, 365, 395, 520, 521
channel blocker   324
decreased   283, 284
dietary   77, 89, 119, 121–124, 126–128, 277, 281, 284, 310, 362, 369–373, 375, 376, 395, 406, 410, 444, 464, 581
excessive   123, 310
intracellular   328
call(s), distress   446, 448
callouses   167
calories   89, 122, 123, 566
decreased   79
excessive   99, 100, 312
calvarium bone   501, 502
cambendazole   226
Campylobacter   198, 528, 547, 565
campylobacteriosis   111, 114, 198
Canada goose/geese   58, 82, 90, 183, 252, 392
canal
central   152
reproductive   277
triosseal (foramen)   136, 137
spinal   153

cancer   84, 185, 383, 385, 394, 399, 411, 420–422, 424–426
Candida albicans   291, 292, 529
candidiasis (mycosis; crop mycosis)   114, 211–213, 290–293, 362, 579
candler   470
candling   227, 287, 470
canker (*Trichomonas gallinae*), crop   211
cannibalism (conspecific consumption)   275, 451
behavior   53, 91, 139, 141, 222, 270, 271, 275–277, 281, 291, 305, 357, 415, 450, 518
cannula
air sac   344, 349, 359, 360, 387
lacrimal duct   406
Cape Barren (breed)   61, 69
Capillaria   211, 212, 293, 299, 529, 573
annulata   293
contorta   212, 293
obsignata   299
capillariasis, crop   212, 213, 292, 293
capillary(ies)
air (terminal bronchus/i)   147, 568
blood   143, 148, 149, 154, 216, 318
clot time   401
pulmonary   325
refill time (CRT)   162, 347
sinusoidal   146
caponizationn (castration)   139, 397, 423, 424
capsule
gland   139, 153, 154
joint   502, 503
kidney   148
liver   224, 302, 311, 312, 334, 487
capture   71, 73, 567
carbohydrates   80
dietary   80, 87

excessive   80, 100, 101
carbonate
crystallized calcium   277, 464
carcass management   6, 112, 113, 460
carcinoma   422, 426
ovarian   250, 525
squamous cell   248, 391
cardiac (heart)   69, 117, 142, 144, 155, 164, 177, 178, 247, 317–319, 321–323, 347, 349, 388, 390, 468, 469, 486–490, 506
abnormality   126, 317, 318, 322–326, 328–330, 333–335, 347
arrest   343, 345, 358, 381
auscultation   162, 164, 165, 172, 318, 343, 470
chamber(s)   321–323, 325
compression   343, 344
disease   32, 164, 271, 317, 323–325, 327–330, 335
distress   71, 72, 334, 344
failure, congestive   318, 324, 325, 332, 333, 335, 351
imaging   320, 321, 323, 325, 329, 333
medication(s)   323
muscle   121, 328, 333
peculiarities, avian   318
rhythm   320
sounds   342
toxicosis   334
troponin T   318
cardiomyopathy
dilated (round heart disease; diluted cardiomyopathy)   324–330, 333, 334
hypertrophic   324, 325, 329
restrictive   325, 326
spontaneous (round heart disease; dilated cardiomyopathy)   324–330, 333, 334
cardiopulmonary
arrest   343

cardiopulmonary (*cont'd*)
  resuscitation (CPR)   343,
    344
cardiovascular system   155,
    317, 318, 329
  radiograph   320, 325, 326
care
  critical   343, 354, 566
  standard of   3
carina
  (keel)   136
  (syrinx)   182
carotid artery   153
carprofen analgesia   355, 356
carrier(s)
  air shipment   13
  disease (asymptomatic)   18,
    110, 198, 200, 222, 246,
    294, 296, 298, 301, 306,
    308
  dog (for transport)   71
cartilage   141, 147, 481, 482
  abnormal   249, 318
  accumulation   249
Cary-Blair transport media   510
caseous
  cecal cores   208–210, 295,
    296, 311
  dermatitis   259, 260, 271
  exudate   222, 278, 280, 281,
    309, 487, 501
  ovary   281
  oviduct   275, 276, 279–281,
    309
  proventriculus   213
  sinus(es)   220, 222, 501
Cassia   334, 378
castration (caponization)   139,
    397, 423, 424
catheter
  coelomic   397
  crop   568
  duodenal   397, 398
  intraosseous (IO)   265, 345,
    350–352, 458, 566–568
  intravenous (IV)   265, 268,
    320, 345, 350–353, 355,
    356, 358, 365, 382, 397,
    406

proventriculus   375
  urinary   359
caudal
  mesenteric vein   148, 149
  vena cava   145, 148, 149,
    410, 418, 419, 421, 423
CAV (chicken anemia virus;
    infectious chicken anemia)
    260, 271, 518, 587
cava
  caudal vena   145, 148, 149,
    410, 418, 419, 421, 423
  cranial vena   318
cavity
  abdominal   125, 303, 312,
    468, 585
  coelomic   147, 150, 154, 166,
    172, 174, 177, 178, 181,
    184, 185, 187, 189, 190,
    222, 235, 249, 268, 278,
    280, 345, 350, 357, 363,
    390, 391, 396, 400, 404,
    410, 415, 416, 418, 420,
    425, 468, 484, 487, 585
  nasal   141, 146
  pharyngeal   141, 142, 146
cecal
  cores, caseous   208–210,
    295, 296, 311
  dropping(s)   160, 289
  gland(s)   144
  worm(s)   209, 210, 215, 293,
    305, 311, 572, 573
cecectomy   399
cecum   144, 294, 295, 299, 305,
    311, 399
celiacartery   155
celiotomy   78, 79, 389, 390, 391,
    396, 397, 400, 402–405,
    410–412, 414, 416, 418,
    420, 422, 424, 425
cell(s)
  air   466, 471
  alpha   146
  beta   146
  C cells (parafollicular cell)
    153, 154
  carcinoma, squamous   248,
    391

culture (viral culture)   200,
    291, 529, 584, 591
  delta   146
  granulosa   248, 422, 462, 465
  Leydig   150, 153
  lymphatic   143, 155, 423
  parafollicular (C cells)   153,
    154
  red blood (RBC; erythrocyte)
    215, 216, 369, 371, 507,
    516–518, 523
  volume, pack (PCV;
    hematocrit)   271, 318,
    325, 326, 347, 348, 375,
    515–518, 523
cellulitis   271, 308, 309
  breast   309
Centers for Disease Control
    (CDC)   195–198, 541
central
  canal   152
  necrosis   216
  nervous system   152, 214,
    234
  nucleus   465
  vein   146
  zone (*area pellucida*)   468
cephalosporins (prohibited
    drug)   547, 564
cereal grain(s)   80, 125
cerebellum   152, 153, 502
  lobe   152
cerebral
  cortex   152
  hemisphere   152, 153, 502
  resuscitation, cardiopulmonary
    (CPCR)   343
  vessels   256, 318
cerebri
  epiphysis (pineal
    gland)   153, 444
  hypophysis (pituitary
    gland)   153, 444, 446
certificates, health   11–14
cervical
  air sac   147, 180, 182
  dislocation   458, 460
  esophagus   142, 392, 394,
    483, 484

muscle (pipping muscle) 586
region 262, 265, 266, 483, 486
spinal nerves 152
vertebrae 135, 142, 177, 460, 483
cessation
egg (of laying) 48, 54, 101, 102, 122, 231, 276, 277, 281, 377, 412
heartbeat 459
cestodes (tapeworms) 215, 287, 288, 299, 573
chain reaction, polymerase (PCR) 198–200, 203, 211, 214, 220, 221, 223–225, 248, 269, 271, 288, 385, 507, 508, 511, 530
real time 231, 232
chalaza(e) 151, 463–465
chalaziferous layers 463
chamber(s)
air 464
anterior 161, 357
cardiac 321–323, 325
infraorbital sinus 383
channel
blocker, calcium 324
crop 142
charter, city(ies) 5–9
checks, body 287
chemical(s)
bulk 544, 548
contraceptives 87, 89, 90
disinfectants 109, 113, 114, 198, 201, 203, 229, 271, 300, 304, 388, 478
feed 117, 118, 128, 286
hazards 538, 542, 553, 554
restraint 74
test interference 510
treatment 299
chemistry (biochemistry) 289, 333, 348, 362, 363, 365, 506, 507, 515, 520, 540
Chemists, Association of Official Analytic (AOAC) 556

chemotherapy 195, 208, 391, 409, 423
chiasma, optic 153
chick
dead-in-shell 472
development 462, 466–470, 472
diseases 172, 208, 219, 245, 249, 257, 309, 472, 529, 571, 574, 575
evaluation 135, 140, 145, 172
learning 437, 441
management 49, 86, 118, 128, 449, 571, 574, 575
monitoring 470
purchasing 12, 45
sex-linked 24
vaccination 113, 248, 291, 584, 589
vocalization 436
chicken
anemia (infectious anemia) 114, 271, 519
virus (CAV) 260, 271, 518, 587
broiler (chicken) 86, 117, 123, 124, 128, 129, 161, 162, 208, 219, 220, 249, 259, 271, 280, 299, 300, 309, 322, 326–328, 333, 407, 452, 537, 569, 570, 572, 574–578
coop 4–6, 8, 45–47, 50, 54, 55, 111, 113, 159, 223, 373, 446, 451
drug use 267, 268, 343, 528, 535, 536, 540–542, 544, 545, 547–549, 552, 556, 557, 562, 565
mite(s) 111, 112, 166, 259, 261–264, 510, 518, 573
Dermanyssus gallinae (chicken mite) 261, 262
Chicken Class (Standard of Perfection breeds) 23, 24, 30, 536, 537, 569

chiggers (larvae of *Neoschongastia americana*) 259, 263, 264
chlamydiosis, avian 195, 199–201, 301, 330, 332, 334
Chinese goose/geese (breed) 57, 63, 66, 67, 70, 186, 384
chirping, excessive 50
Chlamydophila (*Chlamydia*) *psittaci* 195, 199, 301, 331
sp. 360
chloride, potassium 458, 460
chlorinated biphenyls 334
chlorination, drinking water 52, 310, 505
choana 141, 171, 291
cleft 141, 220, 510
granuloma 385
slit 141, 146, 168, 349, 480, 490
choanal papilla(e) 141, 168, 480, 490
Choanotaenia infundibulum 299
chocolate eggers 26, 27, 29, 63, 64
cholera
avian 111
fowl 113, 220, 222, 227, 260, 271, 332, 574, 576, 577, 579
vaccine (bacterin) 113, 587
cholesterol
abnormal accumulation 272
blood 83, 85, 335, 522
clefts 272
intracellular 272
supplementation 335
choline 85, 86, 120
dietary 86
deficiency 86, 120, 240
treatment 240, 312, 362
chondroma 248
chorion 469
choroid plexus(es) 152

chronic
  disease 78, 79, 93, 112, 202,
    289, 297, 363, 412
  respiratory disease (CRD;
    Mycoplasma gallisepticum
    infection) 11, 112,
    219–221, 240, 281, 301,
    309, 331, 383–385, 523,
    525, 574–576, 578, 579
  vaccine 307, 584, 586,
    589–591
Cimex lectularius 263, 264
circovirus 271
circulation, air 47, 378, 461,
  568
city(ies)
  American 5
  charter 5–9
  codes 5–9
  ordinance(s) 4–9
  water 111, 505
Class (Standard of Perfection
  breeds)
  American 24, 25, 31, 37
  Asiatic 24, 25, 31, 37
  Bantam 23–25, 30, 31, 37,
    63, 64, 506
  chicken(s) 23, 24, 30, 536,
    537, 569
  Continental 24, 25, 31, 37
  duck(s) 63, 64
  English 24, 25, 31, 37
  Feathered (leg) 25, 31, 37
  Game 24, 25, 31, 37
  goose/geese 63, 66
  Mediterranean 24, 25, 31, 37
  Rose Comb (clean
    legged) 23–26, 28, 31,
    32, 35–37, 39, 43, 161
  Single Comb (clean
    legged) 23–26, 28, 31,
    32, 34, 36, 37, 39, 40, 161
  Standard 23–25, 31, 37, 62,
    63
classification (poultry),
    FDA 102, 255, 409,
    536, 542, 543, 545, 546,
    562, 563

clavicle(s) bone(s) 136, 137,
  175, 177, 178
clavicular air sac 175,
  180–182, 388
clay
  hematocrit 375
  kaolin 262
  mineral (vermiculite) 88
  print 459
cleft(s)
  choanal 141, 220, 510
  cholesterol 272
  crop (channel) 142
  infundibular 141
  labial 145
clinical examination (physical
    examination) 78, 79,
    112, 159, 161, 165, 166,
    172, 234–236, 248, 249,
    251, 255, 282, 289, 290,
    292, 293, 306, 327, 345,
    347, 356, 357, 363, 364,
    400, 504, 506
clinical history 477, 504, 505,
    515
cloaca (vent) 60, 62, 140,
    144–146, 148, 150–152,
    166, 305, 390, 398, 406,
    410, 415, 444, 463, 464,
    482, 491, 492, 496, 499, 510
  malformations 185
  pasty (pasty vent) 167, 168,
    289, 293–295
cloacal
  bursa (of Fabricius) 155,
    156, 271, 296, 297, 307,
    308, 400, 492
  disease 399, 400, 405, 411, 412
  drinking 210, 311
  egg (egg bound) 184, 250,
    277, 412
  imaging 174, 179–182, 184,
    185, 189, 280, 320, 321,
    323, 349, 361, 405, 406
  migration 287, 415
  prolapse 53, 168, 250, 275,
    305, 306, 362, 363, 400,
    401, 413, 450

surgeries 390, 398–400, 415,
    416, 418, 425, 427
  swabs 231, 303, 305, 401,
    509, 510
  trauma 268, 398, 400, 450
  temperature 348
cloacalith 400
cloacopexy 383, 400
Clostridium
  botulinum 256, 377
  colinum 302, 574
  perfringens 125, 299, 574,
    575, 578
  spores 301
  spp. 208, 210, 300
clot
  blood 120, 401, 509
  fibrin 326
  time, capillary 401
clutch 89, 99, 169, 244, 273,
    284, 415, 435, 436, 446
coaptation, external 253–255
coarse spray droplet 589
cob(s)
  corn 49, 451
  (swan) 58, 68
cobalt 334
Cobb500 24, 161, 162, 167
coccidia 208–210, 214, 297,
    528, 529, 571
  vaccination 297
coccidiosis 89, 125, 206, 208,
    210, 279, 296, 297, 299,
    300, 518, 528, 571, 572,
    576, 577, 586
coccidiostats 287, 297
coccygeal, aponeurotic region
    153
Cochin (breed) 30, 36, 38, 40, 41
code(s)
  city(ies) 5–10
  health 5, 6, 9, 18
Codex Alimentarius
    Commission (FAO/
    WHO Food
    Standards) 540, 555
coelomic
  aspiration 361, 420, 422

catheter 397

cavity 147, 150, 154, 166,
    172, 174, 177, 178, 181,
    184, 185, 187, 189, 190,
    222, 235, 249, 268, 278,
    280, 345, 350, 357, 363,
    390, 391, 396, 400, 404,
    410, 415, 416, 418, 420,
    425, 468, 484, 485, 487,
    585

contamination 396

disease 91, 99, 174, 177,
    179, 182, 190, 222, 235,
    268, 278, 280, 281, 323,
    326–328, 345, 352, 357,
    361, 363, 377, 405, 406,
    410–412, 416–418, 458,
    585

distension 70, 174, 189, 190,
    235, 248, 249, 325, 327,
    345, 346, 377, 412, 415,
    422, 426

endoscopy 349, 404, 405,
    411, 412, 422

fat 78, 88, 424, 425

fluid 166, 189, 190, 249,
    318, 323, 325–329, 345,
    346, 349, 350, 361, 363,
    377, 400–402, 420, 566

imaging 174, 177–179, 181,
    182, 184, 185, 187, 189,
    190, 249, 422

radiograph 179, 249, 279,
    326, 363, 400

surgery 102, 349, 352, 390,
    391, 396, 397, 400, 402,
    404, 407, 413, 414, 417,
    418, 425, 484

coelomitis (peritonitis), egg
    yolk 102, 185, 235, 278,
    279, 303, 362, 363, 411,
    412, 416–418, 516,
    518–520

cold 26, 32, 38, 39, 47, 347,
    363, 436

excessive 47, 48, 50, 139,
    236, 281, 283, 325, 450

excision 421, 426

vaccine 586

coligranuloma 308

colisepticemia 308

collagen
    fiber(s) 153, 155, 327, 335, 413
    patch 396
    supplementation 126

collapse 317, 318, 345
    egg 174, 278, 398
    rib 122
    trachea 388, 389
    vein 506

collar, neck 98, 99

collection
    display 67, 97, 207, 543
    egg 471
    sample 72, 206, 290, 348,
        403, 425, 468, 477, 478,
        487, 504, 506, 507,
        509–511, 515

College of Poultry Veterinarians
    (ACPV), American 3

colliculus, rostral (optic
    tectum) 152

colloid
    accumulation 153, 154
    administration 350–352,
        358, 520

colon (colorectum) 144, 145,
    311, 363, 390, 398–400,
    413, 491, 492

color
    bone 30, 35, 185, 187, 501
    feather 30, 35, 67, 121, 262
    loss, shell 286, 287
    straw 272
    vision
        blue 436
        green 436
        red 436
    yolk 299, 473

colorectum (colon) 144, 145,
    311, 363, 390, 398–400,
    413, 491, 492

colostomy 399

column, vertebral (backbone;
    spine) 142, 177, 234,
    483

comb
    abnormal 162, 163, 231,
        244, 246, 270, 272, 273,
        290, 291, 295, 297, 299,
        303, 304, 308, 317, 325,
        384, 444, 505
    crest 163
    cup (buttercup) 37, 44, 161
    dubbed 38, 139, 163, 357
    examination 133, 134, 139,
        160–164, 172, 347, 470,
        479
    frostbite 48, 139, 236, 243,
        272, 358, 427
    pea 25, 27, 31, 33
    pulse oximeter 240
    rose 23–26, 28, 31, 32,
        35–37, 39, 43, 161
    single 23–26, 28, 31, 32, 34,
        36, 37, 39, 40, 44, 161
    spiked rose 25
    type(s) 23–26, 31, 32, 36, 37,
        39, 139
    V shaped (devil bird) 41
    walnut 36, 37, 42, 44, 161

comfort behavior 91, 440,
    441

commercial hatchery 7, 10,
    12, 13, 113, 198, 226,
    248, 295, 296, 310, 586,
    590

Commission, Codex
    Alimentarius (FAO/
    WHO Food
    Standards) 540, 555
    common iliac vein(s) 148,
        149, 410, 419–421

companion animal 4, 14, 23,
    100, 323, 324, 438, 448,
    546, 547

comparison (to mammals),
    bone 251

complement fixation 523

compliance policy (minor
    species), medicated
    feeds 540, 545

compounding 372, 541,
    547–549

compression 410
  air sac 361
  cardiac 343, 344
  thoracic 458, 460
compromised health 317, 348,
    552, 554, 556
concentration, bone lead
    369–371, 374
condition score 77–79, 123,
    172, 328, 478, 479
Conditions and Restrictions,
    Conditions (CC&R) 4
conditionally approved drugs
    543
conductive disorders 318
congestion 303, 325, 326, 329
  hepatic 318, 320, 323
  passive 325, 329
  pulmonary 361
  oviductal 415
congestive heart (cardiac
    failure) 318, 324, 325,
    332, 333, 335, 351
conjunctivitis 203, 223, 360,
    385, 589
connective tissue disorder
    327, 381
conspecific consumption
    (cannibalism) 275, 451
consumption
  conspecific (cannibalism)
    275, 451
  feed 48, 51, 80, 81, 94, 118,
    295, 304, 355, 446, 551,
    567, 569
    rate 551, 569
  human 8, 10, 13, 15–18,
    199, 288, 323, 334, 373,
    377, 450, 474, 536, 537,
    546, 547, 550, 554, 562, 586
  intermediate host 299
  water 18, 51, 118, 125, 304,
    551, 569, 570, 574, 588
    rate 569, 574
contact dermatitis 124
contamination
  bacterial 309, 426, 471–473,
    510, 586
  coelomic 396

copper 285, 369, 372, 518
  cross 197, 513, 587
  diet 52, 358, 371, 377, 426
  drug 553
  egg 281, 309, 586
  environmental 208, 210,
    212, 361, 365, 401, 460,
    473, 538, 539, 551
  exposure 109, 111
  feed 272
  hatchery 226, 296
  larva 90
  lead 373
  mycotoxin 124, 125, 128
  nicarbazin 87, 89, 209, 232,
    287, 550
  soil 369
  tissue 352
  water 526, 527
  weed seed 125
  yolk 355, 369, 373, 553
content(s)
  abnormal 493
  egg 222, 227, 277, 285, 349,
    363, 473
  gastrointestinal 81, 87, 143,
    210, 256, 362, 377, 391,
    398, 478
  oviductal 412, 416, 420
contour feather 140, 220
contraceptive(s), chemical 87,
    89, 90
contraction
  duodenal 396
  leg 256
  oviductal 445
  ventricular 321, 333, 395
contrast media 177, 349, 395,
    396, 405
  injection 320
control
  animal 5, 6, 9, 12, 54
  Centers for Disease
    (CDC) 195–198, 541
  parasitic (prevention) 51,
    89, 110, 112, 259, 282,
    298
  pest (natural) 434
coop

chicken 4–6, 8, 45–47, 50,
    54, 55, 111, 113, 159,
    223, 373, 446, 451
  hatch 94, 95
copper 119, 121
  contamination 285, 369,
    372, 518
  deficiency 327, 518
  egg 26, 285
  supplementation 127, 292
coprodeum 140, 145, 399, 400
coprourodeal fold 145, 399
copulation 426, 427, 444
  forced 69
copulatory organ (phallus) 60,
    62, 69, 91, 100, 150, 363,
    423, 426, 427
coracoid
  bone 137, 175, 177, 483,
    484, 486
  muscle 136, 137
cord
  branching (islets) 146
  hepatic 146
  spinal 152, 153, 257, 369,
    460
  vascular 425
core
  body temperature 147, 166,
    347, 348, 358, 448, 566
  lipid (atheroma) 335
  caseous cecal 208–210, 295,
    296, 311
cormorants 232
corn cob 49, 451
cornea 155, 587
corneal
  accommodation 156
  moisture 163
  ulcer 358
Cornish
  (breed) 29–33, 164
  cross(es) 569
coronavirus 224, 406
corpus
  hemorrhagicum 462
  luteum 150, 462
cortex
  adrenal 154, 496

bone 251
cerebral 152
kidney 148
olfactory 152
coryza (infectious coryza) 114, 221, 223, 224, 507, 575–577, 579
vaccine 590
corpuscular volume(MCV), mean 516, 517
Cosmetic Act, Federal Food, Drug and 538, 543
Council, National Research (NRC) 76, 77, 81, 86
Covenants, Conditions and Restrictions (CC&R) 4
CPR (cardiopulmonary resuscitation) 343, 344
cranial
nerve(s) 153
vena cava 318
CRD (chronic respiratory disease; *Mycoplasma gallisepticum* infection) 11, 112, 219–221, 240, 281, 301, 309, 331, 383–385, 523, 525, 574–576, 578, 579
vaccine 307, 584, 586, 589–591
cream, silver 567
crest 37
comb 163
feather 39, 43, 44, 67
critical care 343, 354, 566
crop (ingluvies) 70, 118, 133, 135, 137, 140, 142, 163, 172, 328, 362, 394, 483, 484
aspiration 256, 292, 362
candidiasis (mycosis; *Candida albicans*) 291, 292, 293
canker (*Trichomonas gallinae*) 211
capillariasis 212, 213, 292, 293
catheter 568
channel (cleft) 142
esophageal diverticulum (crop) 142, 483, 484

featherless 282
fluid 174, 177, 181, 247, 292, 293, 300, 302
gavage 566
gland(s) 142
impaction 292, 293, 362, 393
injection 585
milk 142
mycosis (candidiasis; mycosis) 114, 211–213, 290–293, 362, 579
pendulous 292, 293
radiograph 177, 181, 292, 362
stasis 246, 292, 362, 369
surgery 385, 388, 392–394
worms (*Capillaria contorta*) 212, 213, 292, 293
cross
agglutination 295
beam 173
contamination 197, 513, 587
Cornish 569
hybrid 24, 26, 27, 63
protection 209
reaction 523
striation 307, 500
Crotalaria 334, 378
crusts 161, 309
Cryptosporidiosis 199, 208, 210, 213
Crytosporidium
baileyi 199, 210, 211, 528
meleagridis 211
parvum 211
crystallized calcium carbonate 277, 464
crystals
calcite 466
hydroxyapatite 118, 119, 122
urate (uric acid) 356, 406
Culclotogaster heterographa (head louse) 260
culture(s) 418

bacterial 198, 199, 201, 220–222, 235, 239, 240, 245, 265, 269, 271, 281, 294–296, 299–301, 310, 318, 333, 349, 356, 362, 364, 385, 398, 401, 402, 412, 413, 416–418, 422, 426, 466, 471, 472, 477–479, 485, 510, 527, 556
cell (viral culture) 200, 291, 529, 584, 591
egg 466, 470, 471
egg roll 471
egg yolk 471, 472
fungal 292, 508, 529
protozoal 211
shell membrane 471
viral (cell culture) 200, 291, 529, 584, 591
cup, biopsy 402, 404, 405
curled toe(s) 169
paralysis (Vitamin B2 deficiency; Riboflavin deficiency) 86, 120, 237, 244
curved keel bone 122, 163, 165, 284, 363
cutaneous
dermatitis 271
lymphoma (Marek's disease) 269, 270
melanoma 272, 273
pox (dry pox) 291
ulnar vein (basilic vein) 163, 165, 348, 509, 566
xanthoma 272
cuticle 464, 466, 497
cygnet 68, 93
cyst(s) 415
feather 272
oral 391
ovarian 420, 422
oviductal 412, 415
pancreatic 404
parasite 214, 331, 528
testicular 424–426
cystic
ovary 189, 410, 417, 420–422

cystic (*cont'd*)
  oviduct 150, 151, 187, 249, 250, 277, 278, 410–412, 420, 495
    right (retained) 151, 187, 277, 278, 410, 411, 419
  testicle 426
  thyroid 330

d

D, vitamin 93, 283, 284, 362
D3, vitamin
  deficiency 118, 284
  toxicity 284, 310, 334
dabbler (ducks) 57, 58, 60, 73, 74, 76, 94, 95
damage 123, 310, 405, 406, 421
dander, feather 111, 204, 246, 306, 478
dark islet 146
day length(s) 100, 101, 279–283, 285
dead-in-shell chick 472
death syndrome, sudden 328–330
debeaking 53, 54, 59, 91, 141, 275, 281, 282, 306, 480
debris, organic
  build-up 111
  removal 113, 198, 201, 466
debulk 388, 403, 420, 421
decreased
  bird(s) 512
  body fat 298, 300
  calcium 283, 284
  egg production 48, 51, 100–102, 108, 122, 224, 231, 257, 262, 263, 270, 280–283, 286–288, 297–299, 303, 304, 308, 363, 369, 376, 405, 407, 409, 446, 505
defensive behavior 446
deferens, ductus (vasdeferens) 145, 150, 423, 425, 426, 499
deficiency(ies)
  biotin 240

calcium 121, 122, 283, 412
choline 240
copper 327, 518
hormone 121
immune 271
iron 518, 581
manganese 240, 249
mineral 121
niacin (nicotinic acid) 86, 120
nicotnic acid (niacin) 86, 120
nutritional 54, 80, 87, 89, 99, 112, 117, 128, 145, 256, 271, 281, 283, 284, 287, 326, 329, 334, 406, 407, 409, 412, 508, 511, 518, 525
potassium 121, 334, 351, 520, 579
riboflavin (vitamin B2 deficiency; curled toe paralysis) 86, 120, 237, 244
selenium 121, 334
vitamin 118, 120, 281, 283, 290
vitamin A 211, 212, 287, 290, 292, 299
vitamin B1 (thiamine) 256, 581
vitamin B2 (riboflavin deficiency; curled toe paralysis) 86, 120, 237, 244
vitamin B3 (niacin) 86, 120
vitamin D 93, 118, 283, 284, 287, 362
vitamin E 126, 256, 257, 334, 472
vitamin K 286
definition, FDA poultry 537
deformities
  beak 257
  bone 86, 240, 249, 251, 284, 308, 363
  congenital 234, 272
  shell 416
  valgus 161, 240, 249–251
  wing 72, 82

degradation
  heat 110, 111, 126, 198
  vitamin 117
dehydrated shell membrane 467
dehydration 121, 163, 165, 208, 210, 248, 295, 296, 300, 306, 308, 334, 347, 350, 351, 362, 499, 505, 518, 523, 554, 566
Delaware (breed) 24, 29, 31–33, 525
delta cell 146
delta-aminolevulinic acid 369
deoxynivalenol 124, 125
depletion
  calcium 283, 284
  Program, Food Animal Residue Avoidance and (FARAD) 261, 323, 528, 539, 541, 542, 550, 553–555, 563–565, 567, 568, 571, 573, 574, 579, 581
Dermanyssus gallinae (chicken mite) 261, 262
dermatitis 120
  caseous 259, 260, 271
  contact 124
  gangrenous (necrotic) 260, 271
  necrotic 271, 296, 427
  syndrome, anemia (CAV) 271
dermatologic disease 259, 260, 269–271, 290
dermatology 236
descending duodenum 143, 397, 404
designated drugs 323, 550
development
  behavioral 437
  chick 462, 466–470, 472
  embryo 463, 465–468, 473
devil bird (V shaped comb) 41
DHA accumulation, brain 84
diagnosis 110, 112, 477, 478, 504, 509, 511, 515, 520, 531, 544

diagnostic
  egg   286, 462, 470, 472, 473
  kidney   369, 370, 402, 554
Diagnosticians (AAVLD),
    American Association of
    Veterinary   541
diarrhea   112, 119, 289, 290,
    293, 294, 362, 403, 405,
    505, 565
  bacterial   239, 294, 296,
    300–302, 308
  green   108, 161, 290, 295,
    301, 303
  nutritional   237
  toxin   374
  viral   230, 248, 271, 303, 304,
    362
  watery   108, 296, 298, 302,
    303
  white   295, 302
diatomaceous earth   261
dichlorvos   262, 263
diencephalon   153
diet
  contamination   52, 358, 371,
    377, 426
  dilution   122
  formulation   76, 80–84,
    86–89, 100, 101,
    117–119, 122–128, 159,
    166, 237, 250, 256, 259,
    335, 354, 362, 395, 451,
    464, 473, 551
  life stages needs   122, 123,
    159, 166, 250, 256, 286,
    287, 312, 326, 334, 354,
    446, 464, 473
  medical   397, 407, 446
dietary
  arginine   81
  calcium   77, 89, 119,
    121–124, 126–128, 277,
    281, 283, 284, 310, 362,
    363, 369–373, 375, 376,
    395, 406, 410, 444, 464,
    581
  carbohydrates   80, 87
  choline   86
  fats   80, 83, 85, 126

fiber   118
methionine   81
nicotinic acid   86
panthothetic acid   86
protein   82, 126
pyridoxine   86
riboflavin   86
zinc   77, 119, 121, 369,
    374
diffusion
  disk   528
  gel   523, 527
  passive   524, 527
digestive system   140, 141, 144,
    145, 289, 291, 292, 304,
    395, 468, 469, 491, 505
digit(s)   139, 470, 566
  entrapment   265
  supernumerary   187
digital región   238, 481
dilated cardiomyopathy
    324–330, 333, 334
dilution, diet   122
dimercaptosuccinic acid
    (DMSA)   370, 372, 581
directional terminology
    (radiograph)   177
Directive, Veterinary Feed
    (VFD)   127, 549, 550,
    565, 566
disc (disk)
  diffusion   528
  germinal   464, 465, 468, 470
  optic   156
discharge
  nasal   108, 161, 200, 202,
    270, 301–303, 505
  oculonasal   163, 221, 301,
    383
discolored yolks   126, 285,
    286
disease   114
  blue wing   271
  cardiac (heart)   32, 164, 271,
    317, 323–325, 327–331,
    335
  carriers (asymptomatic)   18,
    110, 198, 200, 222, 246,
    294, 296, 298, 301, 306, 308

chick   172, 208, 219, 245,
    249, 257, 309, 472, 529,
    571, 574, 575
chronic   78, 79, 93, 112, 202,
    289, 297, 363, 412
chronic respiratory (CRD;
    Mycoplasma gallisepticum
    infection)   11, 112,
    219–221, 240, 281, 301,
    309, 331, 383–385, 523,
    525, 574–576, 578, 579
  vaccine   307, 584, 586,
    589–591
cloacal   399, 400, 405, 411,
    412
coelomic   91, 99, 174, 177,
    179, 182, 190, 222, 235,
    268, 278, 280, 281, 323,
    326–328, 345, 352, 357,
    361, 363, 377, 405, 406,
    410–412, 416–418, 458,
    585
Control, Center for (CDC)
    195–198, 541
dermatologic   259, 260,
    269–271, 290
elimination   11, 53
fatty liver (syndrome)   80,
    100, 312, 328, 407, 518
flip-over   328
gastrointestinal   177, 289,
    292–297, 299–302, 306,
    308, 326, 376, 401, 402,
    411, 520
Gumboro (infectious bursal
    disease; IBD)   114, 250,
    260, 271, 296, 300, 518,
    519, 524, 590
  vaccine   586, 587, 589, 591
hemorrhagic   120
hepatic   324, 326, 401
infectious bursal (IBD;
    gumboro disease)   114,
    250, 260, 271, 296, 300,
    518, 519, 524, 590
  vaccine   586, 587, 589, 591
kidney   85, 216, 247, 249,
    307, 329, 404–406, 416
lower airway   361

disease (*cont'd*)
lung   182, 226, 231, 232, 301, 307, 308, 324, 328, 332, 334, 361, 378, 390
Marek's   3, 11, 113, 114, 161, 167, 170, 187, 233, 246–249, 269, 306–308, 330, 331, 335, 364–365, 393, 394, 500, 507, 518, 519, 523, 525, 584, 590, 591
cutaneous lymphoma   260, 269, 270
vaccine   584–586, 590, 591
monitoring   99, 102, 289, 296, 324, 399, 515, 531
musculoskeletal   234, 237, 255, 309, 482
neurological   67, 214, 246, 257, 307, 364, 374
Newcastle   13, 14, 19, 111, 113, 114, 195, 202, 203, 221, 223, 224, 229, 231, 257, 281, 290, 302–304, 309, 331, 361, 383, 504, 524, 584, 589–591
vaccine   584, 587, 589–591
viscerotropic velogenic (vvND; END; VND)   229, 231–233
nutritional   89, 112, 120
parasitic   89, 206–216, 263, 294, 311, 362, 364, 398, 518, 519, 528
pullorum   11, 18, 114, 294–296, 422, 523, 577
reportable   201–203, 231, 295, 504
reproductive   91, 166, 249, 250, 275–278, 280, 288, 346, 356, 362, 383, 384, 407, 410–416, 418, 421, 422, 426
respiratory   72, 166, 181, 185, 210–213, 218–226, 230–232, 239, 240, 280, 290, 303–305, 329, 349, 360, 361, 383–385, 388, 474, 480, 525, 574–576, 578, 579

round heart (spontaneous cardiomyopathy; dilated cardiomyopathy)   324–330, 333, 334
skin   259
toxin   334, 373, 376
transmission   11, 12, 14, 18, 45, 51, 52, 76, 82, 89, 99, 107–110, 112, 113, 118, 123, 195, 197, 203, 206, 271, 290, 294, 296, 298, 302, 326, 343, 477, 590
waterfowl   202, 203, 229, 230, 256, 304, 363, 375, 422
white muscle (muscular dystrophy)   121
zoonotic   56, 195, 199, 202, 211, 214, 281, 286, 300, 334, 343, 457, 547
disinfectant(s), chemical   109, 113, 114, 198, 201, 203, 229, 271, 300, 304, 388, 478
disinfection   53, 110, 111, 113, 197, 222, 298, 301, 510
dislocation, cervical   458, 460
disorder(s)
behavior   53
bone   118, 121, 464
conductive   318
connective tissue   327, 381
electrolyte   318, 351, 358, 362, 406
hock   120
phallus   91, 426
display collection   67, 97, 207, 543
distension
abdominal   324
coelomic   70, 174, 189, 190, 235, 248, 249, 325, 327, 345, 346, 377, 412, 415, 422, 426
distress   447
calls   446, 448
cardiac   71, 72
emotional   448
respiratory   212, 345, 348, 358, 359, 361, 362, 411, 589

diuretic   317, 324
loop   324
diver (ducks)   58, 59, 73, 76, 94
diverticulum(a)
esophagus (crop)   142, 483, 484
Meckel's (vitelline diverticulum)   143, 145, 468, 494
proctodeum (bursa)   155
rostral (infraorbital sinus)   383, 387
ventricular   395
vitelline (Meckel's diverticulum)   143, 145, 468, 494
DMSA (dimercaptosuccinic acid)   370–372, 375, 581
DNA   197, 199, 270, 290, 306, 530, 531
dogs
attack   54, 55, 252, 265, 356
carrier(s) (for transport)   71
Imprinting   91
Doppler   318, 321, 328, 344, 347
double yolk (double yolking)   277, 283, 285, 475
down feather(s)   50, 437
doxorubicin   334
drake(s)   58–60, 62–64, 67–70, 73, 74, 77, 87, 100, 423
drinking
behavior   94, 118, 160, 447, 570
cloacal   210, 311
monitoring   118
toxicity   375
vaccination   233, 584, 587, 588, 590
water   74, 76, 94, 119, 179, 447, 570
chlorination   52, 310
medication   86, 118, 292, 310, 549, 565, 568, 571–574, 577
droop, wing   255, 345
droplet
coarse   589

size   589
visualization   51
dropping(s)   56, 76, 108, 158, 160, 172, 200, 204, 246, 310, 362, 401, 447, 505, 579
  bloody   297, 298
  cecal   160, 289
  rodent   52
  yellow   402
drug(s)
  anticoccidial   208, 209, 297, 376, 473, 571–573, 580
  antiparasitic   536, 571–573
  antiviral   202, 353, 546, 547
    prohibited   547
  approval   539, 543, 544, 548, 555, 563, 570
  aspiration   567
  conditionally approved   543
  contamination   553
  Cosmetic Act, Federal Food   538, 543
  designated   323, 550
  elimination   536, 552–554
  Evaluation, Office of New Animal (ONADE)   552
  indexed   543, 564
  intake   567
  monitoring   538
  NSAIDs (non-steroidal anti-inflammatory drugs)   355
  prohibited   102, 409, 536, 540, 541, 544–547, 550, 563–565, 568
  residue testing   539, 555, 556
  use
    chicken   267, 268, 343, 528, 535, 536, 540–542, 544, 545, 547–549, 552, 556, 557, 562, 565
    Clarification Act of, 1994 (AMDUCA), Animal Medicinal   536, 540, 541, 544, 545
    extra-label (ELDU)   536, 541, 544–548, 552–555, 558, 562–566, 571

on-label   536, 546, 547, 552, 553, 558
dry
  air   471, 516
  pox (cutaneous pox)   225, 291
dual purpose breed   23, 24, 26, 29, 32, 38, 469
dubbed comb   38, 139, 163, 357
dubbing   139
  Continental Class (Standard of Perfection breeds)   24, 25, 31, 37
duck(s)
  Classes (Standard of Perfection breeds)   63, 64
  dabbler   57, 58, 60, 73, 74, 76, 94, 95
  divers   58, 59, 73, 76, 94
  plague   214
duckling(s)   49, 68, 69, 77, 81, 86, 87, 102, 196–198, 245, 374, 376
duct(s)
  bile   143, 146, 215, 402, 403
  branching (kidney)   148
  cannula, lacrimal   406
  hepatic   403
  hepatocystic   146, 403
  hepatoenteric   146, 403
  lacrimal   406
  Mullerian   277, 409
  pancreatic   146, 403
  uropygial   139
ductule, efferent   150
ductus deferens (vas deferens)   145, 150, 423, 425, 426, 499
duodenal
  aspiration   398
  catheter   397, 398
  contraction   396
  feeding tube   397
  loop   143, 146, 397, 398, 403, 404
  patch   398
  surgery   403
duodenopancreatic fold   146
duodenum

ascending   397
descending   143, 397, 404
dust
  aerosol   310
  bathing   373, 437, 440, 444, 446, 451
  boxes   262
  malathion   262, 263
  medicated   262, 573
dyschondroplasia   249
dysplastic feathers   272
dyspnea   161, 189, 210, 223–225, 270, 317, 323, 325, 327, 332, 359, 363, 389, 403, 422
dystocia   174, 185, 361–363, 400, 401, 412, 413
dystrophy, muscular (white muscle disease)   121

e

E.coli (*Escherichia coli*)   198, 219, 220, 222, 224, 227, 234, 239, 271, 276, 279, 281, 295–298, 303, 304, 308–310, 330, 331, 333, 334, 360, 362, 412, 415, 470, 518, 527, 547, 574–576, 578, 579
ear
  flap   139
  gland(s)   156
  lobe   25, 31, 32, 36, 44, 133, 160, 161, 163, 464
earth, diatomaceous   261
earthworm   209, 212, 226, 293, 305, 311, 312
Easter egg(er)   24, 26
eastern equine encephalomyelitis   195, 204, 257, 331, 333
eating
  egg(s)   54, 450, 451
  feather   293, 362
ECG (electrocardiography)   318–320, 325, 326, 328, 334, 344, 345, 347
  wing   240
Echidnophaga gallinaceae   263

echocardiography 321, 323, 325, 334
ectoderm 468
ectoparasite 262
ectopic
  yolk 411
endoscopy 348, 349, 385, 402
  air sac 349, 360, 361
  coelomic 349, 404, 405, 411, 412, 422
  gastrointestinal 349, 370, 393–395, 397
  lung 349
  reproductive 416, 418, 422, 426
  trachea 386
EDTA (ethylenediaminetetra-acetic acid) 370–372, 375, 376, 506, 507, 509, 581
efferent ductule 150
effusion (fluid) 166, 189, 190, 318, 320, 325, 326, 331
egg(s)
  abnormality 286, 475, 505
  abnormally shaped 186
  anatomy 464, 466
  binding (bound) 184, 250, 277, 362, 411, 412, 415, 418
  blood-strained 275
  breeds 24, 29, 298, 412, 446, 464, 569
  brown 25–27, 29, 32, 37–39, 286, 287, 448, 464, 474
  bound (binding) 184, 250, 277, 412
  breakout 472, 473
  breeds (laying breeds) 23–26, 29, 141, 298
  cessation (of laying) 48, 54, 101, 102, 122, 231, 276, 277, 281, 377, 412
  cloacal (egg bound) 184, 250, 277, 412
  collapse 174, 278, 398
  collection 471
  contamination 281, 309, 586
  contents 222, 227, 277, 285, 349, 363, 473

copper 26, 285
culture 466, 470, 471
diagnostic 286, 462, 470, 472, 473
double yolk 277
drop syndrome (EDS) 281, 284, 286–288
Easter 24, 26
eating 54, 450, 451
excessive laying 91, 99, 102, 410
exploding 472
fertile 462, 466, 467
formation 462
grading 17
green 24, 26, 27, 464
goose/geese 467
handling 464, 471, 473
hatching 39, 120, 121, 304, 376, 377, 466, 467, 471
incubation 460, 467–471, 473, 586
  egg 460, 467–471, 473, 586
  humidity 250, 272, 358, 376, 467, 472, 473
  hypoxia 324, 325
  temperature 272, 462, 467, 468, 472
infection 471, 472, 480
labeling 16, 17
layers 24, 29, 298, 412, 446, 464, 569
management 466
membrane culture 471
misshapen 108, 185, 286, 412, 474
pathology 472, 473
pole 466
production 7, 24, 29, 46, 48, 51, 63, 67, 99–102, 123, 159, 282–284, 303, 363, 395, 418, 446, 462
  decreased 48, 51, 100–102, 108, 122, 224, 231, 257, 262, 263, 270, 280–283, 286–288, 297–299, 303, 304, 308, 363, 369, 376, 405, 407, 409, 446, 505

Products Inspection Act 16, 17
quality 16, 283, 284, 288, 473, 474, 505
residues 553
roll culture 471
sandpaper (rough surface) 287
shell-less 224, 284, 288, 464
shell quality 284, 287, 288, 395
storage 471, 472
  fertile 467
  improper 310
temperature
  (incubation) 272, 462, 467, 468, 472
tooth 141, 470
unaesthetic 462, 473
ventilation 467, 472, 505, 589
visualization 227, 287, 470
washing 466
weight 27
white 463–465, 469, 470, 472, 474, 497, 553
  thin 463–466, 474
withdrawal time 562
worms 287, 474
yolk culture 472
yolk peritonitis 102, 185, 235, 278, 279, 303, 362, 363, 411, 412, 416–418, 516, 518–520
yolkless 474, 475
eggers
  chocolate 26, 27, 29, 63, 64
  Easter 24, 26
eggshell
  soft 278, 279, 287, 398, 412
  ends 287
  gland (uterus; shell gland) 147, 151, 152, 185, 275, 277, 283, 286–288, 409, 410, 413, 415, 416, 418, 445, 463, 474, 495–497
  organic matrix 464, 466
  quality 284, 287, 288, 310, 363, 395

sandpaper (rough surface) 287
Egyptian goose/geese (breed) 63
Eimeria
  acervulina 206
  adenoides 208, 577
  lettyae 209
  maxima 206
  meleagrimitis 208, 577
  necatrix 577
  spp. 206, 208, 209, 297, 529
  tenella 208, 297, 571, 577
ELDU (extra-label drug use) 536, 541, 544–548, 552–555, 558, 562–566, 571
  medical record requirement 548
electrical activity, cardiac 319, 334, 344
electrocardiography (ECG) 318–320, 325, 326, 328, 334, 344, 345, 347
  wing 240
electrocautery 420, 425, 426
electrocution 356, 358
electrolytes 127, 351
  disorder 318, 351, 358, 362, 406
  elimination, disease 11, 53
  supplementation 326
electrophoresis, pulse field 197
elimination
  drug 536, 552–554
  toxin 370
ELISA (enzyme-linked immunosorbent assay) 200, 203, 220, 224, 231, 248, 257, 308, 523–526
embryo
  blood vessel branching 470
  development 463, 465–468, 473
embryonic fluid 469
Embden (breed) 63, 66, 67, 86
emergency care 343, 345
eminence
  median 153

uropygial 139
emotional distress 448
encephalomalacia 120, 256, 257
encephalomyelitis
  avian (epidemic tremor) 113, 257, 331, 524, 587, 590, 591
    vaccine 113, 587, 590, 591
  eastern equine 195, 204, 257, 331, 333
  western equine 195, 204
endocrine system 153
endoderm 468
endoscopy 348, 349, 361, 370, 385, 386, 393–395, 397, 402, 404, 405, 411, 412, 416, 418, 422, 426
endotracheal intubation 388, 389
English Class (Standard of Perfection breeds) 24, 25, 31, 37
enrichment
  behavior 451
  broth 472
  light 92
enteritis
  hemorrhagic 232, 297
  necrotic 125, 296, 299, 300, 574, 575, 578, 580
  ulcerative 301, 302, 574
Enterococcus 330, 331
enterotomy 397
entoglossal 136, 141
entrapment
  digit 265
  intestinal 397
  sublingual 392
environmental
  contamination 208, 210, 212, 361, 365, 401, 460, 473, 538, 539, 551
  factors 49, 77, 79, 99, 123, 154, 200, 203, 212, 227, 281, 293, 303, 324, 325, 328, 329, 409, 412, 441, 445, 448, 451, 520, 527, 569, 570
  modifications 59, 91, 371, 375, 409, 434, 448

safety 17, 439
samples 76, 511
toxins 76, 334, 361, 365, 401, 473, 538
Environmental Protection Agency (EPA) 197, 538, 539, 541
enzyme 87, 395
  additives 87
  linked immunosorbent assay (ELISA) 200, 203, 220, 224, 231, 248, 257, 308, 523–526
  supplementation 87, 125
eosinophil(s) 517, 519
EPA (Environmental Protection Agency) 197, 538, 539, 541
epicardium, hemorrhagic 332
epidemic tremor (avian encephalomyelitis) 257
epididymis 150, 154, 422, 424, 426
epiphysis cerebri (pineal gland) 153, 444
equine encephalomyelitis
  eastern 195, 204, 257, 331, 333
  western 195, 204
erucic acid 334, 379
Erysipelothrix 330, 331
erythroblastosis 248, 308
erythrocyte (red blood cell; RBC) 215, 216, 369, 371, 507, 516–518, 523
erythrocytic protozoa 216
erythromycin 222, 246, 571, 575, 579
Escherichia coli (E. coli) 198, 219, 220, 222, 224, 227, 234, 239, 271, 276, 295–298, 303, 304, 308–310, 330, 331, 333, 334, 360, 362, 412, 415, 470, 518, 527, 547, 574–576, 578, 579
esophageal
  feeding tube 392, 568
  gland(s) 491

esophagostomy 392

esophagus

cervical 142, 392, 394, 483, 484

diverticulum (crop) 142, 483, 484

impaction 393

ethanol 334

ethylenediaminetetraacetic acid (EDTA) 370–372, 375, 376, 506, 507, 509, 581

Eustachian (auditory) tube 142

euthanasia 7, 89, 90, 202, 239, 251, 365, 383, 391, 457–459, 506, 556, 557

evaluation

air sac 348, 349

chick 135, 140, 145, 172

Office of New Animal Drug (ONADE) 552

examination

clinical (physical examination) 78, 79, 112, 159, 161, 165, 166, 172, 234–236, 248, 249, 251, 255, 282, 289, 290, 292, 293, 306, 327, 345, 347, 356, 357, 363, 364, 400, 504, 506

comb 133, 134, 139, 160–164, 172, 347, 470, 479

fecal 112, 198, 199, 207, 208, 210, 212, 215, 292, 293, 297, 298, 348, 362, 507, 528, 529

postmortem (necropsy) 6, 35, 113, 122, 143, 165, 168, 184, 190, 200, 212, 213, 218, 220, 222, 224, 235, 237, 239, 245, 247, 248, 250, 256, 273, 276–279, 290, 296, 298, 300, 301, 303, 307, 326–328, 330–333, 363, 365, 370, 376–378, 382, 389, 391, 397, 400, 415, 459, 473, 477, 478, 502, 510, 511, 520, 523, 528

techniques 477–502

waterfowl 72, 73, 506, 524, 525

excessive

ammonia 47

body fat 80, 362

calcium 123, 310

calories 99, 312

carbohydrates 101

chirping 50

cold 47, 48, 50, 139, 236, 281, 283, 325, 450

egg laying 91, 99, 102, 410

feather loss 51, 282

feather picking 439, 441, 450

heat 47, 48, 93, 281, 283, 295, 358, 361, 589

hemorrhage 297, 327, 404, 418, 519

mating 450

moisture 309

protein 82

sodium bicarbonate 123

training 405

vaccine reaction 589

excision

cold 421, 426

exploding egg 472

export market 107, 505

exposure 109, 110, 112, 113, 196, 256, 257, 263, 270, 271, 276, 280, 297, 298, 302, 304, 307, 312, 461, 523, 525, 571

air 241, 378

contamination 109, 111

light 48, 93, 100, 102, 126, 282, 285, 407, 444, 446

mate 91, 446

predator 46, 54, 112, 113, 269, 437

radiograph 173, 195, 320, 348

surgery 382, 390, 391, 396, 416, 420, 424, 482

toxin 76, 231, 233, 365, 368, 369, 371, 373, 374, 376–378, 460, 480, 481, 507, 538, 550, 553, 554

extensor carpi

radialis muscle 136–138

ulnaris muscle 136, 137

externa, theca 462

external

acoustic meatus 133, 136, 156, 163

coaptation 253–255

fixation 252–255, 354

iliac vein 148, 149

nares 134, 136, 140

tympanic membrane 147

extra-label drug use (ELDU) 536, 541, 544–548, 552–555, 558, 562–566, 571

extracellular fluid 350

exudate(s) 530

accumulation 222, 277, 385

caseous 222, 278, 280, 281, 309, 487, 501

eye 303, 309, 360, 385, 480

fibrinous 304, 311

fibronecrotic 293, 300, 304, 310, 485, 491

fluid 220–222, 275, 278, 280, 281, 293, 300, 309, 332, 360, 480, 491, 501

frothy 220, 221, 505

joint 509

oviductal 275, 276, 279–281, 309

pericardial 332

sinus 220, 501

yellow 220, 278, 309

eye

anatomy 134, 155, 156, 290, 332, 357, 387, 473, 480, 501

exudate 303, 309, 360, 385, 480

gray 247, 248, 309

level 51, 160

protection 203

vaccination (eye drop) 233, 584, 586–588, 590, 591

worm 213

eyelid(s) 160, 270, 291, 347, 480, 587

f

factors
  drug elimination   536,
    552–554
  environmental   49, 77, 79,
    99, 123, 154, 200, 203,
    212, 227, 281, 293, 303,
    324, 325, 328, 329, 409,
    412, 441, 445, 448, 451,
    520, 527, 569, 570
  water intake   118, 127, 218,
    399, 551
failure, hatch   446, 462, 467,
    472, 473, 475
false joint   254
FAO/WHO Food Standards
    (Codex Alimentarius
    Commission)   540,
    555
FARAD (Food Animal Residue
    Avoidance and
    Depletion Program
    261, 323, 528, 539, 541,
    542, 550, 553–555,
    563–565, 567, 568, 571,
    573, 574, 579, 581
farmer(s)'s
  lung   204
  market(s)   10, 17, 18, 546
fatigue, cage layer (osteomalacia)
    283, 363, 464
fat
  abdominal   81, 85, 304, 321
  accumulation   80, 88
  coelomic   78, 88, 424, 425
  dietary   80, 83, 85, 126
  metabolism, hepatic   85
  oils, and   126
fatty acid(s)   82–85, 117, 126,
    127, 326, 335, 379, 424,
    523
  omega-3   82, 83, 85, 326, 335
  omega-6   82, 83
  omega-9   85
fatty liver (disease)
    syndrome   80, 100, 312,
    328, 407, 518
FDA (Food and Drug
    Administration)

Classification (poultry)   102,
    255, 409, 536, 537, 542,
    543, 545, 546, 562, 563
prohibited medications
  list   536, 540, 541,
    544–547, 563–565, 568
fear
  behavior   91, 447, 452
  definition   537
feather   117, 126, 134,
    137–140, 156, 161, 166,
    172, 173, 261, 265, 282,
    307, 345, 349, 354, 414,
    444, 468, 470, 480, 481,
    510, 512, 566, 585, 587,
    588
  abnormal   133
  blood   99, 261
  blood-stained   223, 298, 450
  by-products   536, 546, 552
  color   30, 35, 67, 121, 262
  contour   140, 220
  crest   39, 43, 44, 67
  cysts   272
  dander   111, 204, 246, 306,
    478
  down   50, 437
  dysplastic   272
  eating   293, 362
  follicle   145, 247, 260, 269,
    270, 272, 306, 307
  growth   51, 82, 99, 281–283,
    354
  hair-like   30, 44
  loss   265, 282, 283, 505
    breast   70, 71, 282, 283
    excessive   51, 282
  moth-eaten   260
  picking   141, 439, 441, 450
  preen   76, 437, 439–441
  primary   99, 140, 166, 283
  quality   281, 289
  ruffled (fluffed)   161, 206,
    209, 230, 256, 296, 297,
    302, 308, 311, 324, 444,
    448, 505
  secondary   140, 283
  shaft   112, 140, 166, 261,
    262, 509, 528

soiled (fecal-stained)   262,
    289, 293, 294, 308, 362, 406
stress-lined   167, 479
tail   38, 172, 444, 510
transmission (disease)   246,
    306
trimming   167, 357
wing   138, 140, 167, 172,
    283, 481
Feathered (leg) Class (Standard
    of Perfection
    breeds)   25, 31, 37
featherless, crop   282
fecal
  accumulation   89, 265, 425
  examination   112, 198, 199,
    207, 208, 210, 212, 215,
    292, 293, 297, 298, 348,
    362, 507, 528, 529
  floatation   208, 215, 294,
    298, 362, 528, 529
  quality   293
  sample   348, 507, 508, 528,
    529
fecal-stained (soiled) feather(s)
    262, 289, 293, 294, 308,
    362, 406
Federal Food, Drug and
    Cosmetic Act   538, 543
feed(s)
  additives   77, 87, 88, 124,
    127, 128, 505, 540, 544,
    550, 565, 567, 569
  chemicals   117, 118, 128,
    286
  consumption   48, 51, 80, 81,
    94, 118, 295, 304, 355,
    446, 551, 567, 569
    rate   551, 569
  contamination   272
  Directive, Veterinary
    (VFD)   127, 549, 550,
    565, 566
  ingredients   118, 119,
    124–126, 547, 548
  intake   51, 52, 118, 123, 218,
    259, 277, 281, 283–286,
    312, 326, 362, 374, 395,
    407, 523, 551, 567

feed(s) (*cont'd*)
  labeling   540, 544, 565, 566
  medicated   89, 549, 550, 564
    compliance policy (minor
      species)   540, 545
  moisture (content)   118, 126
  quality   82, 125, 126, 306,
    446, 551
feeding tube   406
  duodenal   397
  esophageal   392, 568
  proventricular   394
feet (foot)   48, 67, 93, 96, 109,
    120, 167, 171, 172, 231,
    234–236, 239, 241, 243,
    260, 270, 272, 273, 304,
    348, 358, 364, 376, 446,
    469, 479, 481
  abnormal   234
  necrosis (footpad)   259
  overgrowths   167
  radiograph   187
female genital system   150, 151
femoral
  artery   138
  fracture(s)   187, 188, 354
  head   255, 482
femur bone   118, 177, 178, 187,
    251, 255, 350, 360, 458,
    499
femorotibial muscles   138
fenbendazole   213, 226, 287,
    293, 299, 565, 572, 573
fence, wire   54
fertile egg(s)   462, 466, 467
fiber(s)
  collagen   153, 155, 327, 335,
    413, 491
  dietary   118
fibrillation, ventricular   326,
    328
fibrin   220, 222–224, 226, 485
  clot   226, 326
fibrinous
  exudates   304, 311
  pericarditis   309, 333
  plaques   291

pneumonia   222, 301
  polyserositis   220, 232
fibroatheroma   335
fibroma   248
fibronecrotic exudate   293,
    300, 304, 310, 485, 491
fibrosarcoma   248
fibrosis, hepatic   403
field electrophoresis, plus   197
figure-of-8 (eight) bandage   82,
    255, 350, 568
filling, abnormal   165
film, blood   506, 509, 529
finding(s), abnormal   133, 159
fine
  needle aspiration   361
  spray droplet   589
fixation
  complement   523
  external   252–255, 354
  tissue   485, 500, 511, 512
fixative   500, 512
flaccid
  neck   246, 306
  paralysis   256
flap, ear   139
flapping, wing   71, 329
flavor (taste), yolk   473
fluffed (ruffled) feather(s)   161,
    206, 209, 230, 256, 296,
    297, 302, 308, 311, 324,
    444, 448, 505
fluoroquinolones (prohibited
    drug)   536, 546, 547,
    557, 563, 565
flush, nasal   361
flea(s)
  market   12, 17, 542
  sticktight   263, 264
flexor carpi ulnaris
    muscle   136–138
flexor crural muscle   137, 138
flip-over disease   328
floor
  área   45, 46, 438, 451
  flotation, fecal   208, 215, 294,
    298, 362, 528, 529

flow, lymphatic   423
flu
  bird   229
  Hong Kong   202
  Spanish   202
fluid
  accumulation   211, 277, 280,
    385, 423
  avoidance air sac   350, 402,
    566
  cerebrospinal   152
  coelomic (ascites)   166, 189,
    190, 249, 318, 323,
    325–329, 345, 346, 349,
    350, 361, 363, 377,
    400–402, 420, 566
  crop   174, 177, 181, 247, 292,
    293, 300, 302
  effusion   166, 189, 190, 318,
    320, 325, 326, 331
  embryonic   469
  extracellular   350
  exudate   220–222, 275, 278,
    280, 281, 293, 300, 309,
    332, 360, 480, 491, 501
  green   400
  intestinal   81, 178, 400
  intraosseous   566
  intravenous, additives   351
  lesions   272, 277–280, 407,
    412, 413, 417, 485, 495,
    498, 505
  mobilization (hemorrhagic)
    347, 352
  pericardial   323, 325, 326,
    329, 331, 358, 488
  retention, abnormal   174
  sampling   211, 278, 363, 412,
    422
  synovial   482, 502, 509
  sinus   220, 303, 383, 385
  therapy   265, 271, 345–347,
    350, 351, 354, 358, 381,
    395, 411, 566, 577
    fluid types   350, 351
    intraosseous (IO)   265, 345,
      350, 351, 458, 566, 568

intravenous (IV)   265, 268, 345, 350, 351, 355, 356, 358, 365, 382, 459, 566

maintenance   351, 566

oral   350

rehydration   268, 351, 352, 362

resuscitation   350, 351, 358

subcutaneous   268, 350, 566

transudate   318

types, fluid therapy   350, 351

warm   375

fluke(s)   215, 391, 415

control   56

fluoroquinolones   536, 546, 547, 557, 563–565

fly strike   265

fold

coprourodeal   145, 399

duodenopancreatic   146

ileocecal (ligament)   143, 399

lymphatic   423

median   141

metatarsal fold   139

patagial   138

peritoneum   143

proctourodeal   145

uroprotodeal   399

folic acid   120, 518

follicle(s)

feather   145, 247, 260, 269, 270, 272, 306, 307

lymphoid   142

ovarian   127, 150, 281, 321, 410, 417–422, 462, 463, 465, 553

preovulatory   417, 419, 420

stimulating hormone (FSH)   444

thyroid   153, 154

folliculitis   260

Food

Animal Residue Avoidance and Depletion Program (FARAD)   261, 323, 528, 539, 541, 542, 550, 553–555, 563–565, 567, 568, 571, 573, 574, 579, 581

Drug

Administration (FDA) Classification (poultry)   102, 255, 409, 536, 542, 543, 545, 546, 562, 563

Cosmetic Act, Federal   538, 543

Safety and Inspection Service (FSIS)   15, 17, 538, 540, 542, 555

Standards, FAO/WHO (Codex Alimentarius Commission)   540, 555

footpad necrosis   259

foraging behavior   54, 76, 122, 437, 446

foramen

optic   136

magnum   502

triosseal (triosseal canal)   136, 137

forced

air incubator   461

copulation   69

forceps, biopsy   400, 402

forces, abnormal   254

formaldehyde   512

formation

bone   84, 283

diet   76, 80–84, 86–89, 100, 101, 117–119, 122–128, 159, 166, 237, 250, 256, 259, 335, 354, 362, 395, 451, 464, 473, 551

egg   462

formulary (medications)   56, 118, 520, 535, 536, 543–545, 547–553, 556, 562, 563, 566–573

fossa

paralumbar   390, 399, 404

renal   147, 499

fowl

cholera   113, 220, 222, 227, 260, 271, 332, 574, 576, 577, 579

vaccine (bacterin)   113, 587

guinea   201, 221, 226, 252, 319, 376, 467, 571

mite, northern (*Ornithonyssus sylviarum*)   261, 262

paralysis   246

plague   229

pox   225, 270, 290, 291, 584

vaccine   113, 587, 588, 591

ticks   263, 264

red jungle   23, 435, 446

fracture(s)

bone   122, 167, 184, 186–188, 251–253, 255, 328, 345, 348, 354, 356, 357, 362, 364, 391, 407, 501

femoral   187, 188, 354

keel   328

liver   312, 362

repair   251–254

frenulum, lingual   141, 392, 393

frostbite, comb   48, 139, 236, 243, 272, 358, 427

frothy exudate   220, 221, 505

FSIS (Food Safety and Inspection Service)   15, 17, 538, 540, 542, 555

FTA card   507, 508, 511, 512

fungal

culture   292, 508, 529

granuloma   182, 183

growth   227, 292

infections   226, 227, 326, 331, 359, 364, 518, 569

pneumonia   326

spores   227

treatment   183, 353, 361, 389, 568

fungus   49, 226, 293, 360, 376, 525

furazolidone   324, 334

furcula (wishbone)   483, 484, 486

furosemide   324, 326, 327, 358

fusidic acid   557

fuzzy growth, air sac   227

g

gall bladder   146, 403, 487–489

gallid
  herpesvirus 1 (infectious laryngotracheitis) 223
  herpesvirus 2 (Marek's disease) 246   330

Game
  Bantam, American (breed) 30, 36, 38, 40
  Class (Standard of Perfection breeds) 24, 25, 31, 37

gander   68

gangrenous dermatitis   260, 271

gape   226

gapeworm   212, 213, 225

gasping for air   108, 211, 212

gastroctemius tendon
  rupture   254, 255
  slipped (perosis)   86, 120, 169, 171, 240, 245

gastrointestinal
  disease   177, 289, 292–297, 299–302, 306, 308, 326, 376, 401, 402, 411, 520
  endoscopy   349, 370, 393–395, 397
  radiograph   362, 370, 371, 375, 396, 397

gazing, star (vitamin B1[thiamine] deficiency)   256

geese/goose
  Asian (breed)   67, 70
  Class (Standard of Perfection breeds)   63, 66

gel
  diffusion   523, 527
    disk   528
  immunodiffusion, agar   203, 231, 305, 523, 527

genital system
  female   150, 151
  male   150

germinal disc   464, 465, 468, 470

Giant, Jersey (breed)   29–32

gizzard (ventriculus; muscular stomach)   88, 117, 126, 127, 140, 142–144, 155, 166, 174, 178–182, 190, 231, 257, 294, 328, 349, 369, 370, 390, 393, 395–397, 486, 488–493

gland(s)
  accessory   150
  adrenal   153, 154, 247, 256, 406, 421, 424, 425, 496
  capsule   139, 153, 154
  cecal   144
  crop   142
  ear   156
  eggshell (uterus; shell gland)   147, 151, 152, 185, 275, 277, 283, 286–288, 409, 410, 413, 415, 416, 418, 445, 463, 474, 495–497
  esophageal   491
  magnum   151, 463
  palatine   141
  pancreatic   146
  parathyroid   153, 154, 487
  pharyngeal   142
  pineal (epiphysis cerebri)   153, 444
  pituitary (hypophysis cerebri)   153, 444, 446
  preen (uropygial)   117, 139, 163, 172, 436, 441
  proventricular   143, 213, 304, 396, 489, 492, 493
  thyroid   153, 154, 487

thymus   155, 483, 484

uropygial (preen)   117, 139, 163, 172, 436, 441

salivary   141

sperm   463, 466, 497

thyroid   153, 154, 487

ultimobranchial   153, 154

glandular stomach (proventriculus)   140, 142–144, 155, 178, 179, 213, 231, 232, 247, 257, 303, 323, 375, 390, 393, 395–397, 489–493

glioma   248

glossa (tongue)   101, 125, 136, 140–142, 171, 225, 240, 392, 393, 478–481, 491, 587, 588

glottis (upper larynx; cranial larynx)   124, 146, 291, 568

glycogen body   153

glycoprotein   230, 304

GnRH (gonadotropin releasing hormone)   444
  agonist(s)   99, 102, 409
  analog   407

gonadal activity   121

gonadotropin releasing hormone (GnRH)   444
  agonist   99, 102, 409
  analog   407

gonorrhea, goose   426

Goose/Geese   68, 100, 178, 188
  African   60, 63, 66, 67, 72, 74, 391
  Canada   58, 82, 90, 183, 252, 392
  Cape Barren   61, 69
  Chinese   57, 63, 66, 67, 70, 186, 384
  Class (Standard of Perfection breeds)   63, 66, 100
  egg(s)   467
  Egyptian   63
  gonorrhea   426
  Graylag   67, 70

Hawaiian 69
Magellan 92
magpie 69
Roman 67
spur-winged 60
swan 67, 70
Toulouse 63, 67, 70, 405
Yangzhao 81
gosling 49, 68, 81, 86, 92
gossypol 126, 285, 378
gout
  articular 310
  visceral (urolithiasis) 122,
      182, 310, 311, 406
grading
  egg(s) 17
  Program, Voluntary 17
grain(s), cereal 80, 125
granuloma 301, 349, 359, 383,
      391, 413, 424, 426
  choanal 385
  fungal 182, 183
  tracheal 360
  tubercules 300
  visceral 300
granulomatous
  infection(s) 78, 201, 226,
      300, 332, 387, 413, 424, 426
  nodules 300
granulosa cell(s) 248, 422, 462, 465
  sarcoma 248
grass, green 392
gray eye 247, 248, 309
Graylag goose/geese 67, 70
grazer 58, 60, 61, 73, 74, 76, 94
green
  algae 56
  color vision 436
  diarrhea 108, 161, 290, 295,
      301, 303
  egg(s) 24, 26, 27, 464
  fluid 400
  grass 392
  koilin (horny layer) 143,
      395, 492, 493
  leafy 80, 88, 90, 159, 198
  muscle 255, 268, 357

onion 378
potato 379
yolk 473
grippe 229
grit 76, 87, 88, 174, 177, 178,
      181, 368, 369
grooming behavior 440, 441
group (social) behaviors 442,
      447
groove, trochlear 168
growth 88
  bone 251
  feather 51, 82, 99, 281–283,
      354
  fungal 227, 292
  microbial 127, 222, 235,
      245, 299, 302, 398, 471,
      472, 478, 527, 528, 537
  mold 110, 127
  ovarian 282
  plant 56
  plate 118, 249
  poor 82, 86, 120, 122, 298,
      324, 325, 377
  promotion 127, 544, 550
  rate 77, 80–82, 86, 87, 89,
      102, 117, 123, 128, 250,
      297, 299, 317, 325, 326,
      328, 470
  vessel 468
guarding behavior 437
guinea fowl 201, 221, 226,
      252, 319, 376, 467, 571
Gumboro disease (infectious
      bursal disease; IBD)
      114, 250, 260, 271, 296,
      300, 518, 519, 524, 590

h
H1N1 202, 230, 231
H3N2 202, 230, 231
H5 19, 202, 203, 230, 231, 304
H5N1 19, 202, 230
H5N2 230
H7 202, 203, 230, 231, 304
hair-like feather(s) 30, 44
Hamburg (breed) 24–28

handling 71, 73, 74, 109, 111,
      165, 195, 197, 201, 203,
      278, 292, 345, 358, 407,
      451, 459, 568, 576
  egg 464, 471, 473
  instructions, safe (eggs) 16
  sample 515, 520, 528
  tissue 382
hard palate 141
hatch 24, 48, 54, 61, 68, 84, 89,
      91, 169, 294, 419, 437,
      446, 467, 469–473, 475,
      537, 571, 586, 590
  coop 94, 95
  failure 446, 462, 467, 472,
      473, 475
hatchability 39, 120, 121, 304,
      376, 377, 467, 471
hatcher 227, 294, 295, 308,
      586
hatchery
  commercial 7, 10, 12, 13,
      113, 198, 226, 248, 295,
      296, 310, 586, 590
  contamination 226, 296
  local 10, 12, 13, 24, 113,
      198, 226, 248, 295, 296,
      310, 586, 590
  NPIP (National Poultry
      Improvement Plan) 10,
      12
  sanitation 471, 473
hatches, abnormal 475
hatching 54, 141, 294, 325,
      419, 437, 466, 467,
      469–472, 537
  egg 39, 120, 121, 304, 376,
      377, 466, 467, 471
  muscle 472
  synchronous 436, 467
hatchling 93, 118, 282, 294,
      296, 309, 591
Hawaiian goose/geese 69
hazards, chemical 538, 542,
      553, 554
head
  femoral 255, 482

head (*cont'd*)
  louse (*Culclotogaster
    heterographa*) 260
healing 77, 265, 352
  air sac 361
  bone 251–255, 356
  wound 121, 235, 242, 267, 268,
    353, 361, 392, 394, 396
health
  Act, Minor Use/Minor
    Species Animal (MUMS)
    542, 543
  bone 83
  certificate(s) 11–14
  code(s) 5, 6, 9, 18
  compromised 554
  Inspection Service, Animal and
    Plant (APHIS) 5, 13–15,
    19, 107, 108, 569, 570
  intestinal 127, 289
  issues 47, 51, 53, 55, 77, 79, 82,
    84, 88, 99, 101, 102, 110,
    112, 117–119, 122, 128,
    139, 145, 154, 208, 289,
    290, 318, 407, 416, 434,
    447, 448, 452, 520, 549, 551
  kidney 85
  Laboratory
    Animal (AHL) 317, 330
    Network, National
    Animal (NAHLN) 231,
    232
  management 107
  monitoring 277, 289, 312,
    345, 347, 348, 351, 477,
    505, 515, 523, 526, 527,
    530, 531, 556
  Organization, World
    (WHO) 203, 555
  public 6, 9–11, 13, 16–19,
    111, 199, 201, 301, 368,
    373, 506, 535, 538,
    546–550, 552, 556, 557,
    563
heart (cardiac) 69, 117, 142,
    144, 155, 164, 177, 178,
    247, 317–319, 321–323,
    347, 349, 388, 390, 468,
    469, 486–490, 506

auscultation 162, 164, 165,
    172, 318, 343, 470
  disease 32, 164, 271, 317,
    323–325, 327–331, 335
    round (spontaneous
      cardiomyopathy; dilated
      cardiomyopathy)
      324–330, 333, 334
  failure, congestive 318, 324,
    325, 332, 333, 335, 351
  infusion
    broth, brain- 471 472
  lesion(s) 294, 307, 308,
    330–332, 377
  muscle(s) 121, 328, 333
  nodule 294, 331
  rate 165, 240, 318–321, 326,
    344, 347, 355, 446
  sound(s) 318, 327
heartbeat, cessation 459
heat 47, 49, 83, 126, 129, 166,
    343, 347, 358
  bulb/lamp 49, 50, 361, 377,
    378, 448, 450
  degradation 110, 111, 126,
    198
  excessive 47, 48, 93, 281,
    283, 295, 358, 361, 589
  removal 46, 358, 450
  stress 48, 358, 589
hemagglutination 203
  inhibition 203, 220, 288, 523
hemagglutinin 202, 230, 304,
    523
hemangioma 248
hematocrit (pack cell volume;
    PCV) 271, 318, 325,
    326, 347, 348, 375,
    515–518, 523
  clay 375
hematology 289, 348, 506,
    507, 515, 516, 520, 529,
    531
hemisphere, cerebral 152, 153,
    502
hemoglobin 347, 464, 489,
    515–517
  imbibition 489
hemopericardium 327, 328, 402

hemorrhage 182, 208, 213,
    216, 231, 232, 235, 241,
    255, 296, 297, 303–305,
    309, 312, 327–330, 332,
    345, 347, 351, 352, 357,
    361, 362, 376–378, 381,
    390, 401, 404, 417–419,
    421, 425, 473, 489, 501,
    518
  excessive 297, 327, 404, 418,
    519
hemorrhagic
  anemia 516, 518
  bursa 296
  disease 120
  enteritis 232, 297
  epicardium 332
  fluid mobilization 347
  lungs 231, 378
  skin 54
  syndrome, fatty liver 328
  trachea 388
  typhlitis 208–210
hen 16, 23, 24, 27, 28, 33–35,
    37, 38, 40–44, 48, 51,
    62–64, 68, 70, 71, 84, 97,
    100, 122, 126, 147, 150,
    154, 166, 168, 170, 224,
    225, 235, 240, 241, 243,
    249, 251, 253, 255,
    264–266, 273, 275, 283,
    284, 305, 309, 332, 345,
    346, 353, 355, 357, 360,
    363, 370, 407, 418, 423,
    436, 438, 441, 444, 446,
    450, 462, 472–474
  broody 29, 54
  infection (hen-to-egg) 18,
    219, 224, 249, 250, 257,
    262, 269, 280, 281, 296,
    471, 472, 474
  laying 7, 46, 48, 54, 100,
    118, 120–124, 126–128,
    150, 151, 153, 159, 167,
    181, 182, 184, 187, 230,
    249, 250, 275, 277–281,
    283–285, 287, 305, 311,
    312, 395, 407, 418, 436,
    444–446, 466, 474

"male" 438
ratio
  nest to   46, 275, 306
  rooster to   466
  spent   585
hepar (liver)   145
heparin   506, 507, 509
hepatectomy   401
hepatic
  biopsy   402
  congestion   318, 320, 323
  cord(s)   146
  diseases   324, 326, 401
  ducts   403
  fat metabolism   85
  fibrosis   403
  imaging   320
  lipidosis   88, 362, 424
  lipogenesis   80, 101
  lobe   145, 146, 390, 402, 403,
    487–489
  lymphoma   269, 307
  necrosis   124, 199, 302, 489
  portal circulation   149
  portal, vein   146, 149
  rupture   362
  sarcoma   330
  steatosis   80, 101
  surgery   402
  system   410
hepatocystic duct   146, 403
hepatoenteric duct   146, 403
hepatomegaly   216, 247,
    306–308, 369, 374, 375,
    402
hepatovirus   257
herding behavior   73
herpesvirus
  1, gallid   223
  2, gallid   246, 330
Heterakis   209, 210, 215, 293,
    573
  gallinarum   305, 311, 572
heterophil   234, 271, 359,
    516–518, 520
high pathogenicity avian
    influenza (HPAI)   19,
    229–231, 304, 305
hinny   63

histology   272, 333, 405, 493,
    525
Histomonas meleagridis   209,
    305, 311, 312
histomoniasis   209, 210, 306,
    311
history, clinical   477, 504, 505,
    515
hock   135
  disorder   120, 171, 221, 235,
    237, 239, 240, 244, 245,
    253–255, 295
Homeowners' Association
    (HOA)   4, 5
Hong Kong flu   202
horizontal
  beam   173, 174, 348
  septum   155
  transmission   245, 257, 308
hormone   520, 539
  androgen   139
  deficiency   121
  gonadotropin releasing
    (GnRH)   444
    agonist(s)   99, 102, 409
    analog   407
  level   139
  pituitary   446
  reproductive   54, 139, 153,
    407, 422–424, 438, 444
  sexual   153
  thyroid   154, 523
horny layer (koilin)   143, 395,
    492, 493
host, intermediate
    (consumption)   56,
    213–215, 293, 299, 311
house
  humidity   47, 219, 462
  temperature   47, 49, 50, 55,
    111, 118, 219, 305, 412,
    505, 537, 551, 569, 586
housing   10, 14, 45, 46, 51–53,
    56, 58, 59, 74, 93, 94,
    112, 123, 159, 310, 343,
    447, 477, 505
HPAI (high pathogenicity avian
    influenza)   19, 229–231,
    304, 305

human consumption   8, 10, 13,
    15–18, 199, 288, 323,
    334, 373, 377, 450, 474,
    536
humerus
  abnormal   179
  bone   118
humidification, air   359
humidity
  egg incubation   250, 272,
    358, 376, 467, 472, 473
  house   47, 219, 462
  level   467
hybrid cross   24, 26, 27, 63
hydropericardium   324, 334
hydrostatic pressure
    325, 390
hydroxyapatite crystal(s)   118,
    119, 122
hygiene   6, 57, 124, 195, 198,
    556, 571
hyoidapparatus (bone)   136,
    141, 391, 481
hyperplasia   292, 330, 411, 412,
    422
hypersensitivity
    pneumonitis   204
hypertension   325–329, 335
  syndrome, pulmonary   325,
    328
hypertrophic
  cardiomyopathy   324, 325,
    329
  kidney   405
hypocalcemia   277, 279, 283,
    351, 363, 364
hypophysis cerebri (pituitary
    gland)   153, 444, 446
hypoxia   318
  egg incubation   324, 325

i

IBD (infectious bursal disease;
    Gumboro disease)   114,
    250, 260, 271, 296, 300,
    518, 519, 524, 590
  vaccine   586, 587, 589, 591
identification   98, 478, 505,
    508, 549, 551

identification (*cont'd*)
  abnormality 177, 187, 328, 359, 470
  agent 220–222, 231, 269, 303, 527, 529, 530
  band 98, 99, 201, 478, 505
  parasite 206, 210, 213, 509, 510, 529
  requirement 16
  rodent 52
  waterfowl 98
ileocecal
  junction 144
  ligament/fold 143, 399
ileum 143, 144, 208, 390, 399, 491, 493, 494
ileus 362
iliac
  artery 147–149, 327, 410, 419–421
  vein
    common 148, 149, 410, 419–421
    external 148, 149
ILT (infectious laryngotracheitis; laryngotracheitis; LT) 113, 114, 223–226, 361, 504, 507, 523, 526, 529, 584, 586, 587, 591
  vaccine 113, 223, 224, 584, 586, 587, 591
imaging
  cardiac 320, 321, 323, 325, 329, 333
  cloacal 174, 179–182, 184, 185, 189, 280, 320, 321, 323, 349, 361, 405, 406
  coelomic 174, 177–179, 181, 182, 184, 185, 187, 189, 190, 249, 422
  hepatic 320
imbibition
  bile 488
  hemoglobin 489
immune 257
  deficiency 196, 271

diffusion, agar gel 523, 527
  system 59, 87, 125, 127, 195, 206, 303, 523, 526, 585, 586
immunohistochemistry 332, 525
immunosorbent assay (ELISA), enzyme-linked 200, 203, 220, 224, 231, 248, 257, 308, 523–526
immunology (serology) 220, 221, 240, 248, 269–271, 287, 298, 305, 306, 506, 507, 515, 523, 531
impaction
  crop 292, 293, 362, 393
  esophageal 393
  oviduct 250, 275, 276, 412, 415, 422, 497
  sublingual 392
  ureteral 406
imprinting
  abnormal 91
  behavior 60, 61
  dog 91
  visual 60
  vocal 60
improper egg storage 471, 472
in egg (worms) 287, 474
in ovo 110, 113, 537, 547, 584, 586, 591
  injection 584, 586
inactivated vaccines 584–586, 590
inactivity 57, 78, 79, 91, 94, 102, 230, 232, 364
  gonadal 121
incubation, egg 460, 467–471, 473, 586
  humidity 250, 272, 358, 376, 467, 472, 473
  hypoxia 324, 325
  temperature 272, 462, 467, 468, 472
incubator 227, 467, 468, 471, 472, 586
  forced air 461
  still air 461
indexed drugs 543, 564

indication for radiograph 348
infection(s)
  bone 300, 308, 385
  cardiac 318, 330, 332, 334
  fungal 226, 227, 326, 331, 359, 364, 518, 569
  hen-to-egg 18, 219, 224, 249, 250, 257, 262, 269, 280, 281, 296, 471, 472, 474
  joint 220, 237, 239, 240, 244–246, 579
  yolk 280, 281, 309, 416
infectious
  anemia, chicken (chicken anemia virus; CAV) 260, 271, 518, 587
  bronchitis 113, 114, 123, 161, 166, 204, 220, 221, 223, 224, 279–284, 286, 287, 305, 309, 310, 359, 383, 406, 463, 474, 494, 510, 523–525
    vaccine 233, 304, 587, 589–591
  bursal disease (IBD) 114, 250, 260, 271, 296, 300, 518, 519, 524, 590
    vaccine 586, 587, 589, 591
  coryza (infectious coryza) 114, 221, 223, 224, 507, 575–577, 579
    vaccine 590
  egg 471, 472, 480
  laryngotracheitis (ILT; laryngotracheitis; LT) 113, 114, 223–226, 361, 504, 507, 523, 526, 529, 584, 586, 587, 591
    vaccine 113, 223, 224, 584, 586, 587, 591
inflammation 78, 85, 167, 204, 210, 213, 215, 226, 234, 260, 271, 280, 281, 300, 311, 363, 383, 385, 388, 405, 411, 415, 416, 426, 489, 492, 587

influenza, avian 10–14, 18, 19,
    108, 111, 202, 203, 223,
    224, 229, 230, 233, 281,
    283, 288, 301, 304, 331,
    332, 361, 504, 510,
    523–525, 529, 530, 547, 564
  high pathogenicity
    (HPAI) 19, 229–231,
    304, 305
  low pathogenicity 19, 230,
    231, 304, 305
infraorbital sinus 162, 222,
    480, 500, 501
  chamber(s) 383
  diverticulum (rostral
    diverticulum) 383, 387
  surgery 383, 385–387
  swelling 383–386
infundibular slit
    (cleft) 141–142
infundibulum 150, 151, 299,
    409–411, 416, 418, 462,
    463, 465, 466, 468, 497
infusion broth, brain-
    heart 471, 472
ingluvial nerves 394
ingluviectomy 394, 395
ingluvies (crop) 70, 118, 133,
    135, 137, 140, 142, 163,
    172, 328, 362, 394, 483,
    484
ingluviotomy 349, 393, 394
ingredients, feed 118, 119,
    124–126, 547, 548
inhibition, hemagglutination
    203, 220, 288, 523
injection 586, 588
  breast 585, 586
  contrast media 320
  crop 585
  in ovo 584, 586
  intra-articular 356
  intracardiac 458, 460
  intracoelomic 458
  intramuscular 149, 265,
    365, 405, 407, 580, 584,
    585

intraosseous 458
intravenous 458, 459
  neck 575, 585
  needle 422
  sinus 580
  subcutaneous 575, 584, 585,
    590, 591
  swelling 202
  wing 585, 581, 590
injury 53, 98, 139, 177, 291,
    352, 358, 436–439, 510
  beak 356, 437
  leg 236, 252
  liver 80
  neck 260, 285, 353, 356,
    359, 389, 450
  nerve 371
  shoulder 173, 255
  soft tissue 186, 255, 265,
    450
  wing 79, 173, 177, 255, 266,
    353, 459
inner tympanic
    membrane 147
insemination, artificial 466
Inspection
  Act
    Egg Products 16, 17
    Poultry Products (PPIA)
    15
  Service
    Animal and Plant
    (APHIS) 5, 13–15, 19,
    107, 108, 569, 570
    Food Safety and
    (FSIS) 15, 17, 538, 540,
    542, 555
instructions, safe (egg)
    handling 16
insufficiency
  nutritional 271
  valvular 321, 325, 330,
    332
insulation 51, 513, 566
insulin 146, 257
intake
  drug 567

feed 51, 52, 118, 123, 218,
    259, 277, 281, 283–286,
    312, 326, 362, 374, 395,
    407, 523, 551, 567
  lipid 80
  water (factors) 118, 127,
    218, 399, 551
integument 269–271
intensity, light 48, 54, 100,
    101, 275, 282, 285, 306,
    328, 436, 447, 450, 470
inter-duodenal ligament 143
interference, chemical
    test 510
interlobular
  septum 139
  vein 148, 149
intermediate
  host consumption 56,
    213–215, 293, 299, 311
  zone 142–144, 153
interna theca 462
internal shell membrane
    464–466, 469
interorbital septum 134
interval, withdrawal
    (WDI) 323, 544, 549,
    553–555
intestinal
  entrapment 397
  fluid 81, 178, 400
  health 127, 289
  lesion(s) 206, 300
  nodule 291, 294, 300, 305
  roundworm 215, 287, 298,
    306, 474, 572
  scraping 299
intestine 125, 140, 143, 190,
    197, 231, 232, 247, 283,
    284, 297–299, 300,
    301, 302, 304, 377,
    397, 398, 400, 489–491,
    493–495
  large 140, 231, 232, 247,
    283, 284, 297, 300, 301,
    304, 377, 397, 398, 400,
    489–491, 493–495

intestine (*cont'd*)
  small   125, 140, 143, 178,
      190, 215, 197, 231, 232,
      247, 283, 284, 297–299,
      300–304, 377, 397, 398,
      489–491, 493–495
intra-articular injection   356
intracardiac
  injection   458, 460
  parasite(s)   331
intracellular
  bacteria (obligate)   301
  calcium   328
  cholesterol   272
  parasite   206
intracoelomic   405, 566
  injection   458
intralobular vein(s)   149
intrameduallary pin   252–255,
      350
intramuscular injection   149,
      265, 365, 405, 407, 580,
      584, 585
intraosseous (IO)
  catheter   265, 345, 350–352,
      458, 566–568
  fluids therapy   265, 345, 350,
      351, 458, 566, 568
  injection(s)   458
intrarenal   148
intravenous (IV)
  catheter (IV)   265, 268, 320,
      345, 350–353, 355, 356,
      358, 365, 382, 397, 406
  fluid additives   351
  fluid therapy   265, 268, 345,
      350, 351, 355, 356, 358,
      365, 382, 459, 566
  injection(s)   458, 459
intubation   361, 382
  air sac   360
  endotracheal   388, 389
ionophore(s)   128, 300
  toxicosis   368, 376
iron   119, 121
  deficiency   518, 581
  dextran   581

Peri's (iron) stain   525
  supplementation   119, 121,
      126, 369, 372
ischiadic (ischiatic; sciatic)
  artery   138, 410
  nerve   120, 136, 138, 237,
      246, 247, 307, 332, 499,
      500
Island Red, Rhode (breed)
      24–26, 164, 410, 569
islet(s)
  alpha   146
  beta   146
  dark   146
  light   146
islet of Langerhans   146, 153
isolation
  broth, virus   511
  health   47, 51, 53, 55, 77, 79,
      82, 84, 88, 99, 101, 102,
      110, 112, 117–119, 122,
      128, 139, 145, 154, 208,
      289, 290, 318, 407, 416,
      434, 447, 448, 452, 520,
      549, 551
isthmus
  oviduct   151, 409, 463, 468,
      497
  stomach   142, 395, 396, 403,
      492, 493
ivermectin   211, 214, 261, 262,
      573

j
jecur (liver)   145
jejunum   143–145, 208, 491,
      493, 494
Jersey Giant (breed)   29–32
joint(s)   177, 178, 239, 254,
      322, 347, 357, 375, 482,
      502
  abnormality   57, 249, 253
  capsule   502, 503
  exudate   509
  false   254
  infection   220, 237, 239, 240,
      244–246, 579

tibiotarsal-tarsometatarsal
      (hock)   120, 135, 167,
      171, 221, 235, 237, 239,
      240, 244, 245, 253, 255,
      295, 579
  urates   310
jugular vein   155, 348, 350,
      458, 459, 483, 484, 490,
      506, 509, 566
junction, 14 (anatomical
      landmarks)   2, 145, 146,
      153, 155, 390, 398, 406,
      416, 418, 421, 424, 485,
      489, 490, 492, 497
  ileocecal   144, 145, 399, 493,
      494
jungle fowl, red   23, 435, 446

k
kaolin clay   262
keel (carina)   136
  bone   112, 136, 272, 289,
      306, 321, 478, 585
    curved keel bone   122,
      163, 165, 284, 363
  fracture   328
kidney   145, 147–150, 154,
      390, 418, 426, 499,
      500
  capsule   148
  cortex   148
  damage   123, 310, 405, 406,
      421
  diagnostic   369, 370, 402,
      554
  disease   85, 216, 247, 249,
      307, 329, 404–406, 416
  health   85
  lobe   147, 150
  stone   123
  surgery   404, 406, 425
  weight   85, 406
Klebsiella   276, 470
Knemidokoptes mutans   261,
      262
koilin   143, 395, 492, 493
  green   492

l

label requirements, prescription 548, 549
labeling
  egg 16, 17
  feed 128, 540, 544, 565, 566
labial cleft 145
labii 145
laboratory 108, 200, 203, 207, 222, 245, 288, 290, 308, 318, 369, 375, 402, 405, 481, 489, 494, 504, 509, 512–515, 523, 527–529, 543, 556
  Animal Health (AHL) 317, 330
  Diagnosticians (AAVLD), American Association of Veterinary 541
  National Veterinary Services (NVSL) 231, 233
  Network, National Animal Health (NAHLN) 231, 232
lacrimal duct 406
  cannula 406
lactams, beta- 554
lactophenol 227
Lakenvelder (breed) 24, 26
lameness 167, 170, 174, 186, 187, 221, 234, 235, 239, 242, 244, 245, 249, 250, 355, 364, 374, 376, 422, 505
lamp/bulb, heat 49, 50, 361, 377, 378, 448, 450
land zone 4, 7, 8, 10
Langerhans, islet of 146, 153
large intestine 140, 232, 400
largyngotracheitis, infectious (ILT; laryngotracheitis; LT) 113, 114, 223–226, 361, 504, 507, 523, 526, 529, 584, 586, 587, 591
  vaccine 113, 223, 224, 584, 586, 587, 591

larvae
  contamination 90
  migration 214, 306
larval migrans
  neural 214
  visceral 214
laryngeal nerve(s) 388
larynx 142, 147, 223, 225, 303
  lower (syrinx; caudallarynx) 142, 146, 147, 182–184, 226, 288, 349, 486, 487, 498
  upper (glottis; cranial larynx) 124, 146, 291, 568
latebra 465
  neck 464, 465
latissimus dorsi muscle 136, 137
layer fatigue, cage 283, 363, 464
layer(s)
  chalaziferous 463
  egg 24, 29, 298, 412, 446, 464, 569
  Easter egg 24, 26
  fatigue, caged (osteomalacia) 283, 363, 464
  horny (koilin) 143, 395, 492, 493
laying
  breeds (egg breeds) 23–26, 29, 141, 298, 412, 446, 464, 569
  cessation of 48, 54, 101, 102, 122, 231, 276, 277, 281, 377, 412
  hen 7, 46, 48, 54, 100, 118, 120–124, 126–128, 150, 151, 153, 159, 167, 181, 182, 184, 187, 230, 249, 250, 275, 277–281, 283–285, 287, 305, 311, 312, 395, 407, 418, 436, 444–446, 466, 474
lead
  concentration, bone 369–371, 374

  contamination 373
  levels, abnormal 370
  toxicosis 368–370
    clinical signs 369
    diagnosis 369
    sources 368
    treatment 370
    weight 368
leafy green(s) 80, 88, 90, 159, 198
leakage, air 390
learning
  chick 437, 441
leg
  abnormality 235
  band 98, 201
  bandage 240, 242, 250, 251
    Robert-Jones 254, 354
    tie-over 268
  bone 172, 442
  contraction 256
  injury 236, 252
  mite, scaly 261, 262
  splay (spraddle) 250
  spraddle (splay) 250
legal requirements, compounding 372, 541, 547–549
legally market 542, 543, 555
Leghorn (breed) 23–26, 28, 29, 84, 161, 164, 237, 238, 246, 298, 319, 322, 327, 446, 448, 459, 516, 518–520, 568, 579, 581
length(s), day 100, 101, 279–283, 285
lentogenic 203, 232, 303
lesion(s)
  beak 91, 118, 120, 125, 172, 257, 270, 273, 356, 385, 392, 437, 473, 480, 481
  cardiac (heart) 294, 307, 308, 330–332, 377
  fluid (-filled) 272, 277–280, 407, 412, 413, 417, 485, 495, 498, 505
  foot 234–236, 241

lesion(s) (*cont'd*)
  intestinal 206, 300
  liver 311
  neurological 234, 246, 247, 364
  respiratory 220, 359, 360, 386
  reproductive 277, 426, 497
  skin 260
leucocyte 518
leukocytic protozoa 216
leucocytozoon 331, 333
leucosis (leukosis) 518, 519
  avian 246, 248–250, 307, 308, 331, 384, 388, 518, 519
  virus 246, 249, 250, 331
levamisole 226, 293
level
  activity 77
  biosafety 200
  eye 51, 160
  hormone 139
  humidity 467
  stress 287, 440
  toxicosis 369, 375, 376
Leydig cell 150, 153
lice 112, 166, 259–261, 573
life
  quality 84
  stages diet needs 122, 123, 159, 166, 250, 256, 286, 287, 312, 326, 334, 354, 446, 464, 473
    nutrient needs 123, 124, 128
ligament
  ileocecal (fold) 143, 399
  interduodenal 143
  ovarian 419
  oviductal 410, 415, 418, 463
  propatagial 138
light
  bulb 50
  enrichment 92
  exposure 48, 93, 100, 102, 126, 282, 285, 407, 444, 446

intensity 48, 54, 100, 101, 275, 282, 285, 306, 328, 436, 447, 450, 470
  magnified 382, 385
  microscope 211
  neuter 62
  red 50, 54
  reflex 358
  white 50
lighting, schedule 277, 286
limberneck (botulism) 76, 113, 114, 214, 233, 256, 284, 368, 377
limbic region 152
lingual
  frenulum 141, 392, 393
  papilla(e) 141
linoleic acid 83, 85
linolenic acid 83
  body temperature 166, 347
lipid
  accumulation 80
  core (atheroma) 335
  intake 80
lipidosis, hepatic 88, 362, 424
lipogenesis, hepatic 80, 101
listeriosis 199
litter 45–47, 49, 51, 53, 54, 88, 110, 125, 219, 234, 236, 246, 297, 298, 300, 302, 308
live vaccines 203, 525, 584, 586–591
liver (hepar; jecur) 145
  capsule 224, 302, 311, 312, 334, 487
  fatty liver (disease)
    syndrome 80, 100, 312, 328, 407, 518
  fracture 312, 362
  injury 80
  lesion(s) 311
  nodules 300
  radiograph 306, 326, 401
  weight 80

lobe(s)
  cerebellar 152
  ear 25, 31, 32, 36, 44, 133, 160, 161, 163, 464
  hepatic 145, 146, 390, 402, 403, 487–489
  kidney 147, 150
  optic 152
  pancreatic 146, 403, 404
  splenic 146, 403
  thymus 155, 483, 484
  uropygial 139, 163
lobule
  renal 149
  pineal 153
local
  analgesia 267, 355, 360, 363
  hatchery 10, 12, 13, 24, 113, 198, 226, 248, 295, 296, 310, 586, 590
  ordinances 4, 5, 8–10
locomotion 94, 445
  wing 170
loop
  diuretic 324
  duodenal 143, 146, 397, 398, 403, 404
  supraduodenal 390
loss
  blood 294, 297, 346, 352, 516
  feather 265, 282, 283, 505
    breast 70, 71, 282, 283
    excessive 51, 282
  moisture 569
  shell color 286, 287
louse (lice)
  head (*Culclotogaster heterographa*) 260
  body (*Menacanthus stramineus*) 259–261
  shaft (*Menopon gallinae*) 260, 261
low
  blood calcium 154, 277, 283, 363, 365, 395, 520, 521

pathogenicity avian influenza (LPAI) 19, 230, 231, 304, 305
lower larynx (syrnx; caudal larynx) 124, 146, 291, 568
LPAI (low pathogenicity avian influenza) 19, 230, 231, 304, 305
LT (laryngotracheitis; infectious laryngotracheitis; ILT) 113, 114, 223–226, 361, 504, 507, 523, 526, 529, 584, 586, 587, 591
  vaccine 113, 223, 224, 584, 586, 587, 591
lucency, air 179
lumbar región 135, 153, 404, 421, 422
  disease 182, 226, 231, 232, 301, 307, 308, 324, 328, 332, 334, 361, 378, 390
  endoscopy 349
  farmer's 204
  hemorrhagic 231, 378
  pigeon breeder's 204
  poultry worker's 204
  radiograph 180, 181, 348, 349
lymph nodes 163
lymphatic
  cell 143, 155, 423
  flow 423
  fold 423
  nodule 143, 155
  system 155
  vessels 155
lymphatic nodules 143
lymphocyte(s) 155, 156, 257, 269, 296, 306, 308, 324, 332, 516, 517, 519
lymphoid
  follicle(s) 142
  leucosis/leukosis 518, 519
  tissue, mural 155
lymphoma

cutaneous (Marek's disease) 269, 270
hepatic 269, 307
ocular 247
skin 259

m

MacConkeys media (agar) 470, 471
Magellan goose/geese 92
maggots 113, 256, 265, 377
magnified light 382, 385
magnum
  foramen 502
  gland(s) 151, 463
magpie goose/geese 69
maintenance fluid therapy 351, 566
malaria, avian 214
malathion dust 262, 263
male
  genital system 150
  hen 438
malformations 468
  cloacal 185
  skeletal 82, 121
Mallard (breed) 57–60, 63, 64, 67, 69–71, 73, 74, 76, 87–90, 94, 99, 182, 184, 389, 581
management 45–55
  Anseriformes 56–106
  chick 49, 86, 118, 128, 449, 571, 574, 575
  carcass 6, 112, 113, 460
  egg 466
  health 107
  pain 99, 102, 381, 382
  waterfowl 45, 69–71, 73, 74, 76, 77, 79–102, 118, 467
  wound 235, 251, 259, 268, 352–354, 357, 364
manganese
  deficiency 240, 249
  supplementation 119, 121, 240, 249
Maran (breed) 24–29

Marek's disease 3, 11, 113, 114, 161, 167, 170, 187, 233, 246–249, 269, 306–308, 330, 331, 335, 364–365, 393, 394, 500, 507, 518, 519, 523, 525, 584, 590, 591
  cutaneous lymphoma 260, 269, 270
  vaccine 584–586, 590, 591
marker, nasal 99
market(s)
  age 537
  export 107, 505
  farmers(s)'s 10, 17, 18, 546
  flea 12, 17, 542
  legally 542, 543, 555
  livebird 18, 304
  weight 30, 537
marrow, bone 125, 185, 187, 300, 519, 538
  nodule 300
mate 91
  cage/pen 59, 110, 260
  exposure 91, 446
  selection 59, 407, 443, 444
material(s), suture 382, 383, 392, 398, 407, 416, 418
mating
  behavior 99, 100, 424, 444, 450, 466
  excessive 450
matrix (eggshell), organic 464, 466
MCV (mean corpuscular volume) 516, 517
mean corpuscular volume (MCV) 516, 517
meal, meat and bone 119, 126, 373
meat
  bird 46, 48, 201, 221
  bone meal, and 119, 126, 373
  to bone ratio 67

meat (*cont'd*)
  breed(s)   23, 29, 31, 32, 272, 469, 569
  spot(s)   285, 286, 473, 474
meatus
  external acoustic   133, 136, 156, 163
mebendazole   226
Meckel's diverticulum (vitelline diverticulum)   143, 145, 468, 494
media
  Aimes transport   507, 508, 510, 511
  bacterial   471, 472
  Cary-Blair transport   510
  contrast   177, 349, 395, 396, 405
    injection   320
  MacConkeys   470, 471
  Mycoplasma transport   478, 479
  Stuart transport media   507, 508, 510, 511
  transport   510–513
  viral transport   478, 479
median
  eminence   153
  fold   141
medical
  Association (AVMA), American Veterinary   457, 545, 565
  diet   397, 407, 446
  record ELDU requirements   548
  Treatment Act, Preservation of Antibiotics for (PAMTA)   550
medicated
  dust   262, 573
  feeds   89, 549, 550, 564
    compliance policy (minor species)   540, 545
  drinking water medication   86, 118, 292, 310, 549, 565, 568, 571–574, 577

medication
  anticoccidial   208, 209, 297, 376, 473, 571–573, 580
  antimicrobial(s)   127, 271, 323, 333, 334, 363, 381, 382, 412, 416, 426, 549, 550, 556–558, 564, 569, 571, 579
  antiparasitic   536, 571–573
  antiviral   202, 353, 546, 547
    prohibited   547
  aspergillosis   579, 580
  cardiac   323
  ELDU (extra-label drug use)   536, 541, 544–548, 552–555, 558, 562–566, 571
  FDA prohibited medications list   536, 540, 541, 544–547, 563–565, 568
  formulary (medications)   56, 118, 520, 535, 536, 543–545, 547–553, 556, 562, 563, 566–573
  routes of administration   536, 544, 545, 547, 549, 552, 553, 564–567, 579
  VFD (Veterinary Feed Directive)   127, 549, 550, 565, 566
medication   563, 573, 579, 580, 581
Medicinal Drug Use Clarification Act of, 1994 (AMDUCA)   536, 540, 541, 544, 545, 548, 549, 552, 554, 556
Mediterranean Class (Standard of Perfection breeds)   24, 25, 31, 37
medium spray droplet   589
medulla oblongata   152, 153
melanoma
  cutaneous   272, 273
  intraosseous   273

melatonin   153
membrane
  culture, egg   471
  dehydrated shell   467
  semilunar   147, 489
  shell   284, 285, 465, 466, 469, 471, 472, 497
    external   151, 464, 466, 474
    internal   464–466, 469
    ruptured   474
  tympanic
    external   147
    internal   147
  yolk   463, 465
Menacanthus stramineus (body louse)   259–261
meninges   152
meningioma   248
Menopon gallinae (shaft louse)   260, 261
mesencephalon   152
mesenteric vein, caudal   148, 149
mesoderm   468
mesogenic   232, 303
mesothelioma   248
mesotubarium   150, 151
metabolism
  calcium   154, 283, 284, 287, 335, 369, 372, 375, 376, 412, 444, 445, 464, 581
  hepatic fat   85
metacarpal bone(s)   177
metatarsal
  artery   347
  fold   139
  region   133, 135, 137, 139, 164, 167, 170, 171, 177, 186–188, 237, 238, 244, 246, 253, 265, 347, 348, 350, 354, 441, 506, 509, 566, 579
  spur   137, 139, 187, 438, 481
  vein   265, 350, 506, 509, 566, 579

methionine (methyl hydroxyl)
  analog   126
  dietary   81
methyl hydroxyl (methionine)
  analog   126
MG (*Mycoplasma
  gallisepticum*)   11, 112,
  219–221, 240, 281, 301,
  331, 383–385, 507, 523,
  525, 574–576, 578, 579
  vaccine   584, 586, 589–591
microbial growth   127, 222,
  235, 245, 299, 302, 398,
  471, 472, 478, 527, 528,
  537
microbiology   471, 506, 515,
  520, 526, 530
microscope
  light   210, 211, 261, 262, 511,
  529
  operating   425
midline
  beak (culmen)   140
  ventral   390, 391, 396–400,
  402, 404, 408, 411, 413,
  416, 418, 420, 424
migration   79, 101
  cloacal   287, 415
  larvae   214, 306
migratory waterfowl, North
  American   102, 108,
  229, 230
milk, crop   142
mineral
  clay (vermiculite)   88, 118
  deficiencies   118, 121, 122,
  141, 281, 287
  supplementation   77, 84,
  118, 119, 121, 126–129,
  174, 177, 178, 181, 190
mineralization
  bone   84, 93, 119, 122, 464
minor
  species, medicated feeds
  compliance policy   540,
  545
  Use

Animal Drug Program
  (MUADP)   541, 543
Minor Species Animal
  Health Act (MUMS)
  542, 543
misshapen egg   108, 185, 286,
  412, 474
mite(s)
  chicken (*Dermanyssus
  gallinae*)   111, 112, 166,
  259, 261–264, 510, 518, 573
  northern fowl (*Ornithonyssus
  sylviarum*)   261, 262
  scaly leg (*Knemidocoptes
  mutans*)   261, 262
mixed breeds   61, 72, 73, 101,
  408, 414
MM (*Mycoplasma meleagridis*)
  11, 240
mobilization, fluid   347, 352
modification
  beak   53, 54, 59, 91, 141,
  275, 281, 282, 306, 480
  behavioral   100, 391, 401,
  424, 438
  environmental   59, 91, 371,
  375, 409, 434, 448
  nutritional   328
modified agglutination test
  (MAT)   214
moisture
  accumulation   47, 259, 471
  air   219
  barrier   236
  corneal   163
  excessive   309
  feed content   118, 126
  loss   569
  removal   46, 47, 49, 119, 219
mold growth   110, 127
molt   26, 51, 54, 99, 101, 122,
  281, 283, 474
  planned   283
molting   54, 67, 282, 283, 296,
  439, 474, 505, 520
monitoring
  anesthetic   240

chick   470
disease   99, 102, 289, 296,
  324, 399, 515, 531
  drinking   118
  drug   538
  health   277, 289, 312, 345,
  347, 348, 351, 477, 505,
  515, 523, 526, 527, 530,
  531, 556
  rodent   53
  Salmonella   11
monocyte   517, 519
moth-eaten feather(s)   260
motor nerve(s)   369
mouth   120, 125, 133, 140, 141,
  146, 168, 171, 196, 211, 212,
  220, 223, 226, 261, 262, 290,
  295, 327, 450, 479, 480, 568
movement, air   46, 360, 390
MS (*Mycoplasma synoviae*)   11,
  220, 221, 237, 239, 240,
  246, 507, 523, 574–576,
  578, 579
MUADP (Minor Use Animal
  Drug Program)   541,
  543
mucosa   143, 152, 208, 226,
  231, 232, 290, 292, 293,
  297–299, 305, 392, 398,
  401, 427, 490–494, 498,
  510
Mullerian duct   277, 409
mule(s)   63, 67, 70, 80
MUMS (Minor Use/Minor
  Species Animal Health
  Act)   542, 543
municipal ordinances   9
mural
  endocarditis   333, 488
  granuloma   305
  lymphoid tissue   155
  thickening   493
muscle(s)
  alular   136
  biceps brachii   136–138
  cardiac (heart)   121, 328,
  333

muscle(s) (*cont'd*)
  cervical (pipping muscle) 586
  disease, white (muscular dystrophy) 121
  extensor carpi radialis 136–138
  extensor carpi ulnaris 136, 137
  femorotibial 138
  flexor carpi ulnaris 136–138
  flexor crural 137, 138
  green muscle 255, 268, 357
  hatching 472
  latissimus dorsi 136, 137
  pectoral (muscle score) 77–79
  pipping (cervical muscle) 586
  pronator 136–138
  quadriceps femoris 136, 138
  sartorius 136, 138
  trachealis 146
  trapezius 136
  wing 82, 137
Muscovy (breed) 57, 58, 60, 62–64, 67, 68, 71, 80, 81, 83, 91, 331, 426, 467
muscular stomach (ventriculus; gizzard) 88, 117, 126, 127, 140, 142–144, 155, 166, 174, 178–182, 190, 231, 257, 294, 328, 349, 369, 370, 390, 393, 395–397, 486, 488–493
muscular dystrophy (white muscle disease) 121
musculoskeletal
  diseases 234, 237, 255, 309, 482
  system 173, 186, 187, 234, 345, 364, 505
    radiograph(s) 173–175, 186, 235, 240, 241, 243, 249, 251, 253, 354, 364, 365, 460

mycelia 226, 227
mycobacteriosis, avian 201, 202, 300, 301, 306, 519
Mycobacterium 331, 360
  avium 201
    subspecies *avium* 300
  genevense 201
Mycoplasma 12, 220, 221, 240, 245, 279, 309, 360, 478, 479, 507, 510, 511, 524, 526, 528
  agglutination 524
  gallisepticum (MG; chronic respiratory disease, CRD) 11, 112, 219–221, 240, 281, 301, 309, 331, 383–385, 507, 523, 525, 574–576, 578, 579
    vaccine 584, 586, 589–591
  meleagridis (MM) 11, 240
  synoviae (MS) 11, 220, 221, 237, 239, 240, 246, 507, 523, 574–576, 578, 579
  transport media 510–513
mycoplasmosis 114, 200, 219, 220–222, 224, 240, 579, 580
mycosis (candidiasis; crop mycosis) 114, 211–213, 290–293, 362, 579
mycotoxicosis 376
mycotoxin(s) 111, 124, 125, 128, 376, 480, 481, 518
  contamination 124, 125, 128
myeloblastosis 308
myelocytomatosis 308
myenteric plexus(es) 395
myiasis 357
myocardium 121, 155, 257, 332, 488
myology 136
myoma 248
myxosarcoma 248

n
NAHLN (National Animal Health Laboratory Network) 231, 232
nails 71, 168
nares
  external 134, 136, 140
NSAIDs (non-steroidal anti-inflammatory drugs) analgesia 355
nasal 133, 134, 136, 500, 501
  arch 133, 134
  cavity 141, 146
  discharge 108, 161, 200, 202, 270, 301–303, 505
  flush 361
  marker 99
  opening 133
  vaccine 586
National
  Animal Health Laboratory Network (NAHLN) 231, 232
  Poultry Improvement Plan (NPIP) 10–12, 18, 113, 195, 220, 242, 281, 294–296
    hatchery 10, 12
  Research
    Council (NRC) 76, 77, 81, 86
    Support Project-7 (NRSP-7) 543
  Residue Program (NRP) 538
  Veterinary Services Laboratory (NVSL) 231, 233
natural
  orifices 133
  pest control 434
ND (Newcastle disease) 13, 14, 19, 111, 113, 114, 195, 202, 203, 221, 223, 224, 229, 231, 257, 281, 290, 302–304, 309, 331, 361, 383, 504, 524, 584, 589–591
  vaccine 584, 587, 589–591

virulent (VND; vvND; END) 229, 231–233

virus 302, 303, 383, 584, 587, 591

neck 31, 36, 38, 41, 42, 67, 74, 78, 79, 117, 133–135, 142, 155, 166, 167, 224, 231, 234, 247, 256, 260, 270, 282, 283, 360, 388, 444, 447, 450, 472, 483, 484, 568, 574, 575

collar 98, 99

flaccid 246, 306

injections 575, 585

injury 260, 285, 353, 356, 359, 389, 450

latebra 464, 465

positions 256

swelling 108, 260, 271, 304

tremors 257

twisted 108, 505

necropsy (postmortem examination) 6, 35, 113, 122, 143, 165, 168, 184, 190, 200, 212, 213, 218, 220, 222, 224, 235, 237, 239, 245, 247, 248, 250, 256, 273, 276–279, 290, 296, 298, 300, 301, 303, 307, 326–328, 330–333, 363, 365, 370, 376–378, 382, 389, 391, 397, 400, 415, 459, 473, 477, 478, 502, 510, 511, 520, 523, 528

techniques 477–502

necrosis

central 216

hepatic 124, 199, 302, 489

footpad 259

necrotic

dermatitis 271, 296, 427

enteritis 125, 296, 299, 300, 574, 575, 578, 580

needle

biopsy 402

injection 422

needs, nutrient (lifestage) 123, 124, 128

negative pressure 353

neighborhood association 4, 5

nematode(s) 209, 212–215, 226, 293, 298, 299, 305, 331, 373, 528

Neoschongastia americana (adult form of chiggers) 263, 264

nephron 85, 148, 149

nerve(s) 84, 234, 256, 306, 352, 357, 396, 436, 581, 585

brachial 237, 255, 256, 307, 581

cervical spinal 152

cranial 153

ingluvial 394

injury 371

ischiatic (ischiadic; sciatic) 120, 136, 138, 237, 246, 247, 307, 332, 499, 500

laryngeal 388

motor 369

myenteric 395

peripheral 307, 369

plexus 246, 255, 256, 395, 421, 422, 499, 581

sacral 421, 422

sciatic (ischiadic; ischiatic) 120, 136, 138, 237, 246, 247, 307, 332, 499, 500

vagus 483

nervous system 149, 232, 303, 371, 468, 505

central 152, 214, 234

peripheral 234, 257

nest

box (nestbox) 45, 46, 53, 54, 100, 159, 275, 281, 282, 443–446, 450, 451, 573

sanitation 471

nest-to-hen ratio 46, 275, 306

nesting área 45, 46, 54, 71, 96, 100, 281, 284, 295, 306, 438, 444–446, 451, 468, 471, 573

Network, National Animal Health Laboratory (NAHLN) 231, 232

neural larval migrans 214

neuraminidase 202, 230, 304, 523, 546, 564

neuritis

optic 216

peripheral 237

neuroendocrine 153

neurological

disease 67, 214, 246, 257, 307, 364, 374

lesion(s) 234, 246, 247, 364

signs 199, 357, 358

neurotropic 232

neuter, light 62

New

Animal Drug Evaluation, Office (ONADE) 552

Hampshire (breed) 24, 29, 31, 32

Newcastle disease (ND; APMV-1; PMV-1) 13, 14, 19, 111, 113, 114, 195, 202, 203, 221, 223, 224, 229, 231, 257, 281, 290, 302–304, 309, 331, 361, 383, 504, 524, 584, 589–591

vaccine 584, 587, 589–591

virus 302, 303, 383, 584, 587, 591

viscerotropic velogenic (vvND) 229, 231–233

Newcastle-upon-Tyne 232

niacin (nicotinic acid) 86

deficiency 86, 120

dietary 86

supplementation 86, 120

nicarbazin 87, 89, 209, 232, 287, 550

contamination 287

nicotinic acid (niacin) 86, 120

deficiency 86, 120

dietary 86

supplementation 86, 120

nitrofuran(s)   334, 546, 558, 564
nodes, lymph   163
nodules   294
  bone marrow   300
  granulomatous   300
  heart   294, 331
  intestinal   291, 294, 300, 305
  liver   300
  lymphatic   143, 155
  oral (plaques)   291
  parathyroid   154
  skin   247, 291, 588
  spleen   300
  ventricular   257
  white   206, 226, 257, 294, 300
non-infectious   195, 384, 415, 508, 525
North American migratory waterfowl   102, 108, 229, 230
northern fowl mite (*Ornithonyssus sylviarum*)   261, 262
nostrils   76, 161, 270
NPIP (National Poultry Improvement Plan)   10–12, 18, 113, 195, 220, 242, 281, 294–296
  hatchery   10, 12
NRC (National Research Council)   76, 77, 81, 86
NRSP-7 *see* National Research Support Project-7
NSAIDs (non-steroidal anti-inflammatory drugs)   355
nucleic acid   531
nucleus, central   465
nutrient needs (lifestage)   123, 124, 128
nutrition   76, 77, 81, 87, 88, 117–129, 153, 206, 269, 283, 289, 310, 330, 354, 363, 397, 462, 472, 473, 477, 520, 556
nutritional

deficiencies   54, 80, 87, 89, 99, 112, 117, 128, 145, 256, 271, 281, 283, 284, 287, 326, 329, 334, 406, 407, 409, 412, 508, 511, 518, 525
diarrhea   237
disease   89, 112, 120
insufficiency   271
modification(s)   328
status   145, 275, 369, 487
support   354, 362, 371
supplementation   52, 77, 87, 122, 123, 128, 145, 545

O
obesity   57, 60, 78, 80, 85, 88, 91, 93, 234, 277, 363, 364, 407, 412
obligate intracellular bacteria   301
oblique septum   155
occipital   135, 152, 506
ochratoxin   124, 125, 518
ocular lymphoma   247
oculonasal discharge   163, 221, 301, 383
Office of New Animal Drug Evaluation (ONADE)   552
Official Analytical Chemists, Association of (AOAC)   556
oils, and fats   126
oleic acid   85
olfactory
  bulb   152
  cortex   152
omega-3 fatty acids   82, 83, 85, 326, 335
omega-6 fatty acids   82, 83
omega-9 fatty acids   85
omphalitis   295, 308, 309, 471, 472
ONADE (Office of New Animal Drug Evaluation)   552
oncovirus(es)   306, 308

type C   308
onion, green   378
on-label drug use   536, 546, 547, 552, 553, 558
oocyte(s)   419, 464, 465, 528, 529
  primary   462
oophoritis   280, 411, 420, 422
opaca, area   468
opening, nasal   133
operating microscope   425
opioid(s) analgesia   355
opisthotonos   231, 256
optic
  chiasma   153
  disk   156
  foramen   136
  lobe(s)   152
  neuritis   216
  tectum (rostral colliculus)   152
  tract   152
oral
  cyst(s)   391
  fluid therapy   350
  nodules (plaques)   291
  region   124, 141, 142, 160, 161, 163, 168, 171, 172, 211, 212, 290, 292, 305, 344, 346, 347, 357, 375, 391–393, 478, 480, 490, 529, 568
  scraping   529
orbital región   133, 134
order, pecking (social order)   39, 62, 438, 467
ordinances
  city(ies)/local   4–10
  municipal   9
organ, copulatory (phallus)   60, 62, 69, 91, 100, 150, 363, 423, 426, 427
organic
  acid   127
  debris
    build-up   111

removal   113, 198, 201, 466

matrix (eggshell)   464, 466

production   18, 571

Organization, World Health (WHO)   203, 555

orifices (natural)   133

Orloff (breed)   30, 36, 39, 42, 236

ornamental breed(s)   23, 26, 30, 36, 38

Ornithobacterium   222

Ornithonyssus sylviarum   261

ornithosis (avian chlamydiosis)   195, 199–201, 301, 330, 332, 334

oropharynx   225, 290–293, 491, 509, 510, 527

Orpington (breed)   29–32, 170, 247

Buff   29–34

Orthomyxoviridae   202, 229

orthomyxovirus   304

osmotic pressure   520

osseous

syringeal bulla(ae)   69, 182, 184, 388, 389

osteogenic sarcoma   248

osteoma   248

osteomalacia (cage layer fatigue)   283, 363, 464

osteomyelitis   186, 187, 234, 235, 240, 241, 245, 251, 364

osteopetrosis   308

outdoor

access   32, 46, 50, 54, 56, 79, 93, 102, 357

lighting   100

outer shell membrane   151, 464, 466, 474

output, cardiac   318, 347

ovarian

artery   419, 421

aspiration   420, 422

carcinoma   250, 525

cyst(s)   420, 422

follicle(s)   127, 150, 281, 321, 410, 417–422, 462, 463, 465, 553

growth   282

ligament   419

stalk   154

ovariectomy   102, 419–423

ovary

abnormal   189

caseous   281

cystic   189, 410, 417, 420–422

misshapen   294

overgrowth

bacterial   398, 478, 527

beak   480

feet   167

yeast   291, 292

oviduct

caseous   276, 279, 280, 309

cystic   150, 151, 187, 249, 250, 277, 278, 410–412, 420, 495

impaction   250, 275, 276, 412, 415, 422, 497

isthmus   151, 409, 463, 468, 497

retained (cystic right)   151, 187, 277–278, 410, 411, 419

oviductal

artery   410, 416

aspiration   412, 416

congestion   415

content(s)   412, 416, 420

contraction   445

cyst(s)   412, 415

exudate   275, 276, 279–281, 309

ligament   410, 415, 418, 463

prolapse   362, 363, 412

ovulation   127, 185, 286, 409, 411, 417, 444, 462

ovum   150, 293, 409, 411, 462, 463, 468

oxalic acid   379

oximeter, pulse (comb)   240

oxyspiruriasis   213

p

pack cell volume (PCV; hematocrit)   271, 318, 325, 326, 347, 348, 375, 515–518, 523

pain   73, 167, 234, 249, 355, 356, 365, 406, 436, 437, 439, 459, 567

analgesia   235, 268, 355, 381, 382

management   99, 102, 381, 382

recognition   355

palate   125, 141

hard   141

palatine gland(s)   141

palpation, abnormal   166

PAMTA (Preservation of Antibiotics for Medical Treatment Act)   550

pancreas   143, 144, 146, 153, 247, 257, 374, 390, 403, 404, 468, 493

pancreatectomy   403, 404

pancreatic

cyst(s)   404

duct   146, 403

gland(s)   146

lobe   146, 403, 404

pandemic   202, 230

pantothenic acid   86, 120

dietary   86

papillae

choanal   141, 168, 480, 490

lingual   141

pharyngeal   141, 142

proventricular   143

urodeum   423

parabronchi (tertiary bronchi)   147

parafollicular cell (C cells)   153, 154

paralumbar fossa   390, 399, 404

paralysis

curled toe   86, 120, 237, 244

paralysis (*cont'd*)
  flaccid   256
  fowl paralysis   246
  range   167, 246, 306
Paramyxoviridae   302
paramyxovirus serotype, 1
    (APMV-1; Newcastle
    disease), avian   203,
    232, 279, 287, 302, 331,
    525
parasite
  cyst(s)   214, 331, 528
  identification   206, 210, 213,
    509, 510, 529
    prevention control   51, 89,
    110, 112, 259, 282, 298
  intracellular   206
parasitic diseases   89, 206–216,
    263, 294, 311, 362, 364,
    398, 518, 519, 528
parasitology   207, 226, 506,
    529, 571
parasympathetic   149
parathormone   154
parathyroid
  accessory   154
  gland(s)   153, 154, 487
  nodules   154
paratyphoid   114, 280, 296
  Salmonella   296
parrot fever (avian chlamydiosis)
    195, 199–201, 301, 330,
    332, 334
partial pressure   521
partridge(s)   25, 30, 84, 225,
    293, 319, 563
passive
  congestion   325, 329
  diffusion   524, 527
Pasteurella
  multocida   222, 231, 233,
    239, 281, 301, 330–332,
    415, 507, 574, 576, 577,
    579, 587
  sp.   360, 507
pasty vent (cloaca)   167, 168,
    289, 293–295

patagial fold   138
patagium   133, 135, 587, 588
  alular   133, 135
patch(es)
  collagen   396
  duodenal   398
pathogenic   11, 19, 203, 220,
    223, 224, 229, 230, 232,
    248, 304, 305, 527
pathogenicity avian influenza,
    high (HPAI)   19,
    229–231, 304, 305
Pathologists (AAAP), American
    Association of Avian   4
pathology, egg   472, 473
patient positioning (radiograph)
    74, 174, 177, 348
pawprint, clay   459
PCR (polymerase chain reaction)
    198–200, 203, 211, 214,
    220, 221, 223–225, 248,
    269, 271, 288, 385, 507,
    508, 511, 530
  real time   231, 232
PCV (packed cell volume;
    hematocrit)   271, 318,
    325, 326, 347, 348, 375,
    515–518, 523
pea
  comb   25, 27, 31, 33
  sweet   379
peas' toxin (β-
    aminopropionitrile)
    327
peafowl   219, 220, 223, 226,
    311, 467, 563, 581
pecking
  behavior   450
  feather(s) (picking)   141,
    439, 441, 450
  vent   450
pecten oculi   156
pectoral(s)   136, 137, 149, 163,
    172, 255, 256, 296, 482,
    483, 485, 486, 585
  girdle (bone)   136, 174, 175,
    178

muscle score   77–79
peculiarities, avian
    cardiac   318
Pekin (breed)   57, 63, 64, 77,
    79–81, 87, 93, 99, 102,
    171, 199, 235, 238, 239,
    252, 266, 318–320, 370,
    382, 403, 404, 413, 417,
    419, 423
pellucida, *area*   468
pelvic   136, 185, 280, 322
pendulous crop   292, 293
penetration
  air sac   399, 416, 424
pen-mate   59, 110, 260
perception
  pressure (touch)   436, 437
  sensory behavior   436
percher(s)   58, 60, 76
pericardial   220, 224, 304, 309,
    311, 320, 323, 325–327,
    329, 331–334, 358,
    488
  exudate   332
  fluid   323, 325, 326, 329,
    331, 358, 488
pericarditis   199, 294, 301, 309,
    330, 331
  fibrinous   309, 333
  restrictive   332
pericardium   155, 485, 488
perihepatitis   306, 309, 332,
    333
peripheral
  nerve(s)   307, 369
  nervous system   234, 257
  neuritis   237
peritoneum   167, 272
  fold   143, 146
peritonitis   294, 301, 302, 308,
    309, 311
  egg yolk   102, 185, 235, 278,
    279, 303, 362, 363, 411,
    412, 416–418, 516,
    518–520
permethrin   262, 263, 573
permitting   5, 9, 18

perosis (slipped gastrocnemius tendon) 86, 120, 169, 171, 240, 245
pest control (natural) 434
pest(s) 56, 89, 90, 107, 109, 111, 434, 542
phalange(s) 139, 177, 186, 470
phallic sulcus, spiral 150
phallus (copulatory organ) 60, 62, 69, 91, 100, 150, 363, 423, 426, 427
 amputation 363
 disorder 91, 426
 prolapse 100, 363, 427
pharyngeal
 cavity 141, 142, 146
 gland(s) 142
 laceration 392
 papilla(e) 141, 142
 pouch 154
 wall 141, 155
pharynx 141, 142, 146
pheasant(s) 201, 204, 208–210, 212, 213, 221, 223, 225, 256, 257, 293, 295, 302, 305, 376, 384, 406, 467, 516, 517, 521, 522, 545, 563, 579
phonation 147
physical examination (clinical examination) 78, 79, 112, 159, 161, 165, 166, 172, 234–236, 248, 249, 251, 255, 282, 289, 290, 292, 293, 306, 327, 345, 347, 356, 357, 363, 364, 400, 504, 506
phytic acid 119, 379
picking (pecking) feather(s) 141, 439, 441, 450
Picornaviridae 257
pigeon 201, 355
 breeder's lung (hypersensitivity pneumonitis) 204
 pox 291

pin
 feathers 82, 261
 intrameduallary 252–255, 350
pine pellet litter 236
pine wood shavings 49
pineal gland (epiphysis cerebri) 153, 444
 lobule 153
pinion 76, 99
pinnae 140
piperacillin 265
pipping (cervical muscle) 586
pituitary gland (hypophysis) 153, 444, 446
 hormone 446
plague
 duck 214
 fowl 229
planned molt 283
plant(s)
 growth 56
 Health Inspection Service, Animal and (APHIS) 5, 13–15, 19, 107, 108, 569, 570
 toxic 378, 379
plantar region 167, 168, 171, 177, 186, 234–239, 241, 242, 252
plaques
 fibrinous 291
 oral (nodules) 291
plasma 83, 85, 88, 125, 156, 324, 334, 347, 350, 351, 355, 365, 369, 422, 444, 465, 506, 507, 509, 520, 523, 553, 554, 581
plate
 agglutination 220, 295
 growth 118, 249
platinum (white) yolk 299
plexus(es) 246, 255, 256, 395, 421, 422, 499, 581
 brachial 255, 256, 581
 avulsion 255, 256

choroid 152
 myenteric 395
 sacral 404, 421, 422
 sciatic 246, 499, 500
pliable (soft) bones 118, 121, 283
plowshare (pygostyle) 135, 177
plucking 441
plumping 463
Plymouth Rock (breed) 23–26, 224, 298, 317
 Barred 24, 25, 28, 161, 163, 169, 224, 244, 273, 307
PMV-1, avian (APMV-1; Newcastle disease) 203, 232, 279, 287, 302, 331, 525
pneumatic bone 179, 187, 251, 350, 458, 566
pneumoencephalitis 231, 233
pneumonia 214, 351, 361
 aspiration 292, 350, 361, 375, 568
 brooder 226
 fibrinous 222, 301
 fungal 326
pneumonitis
 hypersensitivity 204
 toxic 204
pod, bladder 378
pododermatitis (bumblefoot) 57, 60, 93, 171, 186, 187, 234–239, 241, 251, 252, 266, 330, 348, 354, 364, 579
 radiograph 186
pole, egg 466
policy
 compliance (minor species), medicated feeds 540, 545
 visitor policy 109
Polish (breed) 23, 29, 30, 36, 39, 42, 43
polyglycolic acid 392

polymerase chain reaction (PCR)
198–200, 203, 211, 214,
220, 221, 223–225, 248,
269, 271, 288, 385, 507,
508, 511, 530
real time 231, 232
polyserositis, fibrinous 220,
232
polytetrafluoroethylene (PTFE;
Teflon) toxicosis 361,
368, 377, 378
poor growth 82, 86, 120, 122,
298, 324, 325, 377
porphyrins 464
portal
circulation (hepatic) 149
system (renal) 148, 149,
318, 350, 421
venous ring 148, 149
vein (hepatic) 146, 149
position
abnormal 256, 505
neck 256
patient (radiograph) 74,
174, 177, 348
positive pressure 390
postmortem examination
(necropsy) 6, 35, 113,
122, 143, 165, 168, 184,
190, 200, 212, 213, 218,
220, 222, 224, 235, 237,
239, 245, 247, 248, 250,
256, 273, 276–279, 290,
296, 298, 300, 301, 303,
307, 326–328, 330–333,
363, 365, 370, 376–378,
382, 389, 391, 397, 400,
415, 459, 473, 477, 478,
502, 510, 511, 520, 523,
528
techniques 477–502
postorbital region 133, 134,
136
posture
wing 446
potassium 520, 521, 579
chloride 458, 460

deficiency 121, 334, 351,
520, 579
supplementation 119, 121,
127, 327, 376
toxicity 334
potato, green 379
pouch, pharyngeal 154
Poultry
Association (APA),
American 23, 24, 62,
63
APA Standard of Perfection
23, 24, 63
FDA definition 537
Products Inspection Act
(PPIA) 15
Science Association (PSA)
542, 545
Veterinarians (ACPV),
American College
of 3
worker's lung
(hypersensitivity
pneumonitis) 204
pox
avian 113, 114, 171,
211–213, 223–226, 270,
271, 290–292, 384, 391,
507, 523, 567, 584, 588,
590, 591
cutaneous (dry pox) 291
dry (cutaneous pox) 291
fowl 225, 270, 290, 291,
584
vaccine 113, 587, 588, 591
Poxviridae 290
Poxvirus 216, 260, 270, 290,
291
Practitioners (ABVP), American
Board of Veterinary 4
predator 436
avoidance 73, 435, 437, 442
exposure 46, 54, 112, 113,
269, 437
protection 45, 74, 93
recognition 436
trauma 265, 356

preen
feather(s) 76, 437, 439–441
gland (uropygial) 117, 139,
163, 172, 436, 441
pre-mortem aspiration 498
preovulatory follicle(s) 417,
419, 420
prepatagium 133
prescription label
requirements 548, 549
Preservation of Antibiotics for
Medical Treatment Act
(PAMTA) 550
pressure 62, 73, 241, 354, 388,
390, 404, 415, 425, 506, 568
blood 318, 326, 329, 347,
351, 355, 358, 382, 445
hydrostatic 325, 390
negative 353
osmotic 520
partial 521
perception (touch) 436, 437
positive 390
spray 263, 589
prevention control, parasite 51,
89, 110, 112, 259, 282, 298
primary
bronch(us/i) 69, 147, 487,
497, 498
feather(s) 99, 140, 166, 283
oocyte 462
process, uncinate 135, 390
proctodeum diverticulum
(bursa) 155
proctourodeal fold 145
production
egg 7, 24, 29, 46, 48, 51, 63,
67, 99–102, 123, 159,
282–284, 303, 363, 395,
418, 446, 462
decreased 48, 51,
100–102, 108, 122, 224,
231, 257, 262, 263, 270,
280–283, 286–288,
297–299, 303, 304, 308,
363, 369, 376, 405, 407,
409, 446, 505

organic   18, 571
Products Inspection Act
  Egg   16, 17
  Poultry (PPIA)   15
Program
  Food Animal Residue
    Avoidance and
    Depletion (FARAD)
    261, 323, 528, 539, 541,
    542, 550, 553–555,
    563–565, 567, 568, 571,
    573, 574, 579, 581
  National Residue (NRP)   538
  vaccination   590
prohibited drugs   102, 409,
    536, 540, 541, 544–547,
    550, 563–565, 568
  antiviral   547
  cephalosporins   547, 564
  FDA list   536, 540, 541,
    544–547, 563–565, 568
  fluoroquinolones   536, 546,
    547, 557, 563, 565
Project-7, National Research
    Support (NRSP-7)   543
prolapse
  cloacal (vent)   53, 168, 250,
    275, 305, 306, 362, 363,
    400, 401, 450
  oviductal   362, 363, 412
  phallus   100, 363, 427
  uterine   275, 413
prolateral   133, 135
promotion, growth   127, 544,
    550
pronator muscle   136–138
propatagial ligament   138
propionic acid   127
protection
  cross   209
  eye   203
  predator   45, 74, 93
protein
  dietary   82, 126
  excessive   82
  sources   125, 126
Proteus mirabilis   415, 471

protozoa   210, 212, 213, 216,
    398, 529
  erythrocytic   216
  leucocytic   216
protozoal culture   211
proventricular
  feeding tube   394
  gland(s)   143, 213, 304, 396,
    489, 492, 493
  papilla(e)   143
  worm   213
proventriculotomy   182,
    395–397
proventriculus (glandular
    stomach)   140,
    142–144, 155, 178, 179,
    213, 231, 232, 247, 257,
    303, 323, 375, 390, 393,
    395–397, 489, 490–493
  caseous   213
  catheter   375
prussic acid   378
Pseudomonas
  aeruginosa   331, 415, 471,
    472, 575
  sp.   235, 295, 360
psittacosis (avian chlamydiosis)
    195, 199–201, 301, 330,
    332, 334
pterylae   137
PTFE (polytetrafluoroethylene;
    Teflon) toxicosis   361,
    368, 377, 378
pubic bone   99
pudendal, artery   410
pullorum disease   11, 18, 114,
    294–296, 422, 523, 577
pulmo (lungs)   117, 146, 147,
    150, 165, 179, 182, 494–499
  auscultation   165, 166, 172
  disease   182, 226, 231, 232,
    301, 307, 308, 324, 328,
    332, 334, 361, 378, 390
  endoscopy   349
  radiograph   180, 181, 348,
    349
pulmonary

capillaries   325
congestion   361
hypertension syndrome
    325, 328
pulse quality   347
Public
  Health   6, 9–11, 13, 16–19,
    111, 199, 201, 301, 368,
    373, 506, 535, 538,
    546–550, 552, 556, 557,
    563
  Veterinarians, National
    Association of State   199
pulse   347
  field electrophoresis   197
  oximeter, comb   240
purchasing, chick   12, 45
purpose, dual (breed)   23, 24,
    26, 29, 32, 38, 469
pygostyle (plowshare)   135,
    177
pyridoxine
  dietary   86

q
quadrate bone   134
quadriceps femoris
    muscle   136, 138
quail   29, 77, 83, 84, 208–210,
    212, 225, 257, 293, 301,
    302, 335, 376, 394, 396,
    402, 405, 409, 418, 421,
    424, 506, 509, 516, 517,
    521, 545, 563, 574, 579,
    580, 590
quality
  air   283
  bone   84
  egg   16, 283, 284, 288, 473,
    474, 505
  egg shell   284, 287, 288, 310,
    363, 395
  feather   281, 289
  fecal   293
  feed   82, 125, 126, 306, 446,
    551
  life   84

quality (*cont'd*)
  pulse   347
  skin   259
  water   117, 118, 283, 569
quarantine(d)   3, 10, 110, 112,
    200, 220, 590
quill   140, 261

r
rachis   140, 358
radial, artery   240, 347
radiograph(s)   74, 77, 382
  anatomy   177, 179, 187
  cardiovascular   320, 325, 326
  coelomic cavity   179, 249,
      279, 326, 363, 400
  crop   177, 181, 292, 362
  directional terminology   177
  exposure   173, 195, 320, 348
  foot   187
  gastrointestinal   362, 370,
      371, 375, 396, 397
  indication   348
  liver   306, 326, 401
  lung   180, 181, 348, 349
  musculoskeletal system
      173–175, 186, 235, 240,
      241, 243, 249, 251, 253,
      354, 364, 365, 460
  patient positioning   74, 174,
      177, 348
  pododermatitis
      (bumblefoot)   186
  respiratory system   179, 180,
      183, 361, 389
  reproductive   184, 292
  spleen   179
  syringeal bulla   67, 69, 389
  urogenital system   405, 406
  wing   173, 177
radiographic findings,
    abnormal   505
radiosurgery   382, 390, 421
Raillietina cesticillus   299
rales   161, 165, 166, 218, 220,
    221, 224, 229, 230, 232,
    505

rhampotheca   480
range paralysis   167, 246, 306
ranikhet   231
rapeseed (meal)   126, 334, 379
rate
  feed consumption   551,
      569
  growth   77, 80–82, 86, 87,
      89, 102, 117, 123, 128,
      250, 297, 299, 317, 325,
      326, 328, 470
  heart (cardiac)   165, 240,
      318–321, 326, 344, 347,
      355, 446
  respiratory   159, 165, 172,
      240, 355
  water consumption   569,
      574
ratio
  meat to bone   67
  nest to hen   46, 275, 306
  rooster to hen   466
reaction
  cross   523
  polymerase chain (PCR)
      198–200, 203, 211, 214,
      220, 221, 223–225, 248,
      269, 271, 288, 385, 507,
      508, 511, 530
    real time   231, 232
  vaccine   233, 291, 589, 591
real time polymerase chain
    reaction (rtPCR)   231,
    232
recognition
  pain   355
  predator   436
record ELDU requirements,
    medical   548
rectum   144, 148
red
  blood cells (RBC; erythrocytes)
      215, 216, 369, 371, 507,
      516–518, 523
  Book   539, 555
  color vision   436
  jungle fowl   23, 435, 446

light   50, 54
Rhode Island (breed)
      24–26, 164, 410, 569
  Star (cross breed)   24
refill
  blood vessel   347
  time, capillary (CRT)   162, 347
reflex, light   358
region(s)
  aponeurotic   143
    coccygeal   153
  body   133, 135, 510
  cervical   262, 265, 266, 483,
      486
  digital   238, 481
  limbic   152
  lumbar   135, 153, 404, 421, 422
  metatarsal   133, 135, 137,
      139, 164, 167, 170, 171,
      177, 186–188, 237, 238,
      244, 246, 253, 265, 347,
      348, 350, 354, 441, 506,
      509, 566, 579
  oral   124, 141, 142, 160, 161,
      163, 168, 171, 172, 211,
      212, 290, 292, 305, 344,
      346, 347, 357, 375,
      391–393, 478, 480, 490,
      529, 568
  orbital   133, 134
  plantar   167, 168, 171, 177,
      186, 234–239, 241, 242,
      252
  postorbital   133, 134, 136
  suborbital   133, 134
  thoracic   135–137, 142, 147,
      154, 180–182, 226, 320,
      327, 360, 388, 393, 394,
      396, 397, 424, 458, 460,
      483–487, 585
  trunk   133, 177, 335, 487,
      488
regrowth, testicular   424, 425
regulations   3, 5–7, 10–13,
      15–19, 51, 127, 323, 461,
      513, 536, 540, 542, 550,
      562, 563, 591

rehydration, fluid therapy 268, 351, 352, 362

releasing hormone, gonadotropin (GnRH) 444

agonist(s) 99, 102, 409

analog 407

remodeling, bone 122

removal

heat 46, 358, 450

moisture 46, 47, 49, 119, 219

organic debris 113, 198, 201, 466

renal

artery 410, 419, 423

stalk 419

fossa 147, 499

lobule 149

portal system 148, 149, 318, 350, 421

venous ring 148, 149

vein 149, 406, 421

reovirus 114, 239, 255, 331, 524

repair, fracture 251–254

repolarization, artrial 320

reportable disease 201–203, 231, 295, 504

reproduction 69, 117, 120

reproductive

canal 277

diseases 91, 166, 249, 250, 275–278, 280, 288, 346, 356, 362, 383, 384, 407, 410–416, 418, 421, 422, 426

endoscopy 416, 418, 422, 426

hormone(s) 54, 139, 153, 407, 422–424, 438, 444

lesion(s) 277, 426, 497

radiograph 184, 292

reproductive system 234, 282, 419, 422, 423, 426, 474, 494, 495, 505

behaviors 100, 102, 408, 435, 443

dystocia 174, 185, 361–363, 400, 401, 412, 413

egg binding 184, 250, 277, 362, 411, 412, 415, 418

oviductal prolapse 362, 363, 412

requirements

identification 16

medical record ELDU 548

prescription label 548, 549

space 46, 52, 94

Research Support Project-7, National (NRSP-7) 543

resection and anastomosis 388, 389, 394, 397

reservoirs 111, 195, 197, 204, 304, 556

residue

avoidance 261, 323, 350, 550, 563

Depletion Program, Food Animal (FARAD) 261, 323, 528, 539, 541, 542, 550, 553–555, 563–565, 567, 568, 571, 573, 574, 579, 581

egg residues 553

Program (NRP), National 538

testing, drug 539, 555, 556

resorption, bone 84, 121, 122, 127, 464

respiratory

disease 72, 166, 181, 185, 210–213, 218–226, 230–232, 239, 240, 280, 290, 303–305, 329, 349, 360, 361, 383–385, 388, 474, 480, 525, 574–576, 578, 579

disease, chronic (CRD; *Mycoplasma gallisepticum* infection) 11, 112, 219–221, 240, 281, 301, 309, 331, 383–385, 523, 525, 574–576, 578, 579

vaccine 307, 584, 586, 589–591

distress 212, 345, 348, 358, 359, 361, 362, 411, 589

droplets 280, 303, 304

effort, abnormal 165

lesion(s) 220, 359, 360, 386

rate 159, 165, 172, 240, 355

system 47, 146, 179, 180, 210, 361, 486, 487, 505, 566

lower airway disease 361

radiograph 179, 180, 183, 361, 389

restraint

chemical 74

wing 160, 161

Restrictions, Convenants, Conditions, and (CC&R) 4

restrictive

arrest 343

cardiomyopathy 325, 326

pericarditis 332

resuscitation

cardiopulmonary (CPR) 343, 344

cardiopulmonary cerebral (CPCR) 343

fluid therapy 350, 351, 358

retained cystic right oviduct 151, 187, 277, 278, 410, 411, 419

retention, abnormal fluid 174

retractor 390

retrovirus(es), avian 248, 330

rhinotracheitis 220

Rhode Island Red (breed) 24–26, 164, 410, 569

rhomboid 136

rhythm, cardiac 320

riboflavin 88

deficiency (vitamin B2 deficiency; curled toe paralysis) 86, 120, 237, 244

dietary 86

riboflavin (*cont'd*)
supplementation 86, 120, 237
ribonucleic acid (RNA) 124, 229, 232, 297, 302, 308, 530, 531
ribs
bent 284, 363
bone, true 135
collapse 122
right cystic oviduct (retained) 151, 187, 277, 278, 410, 411, 419
ring, static blood 470
RNA (ribonucleic acid) 124, 229, 232, 297, 302, 308, 530, 531
Robert–Jones bandage 254, 354
Rock, Plymouth (breed) 23–26, 224, 298, 317
Barred 24, 25, 28, 161, 163, 169, 224, 244, 273, 307
rodent
droppings 52
identification 52
monitoring 53
rodenticide exposure 368, 377
roll culture, egg 471
Roman (breed) goose/geese 63, 67
rooster(s)
accumulation 47
ratio to hen 466
Rose Comb (clean legged) Class (Standard of Perfection breeds) 23–26, 28, 31, 32, 35–37, 39, 43, 161
spiked 25
rostral
colliculus (optic tectum) 152
diverticulum (infraorbital sinus) 383, 387
Rouen (breed) 63, 68
rough surface (sandpaper) eggshell(s) 287

round heart disease (spontaneous cardiomyopathy; dilated cardiomyopathy) 324–330, 333, 334
roundworms, intestinal 215, 287, 298, 306, 474, 572
routes of administration, medication 536, 544, 545, 547, 549, 552, 553, 564–567, 579
rtPCR (real time polymerase chain reaction) 231, 232
ruffled (fluffed) feather(s) 161, 206, 209, 230, 256, 296, 297, 302, 308, 311, 324, 444, 448, 505
rupture
aortic 327, 335, 518
atrial 327
gastrocnemius tendon 254, 255
hepatic 362
shell membranes 474

S
sac
air 146, 147, 150, 155, 179–182, 220, 381, 390, 391, 397, 485
albumen 469
yolk 143, 145, 309, 468–471, 494
sacral
nerve(s) 421, 422
plexus(es) 404, 421, 422
safe (egg) handling instructions 16
safety, environmental 17, 439
Safety and Inspection Service, Food (FSIS) 15, 17, 538, 540, 542, 555
salicylic acid 356
analgesia 356
salinomycin 209, 334, 376, 571
salivary gland(s) 141, 198

Salmonella 11, 18, 111, 195–198, 276, 280, 281, 290, 294–296, 330, 362, 412, 415, 450, 471, 527, 575, 589
agglutination 524
enteritidis 11, 197, 198, 296
gallinarium 195, 211, 239, 294, 295, 507, 523, 572, 575
monitoring 11
paratyphoid 296
pullorum 11, 12, 18, 195, 294, 295, 422, 507, 523, 524, 577
sp. 111, 195, 276, 280, 281, 290, 294–296, 330, 331, 362, 412, 415, 450, 471, 527, 575
salmonellosis 111, 114, 195–198, 208, 210, 211, 295, 306, 518
salpingitis 280, 308–310, 330, 363, 411–413, 415, 416, 419
salpingohysterectomy 102, 185, 277, 279, 355, 363, 398, 409, 412, 413, 415–418, 420, 421, 423
sample
collection sample 72, 206, 290, 348, 403, 425, 468, 477, 478, 487, 504, 506, 507, 509–511, 515
environmental 76, 511
fecal 348, 507, 508, 528, 529
handling 515, 520, 528
live bird 509, 511
sampling, fluids 211, 278, 363, 412, 422
sandpaper (rough surface) eggshell(s) 287
sanitation
hatchery 471, 473
nest 471
Sarcocystis falcatula 332
sarcoma 248, 330, 384, 388, 405

granulosa cell   248

hepatic   330

sartorius muscle   136, 138

scabs   161, 167, 260, 270, 290, 291, 481, 587, 588

scaly leg mite   261, 262

schedule, lightning   277, 286

schistosomes   331, 333

sciatic (ischiadic; ischiatic)

nerve(s)   120, 136, 246, 247, 307, 332, 499, 500

plexus(es)   246, 499, 500

sclera   155

ring bone   136

score, body condition   77–79, 123, 172, 328, 478, 479

scraping(s)   511, 512

intestinal   299

oral   529

skin   509

Sebastopol (breed)   57, 66

secondary

bronch(us/i)   147

feather(s)   140, 283

seed contamination, weed   125

segments, tapeworm   287

selection

antibiotic   265, 556

breed   12, 23, 47, 53, 317, 323, 325, 329

food   436

genetic   317, 318, 325, 326, 329, 448

mate   59, 407, 443, 444

nest site   444

selenium

deficiency   121, 334

semilunar

membrane   147, 489

valves   489

seminiferous tubule(s)   150, 426

Senate Bill, 27(SB27; Senate Bill)   550

sensory perception behavior   436

sepsis, abdominal   403

septic

arthritis   186, 187, 295

septicemia   222, 224, 227, 231, 232, 265, 271, 278, 295, 296, 306, 308, 309, 318, 332, 415, 422, 426

septum

horizontal   155

interlobular   139

interorbital   134

oblique   155

serology (immunology)   220, 221, 240, 248, 269–271, 287, 298, 305, 306, 506, 507, 515, 523, 531

serotype   197, 222–224, 232, 246, 248, 306, 307, 331, 523

serum   83, 85, 86, 200, 224, 248, 257, 289, 294, 308, 326, 362, 369, 370, 374, 375, 395, 401–403, 458, 506, 507, 509, 520, 523–525, 554

plate agglutination   220

Service(s)

Food Safety and Inspection (FSIS)   15, 17, 538, 540, 542, 555

Laboratory, National Veterinary (NVSL)   231, 233

sex-linked

chicks   24

sexual hormones   153

shaft

feather   112, 140, 166, 167, 261, 262, 509, 528

louse (*Menopon gallinae*)   260, 261

wooden   510

shavings, wood   259, 298

hard   49, 227

pine   49

sheep   15, 374, 564

blood agar   471

shell

abnormal   224

color loss   286, 287

deformities   416

gland (uterus; eggshell gland)   147, 151, 152, 185, 275, 277, 283, 286–288, 409, 410, 413, 415, 416, 418, 445, 463, 474, 495–497

membrane   284, 285, 465, 466, 469, 471, 472, 497

dehydrated   467

culture   471

inner   464–466, 469

outer   151, 464, 466, 474

ruptured   474

quality, egg   284, 287, 288, 395

rough surface (sandpaper)   287

shell-less eggs   224, 284, 288, 464

shipment carriers, air   13

shoulder injury   173, 255

show(s), breed   223

Sicilian Buttercup (breed)   30, 37, 39, 43, 44

signs

neurologic   199, 357, 358

Silkie (breed)   30, 35, 37, 39, 44, 167, 168, 187, 272, 273, 278, 352, 358, 446, 495

silver   24, 25, 27, 28, 31, 34–36

cream   567

toxicity   334

Simuliidae   264, 265, 333

single

bird   56, 61, 71, 89, 94, 100, 435, 466, 568

comb   23–26, 28, 31, 32, 34, 36, 37, 39, 40, 44, 161

ovary   150

Single Comb (clean legged) Class (Standard of Perfection breeds)   23–26, 28, 31, 32, 34, 36, 37, 39, 40, 44, 161

sinus

aspiration   385

caseous   220, 222, 501

sinus (*cont'd*)
  diverticulum, infraorbital
      (rostral diverticulum)
      383, 387
  exudate   220, 501
  fluid   220, 303, 383, 385
  injection(s)   580
sinusitis   203, 220, 240, 360,
      361, 383–386, 578–580
sinusoidal capillaries   146
sinusotomy   385
sizes
  droplet   589
skeletal malformations   82,
      121
skin
  abnormal   166, 167, 505
  breast   269, 271
  disease   259
  hemorrhagic   54
  lesion(s)   260
  lymphoma   247
  nodules   247, 291, 588
  quality   259
  scraping(s), skin   509
skull   37, 57, 134, 136, 167, 187,
      308, 348, 349, 356, 357,
      375, 385, 460, 501, 502
  bone   136
slaughter   6, 15, 16, 199, 200,
      203, 457, 458, 550, 551,
      575, 576, 578
slide, microscope   297
slipped gastrocnemius tendon
      (perosis)   86, 120, 169,
      171, 240, 245
slit
  choanal   141, 146, 168, 349,
      480, 490
  infundibular   141, 142
small
  intestine   125, 140, 143, 178,
      190, 215, 298–300, 302,
      303, 397
  droplets (nebulization)   567,
      568
smear(s)

blood   318, 333, 508, 515,
      516, 529
smell
  abnormal   160, 168
sneeze(s)   218, 220, 221, 229, 304
snick   218, 220, 221, 224, 229,
      230, 232
snoods   48
social/group behavior   442, 447
social order (pecking order)
      39, 62, 438, 467
sodium
  bicarbonate, excessive   123
soft
  bones (pliable)   118, 121, 283
  eggshell   278, 279, 287, 398,
      412
    ends   287
  tissue   174, 177–179, 182,
      183, 186–190, 241, 249,
      251, 334, 348, 349, 381,
      383, 391, 400, 441, 568
    injury   186, 255, 265, 450
    surgery   99, 102, 186, 249,
      381–427
soil
  contamination   369
soiled (fecal-stained) feather(s)
      262, 289, 293, 294, 308,
      362, 406
sounds
  abnormal   165, 505
  cardiac (heart)   318, 327,
      342
sources, protein   125, 126
space requirements   46, 52, 94
Spanish flu   202
special stain   508, 525
species (minor), medicated
      feeds compliance
      policy   540, 545
Speckled Sussex (breed)   34,
      160, 170, 235
spent hen(s)   585
sperm gland(s)   463, 466, 497
spiked rose comb   25
spinal

canal   153
cord   152, 153, 257, 369, 460
nerves
  cervical   152
spine (vertebral column;
      background)   142, 177,
      234, 483
spiral phallic sulcus   150
splay (spraddle) leg   250
spleen
  accessory   155
  nodules   300
  radiograph   179
splenic lobe   146, 403
splint   254
spontaneous
  cardiomyopathy (round heart
      disease; dilated
      cardiomyopathy)
      324–330, 333, 334
  atherosclerosis   335
spores
  Clostridium   301
  fungal   227
spot(s)
  blood   285, 286, 462, 473,
      474
  meat   285, 286, 473, 474
spraddle (splay) leg   250
spray
  droplet
    coarse   589
    fine   589
    medium   589
  pressure   263, 589
  vaccination   588, 589
spur
  bone (metatarsal)   186
spur-winged goose/geese   60
squamous cell carcinoma   248,
      391
stain, special   508, 525
stained eggs, blood   275
stalk
  ovarian   154
  renal artery   419
  yolk   143, 145, 468, 469

stance, abnormal 161, 167, 250, 251

Standard
  Class (Standard of Perfection breeds) 23–25, 31, 37, 62, 63
  Care, of 3
  Perfection, of (American Poultry Association; APA) 23, 24, 62, 63

Standards, FAO/WHO Food (Codex Alimentarius Commission) 540, 555

Staphylococcus
  aureus 239, 276, 333, 471
  sp. 234, 271, 295, 330, 331, 412

star
  Black (crossbreed) 24, 245
  gazing (Vitamin B1[thiamine] deficiency) 256
  Red (crossbreed) 24

stasis
  crop 246, 292, 362, 369

State Public Health Veterinarians, National Association of 199

static blood ring 470

status, nutritional 145, 275, 369, 487

steatosis, hepatic 80, 101

stem, brain 152, 153

sternal bursa 245, 272

sternum 69, 135, 155, 166, 321, 344, 349, 390, 391, 402, 482, 484–486

sticktight flea(s) 263, 264

stigma 151, 420, 462, 463, 497

still air incubator 461

stimulating hormone, follicle (FSH) 444

stomach
  glandular (proventriculus) 142, 489, 492
  isthmus 142, 395, 396, 403, 492, 493

muscular (ventriculus; gizzard) 88, 117, 126, 127, 140, 142–144, 155, 166, 174, 178–182, 190, 231, 257, 294, 328, 349, 369, 370, 390, 393, 395–397, 486, 488–493

stone, kidney 123

stool, abnormal 362

storage
  air 147
  egg 471, 472
  fertile 467
  improper egg 310

straw 49, 254, 259
  colored 272

Streptococcus 331, 415

stress
  heat 48, 358, 589
  level 287, 440

stress-lined feather(s) 167, 479

striation, cross 307, 500

strike, fly 265

Stuart transport media 507, 508, 510, 511

subcutaneous
  air accumulation 361
  fluid therapy 268, 350, 566
  injection 575, 584, 585, 590, 591

sublingual
  entrapment 392
  impaction 392

suborbital región 133, 134

sudden death syndrome 328–330

sulcus, spiral phallic 150

sulfate, zinc 294, 298

sulfonamides 222, 376, 518, 564, 571

sulfur 119, 209, 262, 281

supplements 85, 87, 89, 159, 326, 335, 373

supplementation
  cholesterol 335
  collagen 126
  copper 127, 292

electrolyte 326

enzyme 87, 125

mineral 77, 84, 118, 119, 121, 126–129, 174, 177, 178, 181, 190

potassium 119, 121, 127, 327, 376

riboflavin (vitamin B2) 86, 120, 237

selenium 119, 121, 371

vitamin 118, 120, 122, 286, 505

vitamin A 299, 362

vitamin B3 (niacin) 86

vitamin C 86, 87, 371

vitamin D 362

vitamin E 312, 362

vitamin K 312, 362, 401

support
  nutritional 354, 362, 371
  Project-7, National Research (NRSP-7) 543

supraduodenal loop 390

surgery
  beak 385, 391
  cloacal 390, 398–400, 415, 416, 418, 425, 427
  coelomic 102, 349, 352, 390, 391, 396, 397, 400, 402, 404, 407, 413, 414, 417, 418, 425, 484
  crop 385, 388, 392–394
  duodenal 403
  exposure 382, 390, 391, 396, 416, 420, 424, 482
  hepatic 402
  infraorbital sinus 383, 385–387
  kidney 404, 406, 425
  soft tissue 99, 102, 186, 249, 381–427
  waterfowl 102, 381–383, 385, 386, 389, 391, 394, 395, 397, 400, 403, 407, 409, 412, 415–417, 425, 426, 470

surveillance 16, 18, 197, 214, 230, 317, 330, 331, 477
suspended animation 467
Sussex (breed) 29, 31, 32, 34, 160, 170, 235
suture material(s) 382, 383, 392, 398, 407, 416, 418
swab
  calcium alginate 510
  cloacal 231, 303, 305, 401, 509, 510
swan goose/geese 67, 70
sweet pea 379
swelling
  infraorbital sinus 383–386
  injection 202
  neck 108, 260, 271, 304
sympathetic 149
synchronous hatching 436, 467
syndrome
  anemia dermatitis (CAV) 271
  ascites 317, 318, 326, 330, 333, 334
  egg drop (EDS) 281, 284, 286–288
  fatty liver hemorrhagic (disease) 80, 100, 312, 328, 407, 518
  pulmonary hypertension 325, 328
  sudden death 328–330
Syngamus trachea 212, 213, 226
synovial fluid 482, 502, 509
synsacrum bone 499
syringeal bulla(ae)
  osseous 69, 182, 184, 388, 389
  radiograph 67, 69, 389
syrinx (lower larynx; caudal larynx) 142, 146, 147, 182–184, 226, 288, 349, 486, 487, 498
system
  cardiovascular 155, 317, 318, 329

radiograph 320, 325, 326
  central nervous 152, 214
  digestive 140, 141, 144, 145, 289, 291, 292, 304, 395, 468, 469, 491, 505
  endocrine 153
  genital system
    female 150, 151
    male 150
  hepatic 410
  immune 59, 87, 125, 127, 195, 206, 303, 523, 526, 585, 586
  lymphatic 155
  musculoskeletal 173, 186, 187, 234, 345, 364, 505
    radiograph 173–175, 186, 235, 240, 241, 243, 249, 251, 253, 354, 364, 365, 460
  nervous 149, 232, 303, 371, 468, 505
  renal portal 148, 149, 318, 350, 421
  reproductive 234, 282, 419, 422, 423, 426, 474, 494, 495, 505
  respiratory 47, 146, 179, 180, 210, 361, 486, 487, 505, 566
  urinary 147
  urogenital 145
    radiograph 405, 406

t

T, cardiac troponin 318
T-2 toxin 124
tail 25, 31, 38, 41, 60, 67, 78, 99, 139, 163, 165, 166, 172, 177, 262, 283, 345, 444, 450, 510
  feather(s) 38, 172, 444, 510
tapeworm (Cestodes) 215, 287, 288, 299, 573
  segments 287
tarsometatarsal bone 177, 187, 188, 244

taste (flavor), yolk 473
tectum, optic (rostral colliculus) 152
Teflon (polytetrafluoroethylene; PTFE) 361, 368, 377, 378
temperature
  air 47, 219
  body (core) 147, 166, 347, 348, 358, 448, 566
  cloacal 348
  egg incubation 272, 462, 467, 468, 472
  house 47, 49, 50, 55, 111, 118, 219, 305, 412, 505, 537, 551, 569, 586
  outdoor 49
tendon
  gastrocnemius
    rupture 254, 255
    slipped (perosis) 86, 120, 169, 171, 240, 245
terminal
  aspiration 498
  bronch(us/i) (air capillaries) 147, 568
terminology, directional (radiograph) 177
tertiary bronch(us/i) (parabronchi) 147
test interference, chemical 510
testes(is) 145, 150, 153, 424, 425
  abnormal 425, 426
testicle
  cystic 426
testicular
  artery 423
  aspiration 426
  cyst(s) 424–426
testing, drug residues 539, 555, 556
tetany
  calcium 121, 277, 283
tetrachlorvinphos 262
tetracycline(s) 201, 219–224, 245, 302, 551, 558, 574, 578

theca   153, 462
  externa   462
  interna   462
therapy
  fluid   265, 271, 345–347,
      350, 351, 354, 358, 381,
      395, 411, 566, 577
    fluid types   350, 351
    intraosseous (IO)   265, 345,
      350, 351, 458, 566, 568
    intravenous (IV)   265,
      268, 345, 350, 351, 355,
      356, 358, 365, 382, 459,
      566
  maintenance   351, 566
  oral   350
  rehydration   268, 351, 352, 362
  resuscitation   350, 351, 358
  subcutaneous   268, 350, 566
thiabendazole   213, 226
thick albumen   463–465, 474
thin albumen   463–466, 474
thoracic
  air sac   154, 180, 181, 183,
      226, 360, 397, 424
  compression   458, 460
  girdle   137, 485, 486
  region   135–137, 142, 147,
      154, 180–182, 226, 320,
      327, 360, 388, 393, 394,
      396, 397, 424, 458, 460,
      483–487, 585
threats, health   10, 13, 14, 18,
      544
thrombocyte(s)   401, 516, 519
thymus
  lobes/gland(s)   155, 483, 484
thyroid
  cystic   330
  follicle(s)   153, 154
  gland(s)   153, 154, 487
  hormone   154, 523
tibia bone   118
tibiotarsal-tarsometatarsal joint
      (hock)   120, 135, 167, 171,
      221, 235, 237, 239, 240,
      244, 245, 253, 255, 295, 579

ticks, fowl   263, 264
tie-over   268
time
  capillary clot   401
  capillary refill (CRT)   162, 347
tissue(s)
  abnormal   190, 349, 385,
      393, 404, 410, 420, 427
  adipose   146, 400, 482
  contamination   352
  fixation   485, 500, 511, 512
  handling   382
  injury, soft   186
  mural lymphoid   155
toe(s)
  amputation   243, 267
  curled   169
  paralysis, curled (vitamin B2
      deficiency; riboflavin
      deficiency)   86, 120,
      237, 244
tomia   141
tomium   141
tongue (glossa)   101, 125, 136,
      140–142, 171, 225, 240,
      392, 393, 478–481, 491,
      587, 588
  depressor   479, 500
torsion, oviduct   415
torticollis   199, 231, 232, 246
Toulouse (breed) goose/
      geese   63, 67, 70, 405
toxic   119, 124, 149, 204, 209,
      286, 324, 326, 334, 361,
      365, 368, 374–379, 469,
      508, 518, 538, 563, 571,
      580
toxicity
  drinking water   375
  potassium   334
  selenium   166, 334, 368,
      377
  silver   334
  vitamin D   284, 310, 334
  vitamin E   334
  zinc   178, 182, 362, 365,
      368–370, 372–376, 581

toxicology   368–379, 506–508,
      571
toxicosis
  cardiac   334
  iononphore   368, 376
  lead   368–370
    clinical signs   369
    diagnosis   369
    sources   368
    treatment   370
  polytetrafluoroethylene
      (PTFE; Teflon)   361,
      368, 377, 378
  toxic plants   378, 379
toxin(s)
  alpha   299
  beta   299
  diarrhea   374
  elimination   370
  environmental   76, 334, 361,
      365, 401, 473, 538
  exposure   76, 231, 233,
      365, 368, 369, 371, 373,
      374, 376–378, 460, 480,
      481, 507, 538, 550, 553,
      554
  peas' (β-aminopropionitrilen)
      327
  T-2   124
Toxoplasma gondii   214, 331,
      333
toxoplasmosis   214
trachea
  collapse   388, 389
  endoscopy   386
  hemorrhagic   388
tracheal
  avulsion   389
  granuloma   360
trachealis muscle   146
tracheotomy   388, 389
tract, optic   152
training, excessive   405
tramadol analgesia   356, 581
trapezius muscle   136
transfusion, blood   271, 347,
      352, 370

transmission
  aerosol 220–224, 226, 231,
    232, 303, 304
  disease 11, 12, 14, 18, 45,
    51, 52, 76, 82, 89, 99,
    107–110, 112, 113, 118,
    123, 195, 197, 203, 206,
    271, 290, 294, 296, 298,
    302, 326, 343, 477, 590
  feather(s) (disease) 246, 306
transport media 510–513
  Aimes 507, 508, 510, 511
  Cary-Blair 510
  Mycoplasma 478, 479
  Stuart 507, 508, 510, 511
  viral 478, 479
transportation 12, 13, 18, 195,
    507, 508, 511, 513, 520
transudate (fluid) 318
trauma
  air sac 361, 458
  cloacal 268, 398, 400, 450
  predator 265, 356
treatment
  Act, Preservation of
    Antibiotics for Medical
    (PAMTA) 550
  biotin 240, 312, 362
  chemical 299
  choline 240, 312, 362
  fungal 183, 353, 361, 389,
    568
trematodes 215, 331, 415, 573
tremor 108, 231
  epidemic (avian
    encephalomyelitis) 257
  neck 257
trephination, beak 385
triage 343, 346
Trichomonas gallinae 211,
    529
trichomoniasis 211, 290, 292
trimming
  beak 53, 54, 59, 91, 141,
    275, 281, 282, 306, 480
  feather(s) 167, 357
  wing 58, 72, 99

triosseal canal (foramen) 136,
    137
trochlear groove 168
troponin T
  abnormal 324
  T, cardiac 318
true rib bone 135
trunk region 133, 177, 335,
    487, 488
tube
  Eustachian (auditory) 142
  feeding 406
    duodenal 397
    esophageal 392, 568
    proventricular 394
tubercules (granuloma) 300
tuberculosis, avian 111, 114,
    201, 300, 557
tube agglutination 295
tubule(s)
  seminiferous 150, 426
turkey(s) 11, 25, 29, 31, 37, 45,
    46, 52, 77, 120, 169, 171,
    177–180, 196, 199–202,
    204, 208–211, 213, 215,
    219–223, 225–227, 230,
    231, 240, 242, 244, 245,
    248–250, 256, 257, 264,
    268, 270, 272, 284,
    290–295, 297–299,
    301–306, 309, 311, 312,
    317, 319–325, 327–331,
    333–335, 353, 376, 396,
    399, 410, 413, 423, 459,
    466, 467, 516–519, 521,
    522, 524, 525, 529, 536,
    537, 542, 545–547,
    562–564, 569–572,
    574–580, 584–586
tylosin 220, 221, 246, 578,
    580
tympanic membrane
  external 147
  internal 147
type(s)
  comb 23–26, 31, 32, 36, 37,
    39, 139

C oncoviruses 308
  fluid, fluid therapy 350, 351
typhlitis, hemorrhagic
    208–210

u
ulcer
  corneal 358
ulcerative enteritis 301, 302,
    574
ulnar
  vein, cutaneous (basilic vein
    163, 165, 348, 509, 566
ultimobranchial body
    (gland) 153, 154
ultrasonography 79, 349, 411,
    422
ultraviolet
  vision 436
unaesthetic egg 462, 473
uncinate process 135, 390
upper larynx (glottis; cranial
    larynx) 124, 146, 291,
    568
urate(s)(uric acid)
  accumulation 310
  crystal(s) 356, 406
  joint 310
ureter(s) 145, 147, 148, 295,
    296, 390, 399, 400, 405,
    406, 418, 423, 425, 426,
    499
ureteral impaction 406
ureterotomy 406
uric acid 289, 310, 406, 469,
    522
  crystals 356, 406
urinary
  catheter 359
  system 147
urodeum
  papilla(e) 423
urogenital
  system 145
  tract 182
  radiograph 405, 406
urolith(s)

calcium   406
urolithiasis (visceral gout)
      122, 182, 310, 311, 406
uroprotodeal fold   399
uropygial gland (preen
      gland)   117, 139, 163,
      172, 436, 441
   duct   139
   eminence   139
   lobes   139, 163
usage, whole   202, 285, 506,
      509
use
   chicken drug   267, 268, 343,
      528, 535, 536, 540–542,
      544, 545, 547–549, 552,
      556, 557, 562, 565
   extra-label drug
      (ELDU)   536, 541,
      544–548, 552–555, 558,
      562–566, 571
   on-label drug   536, 546, 547,
      552, 553, 558
   uterus (eggshell gland; shell
      gland)   147, 151, 152,
      185, 275, 277, 283,
      286–288, 409, 410, 413,
      415, 416, 418, 445, 463,
      474, 495–497
uterine   398
   prolapse   275, 413

V
vaccination
   chick   113, 248, 291, 584, 589
   drinking water   233, 584,
      587, 588, 590
   eye (drop)   233, 584,
      586–588, 590, 591
   nasal   586
   program   590
   spray   588, 589
   wing web   584, 587, 588,
      590, 591
vaccine(s)
   aerosol administration   588,
      589

avian encephalomyelitis
      113, 587, 590, 591
chronic respiratory disease
      (CRD; *Mycoplasma
      gallisepticum*
      infection)   11, 584, 586,
      589–591
cold   586
fowl cholera   113, 587
fowl pox   113, 587, 588, 591
inactivated   584–586, 590
infectious
   bronchitis   233, 304, 587,
      589–591
   bursal disease   586, 587,
      589, 591
   coryza (coryza)   590
   laryngotracheitis   113,
      223, 224, 584, 586, 587,
      591
live   203, 525, 584, 586–591
Mycoplasma gallisepticum
      11, 584, 586, 589–591
Marek's disease   584–586,
      590, 591
nasal   586
Newcastle disease (PMV-1;
      APMV-1)   584, 587,
      589–591
reaction   233, 291, 589, 591
   excessive   589
vagal, arrest   345
vagus nerve   483
vagina   60, 69, 151, 152, 277,
      410, 412, 413, 415, 444,
      463, 464, 497
valgus deformities   161, 240,
      249–251
valves, semilunar   489
valvular insufficiency   321,
      325, 330, 332
vane   140, 289
vas deferens (ductus
      deferens)   145, 150,
      423, 425, 426, 499
vascular cord   425
vasculitis   232, 335

vasectomy   425, 426
vein(s)
   adrenal   423
   basilica vein (cutaneous
      ulnar)   163, 165, 348,
      509, 566
   brachial (wing)   506, 509,
      566
   caudal mesenteric   148, 149
   central   146
   caudal vena cava   145, 148,
      149, 410, 418, 419, 421,
      423
   collapse   506
   common iliac   148, 149, 410,
      419–421
   cranial vena cava   318
   cutaneous ulnar (basilic)
      163, 165, 348, 509, 566
   external iliac   148, 149
   hepatic portal   146, 149
   interlobular   148, 149
   intralobular   149
   jugular   155, 348, 350, 458,
      459, 483, 484, 490, 506,
      509, 566
   metatarsal   265, 350, 506,
      509, 566, 579
   renal   149, 406, 421
   ulnar (basilic)   163, 165,
      348, 500, 566
   wing (brachial)   506, 509,
      566
velogenic Newcastle disease,
      viscerotropic (vvND;
      END, VND)   229,
      231–233
vena cava
   caudal   145, 148, 149, 410,
      418, 419, 421, 423
   cranial   318
venous ring (renal portal)   148,
      149
vent
   pasty (cloaca)   167, 168, 289,
      293–295
   pecking   450

vent (*cont'd*)
  prolapse 53, 168, 250, 275, 305, 306, 362, 363, 400, 401, 413, 450
  ventilation 46–48, 55, 204, 219, 325, 344, 376, 387, 390
  egg 467, 472, 505, 589
ventplasty 400, 401
ventral midline 390, 391, 396–400, 402, 404, 408, 411, 413, 416, 418, 420, 424
ventricle(s) 152, 321–326, 328, 329, 333, 488, 489
ventricular
  contraction 321, 333, 395
  diverticula 395
  fibrillation 326, 328
  nodules 257
ventriculotomy 395–397
ventriculus (gizzard; muscular stomach) 88, 117, 126, 127, 140, 142–144, 155, 166, 174, 178–182, 190, 231, 257, 294, 328, 349, 369, 370, 390, 393, 395–397, 486, 488–493
vermiculite (clay mineral) 88, 118
vermis 153
vertebrae, cervical 135, 142, 177, 460, 483
vertebral column (backbone; spine) 142, 177, 234, 483
vessel(s)
  branching blood (embryo) 470
  cerebral 256, 318
  growth 468
  lymphatic 155
  refill, blood 347
Veterinarians
  American College of Poultry (ACPV) 3

Association of Avian (AAV) 4
National Association of State Public Health 199
veterinary
  accreditation 13, 14
  Feed Directive (VFD) 127, 549, 550, 565, 566
  Laboratory Diagnosticians (AAVLD), American Association of 541
  Medical Association (AVMA), American 457, 545, 565
  Practitioners (ABVP), American Board of 4
  Services Laboratory, National (NVSL) 231, 233
VFD (Veterinary Feed Directive) medications 127, 549, 550, 565, 566
viral
  arthritis 524
  culture (cell culture) 200, 291, 529, 584, 591
  diarrhea 230, 248, 271, 303, 304, 362
  transport media 478, 479
virulent Newcastle disease (viscerotrophic velogenic Newcastle disease; exotic Newcastle disease) 229, 231–233
virus
  avian leucosis/leukosis 246, 249, 250, 331
  chicken anemia (infectious chicken anemia; CAV) 260, 271, 518, 587
  Newcastle disease 302, 303, 383, 584, 587, 591
  West Nile 195
viscera, abdominal 150
visceral
  gout (urolithiasis) 122, 182, 310, 311, 406

granuloma 300
viscerotrophic velogenic Newcastle disease (vvND; END, VND) 229, 231–233
vision
  color
    blue 436
    green 436
    red 436
    ultraviolet 436
visitor policy 109
visual imprinting 60
visualization, egg 227, 287, 470
vitamin
  deficiency 118, 120, 281, 283, 290
  degradation 117
  supplementation 118, 120, 122, 286, 505
  A
    deficiency 211, 212, 287, 290, 292, 299
    supplementation 299, 362
  B1 (thiamine)
    deficiency 256, 581
    supplementation 581
  B2 (riboflavin)
    deficiency (curled toe paralysis) 86, 120, 237, 244
  B3 (niacin)
    deficiency 86, 120
    supplementation 86
  D 93, 283, 284
    deficiency 93, 118, 283, 284, 287, 362
    supplementation 362
    toxicity 284, 310, 334
  E
    deficiency 126, 256, 257, 334, 472
    supplementation 312, 362
    toxicity 334
  K
    deficiency 286

supplementation 312, 362, 401

vitelline diverticulum (Meckel's diverticulum) 143, 145, 468, 494

vitellus (yolk) 464, 465, 470

vitreous body 156

VND (virulent Newcastle disease; vvND; END) 229, 231–233

vocal imprinting 60

vocalization
chick 436

volume
air sac 182
pack cell (PCV; hematocrit) 271, 318, 325, 326, 347, 348, 375, 515–518, 523
mean corpuscular (MCV) 516, 517

V-shaped comb (devil bird) 41

vvND (viscerotropic velogenic Newcastle disease; END, VND) 229, 231–233

W

wall
abdominal 145, 150
pharyngeal

walnut comb 36, 37, 42, 44, 161

warm fluid(s) 375

washing eggs 466

water
additive 550, 567
chlorinated 52, 505
city 111, 505
consumption 18, 51, 118, 125, 304, 551, 569, 570, 574, 588
rate 569, 574
contamination 526, 527
drinking 74, 76, 94, 119, 179, 447, 570
chlorination 52, 310

medication 86, 118, 292, 310, 549, 565, 568, 571–574, 577
toxicity 375
vaccination 233, 584, 587, 588, 590

droplet(s) 51

intake factors 118, 127, 218, 399, 551

quality 117, 118, 283, 569

waterfowl 11, 46, 52, 56–63, 67–69, 73, 156–106, 331
analgesia 581
disease 202, 203, 229, 230, 256, 304, 363, 375, 422
examination 72, 73, 506, 524, 525
identification 98
management 45, 69–71, 73, 74, 76, 77, 79–102, 118, 467
medication 563, 573, 579–581
migratory 108
surgery 102, 381–383, 385, 386, 389, 391, 394, 395, 397, 400, 403, 407, 409, 412, 415–417, 425, 426, 470

watery diarrhea 108, 296, 298, 302, 303

wattle(s) 25, 31, 36, 48, 108, 133, 134, 139, 160–163, 172, 202, 222, 231, 260, 271, 290, 291, 297, 299, 303, 304, 317, 357, 358, 479, 505

WDI (withdrawal interval) 323, 544, 549, 553–555

web, wing 587, 588
vaccination 584, 587, 588, 590, 591

weed seed contamination 125

weight
adrenal 154
bearing 170, 364

body 17, 25, 31, 37, 46, 50, 63, 76–81, 84, 86, 93, 94, 101, 102, 117, 123, 125, 147, 168, 177, 201, 206, 209, 211, 212, 226, 234, 235, 237, 240, 245, 246, 251, 256, 259, 262, 270, 275–277, 293, 296, 298, 299, 301, 312, 322, 345, 348, 352, 369, 402, 407, 424, 426, 478, 506, 513, 549–551, 566, 569–572, 574, 580
egg 27
kidney 85, 406
lead 368
liver 80
market 30, 537

Welfare Act (AWA), Animal 14, 15

Welsummer (breed) 24–26, 28, 29, 225, 241

West Nile virus 195

western equine encephalomyelitis 195, 204

white
diarrhea 295, 302
egg (albumen) 463–465, 469, 470, 472, 474, 497, 553
thin 463–466, 474
light 50
muscle disease (muscular dystrophy) 121
nodules 206, 226, 257, 294, 300
yolk (platinum) 299

WHO/FAO Food Standards (Codex Alimentarius Commission) 540, 555

whole blood
agglutination 202, 295
usage 202, 285, 506, 509

widgeon, American (breed) 70, 97

window, acoustic 322, 323

wing   133, 135, 136, 138, 155, 177, 234, 263, 397, 437, 450, 469, 470, 481, 591
   angel   72, 82, 256
   band   478, 505
   bandage   72, 82, 255, 444
   blue (disease)   271
   bone   82, 172, 255
   deformities   72, 82
   diseases   255
   Doppler   240
   droop   255, 345
      ECG   240
   feathers   138, 140, 167, 172, 283, 481
   flapping   71, 329
   injection   581, 585, 590
   injury   79, 173, 177, 255, 266, 353, 459
   joints   167, 173, 177, 328
   locomotion   170
   muscle   82, 137
   posture   446
   radiograph   173, 177
   restraint   160, 161
   teal, blue (breed)   70
wing web vaccination   584, 587, 588, 590, 591
wire fence   54
wishbone (furcula)   483, 484, 486
withdrawal
   interval (WDI)   323, 544, 549, 553–555
   time(s)   261, 265, 267, 323, 562, 567, 568, 571, 573, 574, 579, 581
      egg   562, 571, 573, 574, 579, 581
wood shavings   259, 298

hard   49, 227
   pine   49
worker's lung, poultry   204
World Health Organization (WHO)   203, 555
worm(s)
   cecal   209, 210, 215, 293, 305, 311, 572, 573
   crop (*Capillaria contorta*)   212, 213, 292, 293
   egg   287, 474
   eye   213
   proventricular   213
wound
   healing   121, 235, 242, 267, 268, 353, 361, 392, 394, 396
   management   235, 251, 259, 268, 352–354, 357, 364
Wyandotte (breed)   24, 29–32, 34, 35, 364, 568, 581

x

xanthoma, cutaneous   272
xanthomatosis   260, 272

y

Yangzhao goose/geese   81
yeast(s)   86, 120, 127
   overgrowth   291, 292
yellow
   droppings   402
   exudate   220, 278, 309
yolk   145, 150, 224, 462–468, 471, 472, 553, 554
   blood spot   285, 286, 462, 473, 474
   color   299, 473
   contamination   355, 369, 373, 553

culture, egg   471, 472
discolored   126, 285, 286
double egg   277, 283, 285, 475
ectopic   411
green   473
infection   280, 281, 309, 416
membrane   463, 465
peritonitis (coelomitis)
      egg   102, 185, 235, 278, 279, 303, 362, 363, 411, 412, 416–418, 516, 518–520
   sac   143, 145, 309, 468–471, 494
   stalk   143, 145, 468, 469
   taste (flavor)   473
   white (platinum)   299
yolking, double (double yolk)   277, 283, 285, 475
yolkless egg   474, 475

z

zinc
   dietary   77, 119, 121, 369, 374
   sulfate   294, 298
   toxicity   178, 182, 362, 365, 368–370, 372–376, 581
zone
   central (*area pellucida*)   468
   intermediate   142–144, 153
   land   4, 7, 8, 10
   thermoneutral   47
zoning   5, 7–9
zoonotic disease   56, 195, 199, 202, 211, 214, 281, 286, 300, 334, 343, 457, 547
zygote   468